OXFORD MEDICAL PUBLICATIONS

AN EVIDENCE-BASED RESOURCE
FOR PAIN RELIEF

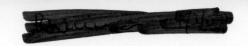

AN EVIDENCE-BASED
RESOURCE FOR PAIN RELIEF

H.J. McQUAY, DM
Clinical Reader in Pain Relief, Nuffield Department of Anaesthetics, Oxford

R.A.MOORE, DSc
Consultant Biochemist, Nuffield Department of Anaesthetics, Oxford

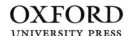

OXFORD
UNIVERSITY PRESS

OXFORD
UNIVERSITY PRESS

Great Clarendon Street, Oxford OX2 6DP

Oxford University Press is a department of the University of Oxford.
It furthers the University's objective of excellence in research, scholarship,
and education by publishing worldwide in

Oxford New York

Athens Auckland Bangkok Bogotá Buenos Aires Calcutta
Cape Town Chennai Dar es Salaam Delhi Florence Hong Kong Istanbul
Karachi Kuala Lumpur Madrid Melbourne Mexico City Mumbai
Nairobi Paris São Paulo Singapore Taipei Tokyo Toronto Warsaw

with associated companies in Berlin Ibadan

Oxford is a registered trade mark of Oxford University Press
in the UK and in certain other countries

Published in the United States
by Oxford University Press Inc., New York

First published 1998
Published new as paperback 1998
Reprinted 1999

A catalogue record for this book is available from the British Library

Library of Congress Cataloging in Publication Data
McQuay, H. J. (Henry J.)
An evidence-based resource for pain / H. J. McQuay, R. A. Moore.
(Oxford medical publications)
Includes bibliographical references.
1. Analgesics—Testing.   2. Evidence-based medicine.   3. Pain—
Chemotherapy—Research.   4. Clinical trials—Design.   I. Moore, R.
A. (R. Andrew)   II. Title.   III. Series.
[DNLM: 1. Pain—therapy.   2. Clinical Trials.   3. Evidence-Based
Medicine.   WL 704 M4795a   1998]
RM319.M38   1998   615'.783—dc21   97–42656

ISBN 0 19 263048 2 (Pbk)

Printed in Great Britain by
The Bath Press Ltd, Bath

Contents

Acknowledgements

We owe a huge debt to our colleagues, who encouraged us in this enterprise. Alejandro Jadad, Dawn Carroll, and our volunteers broke the back of manual searching for randomized trials of pain-relieving interventions. The chapters on finding trials, on appraising their quality, and on existing systematic reviews borrow heavily from the publications which came from Alejandro Jadad's D. Phil. thesis. The Oxford contributions of Dawn Carroll, Sally Collins, David Gavaghan, Jayne Edwards, John Reynolds, Phil Wiffen, Owen Moore and Bethany Nye are gratefully acknowledged. Without their endeavour and their patience much of this book would not have been published. Martin Tramèr (Oxford and Geneva), Eija Kalso (Helsinki), Pascale Picard (Clermont-Ferrand), Clara Faura (Alicante), and Göran Leijon (Linköping) collaborated on particular reviews, and Martin Tramèr applied the same rigorous approach he used on systematic reviews of anti-emetics to reviews of analgesics. Our clinical colleagues, Chris Glynn and Tim Jack, have been helpful, enthusiastic, and protective sounding-boards.

Our thinking over the past six years or so has been informed by discussion and argument with some very talented professionals who were either in Oxford or who have come here to work. They include Muir Gray, Iain Chalmers, David Sackett, and Doug Altman. Many other individuals have acted as sounding boards, such as Douglas Justins, Ed Charlton, and Tony Dickenson. Others have helped and supported, including John Williams, Dick Waite, Ann Southwell, and Aprille Cornell. Our libraries in and around Oxford have been magnificent, especially Claire Abbott here in the Churchill, but also many libraries in academia and industry who have provided us with the raw material for the work.

Financial support for the work has been provided from many different sources for different aspects of the work, including Pain Research Funds, European Union Biomed 2, the National Health Service Research and Development Health Technology Assessment Programme, and NHSE Anglia and Oxford Research and Development Directorate, as well as from pharmaceutical companies.

Finally, it is a pleasure to acknowledge our mentor, John Lloyd. Not only did he start the Oxford Pain Relief Unit, but he set us and many others on a quest for better treatments and greater understanding.

Introduction

What the book aims to be, and what it is not

Our aim in writing this book was to draw together an approach to assessing evidence. When we began in pain research twenty years ago we wanted to know the answers to simple questions, such as: Which was the best analgesic in a particular pain context?

We learned rapidly that this was not an easy question to answer. Our mentors in analgesic trials, Louis Lasagna, Ray Houde, and Stanley Wallenstein, had ploughed this field before, and had found no satisfactory way to take a set of trials and from that data work out which was the most effective analgesic. What they did do was to lay down explicit rules about the design and conduct of pain trials. These rules, including randomization and double-blinding, have stood the test of time. The trials done according to their rules over the following forty years have given us the raw material for our work.

What has changed is that a set of methods has evolved, and is still evolving, to allow us to begin to answer some of the questions. These methods have come from the clinical epidemiologists, who developed them mainly for studying what we would call prophylaxis, such as clot-dispersal treatment after myocardial infarction. In that setting, a success, a prevented cardiac death within the succeeding five weeks, might be 1 in 20, or indeed 1 in 40. A pain patient offered a therapy with a 1 in 20 chance of success might demur. It is the transposition of these methods into the study of treatments, treatments with a chance of success between better than 1 in 2 and 1 in 10, that has made what follows possible.

What we want this book to offer is an explicit approach to this assessment of the evidence. The methods, how to find the papers, criteria by which to judge them, what data to extract and how then to handle that data, are all here. We have had to develop new methods and extend existing ones. The first part of the book documents the methods we use. We make no apology for this, because although the information we all want is the chance of success of a particular intervention, the credibility of that number, the chance of success, rests on the credibility of the methods used to derive it. Using the tables in a particular chapter we hope that the reader could, and will, backtrack and see if they reach the same conclusions as we do.

There are many things which this book is not. The most obvious is that it is not a book of recipes for managing different pain syndromes. We hope that it will be a resource for those who think about the ingredients of the recipes. The second thing the book is not is complete. We have yet to apply this approach to all the different interventions used in managing pain. We have tried to focus on common treatments, and drug treatments are by far the commonest tools used to manage pain in both primary and secondary care. Even then there are omissions, such as oral morphine in cancer pain, multiple (chronic) dosing, and adverse effects. There is still a vast amount to do, so that the third thing the book is not is the final word. As more reviews emerge, and as better methods are developed, we hope that the resource will grow more substantial. Pain specialists may be sad if they find that their favourite treatments do not perform as well as they thought. We suspect that this would be true in many other areas of medicine too, and we hope that people will use and improve these methods in these areas.

Pain: some background information

We are all different, and we ourselves can respond differently

The standard cocktail party conversation with someone who treats pain for a living is about pain threshold. Usually it is a proud boast about how high the individual's threshold is, sometimes it is to complain about others' low thresholds. The concepts of threshold, the point at which you notice pain, and of tolerance, how much pain can you stand before you run away, are often muddled in the conversation, but that does not matter, because the important point is the variability. There are differences between us all, and indeed differences within ourselves depending on circumstances. Figure 1 summarizes some of the sensory, affective, cognitive, and behavioural dimensions that underlie this variability. While this book tries to tease apart the contribution that particular analgesic interventions can make, it would be naïve in the extreme to forget about these other influences. This book should help to decide which interventions should be included in the black bag. Deciding which to take out of the black bag for a particular patient, and when, taking all these other factors into account, is what then constitutes high quality care.

Getting the pain message across

Pain is something we feel. If we want someone else to know about it we have to signal our pain to them—usually we tell them. Pain measurement is necessarily subjective. We do not have any objective measures of pain, no blood tests, no urine dipsticks, no electroencephalograms. At its simplest the patient feels the pain, and it is that report which has to be the yardstick against which we measure the effects of treatment. Despite being subjective, pain measurement can be remarkably

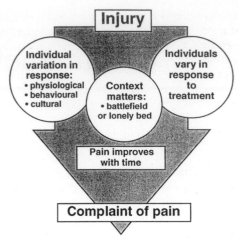

Fig. 1 Factors influencing the pain reported by the patient.

robust. From the research point of view the outcome measures and the necessities of paying attention to trial design, randomization, double-blinding, and comparators, were resolved and emphasized many years ago, so that the rules for pain trials were clear much earlier than in other areas of medicine which also use subjective measures. From the clinical point of view the message is: believe the patient. It also leaves us with a difficult problem, which is how we gauge pain in patients who cannot report it, such as the very young or the unconscious.

Acute and chronic pain

This book has two main sections, acute pain and chronic pain. This conventional division poses a semantic problem—how should chronic pain be defined?—to which an intuitive answer is that chronic pain is pain which recurs or pain which persists beyond the usual duration of an acute injury or disease. The second problem is that many of the analgesic interventions which are used (and are effective) in acute pain are also used and are effective in chronic pain. This means that the acute pain section of the book contains much that is necessary for simple pharmacological management of chronic pain.

Pain days

It is easy to underestimate the burden which chronic pain creates for the individual, for their families, and for society. It affects large numbers of people. Roughly 10% of the population in Western countries say that they suffer from chronic pain (see [1] for UK data), and 30% of disabled adults reported severe, recurring pain limiting normal daily living [2]. This adds up to a huge number of days with pain. In France we know that 10% of the population have a general anaesthetic each year (François Clergue, personal communication). If we allow an average of three pain days after each general anaesthetic (some will have no pain days, others many), then a crude estimate of acute pain incidence would be 10% of 60 million multiplied by 3 (days), or 18 million pain days. Contrast that with an estimate of chronic

pain days, where 10% of the 60 million complain of chronic pain, giving a total of 6 million times 365 chronic pain days—or a huge 2190 million pain days (Table 1).

Although this book shows clearly that there are effective ways to treat pain what it does not say is how to manage those whose pain does not respond, or responds poorly. That is a continuing challenge to us all. Our goal has to be to maximize pain relief at minimal cost in terms of disability (Fig. 2).

Table 1 Number of acute or chronic pain days

	No. of people affected (million)	No. of days	Total pain days (million)
Acute pain	6	3	18
Chronic pain	6	365	2190

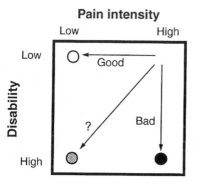

Fig. 2 The goal: maximize pain relief, at minimal disability.

Basing decisions on evidence

> Among stamp collectors letter writers are not always welcome. (George Steiner in *After Babel*, Oxford University Press, 1992, p. xi)

Finding and using the best available evidence should be part of our professional lives. Archie Cochrane said in 1979: 'It is surely a great criticism of our profession that we have not organized a critical summary, by specialty or subspecialty, adapted periodically, of all relevant randomized controlled trials'. We have been slow to grasp this.

There are several interlinked strands:

- finding the evidence
- appraising the evidence
- making the evidence (doing trials or systematic reviews)
- using the evidence

The focus in this book is on systematic reviews of existing trials. Systematic reviews and large randomized trials constitute the most reliable sources of evidence we can muster (Table 2). Put simply, they are the best chance we have to determine what is true (Fig. 3). Early chapters also give details of how to find trials, and how to appraise their quality. Later, there is advice on how to appraise the quality of systematic reviews themselves.

Table 2 Type and strength of efficacy evidence

I. Strong evidence from at least one systematic review of multiple well-designed randomized controlled trials

II. Strong evidence from at least one properly designed randomized controlled trial of appropriate size

III. Evidence from well-designed trials without randomization, single group pre-post, cohort, time series, or matched case-controlled studies

IV. Evidence from well-designed non-experimental studies from more than one centre or research group

V. Opinions of respected authorities, based on clinical evidence, descriptive studies, or reports of expert committees

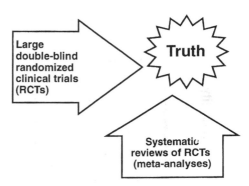

Fig. 3 Getting close to the truth.

Evidence-based medicine

The strident debate between the proponents and the opponents of evidence-based medicine (EBM) has led to clarity. A current definition of EBM is that it is the conscientious, explicit, and judicious use of current best evidence in making decisions about the care of individual patients [3]. The practice of EBM requires the integration of individual clinical expertise with the best available external clinical evidence from systematic research. Decisions that affect the care of patients should be taken with due *weight* accorded to *all* valid, relevant information. There are many factors, as well as the results of randomized controlled trials, which may weigh heavily in both clinical and policy decisions, such as patient preferences and resources, and these must contribute to decisions about the care of patients (*due weight*). Valid, relevant evidence should be considered alongside these other factors in the decision-making process. No one sort of evidence should necessarily be the determining factor in a decision. *All* implies that there should be an active search for that valid, relevant information and that an assessment should be made of the accuracy of the information and the applicability of the evidence to the decision in question (i.e. information should be appraised). EBM is thus what most clinicians have been trying to practise all their working lives.

What is changing is that there is an increasing number of well-conducted randomized controlled trials and systematic reviews, and that there is a political pressure, both from those receiving care and from those who pay for it, to support our treatment choices with high quality evidence. That should not be too irksome, given that professionally, we would all wish to do the best for our patients. What happens, as this book shows, is that the evidence supports some interventions and suggests that others are considerably less effective than some of us believe. This should not make us paranoid. Precisely the same message has emerged in the other areas of medicine which have received similar attention. What is clear is that very often the quality of the trials of invasive interventions is much lower than the quality of drug trials. The onus must be on us to do bigger and better trials if we wish to continue using some of these techniques.

But it is not just trials that are needed. Audit, too, has its part to play—even if it serves to highlight the problems we face. An audit of patients in hospital [4] has demonstrated that at the heart of the UK hospital service, where delivery of good pain relief should be easiest and best, as many as 87% of patients said that they experienced pain of moderate or severe intensity (Table 3). Improving the service to improve these figures is a worthwhile target for us all. Ironically, it is just such moderate or severe pain which is an entry criterion for the rigorous trials whose results we use in the following chapters. Those who refuse to bless or fund trials with such an entry criterion should take note. If 87% of patients endure severe or moderate pain in normal clinical practice then investigators are not out of line to require such a pain level to show that their putative remedies work. The canny reader will spot examples in the following pages where these rules were bent, and no satisfactory answer was forthcoming. To the authors it is unethical to recruit patients into studies that cannot produce an answer.

Table 3 Audit of pain in hospital [4]

	No. of patients	%
Pain was present all or most of the time	1042/3162	33
Pain was severe or moderate	2755/3157	87
Pain was worse than expected	182/1051	17
Had to ask for drugs	1085/2589	42
Drugs did not arrive immediately	455/1085	41

References

1. Rigge M. *Which? Way to Health*, 1990; 66–8.
2. Astin M, Lawton D, Hirst M. The prevalence of pain in a disabled population. *Society of Scientific Medicine*, 1997; **42**:1457–64.
3. Sackett D, Richardson WS, Rosenberg W, Haynes B. *Evidence-based medicine*. London: Churchill Livingstone, 1996.
4. Bruster S, Jarman B, Bosanquet N, Weston D, Erens R, Delbanco TL. National survey of hospital patients. *British Medical Journal*, 1994; **309**:1542–6.

Part I
METHODOLOGY

Finding all the relevant trials

Evidence that is both relevant and valid is necessary for effective care. The randomized controlled trial (RCT) is the most reliable way to estimate the effect of an intervention. The principle of randomization is simple. Patients in a randomized trial have the same probability of receiving any of the interventions being compared. Randomization abolishes selection bias because it prevents investigators influencing who has which intervention. Randomization also helps to ensure that other factors, such as age or sex distribution, are equivalent for the different treatment groups. Inadequate randomization, or inadequate concealment of randomization, lead to exaggeration of therapeutic effect [1].

To produce valid reviews of evidence, the reviews need to be systematic, and to be systematic, qualitative, or quantitative, they need to include all relevant randomized controlled trials (RCTs). Identifying all the relevant trials is a 'fundamental challenge' [2] which is easily underestimated.

The first obstacle faced by any reviewer is finding out how many eligible RCTs exist. Commonly, the total is unknown. Usually only for newer interventions are reviewers likely to be sure that they have found all the RCTs. Otherwise the only way to find how many RCTs there are would be to scan every record in each of the available bibliographic databases, to search by hand all non-indexed journals, theses, proceedings and textbooks, to search the reference lists of all the reports found, and to ask investigators of previous RCTs for other published or unpublished information [3] (Fig. 1).

In practice, constrained by time and cost, reviewers have to compromise, and then hope that what they have found is a representative sample of the unknown total population of trials. The more comprehensive the searching the more trials will be found, and any conclusions will then be stronger.

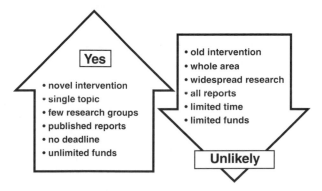

Fig. 1   Is a complete search possible?

Comprehensive searches can be very time consuming and costly, so again this emphasizes the necessary compromise, where the target is the highest possible yield for given resources.

Retrieval bias is the failure to identify reports which could have affected the results of a systematic review or meta-analysis [4]. This failure may be because trials are still ongoing, or completed but unpublished (publication bias) or because although published the search did not find them. Trying to identify unpublished trials by asking researchers had a very low yield [5], and was not cheap. Registers of ongoing and completed trials are another way to find unpublished data, but such registers are rare.

This chapter describes:

- the methods used to identify eligible reports of RCTs published from 1950 to date
- information management

Developing a citation database

The process had three phases: (1) definition of inclusion criteria, (2) identification of reports, and (3) information management.

Inclusion criteria

A report was regarded as eligible if the following criteria were fulfilled:

- Allocation to the intervention was described as randomized (no precise description of the method of randomization was required) or as double-blind or as both, or if it was suggested that the interventions were given at random and/or under double-blind conditions, *and*
- analgesic interventions with pain or adverse effects as outcomes, and/or any intervention using pain as an outcome measure, were compared.
- Reports were excluded which investigated analgesic effectiveness during (as opposed to after) diagnostic or surgical procedures.

Identification of reports

Details of the process are given in Jadad *et al.* 1996 [6]. Since that publication the major changes are the use of other databases as well as MEDLINE. Searching on EMBASE, the Cochrane Library, CINAHL, and PSYCHLIT is now part of our standard operating procedures (Fig. 2).

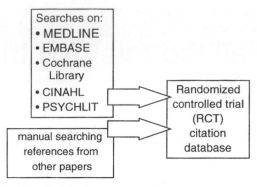

Fig. 2   Finding the citations.

MEDLINE search for randomized controlled trials (RCTs) published from 1966 to date

The records identified by the optimized MEDLINE search strategy were downloaded (Biblio-Link version 1.1, Personal Bibliographic Software, Inc.) and transferred to a reference management program (Pro-Cite, Personal Bibliographic Software, Inc., version 2.1). These records were then sorted in alphabetical order and each of the downloaded records was checked on screen for definite eligibility, probable eligibility or ineligibility, and coded accordingly within each Pro-Cite record. Hard copies of eligible and probable reports were obtained, and if necessary were translated, and eligibility was then confirmed (Table 1).

Manual searching of journals published from 1950 to date

A Pro-Cite file of all the records regarded as eligible and probably eligible (1950–90) was created. This file was used to produce a list of the 50 journals with the highest yield. These journals were searched by hand to find RCTs. These RCTs, either missed by MEDLINE indexing, or in non-indexed journals, are then added to the citation database if perusal of the hard copy confirms that they are indeed RCTs.

Management of the information

The citation database is maintained as a Pro-Cite file. The number in that database is used as the unique identifying number for the hard copy.

Trend in the number of *randomized controlled trials* (RCTs) in pain relief research published 1950–90

From 1956 to 1980, there were twice as many reports published in each successive five year period. From 1980 to 1990 the number of reports increased by more than 1000 per 5-year period. More than 85% of the reports identified were published during the last 15 years. This is illustrated by the trend in the number of RCTs in the journal *Pain* over the past 20 years (Fig. 3).

Table 1   Refined high-yield MEDLINE search strategy

Step no.	Request
1	PAIN*
2	explode PAIN / all subheadings in MeSH
3	ANALG*
4	explode ANALGESIA / all subheadings in MeSH
5	explode ANALGESICS / all subheadings in MeSH
6	CLINICAL
7	TRIALS
8	CLINICAL TRIALS
9	EXPOSE CLINICAL-TRIALS / all subheadings in MeSH
10	RANDOM*
11	RANDOM-ALLOCATION (Term allows no subheadings) in MeSH
12	RANDOMIZED-CONTROLLED-TRIALS / all subheadings in MeSH
13	DOUBLE
14	BLIND
15	DOUBLE BLIND
16	DOUBLE-BLIND-METHOD (Term allows no subheadings) in MeSH
17	META-ANALYSIS
18	META-ANALYSIS (Term allows no subheadings) in MeSH
19	HUMAN
20	(no. 1 or no. 2 or no. 3 or no. 4 or no. 5) and (HUMAN in MeSH)
21	HUMAN
22	(no. 8 or no. 9 or no. 10 or no. 11 or no. 12 or no. 15 or no. 16 or no. 17 or no. 18) and (HUMAN in MeSH)
23	no. 20 and no. 22

MeSH, medical standardized heading.

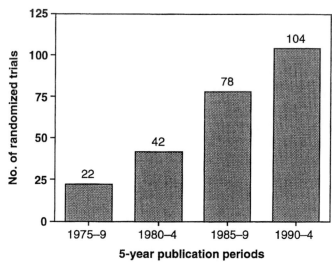

Fig. 3   Randomized controlled trials (RCTs) in the journal *Pain*, 1975–94.

A simple breakdown (Table 2) showed that 54% of all reports were in acute pain, 43% in chronic non-cancer, and 3% in chronic cancer. Pharmacological reports were commonest (75%), with 14% classified as invasive, 7% as

Table 2 Pain trials database, 1950–94

	Acute	Chronic	Cancer	Total	%
Complementary	112	223	10	345	2
Invasive	1697	336	34	2067	14
Pharmacological	5390	4978	337	10 705	75
Physical	402	501	36	939	7
Psychological	100	191	10	301	2
Total	7701	6229	427	14 357	
%	54	43	3		

reports of physical interventions, and 2% each for psychological and complementary.

Conclusions

The importance of basing systematic reviews on the highest quality evidence (randomized trials) is obvious from our experience in the pain field [7], and from the experience of others. This means that very considerable time and effort has to be spent to gather all the relevant material for each review.

The process described here gives an outline of what is a laborious task. The addition of another year's citations, maintaining the existing database (now 15 000 citations), and the associated chores make a full-time job. To make the information accessible to others we have contributed our citations of known RCTs to the Cochrane Library, and to those making sure that MEDLINE (NLM) tags all the RCTs which we could previously find only by manual searching.

References

1. Schulz KF, Chalmers I, Hayes RJ, Altman DG. Failure to conceal treatment allocation schedules in trials influences estimates of treatment effects. *Controlled Clinical Trials* 1994; **15**:S63–4.
2. Chalmers I, Dickersin K, Chalmers T. Getting to grips with Archie Cochrane's agenda. *British Medical Journal* 1992; **305**:786–7.
3. Jadad AR, McQuay HJ. A high-yield strategy to identify randomized controlled trials for systematic reviews. *Online Journal of Current Clinical Trials* [serial online] 1993; Doc No 33:3973 words; 39 paragraphs. 5 tables.
4. Simes RJ. Confronting publication bias: a cohort design for meta-analysis. *Statistics in Medicine* 1987; **6**:11–29.
5. Hetherington J, Dickerson R, Chalmers I, Meinert C. Retrospective and prospective identification of unpublished controlled trials: lessons from a survey of obstetricians and pediatricians. *Pediatrics* 1989; **84**:374–80.
6. Jadad AR, Carroll D, Moore A, McQuay H. Developing a database of published reports of randomised clinical trials in pain research. *Pain* 1996; **66**:239–46.
7. Carroll D, Tramer M, McQuay H, Nye B, Moore A. Randomization is important in studies with pain outcomes: Systematic review of transcutaneous electrical nerve stimulation in acute postoperative pain. *British Journal of Anaesthesia* 1996; **77**:798–803.

3
Judging the quality of trials

Once you have found all the reports of the trials relevant to your question there is another stage in the process. This stage is first to confirm that these reports meet certain *quality standards* and second that, even though a report may pass those quality standards, whether the trial is *valid*. Imagine a situation where you found 40 reports of trials on your question. You then discover that 20 of the reports say that the intervention is terrific, and 20 conclude that it should never be used. Delving deeper you find that the 20 'negative' reports score highly on your quality standards scale. The 'positive' reports score poorly for quality. The quality scale should include measures of bias. Bias is the simplest explanation why poor quality reports give more positive conclusions than high quality reports.

The quality standards that you require cannot be absolute, because for some clinical questions there may not be any randomized trials (RCTs). Setting RCTs as a minimum absolute standard would therefore be inappropriate for all the questions we might want to answer. In the pain world, however, there are two reasons for setting this high standard, and requiring trials to be randomized. The first reason is that we do have, particularly for drug interventions, quite a number of RCTs. The second we would argue is that it is even more important to stress the minimum quality standards of randomization and double-blinding when the outcome measures are subjective.

This chapter describes briefly the development of a quality score which was then used for the systematic reviews which follow. A detailed description of the way the scale was developed and tested has been published [1]. We conclude the chapter with our current views on this and other quality scales.

Developing and validating a quality scale

Previous methods to measure the 'quality' of clinical reports and incorporate the results in systematic reviews may all be criticized because of failure to define quality and because they were not validated [2–16]. The danger is that using these scales might lead to conclusions in the review as inconsistent and unreliable as the component studies.

What makes a trial worthy of the label 'high quality'? Quality could refer to the clinical relevance of the study, to the likelihood of biased results, to the appropriateness of the statistical analysis, to the presentation of the data, or to the ethical implications of the intervention, or to the literary style of the manuscript. We think that quality must primarily indicate the likelihood that the study design reduced bias. Only by avoiding bias is it possible to estimate the effect of a given intervention with any confidence.

The purpose of our scale is to assess the likelihood of the trial design to generate unbiased results and approach the 'therapeutic truth'. This has also been described as 'scientific quality' [17]. Other trial characteristics, such as clinical relevance of the question addressed, data analysis and presentation, literary quality of the report, or ethical implications of the study, are not included in our definition.

The aims of the scale are:

1. To assess the scientific quality of any clinical trial in which pain is an outcome measure or in which analgesic interventions are compared for outcomes other than pain (e.g. a study looking at the adverse effect profile of different opioids).

2. To allow consistent and reliable assessment of quality by raters with different backgrounds, including researchers, clinicians, professionals from other disciplines, and members of the general public.

The judges

We assembled a multidisciplinary panel of six judges (a psychologist, a clinical pharmacologist, a biochemist, two anaesthetists, and a research nurse) with an interest in pain research. We discussed the definition of quality and the purposes of the scale. Each judge then had to produce a list of suggested items to be included on the scale. To generate the items, the judges used both criteria published previously and their own judgement. The suggestions were then combined in a single list (49 items).

Using a modified nominal group approach to reach consensus [18], the judges assessed the face validity of each of the items, according to established criteria [19]. Those items associated with low face validity were deleted. An initial instrument was created from the remaining items.

The initial instrument was pre-tested by three raters on 13 study reports. The raters identified problems in clarity and/or application of each of the items. The panel of judges then modified the wording of the items accordingly and produced detailed instructions describing how each of the items should be assessed and scored. The items were classified by their ability to reduce bias (direct or indirectly) and individual scores were allocated to them by consensus. The frequency of endorsement, consistency, and validity of each item were then assessed (Fig. 1).

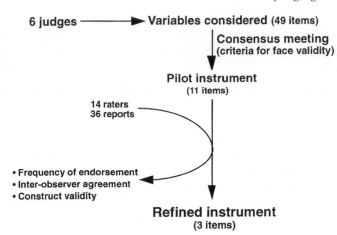

Fig. 1   Developing the scale.

Final version of the scale

The final version of the scale has the three items with highest frequency of endorsement (Fig. 2, see also Tables 1 and 2).

Open vs. blind assessments

A chastening finding during the scale's development was that blind assessment (not knowing authors, journal, year, etc.) of reports produced significantly lower and more consistent quality scores than open assessments [1]. This has important implications, because the cost of organizing truly blind assessment is very considerable.

Table 1   Three-question scale to measure the likelihood of bias in pain research reports

This is not the same as being asked to review a paper. It should not take more than 10 minutes to score a report and there are no right or wrong answers.

Please read the article and try to answer the following questions (see attached instructions):

1. Was the study described as randomized (this includes the use of words such as randomly, random, and randomization)?
2. Was the study described as double-blind?
3. Was there a description of withdrawals and drop-outs?

Scoring the items:

Give a score of 1 point for each 'yes' and 0 points for each 'no'. There are no in-between marks.

Give 1 additional point if:

On question 1, the method of randomization was described *and* it was *appropriate* (table of random numbers, computer-generated, coin-tossing, etc.), *and/or:*

If on question 2 the method of double-blinding was described *and* it was *appropriate* (identical placebo, active placebo, dummy, etc.)

Deduct 1 point if:

On question 1, the method of randomization was described *and* it was *inappropriate* (patients were allocated alternatively, or according to date of birth, hospital number, etc.), *and/or:*

On question 2 the study was described as double-blind but the method of blinding was *inappropriate* (e.g. comparison of tablet vs. injection with no double-dummy)

Table 2   Advice on using the scale

1. Randomization

If the word 'randomized' or any other related words such as random, randomly, or randomization are used in the report, but the method of randomization is not described, give a positive score to this item. A randomization method will be regarded as appropriate if it allowed each patient to have the same chance of receiving each treatment and the investigators could not predict which treatment was next. Therefore, methods of allocation using date of birth, date of admission, hospital numbers, or alternation are not appropriate. Where the score for randomization was zero, the trial should be excluded.

2. Double-blinding

A study must be regarded as double-blind if the word 'double-blind' is used (even without description of the method) or if it is implied that neither the caregiver nor the patient could identify the treatment being assessed.

3. Withdrawals and drop-outs

Patients who were included in the study but did not complete the observation period or who were not included in the analysis must be described. The numbers *and* the reasons for withdrawal must be stated. If there are no withdrawals, it should be stated in the article. If there is no statement on withdrawals, this item must be given a negative score (0 points).

Randomized?	Score
• yes	1
• appropriate?	
– yes (table)	1
– no (alternate)	–1
Double-blind?	
• yes	1
• appropriate?	
–yes (double-dummy)	1
–no	–1
Withdrawals described?	
• yes	1

Fig. 2   Scoring randomized control trials (maximum, 5; minimum, 1).

Comments on the scale

The three-point scale is simple, short, valid, and reliable. Our results suggest that even without clinical or research experience in pain relief people should be able to score the quality of research reports consistently. Our purpose was to allow us to do differential analysis within our systematic reviews based on the quality of the individual primary studies, but the scale may have much wider use.

Chalmers suggested many years ago that the quality of clinical reports should be assessed blind [3]. We found that such blinded assessment produced significantly lower scores. This may be very important if absolute cut-off scores are imposed by systematic reviewers, and if quality scores are used to weight the results of primary studies in subsequent meta-analysis [16, 20]. The results of open evaluations are good enough for busy readers. The improved reliability with blind testing is of more relevance to journal editors for manuscript selection and to systematic reviewers. Quality scales without clinimetric evaluation have already been used in pain work to support the conclusions of systematic reviews [11, 13, 14].

None of the items is specific to pain studies. The three items are very similar to the components of a scale used extensively to assess the effectiveness of interventions during pregnancy and childbirth [8], and also appear in most other scales. Control of selection bias and rater bias is obviously regarded as crucial to quality.

Selection bias is best controlled by allocating patients at random to the different study groups. Each patient should have the same probability of being included in each comparison group, and the allocation should be concealed until after the patient has given consent to take part. Methods of allocation based on alternation, date of birth, or hospital record number cannot be regarded as random. Failure to secure proper randomization increases the likelihood that potential participants in a 'randomized' study will be admitted to the study selectively because of prior knowledge of the group to which they would be allocated or excluded selectively before formal admission in the study [21]. Ideal methods of random-

ization are those in which individuals with no direct relationship to the study participants are in charge of the allocation (e.g. allocation by telephone from a central coordinating office, concealed from the investigators). Appropriate simpler alternatives are coin-tossing, tables of random numbers and numbers generated by computers, but at higher risk of selective selection (Fig. 3).

All these methods are regarded as appropriate for the purposes of our scale, although we are aware that selective selection is still possible even if the group allocation is concealed until after consent has been obtained. We rate the randomization method as inappropriate if the potential participants did not have the same chance of being included in any of the comparison groups (methods based on date of birth, hospital number, or alternation). Even with excellent randomization selection bias may still be introduced if biased and selective withdrawal and drop-outs occur after the allocations have been made [22]. This is why an adequate description of withdrawals and drop-outs is included in the scale. With that information it is possible to analyse on an intention-to-treat basis (all those randomized whether or not they were exposed to the study interventions [23]).

Rater bias can be minimized by blinding the person receiving the intervention, the individual administering it, the investigator measuring the outcome and the analyst. Blinding can be tested by asking the study patients and the researchers which intervention they had. This is not often done. The usual 'best' level of blinding is blinding of the study subject and those making the observations (double-blinding). Double-blinding is often achieved by using control interventions with similar physical characteristics to those of the intervention under evaluation, or by the use of dummies when two or more interventions have to be given by different routes (Fig. 4).

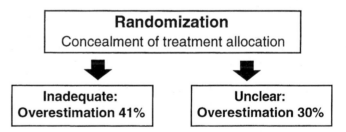

Fig. 3   Effect of randomization on treatment effect. (Schultz *et al.* 1995 [24].)

If not double-blind: Overestimation 17%

Is this important in every setting? (Unconscious) Practicable in every setting? (Surgery)

Fig. 4   Effect of blinding on treatment effect. (Schultz *et al.* 1995 [24].)

Sometimes, however, one of the interventions may produce effects which make blinding very difficult to sustain. Then the use of active placebos or active controls may decrease the likelihood of rater bias. All these precautions are relatively easy to achieve in drug studies. In non-drug studies testing under blind conditions is either difficult or inappropriate (e.g. surgical procedures) or impossible (e.g. acupuncture or transcutaneous electrical nerve stimulation, (TENS). The risk of rater bias limits the confidence with which conclusions can be reached. We know that studies which are not double-blind risk an average exaggeration of treatment effect of 17% [24].

References

1. Jadad AR, Moore RA, Carroll D, Jenkinson C, Reynolds DJM, Gavaghan DJ *et al.* Assessing the quality of reports of randomized clinical trials: is blinding necessary? *Controlled Clinical Trials* 1996; **17**:1–12.

2. Reiffenstein RJ, Schiltroth AJ, Todd DM. Current standards in reported drug trials. *Canadian Medical Association Journal* 1968; **99**:1134–5.

3. Chalmers TC, Smith H, Blackburn B, Silverman B, Schroeder B, Reitmand D *et al.* A method for assessing the quality of a randomized control trial. *Controlled Clinical Trials* 1981; **2**:31–49.

4. Tyson JE, Furzan JA, Reisch JS, Mize SG. An evaluation of the quality of therapeutic studies in perinatal medicine. *Journal of Pediatrics* 1983; **102**:10–13.

5. Andrew A. Method for assessing of the reporting standard of clinical trials with roentgen contrast media. *Acta Radiologica Diagnostica* 1984; **25**:55–8.

6. Evans M, Pollock AV. A score system for evaluating random control clinical trials of prophylaxis of abdominal surgical wound infection. *British Journal of Surgery* 1985; **72**:256–60.

7. Poynard T. Evaluation de la qualité méthodologique des essais thérapeutiques randomisés. *Presse Médicale* 1988; **17**:315–18.

8. Chalmers I, Hetherington J, Elbourne D, Keirse MJN, Enkin M. Materials and methods used in synthesizing evidence to evaluate the effects of care during pregnancy and childbirth. In: Chalmers I, Enkin M, Keirse MJNC, ed. *Effective care in pregnancy and childbirth*. Oxford University Press, 1989; 38–65.

9. Gøtzsche PC. Methodology and overt and hidden bias in reports of 196 double blind trials of nonsteroidal antiinflammatory drugs in rheumatoid arthritis. *Controlled Clinical Trials* 1989; **10**:31–56.

10. Reisch JS, Tyson JE, Mize SG. Aid to the evaluation of therapeutic studies. *Pediatrics* 1989; **84**:815–27.

11. ter Riet G, Kleijnen J, Knipschild P. Acupuncture and chronic pain: a criteria-based meta-analysis. *Journal of Clinical Epidemiology* 1990; **43**:1191–9.

12. Brown SA. Measurement of quality of primary studies for meta-analysis. *Nursing Research* 1991; **40**:352–5.

13. Koes BW, Bouter LM, Beckerman H, van der Heijden G, Knipschild PG. Physiotherapy exercises and back pain: a blinded review. *British Medical Journal* 1991; **302**:1572–6.

14. Koes BW, Assendelft WJ, van der Heijden G, Bouter LM, Knipschild PG. Spinal manipulation and mobilisation for back and neck pain: a blinded review. *British Medical Journal* 1991; **303**:1298–303.

15. Detsky AS, Naylor CD, O'Rourke K, McGeer AJ, L'Abbe KA. Incorporating variations in the quality of individual randomized trials into meta-analysis. *Journal of Clinical Epidemiology* 1992; **45**:255–65.

16. Nurmohamed MT, Rosendaal FR, Buller HR, Dekker E, Hommes DW, Vandenbroucke JP *et al.* Low molecular-weight heparin versus standard heparin in general and orthopaedic surgery: a meta-analysis. *Lancet* 1992; **340**:152–6.

17. Oxman AD, Guyatt GH. Validation of an index of the quality of review articles. *Journal of Clinical Epidemiology* 1991; **44**:1271–8.

18. Fink A, Kosecoff J, Chassin M, Brook RH. Consensus methods: characteristics and guidelines for use. *American Journal Public Health* 1984; **74**:979–83.

19. Feinstein AR. *Clinimetrics*. New Haven CI: Yale University Press, 1987.

20. Fleiss JL, Gross AJ. Meta-analysis in epidemiology, with special reference to studies of the association between exposure to environmental tobacco smoke and lung cancer: a critique. *Journal of Clinical Epidemiology* 1991; **44**:127–39.

21. Chalmers I. Evaluating the effects of care during pregnancy and childbirth. In: Chalmers I, Enkin M, Keirse MJNC, ed. *Effective care in pregnancy and childbirth*. Oxford University Press, 1989; 1–37.

22. Sackett DL, Gent M. Controversy in counting and attributing events in clinical trials. *New England Journal of Medicine* 1979; **301**:1410–12.

23. Peto R, Pike MC, Armitage P, Breslow NE, Cox DR, Howard SV *et al.* Design and analysis of randomised clinical trials requiring prolonged observation of each patient. 1. Introduction and design. *British Journal of Cancer* 1976; **34**:585–612.

24. Schulz KF, Chalmers I, Hayes RJ, Altman DG. Empirical evidence of bias: dimensions of methodological quality associated with estimates of treatment effects in controlled trials. *Journal of the American Medical Association* 1995; **273**:408–12.

4

Pain measurement, study design, and validity

We judge the efficacy of analgesic interventions by the change they bring about in the patient's report of pain. A brief description of methods of pain measurement follows. The second part of the chapter discusses the problems and some solutions when using pain measurement data for systematic reviews.

Pain measurement

Pain is a personal experience which makes it difficult to define and measure (Chapter 1). It includes both the sensory input and any modulation by physiological, psychological, and environmental factors. Not surprisingly there are no objective measures—there is no way to measure pain directly by sampling blood or urine or by performing neurophysiological tests. Measurement of pain must therefore rely on recording the patient's report. The assumption is often made that because the measurement is subjective it must be of little value. The reality is that if the measurements are done properly, remarkably sensitive and consistent results can be obtained. There are contexts, however, when it is not possible to measure pain at all, or when reports are likely to be unreliable. These include impaired consciousness, young children, psychiatric pathology, severe anxiety, unwillingness to cooperate, and inability to understand the measurements. Such problems are deliberately avoided in trials.

Measurement scales

Most analgesic studies include measurements of pain intensity and/or pain relief, and the commonest tools used are categorical and visual analogue scales.

Categorical and visual analogue scales

Categorical scales use words to describe the magnitude of the pain. They were the earliest pain measure [1]. The patient picks the most appropriate word. Most research groups use four words (none, mild, moderate, and severe). Scales to measure pain relief were developed later. The commonest is the five-category scale (none, slight, moderate, good or lots, and complete).

For analysis, numbers are given to the verbal categories (for pain intensity, none = 0, mild = 1, moderate = 2, and severe = 3; and for relief none = 0, slight = 1, moderate = 2, good or lots = 3, and complete = 4). Data from different subjects are then combined to produce means (rarely medians) and measures of dispersion (usually standard errors of means). The validity of converting categories into numerical scores was checked by comparison with concurrent visual analogue scale measurements. Good correlation was found, especially

Categorical verbal rating scales

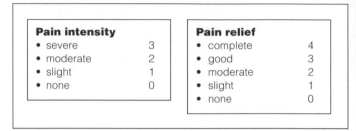

Visual analogue scales

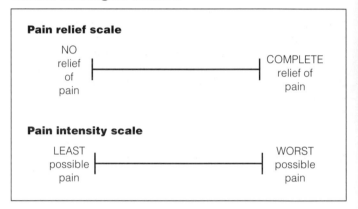

between pain relief scales using cross-modality matching techniques [2–4]. Results are usually reported as continuous data, mean or median pain relief, or intensity. Few studies present results as discrete data, giving the number of participants who report a certain level of pain intensity or relief at any given assessment point. The main advantages of the categorical scales are that they are quick and simple. The small number of descriptors may force the scorer to choose a particular category when none describes the pain satisfactorily.

Visual analogue scales (VAS), lines with the left end labelled 'no relief of pain' and the right end labelled 'complete relief of pain', seem to overcome this limitation. Patients mark the line at the point which corresponds to their pain. The scores are obtained by measuring the distance between the no relief end and the patient's mark, usually in millimetres. The main advantages of VAS are that they are simple and quick to score, avoid imprecise descriptive terms and provide many points from which to choose. More concentration and co-ordination are needed, which can be difficult postoperatively or with neurological disorders.

Pain relief scales are perceived as more convenient than pain intensity scales, probably because patients have the same baseline relief (zero) whereas they could start with different baseline intensity (usually moderate or severe). Relief scale results are then easier to compare. They may also be more sensitive than intensity scales [4, 5]. A theoretical drawback of relief scales is that the patient has to remember what the pain was like to begin with.

Other tools

Verbal numerical scales and global subjective efficacy ratings are also used. Verbal numerical scales are regarded as an alternative or complementary to the categorical and VAS scales. Patients give a number to the pain intensity or relief (for pain intensity 0 usually represents no pain and 10 the maximum possible, and for pain relief 0 represents none and 10 complete relief). They are very easy and quick to use, and correlate well with conventional visual analogue scales [6].

Global subjective efficacy ratings, or simply global scales, are designed to measure overall treatment performance. Patients are asked questions like 'How effective do you think the treatment was?' and answer using a labelled numerical or a categorical scale. Although these judgements probably include adverse effects they can be the most sensitive discriminant between treatments. One of the oldest scales was the binary question 'Is your pain half gone?' Its advantage is that it has a clearer clinical meaning than a 10 mm shift on a VAS. The disadvantage, for the small trial intensive measure pundits at least, is that all the potential intermediate information (1% to 49% or greater than 50%) is discarded.

Analgesic requirements (including patient-controlled analgesia, PCA), special paediatric scales, and questionnaires like the McGill are also used. The limitation to guard against is that they usually reflect other experiences as well as or instead of pain [7]

Judgement of the patient rather than by the carer is the ideal. Carers overestimate the pain relief compared with the patient's version.

Analysis of scale results: summary measures

In the research context, pain is usually assessed before the intervention is made and then on multiple occasions. Ideally the area under the time–analgesic effect curve for the intensity (summed pain intensity differences, SPID) or relief (total pain relief, TOTPAR) measures is derived.

$$SPID = \sum_{t=0-6}^{n} PID_t$$

$$TOTPAR = \sum_{t=0-6}^{n} PR_t$$

Where at the t th assessment point (t = 0, 1, 2, n), P_t and PR_t are pain intensity and pain relief measured at that point respectively, P_0 is pain intensity at t = 0, and PID_t is the pain intensity difference calculated as $(P_0 - P_t)$.

These summary measures reflect the cumulative response to the intervention. Their disadvantage is that they do not provide information about the onset and peak of the analgesic effect. If onset or peak are important then time to maximum pain relief (or reduction in pain intensity) or time for pain to return to baseline are necessary.

Using pain measurement data for systematic reviews

Standardizing the summary measures

Figure 1 shows the method we use to standardize TOTPAR values derived from a categorical verbal rating scale of relief (catPR). The actual TOTPAR is divided by the maximum possible TOTPAR score (maximum duration in hours multiplied by the maximum pain relief score) and converted to a percentage.

This calculation presumes that categorical relief score data is available. One major problem we faced is that not all trials use this classic scale. In order to include trials which used different scales we had to develop ways to convert those different scales back to the common denominator of %maxTOTPAR. The development and validation of those methods are discussed in Chapter 5. We still cannot include trials which use analgesic drug consumption (e.g. PCA), or trials which use non-standard scales.

The hazard for meta-analysis is that if a large number of papers has to be discarded because they do not use standard scales, are the remaining trials representative? For most drug interventions this has not proved to be a major problem, because the majority of trials used standard methods. There are exceptions. For some old drugs, such as dihydrocodeine, we could find remarkably few trials which used standard methods. For academically inspired investigations, as opposed to trials required for drug registration, we have had to exclude many trials which use non-standard methods.

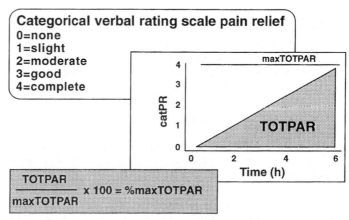

Fig. 1 Calculating percentage of maximum possible pain relief score.

Restricting to moderate and severe initial pain intensity

The trail blazers of analgesic trial methodology found that if patients had no pain to begin with, it was impossible to assess analgesic efficacy, because there was no pain to relieve. To optimize trial sensitivity a rule developed, which was that only those patients with moderate or severe pain intensity at baseline would be studied. Those with mild or no pain would not.

We have stayed true to this rule, so that we excluded trials of a given intervention if the trials studied patients with mild or no initial pain. As with exclusions because of non-standard methods, there have been few pharmacological trials where this rule about baseline pain has led to exclusion, but with pre-emptive techniques and local anaesthetic blocks it has been a major problem.

How do you know what is moderate or severe pain on a visual analogue pain intensity scale?

The usual criterion to ensure adequate sensitivity for analgesic trials is to test the intervention on patients who have established pain of moderate to severe intensity. When visual analogue scales (VAS) are the only pain measure in a trial we need to know what point on a VAS represents moderate pain, so that we can include the trial in a meta-analysis which has an inclusion criterion of baseline pain of at least moderate intensity.

To answer this question we used individual patient data from 1080 patients from randomized controlled trials of various analgesics [8]. Baseline pain had been measured using both a four-point categorical pain intensity scale and a VAS pain intensity scale. We checked the distribution of the VAS scores for 736 patients reporting moderate pain and for 344 reporting severe pain. We also checked the VAS scores corresponding to moderate or severe pain by gender.

Baseline VAS scores for patients reporting moderate pain were significantly different from those of patients reporting severe pain (Table 1 and Fig. 2). Of the patients reporting moderate pain 85% scored over 30 mm on the corresponding VAS, with a mean score of 49 mm. For those reporting severe pain 85% scored over 54 mm with a mean score of 75 mm. There was no difference between the corresponding VAS scores of men and women. Our results indicate that if a patient records a baseline VAS score in excess of 30 mm they would probably have recorded at least moderate pain on a four-point categorical scale.

Study design and validity

Pain measurement is one of the oldest and most studied of the subjective measures, and pain scales have been used for over 40 years. Even in the early days of pain measurement

Table 1 Descriptive statistics for the distribution of visual analogue scale (VAS) pain intensity scores

| | Baseline pain (using a 4-point categorical scale) | |
	Moderate	Severe
Number	736	344
Mean (mm)	49	75
Standard deviation	17	18
Median (mm)	49	76
90% patients > (mm)	26	49
85% patients > (mm)	30	54

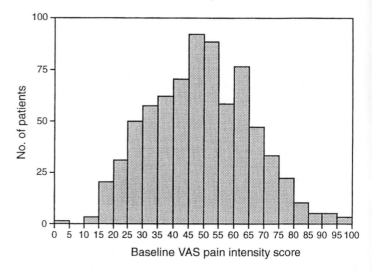

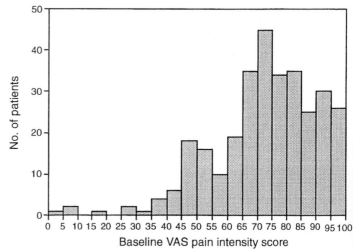

Fig. 2 Frequency distributions of initial visual analogue scale (VAS) pain intensity scores by initial categorical verbal pain intensity.

there was understanding that the design of studies contributed directly to the validity of the result obtained. Trial designs which lack validity produce information that is at best difficult to use, and at worst is useless.

Placebo

People in pain respond to placebo treatment. Some patients given placebo obtain 100% pain relief (see Chapter 5). The effect is reproducible, and some work has been done to try and assess the characteristics of the 'placebo responder', by sex, race, and psychological profile. None has succeeded, but we do know that women have better responses to some analgesics than men, getting more analgesia from the same plasma concentration of drug.

Randomized controlled trials (RCTs)

Because the placebo response was an established fact in analgesic studies, randomization was used early in studies to try to avoid any possibility of bias from placebo responders, and to equalize their numbers in each treatment group. This was true even in studies without placebo, since an excess of placebo responders in an active treatment arm of a study might inflate the effects of an analgesic.

Sensitivity

Particularly for a new analgesic, a trial should prove its internal sensitivity (i.e. that the study was an adequate analgesic assay). This can be done in several ways. For instance, if a known analgesic (paracetamol) can be shown to have statistical difference from placebo, then the analgesic assay should be able to distinguish another analgesic of similar effectiveness. Alternatively, two different doses of a standard analgesic (e.g. morphine) could be used—showing the higher dose to be statistically superior to the lower dose again provides confidence that the assay is sensitive.

Failure to demonstrate sensitivity in one assay invalidates the results from that particular assay. The results could still be included in meta-analysis.

Equivalence

Studies of analgesics of an A versus B design are notoriously difficult to interpret (Fig. 3). If there is a statistical difference, then that suggests sensitivity. Lack of a significant difference (Fig. 3, top panel) means nothing—there is no way to determine whether there is an analgesic effect which is no different between A and B, or whether the assay lacks the sensitivity to measure a difference that is actually present.

This is not just a problem for pain studies [9, 10]. Designs which minimize these problems include using two doses of a standard analgesic, plus placebo to establish sensitivity (Fig. 3 middle and bottom panels). Simple calculations could show what dose of the new analgesic was equivalent to the usual dose of the standard analgesic.

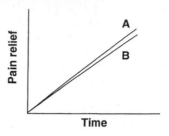

Equivalence: danger of A vs. B negatives
- Was there no difference?
- Was there a difference which was missed?

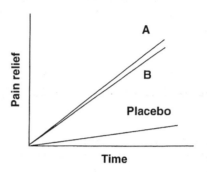

protection: negative control (placebo)

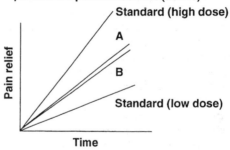

protection: positive control (active)

Fig. 3 Using placebo or active comparators to protect against A vs. B negative results.

Problems

The correct design of an analgesic trial is situation-dependent. In some circumstances very complicated designs have to be used to ensure sensitivity and validity

No 'gold standard'

There may be circumstances in which there is no established analgesic treatment of sufficient effectiveness to act as a 'gold standard' against which to measure a new treatment, often the case in chronic pain. Clearly, the use of placebo or no treatment controls is of great importance, especially when effects are to be examined over prolonged periods of weeks or months.

But it is paradoxically these very circumstances in which ethical constraints act against using placebo or non-treatment controls because of the need to do *something*. In acute pain studies, conversely, there is little problem with using placebos, since the failure of placebo (or any treatment) can be dealt with by prescribing additional analgesics which should work.

When there is no pain to begin with

Clearly, where there is no pain it is difficult to measure an analgesic response. Yet a number of studies seek to do this by pre-empting pain, or using an intervention where there is no pain (intraoperatively, for instance) to produce analgesia when pain is to be expected.

These are difficult, but not impossible, circumstances in which to conduct research. Meticulous attention to trial design is necessary to be able to show differences.

References

1. Keele KD. The pain chart. *Lancet* 1948; 2:6–8.
2. Scott J, Huskisson EC. Graphic representation of pain. *Pain* 1976; 2:175–84.
3. Wallenstein SL, Heidrich IG, Kaiko R, Houde RW. Clinical evaluation of mild analgesics: The measurement of clinical pain. *British Journal of Clinical Pharmacology* 1980; 10:319S–27.
4. Littman GS, Walker BR, Schneider BE. Reassessment of verbal and visual analogue ratings in analgesic studies. *Clinical Pharmacology and Therapeutics* 1985; 38:16–23.
5. Sriwatanakul K, Kelvie W, Lasagna L. The quantification of pain: an analysis of words used to describe pain and analgesia in clinical trials. *Clinical Pharmacology and Therapeutics* 1982; 32:141–8.
6. Murphy DF, McDonald A, Power C, Unwin A, MacSullivan R. Measurement of pain: a comparison of the visual analogue with a nonvisual analogue scale. *Clinical Journal of Pain* 1988; 3:197–9.
7. Jadad AR, McQuay HJ. The measurement of pain. In: Pynsent P, Fairbank J, Carr A, ed. *Outcome measures in orthopaedics*. Oxford: Butterworth Heinemann, 1993:16–29.
8. Collins SL, Moore RA, McQuay HJ. The visual analogue pain intensity scale: what is moderate pain in millimetres? *Pain* 1997; 72:95–7.
9. Jones B, Jarvis P, Lewis JA, Ebbutt AF. Trials to assess equivalence: the importance of rigorous methods. *British Medical Journal* 1996; 313:36–9.
10. McQuay H, Moore A. Placebos are essential when extent and variability of placebo response are unknown. *British Medical Journal* 1996; 313:1008.

5

Estimating relative effectiveness

Minor analgesics—paracetamol, ibuprofen, and combinations with opioids like codeine or dextropropoxyphene—are used often to treat pain. There are few direct comparisons, one with another, but most trials contain a placebo, and it has the potential to be the universal comparator. Instead of measuring relative effectiveness through multiple comparisons of different drugs, it should be possible to compare the absolute effectiveness of analgesics against placebo.

This chapter examines some aspects of clinical trial methods relating to the placebo response in clinical trials of single doses of analgesics using classical methods. It then determines ways in which data can be extracted from published studies for use in meta-analysis.

Placebo responses in analgesic trials

The placebo response is confusing [1]. Two common misconceptions are that a fixed fraction (one-third) of the population responds to placebo, and that the extent of the placebo reaction is also a fixed fraction (again about one-third of the maximum possible [2]). As Wall points out, these ideas stem from a misreading of Beecher's work of years ago [1].

In Beecher's five acute pain studies, 139 patients (31%) of 452 given placebo had 50% or more relief of postoperative pain at two checked intervals [3]. The proportion of patients who had 50% or more relief of pain varied across the studies, ranging from 15% to 53%. There was neither a fixed fraction of responders, nor a fixed extent of response.

Placebo responses have also been reported as varying systematically with the efficacy of the active analgesic medicine. Evans pointed out that in seven studies the placebo response was always about 55% of the active treatment, whether that was aspirin or morphine: the stronger the drug, the stronger the placebo response [4].

Randomized, double-blind trials are meant to eliminate (or at least minimize) both selection bias and observer bias; Evans' observation suggests that significant observer bias occurs. Wall [1] rightly questions the blindness of these trials if this result were true, and elegantly dissects the areas where 'leakage' of blinding can occur (patient–patient, patient–doctor, patient–nurse).

Both these observations call into question the validity of the methods used to gather the data. If the methods are faulty, how reliable are the answers? The first part of this chapter therefore examines the nature of the variation in placebo responses in five randomized, double-blind, parallel-group trials in postoperative pain, and the relationship of the variation to the analgesic effectiveness of the active treatments.

Methods

Individual patient data was used from five placebo controlled double-blind randomized trials which investigated the analgesic effects of various drugs in postoperative pain [5–9] done over a 10-year period by the Pain Research group in Oxford. All were randomized, double-blind, and parallel-group trials of single doses of drugs given orally. Randomization was made from random number tables. Drugs were prepared outside the hospital in which the studies were done. Treatment codes were not broken until the studies were finished. All drugs within a study were identical. Drugs were given in a standardized way by the nurse observer. The methods used by the trained nurse observers to measure pain were identical. Patients were asked a standardized battery of questions in a fixed order at each assessment time in the studies. All patients knew that a placebo was one of several possible treatments. All patients had moderate or severe pain within 72 hours of surgery, and all were aware that they could withdraw from the study at any time for any reason.

Each study used five scales for pain; three for pain intensity and two for pain relief. Of these the five-point categorical verbal rating scale for pain relief (catPR: 0 = none, 1 = slight, 2 = moderate, 3 = good, 4 = complete) was chosen for this analysis because it was closest to Beecher's original method. For each patient the area under the curve of pain relief (categorical scale) against time was calculated (TOTPAR). The percentage of the maximum possible for this summary measure was then calculated (%maxTOTPAR) [10].

Results

In the five trials 130 patients had a placebo. Individual patients' scores with placebo varied from 0% to 100% of the maximum possible pain relief.

Figure 1 shows the distribution of these %maxTOTPAR scores. In the five trials 395 patients had active drugs. Individual patients' scores with different active drugs varied from 0% to 97% of the maximum possible pain relief. Figure 1 shows the distribution of these %maxTOTPAR scores for the active drugs.

The mean %maxTOTPAR scores for the five placebo groups varied from 11% to 29%, and the mean scores for the active drugs varied from 12% to 49%. The relationship between the mean scores for the actives and the mean placebo scores is shown in Fig. 2. Mean placebo scores were related to the mean score for the active in each trial such that the higher the active score, the higher the placebo score. A

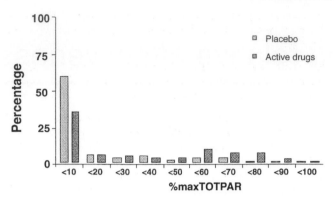

Fig. 1   Distribution of %maxTOTPAR scores for the 130 patients given placebo and for the 395 patients given active drugs.

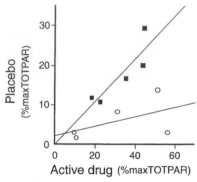

Fig. 2   %maxTOTPAR placebo and active drug scores for the 5 trials. ○ = median, ■ = mean.

similar relationship obtained for the best active and for the worst active from each of the five trials. On average, the mean placebo results were 54% of the mean active results based on a slope of 0.54; 95% confidence intervals around the slope were 0.03 to 1.08.

Figure 2 also shows the relationship between the median scores for active and the placebo treatments. There was little relationship between the two, and, on average, the median placebo score was less than 10% of the median active score. The slope to the regression line was 0.12, but with 95% confidence intervals of –0.24 to 0.48, and included no relationship between placebo response and extent of the response to active analgesic.

The same pattern of results was also found when the analysis was repeated using the results from the visual analogue scale for pain relief.

Comment

The variation of the placebo response in the acute pain setting found by Beecher 40 years ago is confirmed by these results. Using the dichotomous measure of greater than 50% pain relief at 45 and 90 minutes, Beecher found a range of 15% to 53% of patients given placebo had greater than 50% relief in five acute pain studies [3]. Here, using the derived dichotomous measure of 50% maximum pain relief, a range of 7% to 37% of patients given placebo achieved greater than 50% relief across the five studies (Table 1).

In analgesic trials the response of a group of patients to a treatment is usually described not as a dichotomous variable (like the proportion of patients with at least 50% relief), but rather as a continuous variable (the mean extent of the response). The common description of pain intensity difference or pain relief is thus as the mean with standard deviations or standard errors of the mean, as if the data were normally distributed.

Patient responses were not normally distributed, either for patients given placebo or for those given an active treatment (Fig. 1). The predominant group was that getting less than 10% of maximum relief—62% of patients given placebo and 37% of those given an active treatment. In these circumstances, the use of a mean as a description is not valid, and the use of a median is more sensible. Averaging results to describe them is an historic hangover.

In describing the placebo groups, therefore, the range of mean placebo response of 11% to 29% of maximum (Table 1) becomes a range of median placebo response of 2% to 14% and a range of the proportion of patients with at least 50% of %maxTOTPAR of 7% to 37%. Regressing median placebo response against median active response from the same five trials yielded a poor correlation, with a regression line no different from the horizontal, which would be the expected result if there was no bias. The idea that there is a constant relationship between active analgesic and placebo response is therefore an artefact of using an inappropriate statistical description.

It is the comparison of the mean data from placebo and active treatments which led to the observation [4] that

Table 1   Results with placebo: mean (standard deviation, SD), median (interquartile range), and number of patients with at least 50% of %maxTOTPAR in the 5 studies

Ref.	No. of patients	Mean %maxTOTPAR	Median %maxTOTPAR (interquartile range)	No. of patients with at least 50% of %maxTOTPAR	% of patients with at least 50% of %maxTOTPAR
[5]	21	11.9 (19.3)	3.1 (16.4)	2	10
[6]	30	29.4 (29.1)	14.0 (53.0)	11	37
[7]	19	20.1 (29.1)	3.1 (27.3)	4	21
[8]	30	10.7 (17.8)	2.1 (8.3)	2	7
[9]	30	16.9 (21.2)	8.3 (25.0)	2	7

placebo is about 55% as effective as an active treatment, whatever active treatment is used. In the five trials here, comparison of the mean placebo response with the mean active treatment (Fig. 2) produced a regression with a slope of 0.54—exactly the same result!

This defies logic unless there was considerable bias despite randomization and the use of double-blind methods, and if true would undermine the confidence placed in analgesic trial results. But is it true?

Randomization controls for selection bias, and the double-blind design is there to control observer bias. Patients knew a placebo was one possible treatment, and the investigators knew the study design and active treatments; it has been suggested that this can modify patients' behaviour [11, 12]. A small number of patients may have had opportunities to communicate with each other. Doctors who knew the trial design consented the patients, and this may also be a source of bias [13]. The nurse observer spent most time with the patients, but in standardized situations. This would be the most likely source of bias, as the nurse might be able to influence a patient's response by his/her demeanour based on his/her experience of other patients' reactions. That would produce time-dependent changes in study results as has been seen before [14].

Bias may still occur, but its effects are slight. That has important consequences. It means that results obtained over a range of clinical conditions and times may be combined in metanalyses with confidence. Gøtzsche has confirmed similar magnitudes of effect for non-steroidal anti-inflammatory drugs in active and placebo controlled studies [15], showing that the presence of a placebo does not affect the active treatment—the alternative hypothesis.

Deriving dichotomous outcome measures from continuous data in randomized controlled trials (RCTs) of analgesics

The problem is that in most published trial reports the only value available which describes the magnitude of analgesic effect is the mean and standard deviation of the SPID or TOTPAR. Is it possible, then, to use this to generate other, more useful data with which meta-analysis can work with confidence? Meta-analytic outcomes using mean values from different trials have been explored [16, 17], but the result is complicated analysis which is not intuitively accessible to doctor or patient. If individual patient information was available from every randomized controlled trial of analgesics, dichotomous data could be extracted for number-needed-to-treat NNT calculations. The reality is that individual patient data is not available, so that the problem is how to derive dichotomous outcomes from the published mean data. A full version of these arguments is published in Moore *et al.* 1996 [18].

A proposed solution

We examined the hypothesis that, in pharmacological interventions in acute pain:

1. A relationship exists between the descriptive mean value for pain relief and a dichotomous description of the same data set.

2. Knowing that relationship allows the conversion of descriptive mean values for pain relief into dichotomous data that can be used with confidence for meta-analysis.

Relationships that exist between treatment group means and some simple extractable variables from a known data set are an obvious place to start. What is required as an extractable variable is a single value, for instance the proportion or number of patients who have achieved 50% pain relief. If treatment group means reliably predict the proportion with half relief, this suggests that the relationship between the two variables is a product of the underlying distribution. One benefit of using the proportion of patients who have achieved at least 50% pain relief is that it is clinically intuitive.

How robust such a relationship might be can be tested in various ways. The gold standard would be to test relationships between mean and dichotomous variables developed from one set of trials using data from other trials.

In the absence of available information from real trials, surrogate trials can be obtained through simulation. Simulation methods have been used to generate individual patient data for large numbers of trials using the underlying distribution from randomized trials of pharmacological interventions performed in Oxford over about 15 years with standard methods. Such an approach generates precision in defining the underlying distribution of the data and tests assumptions made in deriving the technique for converting mean pain relief data into dichotomous data.

Although simulation methods can give a degree of confidence that the general approach has validity, it is testing against other, real, data sets which will allow the method to be used in meta-analysis.

Methods for converting mean to dichotomous data from clinical trials of analgesics, given in single doses using classical analgesic methodology, have been determined in three stages, all of which use at least 50% maxTOTPAR as a final dichotomous outcome.

Stage 1 Use of Oxford data from about 1500 patients combined with mathematical modelling using TOTPAR scales.

Stage 2 Verification with an external data set of 3500 patients using TOTPAR scales.

Stage 3 Examination of the use of other scales.

For each stage, methods and results are shown separately, and then discussed together.

Stage 1 methods

Actual patient data

Individual patient data was used from 12 placebo and active controlled double-blind randomized trials which investigated the analgesic effects of various drugs in postoperative pain [5–9, 19–26]. These trials were done over a 15-year period by the Pain Research Group in Oxford. Complete individual patient information was available over four or six hours for a number of pain and pain relief scales. Drugs were given orally, except sublingual buprenorphine [20], and intramuscular opioids [26].

Characteristics of the studies were that all were randomized, double-blind and parallel-group. Patients were told about the study by the nurse observer the day before surgery. Informed consent was obtained by the doctor that evening. Randomization was made from random number tables. Drugs were prepared outside the hospital in which the studies were done. Treatment codes were not broken until the studies were finished. All drugs within a study were identical in appearance and double-dummy methods were used when different routes of administration were compared. Drugs were given in a standardized way by the nurse observer. The methods used by the trained nurse observers to measure pain were identical.

Patients were asked a standardized battery of questions in a fixed order at each assessment time in the studies. In placebo controlled trials, all patients knew that a placebo was one possible treatment. All patients had moderate or severe pain within 72 hours of surgery, and all were aware that they could withdraw from the study at any time for any reason. At the start of the assessments the nurse observer made sure that patients had recovered sufficiently from the anaesthetic and were able to communicate reliably. Studies with more than one nurse observer were block randomized with one nurse responsible for each block. Only one nurse did the assessments for any one patient. If no pain relief was obtained from the test medication by 1 hour, or if the pain intensity subsequently reverted to the initial value before the end of the 6-hour study, patients were given analgesia ('escape analgesia').

Each study used five scales for pain; three for pain intensity and two for pain relief. In this study, the categorical measurement of pain relief with a five-point categorical verbal rating scale (catPR 0 = none, 1 = slight, 2 = moderate, 3 = good, 4 = complete) was used because it has been shown that with this scale placebo responses are independent of active treatment efficacy [27].

For each patient the area under the curve of pain relief (categorical scale) against time was calculated (TOTPAR). The percentage of the maximum possible for this summary measure was then calculated (%maxTOTPAR), as well as the numbers and proportion of each group with at least 50%maxTOTPAR (or %>50%maxTOTPAR to accommodate unequal group sizes). The dichotomous descriptor of at least 50%maxTOTPAR was chosen because it is a simple clinical endpoint of pain half relieved, easily understood by professionals and patients.

The relationship between the mean %maxTOTPAR and the actual number of patients with at least 50%maxTOTPAR was examined by linear regression analysis. Using the equation to the regression line, the calculated number of patients with at least 50%maxTOTPAR was then compared with the actual number.

Odds ratios and their 95% confidence intervals were calculated using standard formulae using a fixed-effects model and numbers-needed-to-treat using the method of Cook and Sackett [28]. Where the same treatment (placebo or active) had been given in different trials, data from individual treatment arms were combined.

Simulations

The underlying distribution using %maxTOTPAR for individual real patients in the actual 45 treatments was approximately uniform over the range 10–100% of %maxTOTPAR with a spike in the range 0–10% of %maxTOTPAR. This was an amalgamation of patient data from all the treatments and was unlikely to reflect the actual distribution within any one treatment.

Because the possibility exists that statistical differences in distribution could occur in treatment arms with relatively small patient numbers, simulations were conducted to test how robust the relationships developed with actual treatments and real patients might be. Simulations had three main aims:

1. To generate a very large number of simulated active treatments (10 000) with a mean of 30 simulated patients (standard deviation, 3 patients; minimum group size, 15 patients) in each, where the %maxTOTPAR for each simulated patient was generated randomly from a distribution similar to the real data. Comparable results from real and simulated data would allow the conclusion that the conversion technique was dependent only on the amalgamated distribution of %maxTOTPAR from all trials, and not on the underlying distribution of %maxTOTPAR within each trial.

2. To show that for each simulated treatment, mean %maxTOTPAR could be converted to the calculated number with at least 50%maxTOTPAR using the techniques developed for the 45 actual treatments, and, for these simulated treatments, to compare the calculated number with at least 50%maxTOTPAR to the number generated in the simulation. This would provide an indication of how accurate the conversion technique was likely to be for a large data set with this underlying distribution.

3. To generate simulated individual patient data using two different underlying distributions (normal distribution and a uniform distribution, ensuring in each case that the mean was similar to that for the real data), in order to test the extent to which the accuracy of the conversion technique was dependent on the underlying distribution.

Computer codes were written in Fortran and run on the Oxford University DEC Vax Cluster. Uniform random numbers in the range 0 to 1 (U [0, 1]) were obtained using the intrinsic function 'ran', and these were then used to calculate both random treatment sizes and individual patient data with the appropriate underlying distribution as described below.

(i) Treatment sizes were assumed to be normally distributed with a mean of 30 and a standard deviation of 3. These were calculated by transforming the U [0, 1] values into normal values with the required mean and standard deviation using the Box–Mueller algorithm [29]. If any generated value of the group size was below 15 it was discarded and a new value generated which fell in the appropriate range.

(ii) For generation of the 'simulated actual' distribution the $U[0, 1]$ value generated was first multiplied by 140 (giving a $U[0, 140]$ distribution), but for any values greater than 100 the value was discarded and a new value generated which was multiplied by 10. This process ensured that 50/140 (36%) of patients were uniformly distributed in the range 0% to 10%maxTOTPAR, and the remaining 64% were uniformly distributed in the range 10% to 100%. Standard techniques were then used to show that a distribution generated in this way had a theoretical mean of 37.1 and a standard deviation of 31.7.

(iii) For generation of the 'normal' distribution the Box–Mueller algorithm was again used to generate the appropriate values, but in this case it was necessary to restrict generated values to the range 0–100 %maxTOTPAR. Since this restriction process altered the mean of the underlying distribution, the appropriate values to be used in the simulation to give a mean of 37 were determined by iteration.

(iv) For the generation of the 'uniform' distribution the value $U[0, 1]$ was multiplied by 74.0 to obtain a distribution which was uniform on $[0, 74]$, with a mean of 37.

Stage 1 results

The actual trials used in the analysis, the treatments, numbers in each group, mean %maxTOTPAR, and numbers of patients with at least 50%maxTOTPAR are shown in Table 2. The calculated number of patients in each treatment with at least 50%maxTOTPAR was derived from 45 actual treatments using the relationship between mean %maxTOTPAR and %>50%maxTOTPAR. Mean %maxTOTPAR for each study was entered into the equation to the regression to derive the proportion with more than half relief. This proportion was then combined with the number of patients to generate the actual number of patients in each group predicted to have more than half relief. Numerical values were rounded up or down to the nearest integer.

Actual mean and proportion with at least 50%maxTOTPAR

The relationship between mean %maxTOTPAR and proportion with at least 50%maxTOTPAR is shown in Fig. 3; the equation to the regression line was:

%>50%maxTOTPAR – 1.41 × %maxTOTPAR – 14.1 ($r^2 = 0.89$)

Calculated number of patients with at least 50%maxTOTPAR

The actual and calculated numbers of patients in each group with at least 50%maxTOTPAR are shown in Table 2. The equation to the regression line was:

Calculated number with at least 50%maxTOTPAR = 0.93 × actual + 0.93 ($r^2 = 0.88$)

In 36 of 45 treatments the agreement between actual and calculated was within 2 patients, in 42 of 45 agreement was within 3 patients, and in 43 of 45 agreement was within 4 patients. The two most aberrant results occurred in the same trial [22].

Simulated actual distribution: mean and proportion with at least 50%maxTOTPAR

A simulated distribution, similar to that of the actual data ('simulated actual' distribution) was used to produce 10 000 simulated treatments. This generated a regression of mean %maxTOTPAR against %>50%maxTOTPAR which was very similar to that obtained for the actual data from 45 treatments:

%>50%maxTOTPAR = 1.34 × mean %maxTOTPAR – 14.1 ($r^2 = 0.79$)

Simulated actual distribution: calculated numbers at least 50% maxTOTPAR

This equation was used to obtain the calculated %>50%maxTOTPAR which was then regressed against the actual %>50%maxTOTPAR. The equation to the regression line was very similar to that obtained for the actual data from 45 treatments:

Calculated number with at least 50%maxTOTPAR = 0.82 × actual + 1.92 ($r^2 = 0.83$)

Table 3 shows that using the underlying distribution the difference between calculated and actual number of patients with at least 50%maxTOTPAR was 0–2 in 90% of the simulated studies, and in 99% it was in the range 0–3. These results are very similar to those obtained with the actual data, and again this suggests strongly that provided the underlying actual amalgamated distribution is a reasonable reflection of the assumed 'true' underlying distribution of pain relief, then the conversion technique is accurate and robust.

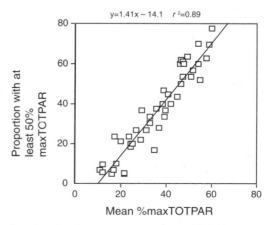

Fig. 3 Relationship between mean %maxTOTPAR and proportion with at least 50% maxTOTPAR.

Table 2 Studies used for calculations

Ref.	Treatment (No.)	Mean %maxTOTPAR	Actual no. with at least 50%maxTOTPAR	Calculated no. with at least 50%maxTOTPAR
[6]	650 mg paracetamol + 65 mg dextropropoxyphene (30)	46.0	18	15
	Placebo (30	29.4	11	8
	Zomepirac 100 mg (30)	38.4	12	12
	Zomepirac 50 mg (30)	49.4	19	17
[21]	Paracetamol 500 mg (30)	31.0	8	9
	Ketorolac 5 mg (30)	39.5	11	12
	Ketorolac 10 mg (30)	47.0	16	15
	Ketorolac 20 mg (30)	54.0	18	19
	Paracetamol 1000 mg (30)	41.9	12	14
[8]	Aspirin 650 mg (30)	23.4	7	6
	Fluradoline 150 mg (30)	17.3	7	3
	Fluradoline 300 mg (30)	26.9	8	7
	Placebo (30)	10.7	2	0
[5]	Bicifadine 100 mg (19)	12.0	1	1
	Bicifadine 150 mg (20)	17.8	2	2
	Placebo (21)	11.9	2	1
	Codeine 60 mg (20)	25.0	4	4
[9]	Bromfenac 5 mg (30)	25.4	6	0
	Bromfenac 10 mg (30)	38.9	4	12
	Bromfenac 25 mg (30)	46.3	15	15
	Placebo (30)	16.9	2	3
	Paracetamol 1000 mg (30)	32.9	10	10
[20]	Bromfenac 10 mg (23)	58.6	16	16
	Bromfenac 25 mg (21)	46.4	13	11
	Buprenorphine 0.2 mg (22)	21.7	1	4
	Buprenorphine 0.4 mg (24)	35.5	9	9
[19]	Paracetamol 1000 mg (30)	51.7	17	18
	Paracetamol 1000 mg + buprenorphine 1.0 mg (30)	47.8	18	16
	Paracetamol 1000 mg + buprenorphine 1.5 mg (29)	54.9	15	18
	Paracetamol 1000 mg + buprenorphine 2.0 mg (30)	50.8	16	17
[7]	Dihydrocodeine 30 mg (18)	40.6	8	8
	Placebo (19)	20.1	4	3
	Zomepirac 100 mg (18)	47.4	11	9
[24]	Paracetamol 1000 mg + codeine 16 mg + caffeine 60 mg (30)	39.1	10	12
	Ibuprofen 400 mg + codeine 25.6 mg (30)	54.0	21	19
[25]	Dihydrocodeine 30 mg (41)	28.7	9	11
	Dihydrocodeine 60 mg (43)	32.8	13	14
	Ibuprofen 400 mg (40)	60.0	31	28
[23]	Ibuprofen 400 mg (23)	44.8	10	11
	Ibuprofen 400 mg + codeine 20 mg (24)	57.7	15	16
[22]	Aspirin 500 mg + paracetamol 500 mg (47)	36.6	13	18
	Aspirin 500 mg + paracetamol 500 mg + codeine 13.6 mg (48)	34.8	8	17
[26]	Pethidine 100 mg (21)	16.1	1	2
	Meptazinol 100 mg (20)	21.8	1	3
	Morphine 15 mg (22)	24.4	4	4

Normal and uniform distributions

In order to test the effect of different underlying distributions, the process of obtaining the number of patients with at least 50%maxTOTPAR was repeated with two further distributions. The results obtained for the 'normal' and 'uniform' distributions (Table 3) were less accurate. Even so, these levels of agreement indicate that the conversion technique is robust even to these gross differences in underlying distribution, and

Table 3 Accuracy of the conversion in actual and simulated treatments

Difference between actual and calculated numbers	45 actual treatments (%)	Simulated actual distribution (%)	Simulated normal distribution (%)	Simulated uniform distribution (%)
≤ 1	57.7	60.3	21.3	40.7
≤ 2	82.1	90.8	44.4	71.2
≤ 3	93.2	98.8	68.2	89.0
≤ 4	95.4	99.8	87.1	97.1
≤ 5	97.7	100.0	96.5	99.3
≤ 6	97.7	100.0	99.4	99.9

Comparison of {actual – calculated} (irrespective of sign) number of patients with at least 50%maxTOTPAR as percentages for the 45 actual treatments and the simulated treatments of 10 000, each using the simulated actual, normal, and uniform distributions. Cumulative percentages are shown at different levels of agreement.

suggests that it will be very robust to the smaller differences that are likely to be encountered in practice.

Numbers-needed-to-treat (NNTs)

NNTs were calculated for paracetamol 1000 mg, zomepirac 100 mg, bromfenac 10 mg, bromfenac 25 mg, dihydrocodeine 30 mg, ibuprofen 400 mg, and ibuprofen 400 mg plus codeine 24.6 mg; for these, and for placebo, there was information from at least two trials (Table 4). NNT values derived from the actual and the calculated data, as well as odds ratios and confidence intervals (CIs), were very similar or identical.

Single treatment arms from the individual reports were combined to obtain odds ratio estimates with 95% con-

fidence intervals using a fixed-effects model and to derive NNT for analgesic effectiveness [28]. At least two identical treatments from different trials were required. Of the 130 patients who received placebo, 21 actually had at least 50%maxTOTPAR and 15 were calculated to have at least 50%maxTOTPAR.

Verification from independent data

Stage 2 methods

Individual patient data from 18 primary randomized control trials (RCTs) was made available by Grünenthal GmbH, Aachen, Germany and Robert Wood Johnson Pharmaceutical Research Institute, Spring House, Pennsylvania, USA.

Study protocols for post-surgical pain (including gynaecological procedures) and pain due to the extraction of impacted third molars were essentially identical. Trials were double-blind, single dose, parallel-group studies; randomization was by computerized random-number generation, stratified on pre-treatment pain. Criteria for patient selection were moderate or severe pain and that the patient's condition was appropriate for management with a centrally acting analgesic or paracetamol combined with centrally acting analgesics.

Ages ranged from 18 to 70 years. Patients had to be co-operative, reliable, and motivated, and be able to take oral medication. Exclusion criteria included patients with mild or no pain, those who had taken analgesic drugs within three hours of study drug administration, those needing sedatives during the observation period, and those with known contra-indications or medical conditions which might interfere with observations.

Drugs were given as single oral doses. They were placebo (695 evaluable patients), codeine 60 mg (649), tramadol 50 mg

Table 4 Number-needed-to-treat (NNT)

Treatment		Active drug at least 50%maxTOTPAR/Total	NNT (95% CI)	Odds ratio (95% CI)
Dihydrocodeine 30 mg	Actual	17/59	7.9 (3.9–∞)	2.2 (1.0–4.7)
	Calculated	19/59	4.8 (3.0–13.3)	4.0 (1.8–9.0)
Paracetamol 1000 mg	Actual	39/90	3.7 (2.6–6.6)	3.9 (2.1–7.1)
	Calculated	42/90	2.9 (2.1–4.3)	6.2 (3.4–11.4)
Zomepirac 100 mg	Actual	23/48	3.2 (2.1–6.1)	5.5 (2.5–11.7)
	Calculated	21/48	3.1 (2.1–5.8)	7.3 (3.2–16.6)
Bromfenac 10 mg	Actual	30/53	2.5 (1.8–3.9)	7.4 (3.6–15.1)
	Calculated	28/53	2.4 (1.8–3.7)	9.8 (4.6–20.8)
Bromfenac 25 mg	Actual	28/51	2.6 (1.9–4.2)	7.0 (3.4–14.6)
	Calculated	26/51	2.5 (1.8–4.1)	9.4 (4.3–20.3)
Ibuprofen 400 mg	Actual	41/63	2.0 (1.6–2.8)	9.3 (4.9–17.7)
	Calculated	39/63	2.0 (1.6–2.7)	12.0 (6.2–23.4)
Ibuprofen 400 mg + codeine 24.6 mg	Actual	36/54	2.0 (1.6–2.7)	10.5 (5.3–20.8)
	Calculated	35/54	1.9 (1.5–2.5)	14.6 (7.1–29.6)

CI, confidence interval. Where the confidence interval of the NNT includes ∞, this indicates no difference between treatment and control.

(409), tramadol 75 mg (281), tramadol 100 mg (468), tramadol 150 mg (279), tramadol 200 mg (50), aspirin 650 mg plus codeine 60 mg (305), and paracetamol 650 mg plus propoxyphene 100 mg (316).

Patients were given the study drug if they had moderate or severe pain on a four-point categorical scale (0 = no pain, 1 = slight, 2 = moderate, 3 = severe). Thereafter, observations were made at 30 minutes, and 1,2,3,4,5, and 6 hours after administration. Pain intensity was measured using the same categorical scale, together with a five-point categorical scale of pain relief (0 = no relief, 1 = a little, 2 = some, 3 = a lot, 4 = complete). Time of remedication was also recorded, as well as a global assessment of therapy (excellent, very good, good, fair, or poor) at the final evaluation. At remedication, pain relief scores reverted to zero and pain intensity scores to the initial value; adverse event recording, but not pain evaluations, continued after remedication.

For each patient the area under the curve of pain relief (categorical scale) against time (TOTPAR) was calculated for 6 hours after the study drug was given. The percentage of the maximum possible for this summary measure was then calculated for each patient (%maxTOTPAR [10]), mean TOTPAR for all patients in each treatment arm was calculated and the number of patients on each treatment achieving at least 50%maxTOTPAR was noted.

The mean TOTPAR value was then used to calculate the theoretical number of patients with at least 50%maxTOTPAR using a relationship established in clinical trials of analgesics in Oxford with 1283 patients with 45 treatments (percentage of patients with at least 50%maxTOTPAR = 1.41 × mean %maxTOTPAR − 14.1). Actual and calculated numbers were then compared using unweighted linear regression analysis.

Stage 2 results

Individual patient information was available from over 3400 patients in 85 different treatment arms in nine studies involving dental surgery (mostly third molar extraction) and nine involving general postoperative pain (including gynaecological procedures). Studies involved between 21 and 58 patients in each treatment (mean 40 patients). The distributions of %maxTOTPAR for all active and all placebo patients in these groups are shown in Fig. 4.

The relationship between actual and calculated numbers of patients with at least 50% maxTOTPAR in each treatment arm is shown in Fig. 5 and the equation to the regression line for this is compared in Table 5 with 45 treatments from trials in Oxford, using both the relationship for the actual data and that from a 10 000 treatment simulation.

Of the 85 treatment arms, 80 (94%) were within four patients per treatment and 74 (87%) within three (Table 6). These proportions were comparable to those obtained previously for actual and simulated treatments (Table 3). Summing the positive and negative differences between actual and calculated numbers of patients with at least 50%maxTOTPAR gave an average difference of 0.30 patients per treatment arm.

Combining the 85 treatments in this data set with earlier 45 treatments [18] produced a new relationship to be used in future conversions:

Proportion of patients with at least 50%maxTOTPAR = 1.33 × mean %maxTOTPAR − 11.5 (r^2 = 0.89)

Use of pain intensity and visual analogue scales

Stage 3 methods

Data for the study were from individual patient data from 13 randomized controlled trials (1283 patients with 45 treatments, Oxford data [18]) and 18 randomized controlled trials (3453 patients with 87 treatments, RWJ data) described in stages 1 and 2.

For each patient the summed pain intensity difference (SPID) was calculated for categorical pain intensity, and the equivalent VAS-SPID for visual analogue scales. For each individual patient the 4-hour or 6-hour SPID was divided by the maximum possible SPID; for example, a patient with a SPID of 6 and initial pain intensity of 3 would have a theoretical maximum SPID of 18, and the %maxSPID would be 33%. The area under the curve of pain relief against time

Table 5 Regression equations for calculated and actual number of patients in each treatment with > 50%maxTOTPAR

Study	Slope	Intercept	Coefficient of determination (r^2)
45 treatment arms from RCTs in Oxford (1)	0.93	0.93	0.88
45 treatment arms from RCTs in Oxford (2)	0.82	1.92	0.83
85 treatment arms from Robert Woods Johnson RCTs (3453 patients) (3)	0.94	0.33	0.89

Results for solutions to the equation: calculated = (actual × slope) + intercept using the relationship between %>50%maxTOTPAR and mean %maxTOTPAR derived from:

(1) 45 actual treatments (Oxford RCTs).
(2) a 10 000 treatment arm simulation.
(3) 85 actual treatments (Robert Woods Johnson RCTs).

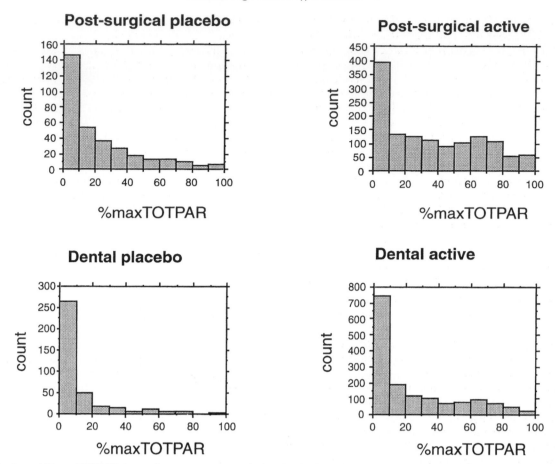

Fig. 4 Distribution of %maxTOTPAR for active treatments and placebo in dental and post-surgical pain.

was calculated for the categorical (TOTPAR) and visual analogue pain relief scale (VAS-TOTPAR). The percentage of the maximum possible for each summary measure was then calculated for each patient [10]. Rules for calculation included that in the event of remedication within 6 hours, pain relief scores reverted to zero and pain intensity scores to their initial value. The mean summary measure for all patients in each treatment arm was calculated. The number of patients on each treatment achieving at least 50%maxTOTPAR was noted.

The relationship between the mean %maxSPID, %maxVAS-SPID and %maxVAS-TOTPAR and the actual number of patients with at least 50%maxTOTPAR was examined by linear regression analysis. Using the equation to the regression line, the calculated number of patients with at least 50%maxTOTPAR was then compared with the actual number using unweighted linear regression analysis.

Stage 3 results

Individual patient scores for categorical pain intensity, visual analogue pain intensity, and pain relief scales (Fig. 6) were asymmetrically distributed, much as was seen for TOTPAR.

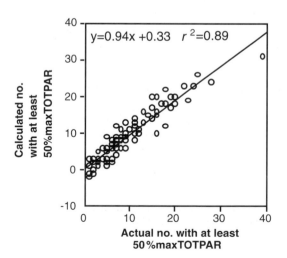

Fig. 5 Relationship between actual and calculated number with at least 50%maxTOTPAR for 3400 patients with 85 treatments.

Table 6   Accuracy of the conversion in actual and simulated treatments

Difference between actual and calculated numbers	45 Oxford actual treatments (%)	Simulated actual distribution (%)	Simulated normal distribution (%)	Simulated uniform distribution (%)	85 RWJ actual treatments (%)
≤ 1	57.7	60.3	21.3	40.7	50.6
≤ 2	82.1	90.8	44.4	71.2	70.6
≤ 3	93.2	98.8	68.2	89.0	87.1
≤ 4	95.4	99.8	87.1	97.1	94.1
≤ 5	97.7	100	96.5	99.3	96.6
≤ 6	97.7	100	99.4	99.9	98.8

Comparison of {actual – calculated, irrespective of sign} number of patients with at least 50%maxTOTPAR as percentages for the 45 actual treatments and 10 000 simulated treatments was done using the simulated actual, normal, and uniform distributions [18]. Cumulative percentages are shown at different levels of agreement. The final column adds the 85 treatment arms from the Robert Woods Johnson (RWJ) trials.

Categorical pain intensity scale

Data were available from 132 treatments with 4713 patients. Individual patient distribution of %maxSPID was asymmetric (Fig. 6A). Linear regression analysis performed for the Oxford and RWJ data sets separately showed similar relationships, so the data sets were combined for all 132 treatments.

Results from Oxford and RWJ data sets and the combined data for the regression of number of patients per treatment with at least 50%maxTOTPAR against mean %maxSPID (with 95% confidence interval).

For all 132 treatments the regression line was:

%>50%maxTOTPAR = 1.36 × mean %maxSPID – 2.3 (r^2 = 0.85)

There was good agreement between the actual number of patients with at least 50%maxTOTPAR in each treatment arm and the calculated number using the relationship derived with %maxSPID (Fig. 7A):

Calculated number with at least 50%maxTOTPAR = 0.86 × actual + 1.37 (r^2 = 0.86)

For 92% of treatments the actual and the calculated numbers with at least 50%maxTOTPAR were within four patients per treatment. Agreement (actual – calculated) was normally distributed around zero (Fig. 8). Summing the positive and negative differences between actual and calculated numbers of patients with at least 50%maxTOTPAR gave an average difference of –0.03 patients per treatment arm.

Visual analogue pain intensity scale

Data were available from 40 treatments within the Oxford data set with 1059 patients. Individual patient distribution of %maxVAS-SPID was asymmetric (Fig. 6B). The regression line between %>50%maxTOTPAR and mean %maxVAS-SPID was:

%>50%maxTOTPAR = 1.18 × mean %maxVAS-SPID – 2.2 (r^2 = 0.87)

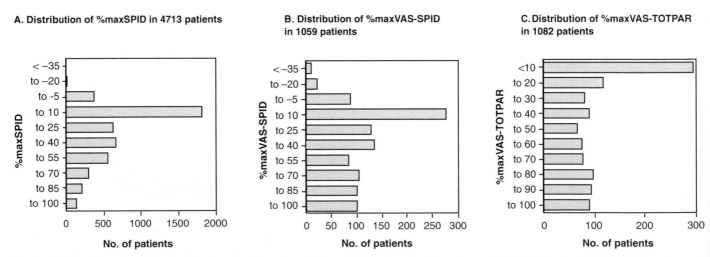

Fig. 6   Distribution of individual patient scores for categorical pain intensity, visual analogue pain intensity, and pain relief scores.

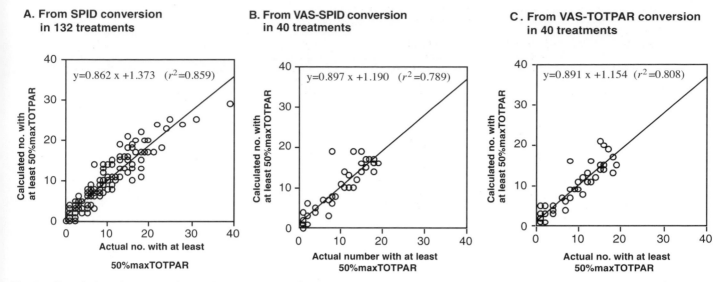

A. From SPID conversion in 132 treatments

$y=0.862 \, x +1.373 \quad (r^2=0.859)$

B. From VAS-SPID conversion in 40 treatments

$y=0.897 \, x +1.190 \quad (r^2=0.789)$

C. From VAS-TOTPAR conversion in 40 treatments

$y=0.891 \, x +1.154 \quad (r^2=0.808)$

Fig. 7   Correlation of actual and calculated numbers of patients with at least 50%maxTOTPAR in each treatment for calculations using categorical pain intensity and VAS pain intensity and relief scores.

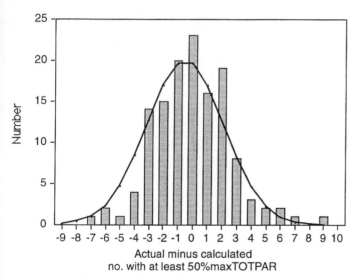

Fig. 8   Distribution of actual minus calculated number of patients with at least 50%maxTOTPAR in each treatment using SPID data. (Columns showing the actual minus calculated number of patients with at least 50%maxTOTPAR in each treatment using SPID. The line shows the normal distribution calculated for these data.)

There was good agreement between the actual number of patients with at least 50%maxTOTPAR in each treatment arm and the calculated number using the relationship derived with %maxVAS-SPID (Fig. 7B):

Calculated number with at least 50%maxTOTPAR = 0.90 × actual + 1.19 ($r^2 = 0.79$)

For 95% of treatments the actual and the calculated numbers with at least 50%maxTOTPAR were within 4 patients per treatment. Summing the positive and negative differences between actual and calculated numbers of patients with at

least 50%maxTOTPAR gave an average difference of −0.23 patients per treatment arm.

Visual analogue pain relief scale

Data were available from 40 treatments with 1082 patients. Individual patient distribution of %maxVAS-TOTPAR was asymmetric (Fig. 6C). The regression line between %>50%maxTOTPAR and mean %maxVAS-TOTPAR was:

%>50%maxTOTPAR = 1.15 × mean %maxVAS-TOTPAR − 8.51 ($r^2 = 0.81$)

There was good agreement between the actual number of patients with at least 50%maxTOTPAR in each treatment arm and the calculated number using the relationship derived with %maxVAS-TOTPAR (Fig. 7C):

Calculated number with at least 50%maxTOTPAR = × 0.89 actual + 1.15 ($r^2 = 0.81$)

For 95% of treatments the actual and the calculated numbers with at least 50%maxTOTPAR were within 4 patients per treatment. Summing the positive and negative differences between actual and calculated numbers of patients with at least 50%maxTOTPAR gave an average difference of −0.11 patients per treatment arm.

Overall comments

For SPID it was possible to use the gold standard of verification by independent data sets. Regressing %>50%maxTOTPAR against mean %maxSPID independently for Oxford and RWJ data sets produced very similar results (Table 7). Using the combined regression analysis, there was excellent agreement between actual and calculated numbers of patients with at least 50%maxTOTPAR in each treatment (Fig. 7A), and the

Table 7 Summary report on SPID calculations on 132 treatments

Data set	No.	Intercept (95% CI)	Slope (95% CI)	Coefficient of determination (r^2)
Oxford	45	−2.3 (−8.3, 3.6)	1.44 (1.24, 1.64)	0.83
RWJ	87	−1.7 (−4.3, 1.0)	1.27 (1.16, 1.38)	0.86
Combined data	132	−2.3 (−4.9, 0.2)	1.36 (1.26, 1.45)	0.85

CI, confidence interval.

sum of the difference over all 132 treatments was −0.03 patients per treatment, with the differences distributed normally around zero (Fig. 8). This is firm evidence for the reliability of the conversion method.

Only 40 treatments from the Oxford data set were available for calculating relationships between patients with at least 50%maxTOTPAR and mean %maxVAS-SPID and mean %maxVAS-TOTPAR. Despite this, the agreement between actual and calculated numbers with at least 50%maxTOTPAR was good (Fig. 7B,C, Table 8), so that over the 40 treatments the sum of actual—calculated was less than a quarter of a patient per treatment arm using either measure.

Although no independent verification was possible for visual analogue scales, the similarity of the results to those independently verified for TOTPAR [18, 30] and SPID buttresses the approach to using mean data from previously published reports to derive dichotomous data for meta-analysis [18].

Comment

There is an asymmetric distribution of summary values of pain relief in clinical trials of analgesics using standard trial methods. Using mean values to describe these summary values is inappropriate and may result in erroneous conclusions [27]. To use information from RCTs of analgesic drugs reporting mean data, conversion to some form amenable to meta-analysis is necessary—and preferably some dichotomous measurement. The alternative may be to discard the many thousands of studies of analgesic interventions in the literature.

Some possible methods of conversion have been subjected to the gold standard of verification by an independent data set. There were many patients, in many studies, with different clinical settings, using placebo and several different active analgesics. The result—the relationship between the calculated and actual number of patients with at least 50%maxTOTPAR—was essentially the same as that obtained originally using the relationship for the actual data and from a 10 000 treatment arm simulation. Verification was also possible for SPID, but not for visual analogue scales, although there is no obvious reason to suspect that conversions explored here should not be accurate.

From the categorical pain relief scale and its summary TOTPAR measure, dichotomous data (the proportion of patients achieving at least 50% of %maxTOTPAR and the corollary, those not achieving 50% relief) can now be derived with some confidence. Categorical pain relief data can also be used with confidence.

Other data may be used as it becomes available to further validate these relationships (Table 9), based on a wide variety of acute pain conditions with different analgesics, including simple analgesics, non-steroidal anti-inflammatory drugs, combinations, and sublingual and intramuscular opioids. The only caution is that the validity of these relationships has been demonstrated only in short-term single dose studies in acute pain models.

References

1. Wall PD. The placebo and the placebo response. In: Wall PD, Melzack R, ed. *Textbook of pain*, (3rd edn). Edinburgh: Churchill-Livingstone, 1994:1297–308.

Table 8 Accuracy of the conversion in actual and simulated treatments. Actual minus calculated percentage of patients with at least 50%maxTOTPAR for treatment arms: agreement to within:

Data sets	Scale	≤ 1	≤ 2	≤ 3	≤ 4	≤ 5	≤ 6
45 Oxford	TOTPAR	58	82	93	95	98	98
85 RWJ	TOTPAR	52	75	85	94	96	100
132 Oxford	SPID	45	70	87	92	95	98
40 Oxford	VAS-SPID	65	75	85	95	95	98
40 Oxford	VAS-TOTPAR	65	73	85	95	98	98

Comparison of actual minus calculated (irrespective of sign) percentage of patients with at least 50%maxTOTPAR as cumulative percentages for the 45 Oxford treatments using TOTPAR [18], and 85 RWJ treatments using TOTPAR [30]. Cumulative percentages are shown at different levels of agreement. The final three rows show comparisons using SPID, VAS-SPID, and VAS-TOTPAR as basis of calculations in Oxford and RWJ data sets.

Table 9 Summary of formulae to derive proportion of patients achieving at least 50% pain relief from mean data using different measures

Outcome measure		Formula
Categorical pain relief		= 1.33 × mean %maxTOTPAR −11.5
Categorical pain intensity	*Proportion of patients*	= 1.36 × mean %maxSPID −2.3
VAS pain relief	*achieving at least 50% relief*	= 1.15 × mean %maxVAS-TOTPAR −8.5
VAS pain intensity		= 1.18 × mean %maxVAS-SPID −2.2

2. Wall PD. The placebo effect: an unpopular topic. *Pain* 1992; **51**:1–3.

3. Beecher HK. The powerful placebo. *Journal of American Medical Association* 1955; **159**:1602–6.

4. Evans FJ. The placebo response in pain reduction. In: Bonica JJ, ed. *Advances in neurology*, Vol. 4. New York: Raven Press, 1974:289–96.

5. Porter EJB, Rolfe M, McQuay HJ, Moore RA, Bullingham RES. Single dose comparison of bicifadine, codeine and placebo in postoperative pain. *Current Therapeutic Research* 1981; **30**:156–60.

6. Evans PJ, McQuay HJ, Rolfe M, O'Sullivan G, Bullingham RE, Moore RA. Zomepirac, placebo and paracetamol/dextropropoxyphene combination compared in orthopaedic postoperative pain. *British Journal of Anaesthesia* 1982; **54**:927–33.

7. McQuay HJ, Bullingham RE, Moore RA, Carroll D, Evans PJ, O'Sullivan G et al. Zomepirac, dihydrocodeine and placebo compared in postoperative pain after day-case surgery. The relationship between the effects of single and multiple doses. *British Journal of Anaesthesia* 1985; **57**:412–19.

8. McQuay HJ, Carroll D, Poppletion P, Summerfield RJ, Moore RA. Fluradoline and aspirin for orthopedic postoperative pain. *Clinical Pharmacology and Therapeutics* 1987; **41**:531–6.

9. McQuay HJ, Carroll D, Frankland T, Harvey M, Moore A. Bromfenac, acetaminophen, and placebo in orthopedic postoperative pain. *Clinical Pharmacology and Therapeutics* 1990; **47**:760–6.

10. Cooper SA. Single-dose analgesic studies: the upside and downside of assay sensitivity. In: Max MB, Portenoy RK, Laska EM, ed. *The design of analgesic clinical trials (Advances in pain research and therapy*, Vol. 18). New York: Raven Press, 1991:117–24.

11. Gracely RH, Dubner R, Deeter WR, Wolskee PJ. Clinicians' expectations influence placebo analgesia. *Lancet* 1985; **1**:43.

12. Wall PD. Pain and the placebo response. Experimental and theoretical studies of consciousness. *CIBA Foundation Symposium* 174. Chichester: Wiley, 1993:187–216.

13. Bergmann J, Chassany O, Gandiol J, Deblois P, Kanis JA, Segrestaa J et al. A randomised clinical trial of the effect of informed consent on the analgesic activity of placebo and naproxen in cancer pain. *Clinical Trials and Meta-Analysis* 1994; **29**:41–7.

14. Shapiro AP, Myers T, Reiser MF, Ferris EB. Comparison of blood pressure response to veriloid and to the doctor. *Psychosomatic Medicine* 1954; **16**:478–88. [11486]

15. Gøtzsche PC. Meta-analysis of NSAIDs: contribution of drugs, doses, trial designs, and meta-analytic techniques. *Scandinavian Journal of Rheumatology* 1993; **22**:255–60.

16. Moertel CG, Ahmann DL, Taylor WF, Schwartau N. Relief of pain by oral medications. *Journal of the American Medical Association* 1974; **229**:55–9.

17. Jadad AR. Meta-analysis of randomised clinical trials in pain relief. University of Oxford: D.Phil. thesis, 1994.

18. Moore A, McQuay H, Gavaghan D. Deriving dichotomous outcome measures from continuous data in randomised controlled trials of analgesics. *Pain* 1996; **66**:229–37.

19. Bullingham RE, McQuay HJ, Moore RA, Weir L. An oral buprenorphine and paracetamol combination compared with paracetamol alone: a single dose double-blind postoperative study. *British Journal of Clinical Pharmacology* 1981; **12**:863–7.

20. Carroll D, Frankland T, Nagle C, McQuay H. Oral bromfenac 10 and 25 mg compared with sublingual buprenorphine 0.2 and 0.4 mg for postoperative pain relief. *British Journal of Anaesthesia* 1993; **71**:814–7.

21. McQuay HJ, Poppleton P, Carroll D, Summerfield RJ, Bullingham RE, Moore RA. Ketorolac and acetaminophen for orthopedic postoperative pain. *Clinical Pharmacology and Therapeutics* 1986; **39**:89–93.

22. McQuay HJ, Carroll D, Watts PG, Juniper RP, Moore RA. Does adding small doses of codeine increase pain relief after third molar surgery? *Clinical Journal of Pain* 1987; **2**:197–201.

23. McQuay HJ, Carroll D, Watts PG, Juniper RP, Moore RA. Codeine 20 mg increases pain relief from ibuprofen 400 mg after third molar surgery. A repeat-dosing comparison of ibuprofen and an ibuprofen-codeine combination. *Pain* 1989; **37**:7–13.

24. McQuay HJ, Carroll D, Guest P, Juniper RP, Moore RA. A multiple dose comparison of combinations of ibuprofen and codeine and paracetamol, codeine and caffeine after third molar surgery. *Anaesthesia* 1992; **47**:672–7.

25. McQuay HJ, Carroll D, Guest PG, Robson S, Wiffen PJ, Juniper RP. A multiple dose comparison of ibuprofen and dihydrocodeine after third molar surgery. *British Journal of Oral and Maxillofacial Surgery* 1993; **31**:95–100.

26. McQuay HJ, Moore RA, Poppleton P, Uppington J, Bullingham RES, Lammer P. Postoperative single-dose comparison of intramuscular meptazinol, morphine and pethidine, compared in the same patients with intravenous meptazinol, morphine and pethidine given by PCA. unpublished.

27. McQuay H, Carroll D, Moore A. Variation in the placebo effect in randomised controlled trials of analgesics: All is as blind as it seems. *Pain* 1996; **64**:331–5.

28. Cook RJ, Sackett DL. The number needed to treat: a clinically useful measure of treatment effect. *British Medical Journal* 1995; **310**:452–4.

29. Dudewicz EJ, Mishra SM. *Modern mathematical statistics*. New York: Wiley, 1988.

30. Moore A, McQuay H, Gavaghan D. Deriving dichotomous outcome measures from continuous data in randomised controlled trials of analgesics: Verification from independent data. *Pain* 1997; **69**:127–30.

6
Combining data and interpreting the results

As professionals we want to use the best treatments and, as patients, to be given them. Knowing that an intervention works (or does not work) is fundamental to clinical decision-making.

When is the evidence strong enough to justify changing practice? Some of the decisions we make are based on individual studies, often on small numbers of patients, which, given the random play of chance, may lead to incorrect decisions. Systematic reviews identify and review all the relevant studies, and are more likely to give a reliable answer. They use explicit methods and quality standards to reduce bias. Their results are the closest we are likely to get to the truth in the current state of knowledge.

The questions a systematic review should answer for us are:

- How well does an intervention work (compared with placebo, no treatment or other interventions in current use)—or can I forget about it?
- Is it safe?
- Will it work and be safe for the patients in my practice?

Clinicians live in the real world and are busy people, and need to synthesize their knowledge of a particular patient in their practice, their experience and expertise, and the best external evidence from systematic review. They can then be pretty sure that they are doing their best. But the product of systematic review and particularly meta-analysis—often some sort of statistical output—is not usually readily interpretable or usable in day-to-day clinical practice. A common currency to help make the best treatment decision for a particular patient is what is needed. We think that common currency is the number-needed-to-treat (NNT).

Quality control

Systematic reviews of inadequate quality may be worse than none, because faulty decisions may be made with unjustified confidence. Quality control in the systematic review process, from literature searching onwards, is vital. How to judge the quality of a systematic review is encapsulated in the following questions [1], which are explained in more detail in Chapter 7:

- Were the question(s) and methods stated clearly?
- Were the search methods used to locate relevant studies comprehensive?
- Were explicit methods used to determine which articles to include in the review?
- Was the methodological quality of the primary studies assessed?

- Were the selection and assessment of the primary studies reproducible and free from bias?
- Were differences in individual study results explained adequately?
- Were the results of the primary studies combined appropriately?
- Were the reviewers' conclusions supported by the data cited?

When systematic reviews use data from different numbers of papers (see [2] for an excellent discussion of eligibility criteria for trials of head lice infection), reasons should be sought. Reviews can use criteria which exclude information important to individual clinicians, or may be too lax by including studies with inadequate trial design. The defence against either mistake is to read the inclusion and exclusion criteria critically to see if they make sense in your clinical circumstance.

Outcome measures chosen for data extraction should also be sensible. Usually, this is not a problem, but again it is a part of the methods that needs to be read carefully to see if you agree with the outcome measure extracted. The reviewer may have used all that is available, and any problems were due to the original trials, but it is a determinant of the clinical utility of the review. Examples in antibiotic treatment of *Helicobacter pylori* infection and peptic ulcer would be outcome measures of short-term bacterial kill rates and long-term remission.

Therapeutic interventions: which study architectures are admissible?

For a systematic review of therapeutic efficacy the gold standard is that eligible studies should be randomized controlled trials (RCTs). If trials are not randomized estimates of treatment effect may be exaggerated by up to 40% [3]. In a systematic review of transcutaneous electrical nerve stimulation (TENS) in postoperative pain, 17 reports on 786 patients could be regarded unequivocally as RCTs in acute postoperative pain. Fifteen of these 17 RCTs demonstrated no benefit of TENS over placebo. Nineteen reports had pain outcomes but were not RCTs; in 17 of these 19, TENS was considered by their authors to have had a positive analgesic effect [4]. When appropriate, and particularly with subjective outcomes, the gold standard for an efficacy systematic review is studies which are both randomized and double-blind. The therapeutic effect may be exaggerated by up to 20% in trials with deficient blinding [3].

Systematic reviews should eliminate bias	
	Overestimation of treatment effect
• Randomization	40%
• Double-blind	17%
• Duplicates	20%
• Small trials	30%

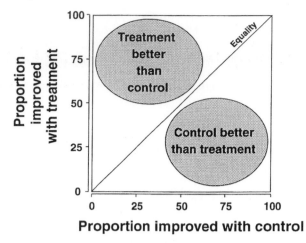

L'Abbé plot for treatment

Not all data can be combined in a meta-analysis: qualitative systematic reviews

It is often not possible or sensible to combine (pool) data, resulting in a qualitative rather than a quantitative systematic review. Combining data is not possible if there is no quantitative information in the component trials of the review. Combining data may not be sensible if trials used different clinical outcomes or followed the patients for different lengths of time. Combining continuous rather than dichotomous data may be difficult. Even if trials measure and present dichotomous data, if the trials are otherwise of poor quality [5] it may not be sensible to combine the data.

Making decisions from qualitative systematic reviews

Making decisions about whether or not a therapy works from such a qualitative systematic review may look easy. In the example above, 15 of the 17 RCTs of TENS in acute pain showed no benefit compared with control. The thinking clinician will catch the Bayesian drift, that TENS in acute pain is not effective. The problem with this simple vote counting is that it may mislead. It ignores the sample size of the constituent studies, the magnitude of the effect in the studies and the validity of their design even though they were randomized.

Combining data: quantitative systematic reviews

There are also two parts to the 'Does it work?' question: how does it compare with placebo and how does it compare with other therapies. Whichever comparison is being considered, the three stages of examining a review are a L'Abbé plot, statistical testing (odds ratio or relative risk), and a clinical significance measure such as NNT.

L'Abbé plots [6]

For therapies a first stage is to look at a simple scatter plot, which can yield a surprisingly comprehensive qualitative view of the data. Even if the review does not show the data

in this way you can do it from information on individual trials presented in the review tables. Figure 1 contains data extracted from three different systematic reviews of treatments for painful diabetic neuropathy [7–9]. Each point on the graph is the result of a single trial, and what happens with the intervention in question (experimental event rate, EER) is plotted against the event rate in the controls (control event rate, CER).

Trials in which the experimental treatment proves better than the control (EER > CER) will be in the upper left of the plot, between the y-axis and the line of equality. All three interventions in Fig. 1 were effective; the Figure does not indicate how effective. If experimental is no better than control then the point will fall on the line of equality (EER = CER), and if control is better than experimental then the point will be in the lower right of the plot, between the x-axis and the line of equality (EER < CER).

Visual inspection gives a quick and easy indication of the level of agreement among trials. Heterogeneity is often assumed to be due to variation in the experimental event

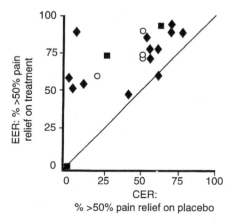

Fig. 1 L'Abbé plot of experimental event rate (EER) vs. control event rate (CER). (RCTs of anticonvulsants, ■; antidepressants, ◆; and topical capsaicin, ○ in diabetic neuropathy [7–9].)

rate, the effect of the intervention. Figure 1 shows that variation in the control event rate can also be a source of heterogeneity, and in this case the controls were all matched placebo in a relatively homogeneous chronic condition with treatments over several weeks to several months.

L'Abbé plots are not yet widely used. They do have several benefits: the simple visual presentation is easy to assimilate. They make us think about the reasons why there can be such wide variation in (especially) placebo responses, and about other factors in the overall package of care that can contribute to effectiveness. They explain the need for placebo controls if ethical issues about future trials arise. They keep us sceptical about overly good or bad results for an intervention in a single trial where the major influence may be how good or bad was the response with placebo.

Variation in control (placebo) response rates

The large variation in CER (from 0% to 80%) is not unusual. Similar variation was seen in trials of anti-emetics in postoperative vomiting [10], and in six trials of prophylactic natural surfactant for preterm infants the CER for bronchopulmonary dysplasia was 24–69% [11]. Such variation would not be expected in other circumstances, like use of antimicrobials. Rates of eradication of *H. pylori* with short-term use of ulcer healing drugs were 0–17% in 11 RCTs (with 10 of 11 below 10%) [12].

The reason for large variations in event rates with placebo may have something to do with trial design and population. The overwhelming reason for large variations in placebo rates in pain studies (and probably studies in other clinical conditions) is the relatively small group sizes in trials. Group sizes are chosen to produce statistical significance through power calculations—for pain studies the usual size is 30–40 patients for a 30% difference between placebo and active.

An individual patient can have no pain relief or 100% pain relief. Random selection of patients can therefore produce groups with low placebo response rate or high placebo response rate, or somewhere in between. Ongoing mathematical modelling based on individual patient data is showing that while group sizes of up to 50 patients are likely to show a statistical difference 80–90% of the time, to generate a close approximation to the 'true' clinical impact of a therapy requires as many as 500 patients per group (or more than 1000 patients in a trial). This is part of the rationale of systematic review.

Examples of the way group size can be a source of variation are important in understanding how pooling of information in pain trials can be of help. One example is given in Fig. 2, of trials in diabetic neuropathy where the proportion of patients given placebo is plotted against the number given placebo.

A similar pattern of an inverted 'V' can also be seen for topical NSAID trials, and indicates that almost all of the variability in placebo responses occurs in trials of small size. In rheumatoid arthritis, Gøtzsche [13] found a similar variability in estimates of change in erythrolyte sedimentation rate (ESR) and joint size by sample size.

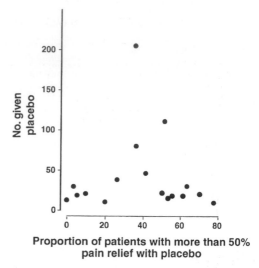

Fig. 2   Relationship between placebo response and trial size for pharmacological interventions in diabetic neuropathy.

The lessons are that information from individual trials of small size should be treated with circumspection in pain and probably other therapeutic areas, and that variation in outcomes seen in trials of small size is probably artefactual, especially in the absence of any Bayesian drift.

Indirect comparisons

Indirect comparisons of efficacy of different interventions, for example, by trying to compare treatments which have each been compared with placebo rather than with each other, may not be viable if the control event rates are dissimilar. *Posthoc* approaches, taking all the trials, then using only those that have a low or a high CER, are frowned on, although using particular clinical settings and anticipating less control event rate spread may be more acceptable [14]. In some circumstances, for instance in prophylaxis for nausea and vomiting, particular control event rate spreads may be determinants of trial validity [15].

In most pain studies neither of these apply.

Statistical significance

Odds ratios

When it is legitimate and feasible to combine data the odds ratio and relative risk are the accepted statistical tests to show that the intervention works significantly better than the comparator. As systematic reviews are used more to compare therapies clinicians need to grip these clinical epidemiological tools, which present the results in an unfamiliar way.

Figure 3 shows the odds ratios for the trials of antidepressants in diabetic neuropathy mentioned above. Some of the component trials did not show statistical significance; the lower 95% confidence interval of the odds ratio was less than 1. Conversely other trials, and the combined analysis,

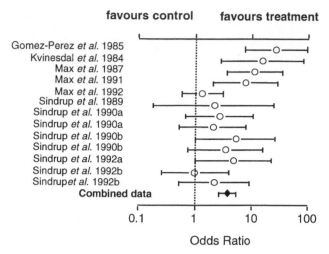

Fig. 3 Odds ratios for antidepressants in diabetic neuropathy. (references in Chapter 31)

did show statistical significance, with the lower 95% confidence interval being greater than 1, which means that 19 times out of 20 the 'true' value will be greater than 1.

The odds ratio can give a distorted impression when analyses are conducted on subgroups which differ substantially in baseline risk [14]. Where control event rates are high (certainly when they are above 50%), odds ratios should be interpreted with caution.

Relative risk or benefit

The fact that it is the odds ratio rather than relative risk or benefit which is used as the test of statistical significance for systematic reviews seems to be due to custom and practice rather than any inherent intellectual advantage [14]. Relative risk or benefit may be better than odds ratios because it is more robust in situations where control event rate is high [16]. With event rates above 10% relative risk produces more conservative figures [17].

In following chapters we try to use relative benefit and relative risk (of harm), despite the uncertainty and disagreement among statisticians and reviewers. In all cases the actual numbers are given so that when the dust has settled calculations can be re-done according to the prevailing opinion.

Heterogeneity

Clinicians making decisions on the basis of systematic reviews need to be confident that apples are not being compared with oranges. The L'Abbé plot is a qualitative defence against this spectre. Statistical testing provides a quantitative rampart, and is available in standard software [18]. Unfortunately, all these tests lack power, so that, while a test positive for heterogeneity suggests mixed fruits are being compared, a negative test does not provide complete reassurance that there is no heterogeneity.

Heterogeneity will also appear to occur because of variations in control and experimental event rates due to the random play of chance in trials of small size. Generally, trials of fewer than 10 patients per group have been omitted in reviews in this report, but considerable variability will occur in group sizes below 50 patients.

How well does the intervention work?

Although odds ratios and relative risks can show that an intervention works compared with control they are of limited help in saying how well the intervention works—the size of the effect or its clinical significance.

Effect size

The classic method of estimating effect size was to use the standardized mean difference [19]. The advantages of this approach are that it can be used to compare the efficacy of different interventions measured on continuous rather than dichotomous scales, and even using different outcome measures. The z-score output is in standard deviation units, and therefore is scale-free.

The disadvantage of effect size is that it is not intuitive for clinicians.

Number-needed-to-treat (NNT)

The NNT concept is proving to be a very effective alternative as the measure of clinical significance from quantitative systematic reviews. It has the crucial advantage of applicability to clinical practice, and shows the effort required to achieve a particular therapeutic target. The NNT is given by the equation

$$NNT = \frac{1}{(IMP_{act}/TOT_{act}) - (IMP_{con}/TOT_{con})}$$

where:
IMP_{act} = number of patients given active treatment achieving the target
TOT_{act} = total number of patients given the active treatment
IMP_{con} = number of patients given a control treatment achieving the target
TOT_{con} = total number of patients given the control treatment

NNT is also 1 divided by the proportion obtaining a particular effect with treatment *minus* the proportion obtaining the same effect with control, when those proportions are expressed as a decimal fraction. Because we have just described the absolute risk reduction, so NNT is also the reciprocal of the absolute risk reduction.

Treatment-specific

NNT is treatment-specific. It describes the *difference* between active treatment and control. The threshold used to calculate

NNT can vary, but NNT is likely to be relatively unchanged because changing threshold changes results for both active and control.

For example, an individual patient data meta-analysis of postoperative pain relief calculated NNTs compared with placebo for paracetamol 650 mg plus propoxyphene 100 mg (APAP/P) between 20% and 80% relief of pain (Fig. 4). With placebo the proportion of patients achieving a particular level of pain relief fell quickly as the target was raised. For an effective analgesic, this proportion fell slowly until high relief targets were reached. The difference remained largely unaltered over a wide range of targets—generating stable NNTs.

An NNT of 1 describes an event which occurs in every patient given the treatment but in no patient in a comparator group. This could be described as the 'perfect' result in, say, a therapeutic trial of an antibiotic compared with placebo. For therapeutic benefit the NNT should be as close as possible to 1; there are few circumstances in which a treatment is close to 100% effective and the control or placebo completely ineffective, so NNTs of 2 or 3 often indicate an effective intervention. For unwanted effects, NNT becomes the NNH (number-needed-to-harm), which should be as large as possible.

It is important to remember that the NNT is always relative to the comparator and applies to a particular clinical outcome. The duration of treatment necessary to achieve the target should be specified. The NNT for cure of head lice at two weeks with permethrin 1% compared with control vehicle was 1.1 (95% CI 1.0 – 1.2) [2, 20].

Confidence intervals

The confidence intervals of the NNT are an indication that 19 times out of 20 the 'true' value will be in the specified range. If the odds ratio or relative risk/benefit is not statistically significant then the NNT is infinite, indicating no difference from control. An NNT with an infinite confidence interval is then but a point estimate. It may still have clinical importance as a benchmark until further data permits finite confidence intervals, but decisions must take account of this parlous state.

Disadvantages

The disadvantage of the NNT approach, apparent from the formula, is that it needs dichotomous data. Continuous data can be converted to dichotomous for acute pain studies so that NNTs may be calculated, by deriving a relationship between the two from individual patient data [21]. Because of the way it is calculated, NNT will also be sensitive to trials with high control event rates. As control event rate (CER) rises the potential for treatment-specific improvement decreases: higher (and apparently less effective) NNTs result. So, as with any summary measure from a quantitative systematic review, NNT needs to be treated with caution, and comparisons can only be made confidently if CERs are in the same range.

Calculating NNTs when they are not provided

Odds ratios

If a quantitative systematic review produces odds ratios but no NNTs, you can derive NNTs from Table 1.

A caveat here is that odds ratios should be interpreted with caution when events occur commonly, as in treatments, and odds ratios may overestimate the benefits of an effect when event rates are above 50%. They are likely to be superseded by relative risk or benefit because it is more robust in situations where event rates are high [14, 22].

Is it safe?

Estimating the risk of harm is a critical part of clinical decisions. Systematic reviews should report adverse events as well as efficacy, and consider the issue of rare but important adverse events. Large RCTs apart, most trials study limited patient numbers. New medicines may be launched after trials on 1500 patients [23], missing these rare but important adverse events. The rule of three is important here. If a particular serious event does not occur in 1500 patients given the treatment, we can be 95% confident that the chance of it occurring is at most 3/1500 [24].

Much the same rules apply to harm as to efficacy, but with some important differences, the number-needed-to-harm (NNH) rather than to-treat (NNT) and the rules of admissible evidence.

Number-needed-to-harm (NNH)

For minor adverse effects reported in RCTs, NNH may be calculated in the same way as NNT. When there is low incidence it is likely that point estimates alone will emerge (infinite confidence intervals). Major harm may be defined in a set of RCTs as intervention-related study withdrawal, and

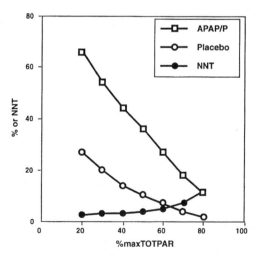

Fig. 4   Effect of different thresholds of pain relief on NNT.

Table 1　Table for estimating NNT when odds ratio (OR) and control event rate (CER) are known, published for prophylactic interventions in [16]

Control event rate (CER)	Odds ratio (OR)																	
	Prophylaxis									Treatment								
	0.5	0.55	0.6	0.65	0.7	0.75	0.8	0.85	0.9	1.5	2	2.5	3	3.5	4	4.5	5	10
0.05	41	46	52	59	69	83	104	139	209	43	22	15	12	9	8	7	6	3
0.1	21	24	27	31	36	43	54	73	110	23	12	9	7	6	5	4	4	2
0.2	11	13	14	17	20	24	30	40	61	14	8	5	4	4	3	3	3	2
0.3	8	9	10	12	14	18	22	30	46	11	6	5	4	3	3	3	3	2
0.4	7	8	9	10	12	15	19	26	40	10	6	4	4	3	3	3	3	2
0.5	6	7	8	9	11	14	18	25	38	10	6	5	4	4	3	3	3	2
0.7	6	7	9	10	13	16	20	28	44	13	8	7	6	5	5	5	5	4
0.9	12	15	18	22	27	34	46	64	101	32	21	17	16	14	14	13	13	11

Formula for *prophylaxis*:　$$NNT = \frac{1-[CER \times (1-OR)]}{(1-CER) \times CER \times (1-OR)}$$

Formula for *treatment*:　$$NNT = \frac{CER(OR-1)+1}{CER(OR-1) \times (1-CER)}$$

Choose the column which is closest to the published odds ratio (*prophylaxis* left side, *treatment* right side), and the row which is closest to the event rate expected, then read off the corresponding NNT. You can also use this table to see how different values for event rate or expected event rate for an individual patient affect the NNT at a given odds ratio.

be calculated from those numbers. Precise estimates of major harm will require much wider literature search to trawl for case reports or series. The absence of information on adverse effects in systematic reviews reduces their usefulness.

Rules of admissible evidence

The gold standard of evidence for harm, as for efficacy, is the RCT. The problem is that in the relatively small number of patients studied in RCTs rare serious harm may not be spotted. For an adverse effect systematic review, study architectures of lower intrinsic quality may therefore be admissible. An extreme example is that observer blinding is superfluous if the outcome is death. Such rare and serious harm cannot and should not be dismissed just because it is reported in a case report rather than in an RCT. The 'process rules' in this area have yet to be determined.

Using NNTs

In the ideal world you will have three numbers for each intervention, an NNT for benefit and NNHs for minor and major harm.

The thrust of this book is to establish the effectiveness or otherwise of a range of interventions, and if effective, to use the NNT as a benchmark of how effective is a particular intervention.

This then becomes the yardstick against which alternative interventions should be judged, and is the pivot for the clinical decision on whether or not to use the intervention for an individual patient.

References

1. Oxman AD, Guyatt GH. Guidelines for reading literature reviews. *Canadian Medical Association Journal* 1988; **138**:697–703. [10169]
2. Vander Stichele RH, Dezeure EM, Bogaert MG. Systematic review of clinical efficacy of topical treatments for head lice. *British Medical Journal* 1995; **311**:604–8.
3. Schulz KF, Chalmers I, Hayes RJ, Altman DG. Empirical evidence of bias: dimensions of methodological quality associated with estimates of treatment effects in controlled trials. *Journal of the American Medical Association* 1995; **273**:408–12.
4. Carroll D, Tramer M, McQuay H, Nye B, Moore A. Randomization is important in studies with pain outcomes: Systematic review of transcutaneous electrical nerve stimulation in acute postoperative pain. *British Journal of Anaesthesia* 1996; **77**:798–803.
5. Jadad AR, Moore RA, Carroll D, Jenkinson C, Reynolds DJM, Gavaghan DJ *et al.* Assessing the quality of reports of randomized clinical trials: is blinding necessary? *Controlled Clinical Trials* 1996; **17**:1–12.
6. L'Abbé KA, Detsky AS, O'Rourke K. Meta-analysis in clinical research. Ann Intern Med 1987; **107**:224–33.
7. Zhang WY, Li Wan Po A. The effectiveness of topically applied capsaicin. A meta-analysis. *European Journal of Clinical Pharmacology* 1994; **46**:517–22.
8. McQuay H, Carroll D, Jadad AR, Wiffen P, Moore A. Anticonvulsant drugs for management of pain: a systematic review. *British Medical Journal* 1995; **311**:1047–52.
9. McQuay HJ, Tramer M, Nye BA, Carroll D, Wiffen PJ, Moore RA. A systematic review of antidepressants in neuropathic pain. *Pain* 1996; **68**:217–27.
10. Tramer M, Moore A, McQuay H. Prevention of vomiting after paediatric strabismus surgery: a systematic review using the numbers-needed-to-treat method. *British Journal of Anaesthesia* 1995; **75**:556–61.

11. Soll JC, McQueen MC. Respiratory distress syndrome. In: Sinclair JC, Bracken ME, ed. *Effective care of the newborn infant*. Oxford University Press, 1992: Ch. 15, 333.

12. Moore RA. Helicobacter pylori *and peptic ulcer. A systematic review of effectiveness and an overview of the economic benefits of implementing that which is known to be effective* (http://www.jr2.ox.ac.uk/ Bandolier/bandopubs/hpyl/hp0.html). Oxford: Health Technology Evaluation Association, 1995.

13. Gøtzsche PC. Sensitivity of effect variables in rheumatoid arthritis: a meta analysis of 130 placebo controlled NSAID trials. *Journal of Clinical Epidemiology* 1990; **43**:1313–18.

14. Sinclair JC, Bracken MB. Clinically useful measures of effect in binary analyses of randomized trials. *Journal of Clinical Epidemiology* 1994; **47**:881–9.

15. Tramèr M, Moore RA, McQuay HJ. A rational approach to sensitivity analyses in meta-analysis: factors influencing propofol's effect on postoperative nausea and vomiting. submitted.

16. Sackett DL, Deeks JJ, Altman DG. Down with odds ratios! *Evidence based medicine* 1996; **1**:164–6.

17. Deeks J. What the heck's an odds ratio? *Bandolier* (issue 25) 1996; **3**:6–7.

18. Revman. The Cochrane Collaboration Review Manager Software (RevMan), 1996.

19. Glass GV. Primary, secondary, and meta-analysis of research. *Education Research* 1976; **5**:3–8.

20. Moore RA, McQuay H, Gray M. *Bandolier—the first 20 issues*. Oxford: Bandolier, 1995.

21. Moore A, McQuay H, Gavaghan D. Deriving dichotomous outcome measures from continuous data in randomised controlled trials of analgesics. *Pain* 1996; **66**:229–37.

22. Sackett D, Richardson WS, Rosenberg W, Haynes B. *Evidence based medicine*. London: Churchill Livingstone, 1996.

23. Moore TJ. *Deadly medicine*. New York: Simon & Schuster, 1995.

24. Eypasch E, Lefering R, Kum CK, Troidl H. Probability of adverse events that have not yet occurred: a statistical reminder. *British Medical Journal* 1995; **311**:619–20.

7

Existing systematic reviews

As part of the evidence-gathering exercise we set out to find all the previous systematic reviews of analgesic interventions.

This was done in two stages. In the first stage we sought all systematic reviews published up to 1993–4. We found 80, and two judges assessed their quality using Oxman and Guyatt's index [1]. Most of the reviews looked at drug interventions for chronic pain conditions. Two-thirds were published after 1990. Most had methodological flaws, such as insufficient information on retrieval methods and on validity assessment and design of the primary studies. Poor quality systematic reviews reached significantly more positive conclusions. Making life even more difficult, when there was more than one systematic review of a particular topic the results did not always agree. A full account of this first stage is published in [2].

The second stage was (and is) a prospective exercise to maintain an up-to-date database of systematic reviews in pain relief.

Introduction

Systematic reviews can potentially resolve conflicts when reports of primary studies disagree, and increase the likelihood of detecting small but clinically important effects [3–5]. They can also be easily misused to produce misleading estimates of effectiveness.

We used a systematic search of the literature to identify the highest possible proportion of systematic reviews assessing analgesic interventions. Our objectives were:

1. To produce a citation database of all available reviews
2. To assess the quality of systematic reviews in pain relief
3. To establish whether or not quality scores are useful to resolve conflicts between different systematic reviews

Methods

Inclusion criteria

Reports had to meet the following criteria:

1. They had to be described as systematic reviews or, if not, they had to include pooled analysis of the results of several independent primary studies. Studies in which statistical synthesis had been planned but was deemed to be inappropriate were also included.
2. They had to incorporate trials in which pain was an outcome measure or in which analgesic interventions were compared for outcomes other than pain within the context of a painful condition (e.g. a study looking at the validity of grip strength to assess the effectiveness of NSAIDs in rheumatoid arthritis).
3. They had to be published or accepted for publication.

Search strategy

A MEDLINE (Silver Platter MEDLINE versions 3.0, 3.1, and 3.11) search was done from 1966 to October 1993. This MEDLINE strategy had been developed to identify the maximum possible number of randomized, double-blind studies or meta-analyses in pain research, and contained text words, 'wild cards', and MeSH terms [6]. We searched 40 journals by hand. We checked the register of systematic reviews at the UK Cochrane Centre for eligible studies, and asked lead authors of abstracts for full manuscripts. We scanned the reference lists for citations of other systematic reviews.

Methodological evaluation

Each study was evaluated twice, using Oxman and Guyatt's index [1, 7], with the name of the journal, the authors, the date of publication, and the source of financial support of the reports obscured. A consensus score was obtained.

Statistical analysis

The chi-square test was used to test the relationship between the direction of the conclusion of the systematic reviews (positive vs. negative/uncertain) and the overall quality scores, and the influence of study architecture on systematic reviews which included study designs other than randomized controlled trials (RCTs) Prior hypotheses were that poor quality reviews and those including designs other than RCTs would be more likely to produce positive conclusions.

Results

Stage 1: Quality assessment of reviews to 1993–4

Seventy of the 84 reports we found were included in the quality assessment (Table 1). The exclusions are specified in [2]. The earliest report was from 1980. Over two-thirds appeared after 1990. Reviews considered between and

Table 1 Details of the systematic reviews

	No.	(%)
Setting		
Chronic	58	(72)
Acute	14	(19)
Mixed	6	(7)
Unclear	2	(2)
Intervention		
Drug	42	(54)
Psychological	16	(20)
Physical	10	(13)
Diagnostic	3	(4)
Complementary	2	(2)
Non-surgical invasive	2	(2)
Multidisciplinary	2	(2)
Surgical	1	(1)
Preventive	1	(1)
Not specified	1	(1)
Outcomes		
Pain	63	(79)
Adverse effects	11	(14)
Validity	3	(4)
Patient preference	1	(1)
Return to work	1	(1)
Pulmonary function	1	(1)
Primary studies		
Randomized only	24	(30)
Randomized and double-blind	7	(9)
Double-blind only	3	(4)
Combination of observational and any above	25	(31)
Observation only	4	(5)
Not reported	17	(21)

Table 2 Pooling methods used in the systematic reviews

Method	No.	(%)
Standardized mean differences	26	(32)
Odds ratios/Mantel–Haenszel	10	(13)
Percentage change comparison	15	(20)
Simple addition	7	(9)
Criteria-based	4	(5)
Weighted means	3	(4)
Mean risk differences	2	(2)
Random effects	2	(2)
Kendal's correlation	1	(1)
Log rank test	1	(1)
Relative potency	1	(1)
Not reported	5	(6)
Pooling considered inappropriate	3	(4)

Table 3 Meta-analyses: quality and conclusions

Overall quality score	Conclusions	
	Positive	Negative/Uncertain
1	11	1
2	12	0
3	6	1
4	11	1
5	8	3
6	8	9
7	4	4

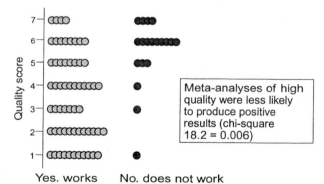

Systematic reviews: quality and estimate of efficacy

Meta-analyses of high quality were less likely to produce positive results (chi-square 18.2 = 0.006)

Efficacy as stated in original review

(Jadad and McQuay 1996 [2].)

196 primary studies (median 28). Sixty reviews reached positive conclusions, 7 negative, 12 uncertain, and 1 did not manage any conclusion. They used different pooling methods (Table 2). All were based on published data only (no individual patient data analysis), without validity checks with the study investigators.

Overall quality scores (item 10)

The median agreed overall score for the systematic reviews was 4 (range 1–7). Systematic reviews of high quality were significantly less likely to produce positive results (Table 3; chi-square 18.2, $P = .006$).

Sixteen of 19 systematic reviews with negative or uncertain results had overall quality scores above the median, compared with only 20 of the 60 with positive results. Systematic reviews restricted to RCTs were significantly less likely to produce positive conclusions (19 of 31) than those which included other study architectures (41 of 49; chi-square = 5.07; $P = 0.024$). All conclusions from systematic reviews of psychological interventions were positive. In only one of those reviews was quality scored above the median. All abstracts scored below the median, and six out of eight abstracts received the minimum possible score.

Interventions evaluated by multiple systematic reviews

There was more than one systematic review for six interventions (Table 4). For acupuncture and non-steroidal anti-inflammatory drugs (NSAIDs) the conclusions of the reviews were the same. Two reviews of acupuncture in chronic pain concluded that the evidence was flawed and that acupuncture

Table 4 Multiple systematic reviews on a particular intervention: quality and conclusions

Intervention	Ref.	Quality	Conclusion
Acupuncture	[9]	6	Uncertain
	[8]	5	Uncertain
Gastrointestinal effects of NSAIDs	[10]	7	Positive
	[11]	6	Positive
	[12]	5	Positive
Manipulation	[19]	6	Uncertain
	[13]	6	Positive
	[14]	4	Positive
	[15]	3	Positive
Second-line drugs for rheumatoid arthritis	[20]	7	Uncertain
	[17]	6	Positive
	[16]	4	Positive
	[18]	4	Positive
Prevention of post-herpetic neuralgia	[23]	7	Uncertain
	[24]	5	Positive
	[26]	3	Positive
	[25]	3	Negative
Laser for musculoskeletal pain	[22]	6	Negative
	[21]	6	Positive

was of uncertain value [8, 9]. These reviews confirmed that the risk of gastrointestinal complications was increased by NSAIDs [10–12].

Most systematic reviews of manipulation for chronic back pain concluded it was useful [13–15], as did reviews of second-line drugs for rheumatoid arthritis [16–18], but for both interventions one review questioned the validity of the findings because of high risk of bias in the primary studies [19, 20].

Systematic reviews produced conclusions in opposite directions for lasers in musculoskeletal pain [21, 22] and for interventions to prevent postherpetic neuralgia [23–26]. Both systematic reviews evaluating laser treatment were given the same quality score.

Comment

The use of systematic reviews to assess analgesic interventions is increasing, but most of the reviews we found had methodological flaws which may threaten their conclusions. Only 8 of the 80 satisfied all the Oxman and Guyatt criteria and 16% were given the lowest possible score. The relationship between methodological rigour, type of primary studies included, and the direction of the conclusions under-scores the importance of review quality. Systematic reviews including only RCTs were less likely to produce positive conclusions.

Reviewers have to work hard to reduce bias. The search for evidence must be comprehensive, decisions about which studies to include or exclude have to be overt, and validity criteria need to be stated. Equally, readers need to be aware of the pitfalls.

We found several examples of reviews of the same intervention producing conflicting results, despite similar quality scores. This occurred despite the concept that systematic reviews can resolve conflicting results between primary studies.

Using the Oxman and Guyatt scoring system for reviews

The purpose of this index is to evaluate the scientific quality (i.e. adherence to scientific principles) of research overviews (review articles) published in the medical literature. It is not intended to measure literary quality, importance, relevance, originality, or other attributes of overviews.

The index is for assessing overviews of primary ('original') research on pragmatic questions regarding causation, diagnosis, prognosis, therapy, or prevention. A research overview is a survey of research. The same principles that apply to epidemiological surveys apply to overviews; a question must be clearly specified, a target population identified and accessed, appropriate information obtained from that population in an unbiased fashion, and conclusions derived, sometimes with the help of formal statistical analysis, as is done in 'meta-analyses'. The fundamental difference between overviews and epidemiological surveys is the unit of analysis, not the scientific issues that the questions in this index address.

Since most published overviews do not include a methods section it is difficult to answer some of the questions in the index. Base your answers, as much as possible, on information provided in the overview. If the methods that were used are reported incompletely relative to a specific item, score that item as 'partially'. Similarly, if there is no information provided regarding what was done relative to a particular question, score it as 'can't tell', unless there is information in the overview to suggest either that the criterion was or was not met.

For Question 8, if no attempt has been made to combine findings, and no statement is made regarding the inappropriateness of combining findings, check 'no'. If a summary (general) estimate is given anywhere in the abstract, the discussion, or the summary section of the paper, and it is not reported how that estimate was derived, mark 'no' even if there is a statement regarding the limitations of combining the findings of the studies reviewed. If in doubt mark 'can't tell'.

For an overview to be scored as 'yes' on Question 9, data (not just citations) must be reported that support the main conclusions regarding the primary question(s) that the overview addresses.

The score for Question 10, the overall scientific quality, should be based on your answers to the first nine questions. The following guidelines can be used to assist with deriving a summary score: If the 'can't tell' option is used one or more times on the preceding questions, a review is likely to have minor flaws at best and it is difficult to rule our major flaws (i.e. a score of 4 or lower). If the 'no' option is used on Questions 2, 4, 6, or 8, the review is likely to have major flaws (i.e. a score of 3 or lower, depending on the number and degree of the flaws).

The Oxman and Guyatt index of scientific quality

Question			Answers	
1. Were the search methods used to find evidence on the primary question(s) stated?	No	Partially	Yes
2. Was the search for evidence reasonably comprehensive?	No	Can't tell	Yes
3. Were the criteria used for deciding which studies to include in the overview reported?	No	Partially	Yes
4. Was bias in the selection of studies avoided?	No	Can't tell	Yes
5. Were the criteria used for assessing the validity of the included studies reported?	No	Partially	Yes
6. Was the validity of all the studies referred to in the text assessed using appropriate criteria?	No	Can't tell	Yes
7. Were the methods used to combine the findings of the relevant studies (to reach a conclusion) reported?	No	Partially	Yes
8. Were the findings of the relevant studies combined appropriately relative to the primary question of the overview?	No	Can't tell	Yes
9. Were the conclusions made by the author(s) supported by the data and/or analysis reported in the overview?	No	Partially	Yes
10. How would you rate the scientific quality of this overview?			

Flaws

Extensive		Major		Minor		Minimal
1	2	3	4	5	6	7

References

1. Oxman AD, Guyatt GH. Validation of an index of the quality of review articles *Journal of Clinical Epidemiology* 1991; **44**:1271–8.
2. Jadad AR, McQuay HJ. Meta-analyses to evaluate analgesic interventions: a systematic qualitative review of their methodology. *Journal of Clinical Epidemiology* 1996; **49**:235–43.
3. Sacks HS, Berrier J, Reitman D, Ancona-Berk VA, Chalmers TC. Meta-analyses of randomized controlled trials. *New England Journal of Medicine* 1987; **316**:450–5.
4. Gerbarg ZB, Horwitz RI. Resolving conflicting clinical trials: Guidelines for meta-analysis. *Journal of Clinical Epidemiology* 1988; **41**:503–9.
5. Kassirer JP. Clinical trials and meta-analysis: What do they do for us? *New England Journal of Medicine* 1992; **327**:273–4.
6. Jadad AR, McQuay HJ. A high-yield strategy to identify randomized controlled trials for systematic reviews. *Online Journal of Current Clinical Trials* [serial online] 1993; Doc No 33:3973 words; 39 paragraphs. 5 tables.
7. Oxman AD, Guyatt GH, Singer J, Goldsmith CH, Hutchison BG, Milner RA *et al.* Agreement among reviewers of review articles. *Journal of Clinical Epidemiology* 1991; **44**:91–8.
8. Patel M, Gutzwiller F, Paccaud F, Marazzi A. A meta-analysis of acupuncture for chronic pain. *International Journal of Epidemiology* 1989; **18**:900–6.
9. ter Riet G, Kleijnen J, Knipschild P. Acupuncture and chronic pain: a criteria-based meta-analysis. *Journal of Clinical Epidemiology* 1990; **43**:1191–9.
10. Chalmers TC, Berrier J, Hewitt P, Berlin J, Reitman D, Nagalingam R *et al.* Meta-analysis of randomized controlled trials as a method of estimating rare complications of non-steroidal anti-inflammatory drug therapy. *Alimentation Pharmacology and Therapeutics* 1988; **2**:9–26.
11. Gabriel SE, Jaakkimainen L, Bombardier C. Risk for serious gastrointestinal complications related to use of nonsteroidal anti-inflammatory drugs. A meta-analysis. *Annals of Internal Medicine* 1991; **115**:787–96.
12. Bollini P, García Rodríguez LA, Pérez Gutthann S, Walker AM. The impact of research quality and study design on epidemiologic estimates of the effect of nonsteroidal anti-inflammatory drugs on upper gastrointestinal tract disease. *Archives of Internal Medicine* 1992; **152**:1289–95.
13. Shekelle PG, Adams AH, Chassin MR, Hurwitz EL, Brook RH. Spinal manipulation for low-back pain. *Annals of Internal Medicine* 1992; **117**:590–8.
14. Ottenbacher K, DiFabio RP. Efficacy of spinal manipulation/ mobilization therapy. A meta analysis. *Spine* 1985; **10**:833–7.
15. Anderson R, Meeker WC, Wirick BE, Mootz RD, Kirk DH, Adams A. A meta-analysis of clinical trials of spinal manipulation. *Journal of Manipulative Physiological Therapy* 1992; **15**:181–94.
16. Capell HA, Porter DR, Madhok R, Hunter JA. Second line (disease modifying) treatment in rheumatoid arthritis: which drug for which patient? *Annals of Rheumatic Disease* 1993; **52**:423–8.
17. Felson DT, Anderson JJ, Meenan RF. The comparative efficacy and toxicity of second-line drugs in rheumatoid arthritis. *Arthritis and Rheumatism* 1990; **33**:1449–61.
18. Felson DT, Anderson JJ, Meenan RF. Use of short-term efficacy/ toxicity tradeoffs to select second-line drugs in rheumatoid arthritis. *Arthritis and Rheumatism* 1992; **35**:1117–25.
19. Koes BW, Assendelft WJ, van der Heijden G, Bouter LM, Knipschild PG. Spinal manipulation and mobilisation for back

and neck pain: a blinded review. *British Medical Journal* 1991; **303**:1298–303.

20. Gøtzsche PC, Pødenphant J, Olesen M, Halberg P. Meta-analysis of second-line antirheumatic drugs: sample bias and uncertain benefit. *Journal of Clinical Epidemiology* 1992; **45**:587–94.

21. Beckerman H, de Bie RA, Bouter LM, De Cuyper HJ, Oostendorp RA. The efficacy of laser therapy for musculoskeletal and skin disorders: a criteria-based meta-analysis of randomized clinical trials. *Physical Therapy* 1992; **72**:483–91.

22. Gam AN, Thorsen H, Lonnberg F. The effect of low-level laser therapy on musculoskeletal pain: a meta-analysis. *Pain* 1993; **52**:63–6.

23. Schmader K, Studenski S. Are current therapies useful for the prevention of postherpetic neuralgia? A critical analysis of the literature. *Journal of General Internal Medicine* 1989; **4**:83–9.

24. Lycka BA. Postherpetic neuralgia and systemic corticosteroid therapy. Efficacy and safety. *International Journal of Dermatology* 1990; **29**:523–7.

25. Naldi L, Zucchi A, Brevi A, Cavalieri D'Oro L, Cainelli T. Corticosteroids and post-herpetic neuralgia. *Lancet* 1990; **336**:947.

26. Crooks RJ, Jones Da, Fiddian P. Zoster-associated chronic pain: an overview of clinical trials with acyclovir. *Scandinavian Journal of Infection* 1991; **78**(suppl.):62–8.

Pain reviews

Abenhaim L, Bergeron AM. Twenty years of randomized clinical trials of manipulative therapy for back pain: a review. *Clinical and Investigative Medicine* 1992; **15**:527–35.

Abram SE. 1992 Bonica Lecture. Advances in chronic pain management since gate control. *Regional Anesthesia* 1993; **18**:66–81.

Adamson GD, Nelson HP. Medical and surgical treatment of endometriosis. *Endocrinologist* 1996; **6**:384–91.

Aker PD, Gross AR, Goldsmith CH, Peloso P. Conservative management of mechanical neck pain: Systematic overview and meta-analysis. *British Medical Journal* 1996; **313**:1291–6.

Ali NMK. Does sympathetic ganglionic block prevent postherpetic neuralia? *Regional Anesthesia* 1995; **20**:227–33.

Allegrante JP. The role of adjunctive therapy in the management of chronic nonmalignant pain. *American Journal of Medicine* 1996; **101**:S33–9.

Altman GB, Lee CA. Strontium-89 for treatment of painful bone metastasis from prostate cancer. *Oncology Nursing Forum* 1996; **23**:523–7.

Amery WK. Onset of action of various migraine prophylactics. *Cephalalgia* 1988; **8**:11–13.

Amery WK. Prophylactic and curative treatment of migraine with calcium antagonists. *Drug Design and Delivery* 1989; **4**:197–203.

Anderson R, Meeker WC, Wirick BE, Mootz RD, Kirk DH, Adams A. A meta-analysis of clinical trials of spinal manipulation [see comments]. *Journal of Manipulative and Physiological Therapeutics* 1992; **15**:181–94.

Antczak-Bouckoms A, Tung F, Chalmers TC, Bouckoms A. Quality assessment and meta-analysis of randomized control trials of ibuprofen. *Pain* 1987; (suppl.):S51.

Assendelft WJJ, Hay EM, Adshead R, Bouter LM. Corticosteroid injections for lateral epicondylitis: a systematic overview. *British Journal of General Practice* 1996; **46**:209–16.

Assendelft WJJ, Koes BW, Van der Heijden GJM, Bouter LM. The effectiveness of chiropractic for treatment of low back pain: An update and attempt at statistical pooling. *Journal of Manipulative and Physiological Therapeutics* 1996; **19**:499–507.

Assendelft WJ, Koes BW, Van der Heijden GJ, Bouter LM. The efficacy of chiropractic manipulation for back pain: blinded review of relevant randomized clinical trials. *Journal of Manipulative and Physiological Therapeutics* 1992; **15**:487–94.

Aylward M. Clinical studies on alclofenac in the treatment of rheumatic diseases: a drug in question. *Current Medical Research Opinion* 1975; **3**:274–85.

Ballantyne JC, Carr DB, Berkey CS, Chalmers TC, Mosteller F. Comparative efficacy of epidural, subarachnoid, and intracerebroventricular opioids in patients with pain due to cancer. *Regional Anesthesia* 1996; **21**:542–56.

Ballantyne JC, Carr DB, Chalmers TC, Dear KB, Angelillo IF, Mosteller F. Postoperative patient-controlled analgesia: meta-analyses of initial randomized control trials. *Journal of Clinical Anaesthesia* 1993; **5**:182–93.

Bamberg P, Caswell CM, Frame MH, Lam SK, Wong EC. A meta-analysis comparing the efficacy of omeprazole with H2-receptor antagonists for acute treatment of duodenal ulcer in Asian patients. *Journal of Gastroenterology and Hepatology* 1992; **7**:577–85.

Baron JC, Bousser MG. [Controlled therapeutic trials in migraine: methodology and results] Essais therapeutiques controles dans la migraine. Organisation et resultats. *Revue Neurologique* 1982; **138**:279–95.

Basinski A, Naylor CD. Aspirin and fibrinolysis in acute myocardial infarction: meta-analytic evidence for synergy. *Journal of Clinical Epidemiology* 1991; **44**:1085–96.

Beckerman H, de Bie RA, Bouter LM, De Cuyper HJ, Oostendorp RA. The efficacy of laser therapy for musculoskeletal and skin disorders: a criteria-based meta-analysis of randomized clinical trials. *Physical Therapy* 1992; **72**:483–91.

Beecher HK. The powerful placebo. *Journal of American Medical Association* 1955; **159**:1602–6.

Belcon MC, Rooney PJ, Tugwell P. Aspirin and gastrointestinal haemorrhage: a methodologic assessment. *Journal of Chronic Disease* 1985; **38**:101–11.

Bernstein J. Overview of efficacy of fenbufen in rheumatoid arthritis and osteoarthritis. *American Journal of Medicine* 1983; **75**:70–4.

Bertagna C, De Gery A, Hucher M, Francois JP, Zanirato J. Efficacy of the combination of nilutamide plus orchidectomy in patients with metastatic prostatic cancer. A meta-analysis of seven randomized double-blind trials (1056 patients). *British Journal of Urology* 1994; **73**:396–402.

Bhatt Sanders D. Acupuncture for rheumatoid arthritis: an analysis of the literature. *Seminars in Arthritis and Rheumatism* 1985; **14**:225–31.

Blanchard EB, Andrasik F, Ahles TA, Teders ST, O'Keefe D. Migraine and tension headache: a meta-analytic review. *Behavioral Therapy* 1980; **11**:613–31.

Blanchard EB, Andrasik F. Psychological assessment and treatment of headache: recent developments and emerging issues. *Journal of Consulting Clinical Psychology* 1982; **50**:859–79.

Bloomfield SS, Mitchell J, Cissell G, Barden TP. Analgesic sensitivity of two post partum pain models. *Pain* 1986; **27**:171–9.

Bogaards MC, ter Kuile MM. Treatment of recurrent tension headache: a meta-analytic review. *Clinical Journal of Pain* 1994; **10**:174–90.

Bollini P, García Rodríguez LA, Pérez Gutthann S, Walker AM. The impact of research quality and study design on epidemiologic estimates of the effect of nonsteroidal anti-inflammatory drugs on upper gastrointestinal tract disease. *Archives of Internal Medicine* 1992; **152**:1289–95.

Bosi Ferraz M, Atra E. Metaanálise: nova opcao em pesquisa clínica. Prinípos básicos e um exemplo clínico. *Revista Paulista de Medicina* 1989; **107**:5–9.

Bosi-Ferraz M, Tugwell P, Goldsmith CH, Atra E. Meta-analysis of sulfasalazine in ankylosing spondylitis. *Journal of Rheumatology* 1990; **17**:1482–6.

Broome ME, Lillis PP. A descriptive analysis of the pediatric pain management research. *Applied Nursing Research* 1989; **2**:74–81.

Broome ME, Lillis PP, Smith MC. Pain interventions with children: a meta analysis of research. *Nursing Research* 1989; **38**:154–8.

Brown BWJ. Meta-analysis and patient-controlled analgesia [editorial; comment]. *Journal of Clinical Anesthesia* 1993; **5**:179–81.

Brunarski DJ. Clinical trials of spinal manipulation: a critical appraisal and review of the literature. *Journal of Manipulative and Physiological Therapy* 1984; **7**:243–9.

Capell HA, Porter DR, Madhok R, Hunter JA. Second line (disease modifying) treatment in rheumatoid arthritis: which drug for which patient? *Annals of Rheumatic Disease* 1993; **52**:423–8.

Capurso L, Koch M. [Prevention of NSAID-induced gastric lesions: H2 antagonists or misoprostol? A meta-analysis of controlled clinical studies] La prevenzione del danno gastrico da FANS: H2 antagonisti o misoprostol? Una meta-analisi degli studi clinici controllati. *Clinica Terapeutica* 1991; **139**:179–89.

Carr D, Eisenberg E, Chalmers TC. Neurolytic celiac plexus block for cancer pain—a meta-analysis. *Abstracts—7th World Congress on Pain* 1993; **338**.

Carroll D, Moore RA, Tramer MR, McQuay HJ. Transcutaneous electrical nerve stimulation does not relieve labour pain-updated systematic review. *Contemporary Reviews in Obstetrics and Gynaecology* Sept 1997; 195–205.

Carroll D, Tramer M, McQuay H, Nye B, Moore A. Randomization is important in studies with pain outcomes: Systematic review of transcutaneous electrical nerve stimulation in acute postoperative pain. *British Journal of Anaesthesia* 1996; **77**:798–803.

Carroll D, Tramer M, McQuay H, Nye B, Moore A. Transcutaneous electrical nerve stimulation in labour pain: A systematic review. *British Journal of Obstetrics and Gynaecology* 1997; **104**:169–75. [

Chalmers TC, Ballantyne JC, Carr DB, Dear KBG, Angelillo IF, Mosteller F. Comparative effects of analgesic therapies upon postoperative pulmonary function: meta-analyses. *Abstracts—7th World Congress on Pain* 1993; **136**.

Chalmers TC, Berrier J, Hewitt P, Berlin J, Reitman D, Nagalingam R *et al*. Meta-analysis of randomized controlled trials as a method of estimating rare complications of non-steroidal anti-inflammatory drug therapy. *Alimentation Pharmacology Therapeutics* 1988; **2**:9–26.

Christensen E, Juhl E, Tygstrup N. Treatment of duodenal ulcer. Randomized clinical trials of a decade (1964 to 1974). *Gastroenterology* 1977; **73**:1170–8.

Cohen JE, Goel V, Frank JW, Bombardier C, Peloso P, Guillemin F. Group education interventions for people with low back pain. An overview of the literature. *Spine* 1994; **19**:1214–22.

Collins SL, Edwards J, Moore A, McQuay HJ. Oral dextropropoxyphene in postoperative pain: a quantitative systematic review. European Journal of Clinical Pharmacology. in press.

Collins SL, Moore A, McQuay H.J., Wiffen PJ. Oral ibuprofen and diclofenac in postoperative pain: a quantitative systematic review. submitted.

Collins S, Moore A, McQuay H. Paracetamol-codeine combinations versus paracetamol alone. Actual size of increase needs to be measured (letter). *British Medical Journal* 1996; **313**:1209.

Cooper SA. Five studies on ibuprofen for postsurgical dental pain. *American Journal of Medicine* 1984; (suppl):70–7.

Cooper SA, Berrie R, Cohn P. Comparison of ketoprofen, ibuprofen, and placebo in a dental surgery pain model. *Advances in Therapeutics* 1988; **5**:43–53.

Cooper SA, Gross DJ, Vogel R, Berrie P. Relative analgesic efficacy of ibuprofen and zomepirac Na in periodontal and oral surgery. *Clinical Pharmacology and Therapeutics* 1983; **33**:194.

Cooper SA, Needle SE, Kruger GO. Comparative analgesic potency of aspirin and ibuprofen. *Journal of Oral Surgery* 1977; **35**:898–903.

Cooper SA, Precheur H, Rosenbeck R, Engel J. The analgesic efficacy of ibuprofen compared to acetaminophen with codeine. *Clinical Pharmacology Therapeutics* 1984; **35**:232.

Crooks RJ, Jones DA, Fiddian P. Zoster-associated chronic pain: an overview of clinical trials with acyclovir. *Scandinavian Journal of Infection* 1991; (suppl.)**78**:62–8.

Cutler R, Fishbain D, Rosomoff H, Abdel-Moty E, Khalil T, Steele-Rosomoff R. Does non-surgical pain treatment of chronic pain return patients to work? A review and meta-analysis of the literature. *Proceedings of the American Pain Society Meeting* 1992:83.

Cutler RB, Fishbain DA, Rosomoff HL, Abdel-Moty E, Khalil TM, Rosomoff RS. Does nonsurgical pain center treatment of chronic pain return patients to work? A review and meta-analysis of the literature. *Spine* 1994; **19**:643–52.

Dahl JB, Moiniche S, Kehlet H. Wound infiltration with local anaesthetics for postoperative pain relief [see comments]. *Acta Anaesthesiologica Scandinavica* 1994; **38**:7–14.

Dahl SL. Nabumetone: a 'nonacidic' nonsteroidal antiinflammatory drug. *Annals of Pharmacotherapentics* 1993; **27**:456–63.

de Craen AJM, Di Giulio G, LampeSchoenmaeckers AJE, Kessels AGH, Kleijnen J. Analgesic efficacy and safety of paracetamol-codeine combinations versus paracetamol alone: A systematic review. *British Medical Journal* 1996; **313**:321–5.

Devine EC. Effects of psychoeducational care for adult surgical patients: a meta-analysis of 191 studies. *Patient Education and Counseling* 1992; **19**:129–42.

Devine EC, Cook TD. Clinical and cost saving effects of psychoeducational interventions with surgical patients: a meta analysis. *Res Nurs Health* 1986; **9**:89–105.

Devine EC, Westlake SK. The effects of psychoeducational care provided to adults with cancer: metapanalysis of 116 studies. *Oncology Nursing Forum* 1995; **23**:1369–81.

Dexter F. Analysis of statistical tests to compare doses of analgesics among groups. *Anesthesiology* 1994; **81**:610–5.

Di Fabio RP. Efficacy of manual therapy. *Physical Therapy* 1992; **72**:853–64.

Di Fabio RP. Efficacy of comprehensive rehabilitation programs and back school for patients with low back pain: a meta-analysis. *Physical Therapy* 1995; **75**:865–78.

Dickersin K. Pharmacological control of pain during labour. In: Chalmers I, Enkin M, Keirse MJNC (ed) *Effective care in pregnancy and childbirth*. Oxford University Press, 1989:913–50.

Dordain G, Aumaitre O, Eschalier A, Decamps A. [Vitamin B12, an analgesic vitamin? Critical examination of the literature] La vitamine B12, une vitamine antalgique? Etude critique de la litterature. *Acta Neurologica Belgica* 1984; **84**:5–11.

Downie WW. Diclofenac/misoprostol. A review of the major clinical trials evaluating its clinical efficacy and upper gastrointestinal tolerability in rheumatoid arthritis and osteoarthritis. *Drugs* 1993; **45**:1–6.

Duckro PN, Cantwell-Simmonds E. A review of studies evaluating biofeedback and relaxation training in the management of pediatric headache. *Headache* 1989; **29**:428–33.

Eandi M, della Pepa C, Rubinetto MP. [Piroxicam in analgesia] Il piroxicam in analgesia. *Clinica Terapeutica* 1991; **136**:107–35.

Edwards JE, McQuay HJ, Moore RA. Systematic review: dihydrocodeine in postoperative pain. submitted.

Einarson TR, McGhan WF, Bootman JL, Sabers DL. Meta-analysis: Quantitative integration of independent research results. *American Journal of Hospital Pharmacy* 1985; **42**:1957–64.

Eisenberg E, Berkey CS, Carr DB, Mosteller F, Chalmers TC. Efficacy and safety of nonsteroidal antiinflammatory drugs for cancer pain: a meta-analysis. *Journal of Clinical Oncology* 1994; **12**:2756–65.

Eisenberg E, Carr DB, Chalmers TC. Neurolytic celiac plexus block for treatment of cancer pain: a meta-analysis. *Anesthesia and Analgesia* 1995; **80**:290–5.

Ernst E, Fialka V. [Low-dose laser therapy: critical analysis of clinical effect] Low-Dose-Lasertherapie: eine kritische Prufung der klinischen Wirksamkeit. *Schweiz Medizinische Wochenschrift* 1993; **123**:949–54.

Ernst E, Fialka V. A review of the clinical effectiveness of exercise therapy for intermittent claudication. *Archives of Internal Medicine* 1993; **153**:2357–60.

Ernst E, Nielsen GL, Schmidt EB. [Fish oils and rheumatoid arthritis]. Fiskeolie og reumatoid artrit. *Ugeskrift for Laeger* 1994; **156**:3490–5.

Felson DT, Anderson JJ, Boers M, Bombardier C, Chernoff M, Fried B *et al.* The American College of Rheumatology preliminary core set of disease activity measures for rheumatoid arthritis clinical trials. *Arthritis and Rheumatism* 1993; **36**:729–40.

Felson DT, Anderson JJ, Meenan RF. The comparative efficacy and toxicity of second-line drugs in rheumatoid arthritis. *Arthritis and Rheumatism* 1990; **33**:1449–61.

Felson DT, Anderson JJ, Meenan RF. The efficacy and toxicity of combination therapy in rheumatoid arthritis. A meta-analysis. *Arthritis and Rheumatism* 1994; **37**:1487–91.

Felson DT, Anderson JJ, Meenan RF. Use of short-term efficacy/toxicity tradeoffs to select second-line drugs in rheumatoid arthritis. *Arthritis and Rheumatism* 1992; **35**:1117–25.

Fernandez E, Turk DC. The utility of cognitive coping strategies for altering pain perception: a meta analysis. *Pain* 1989; **38**:123–35.

Ferraz MB, Atra E. [Meta analysis: a new option in clinical research. Basic principles and a clinical example] Metaanalise: nova opÄcao em pesquisa clinica. Principios basicos e um exemplo clinico. *Rev Paul Med* 1989; **107**:5–9.

Ferraz MB, Tugwell P, Goldsmith CH, Atra E. Meta-analysis of sulfasalazine in ankylosing spondylitis. *Journal of Rheumatology* 1990; **17**:1482–6.

Finley GA, McGrath PJ, Forward SP, McNeill G, Fitzgerald P. Parents' management of children's pain following 'minor' surgery. *Pain* 1996; **64**:83–87.

Fleet RP, Dupuis G, Marchand A, Burelle D, Beitman BD. Panic disorder, chest pain and coronary artery disease: literature review. *Canadian Journal of Cardiology* 1994; **10**:827–34.

Flor H, Fydrich T, Turk DC. Efficacy of multidisciplinary pain treatment centers: a meta-analytic review. *Pain* 1992; **49**:221–30.

France RD, Houpt JL, Ellinwood EH. Therapeutic effects of antidepressants in chronic pain. *General Hospital Psychiatry* 1984; **6**:55–63.

Fullerton T, Gengo FM. Sumatriptan: a selective 5-hydroxytryptamine receptor agonist for the acute treatment of migraine. *Annals of Pharmacotherapeutics* 1992; **26**:800–8.

Furcy SA, Waksman JA, Dash BH. Nonprescription ibuprofen: side effect profile. *Pharmacotherapy* 1992; **12**:403–7.

Gabriel SE, Jaakkimainen L, Bombardier C. The cost-effectiveness of misoprostol for nonsteroidal antiinflammatory drug-associated adverse gastrointestinal events. *Arthritis and Rheumatism* 1993; **36**:447–59.

Gabriel SE, Jaakkimainen L, Bombardier C. Risk for serious gastrointestinal complications related to use of nonsteroidal anti-inflammatory drugs. A meta-analysis. *Annals of Internal Medicine* 1991; **115**:787–96.

Gadsby JG, Flowerdew MW. The effectiveness of transcutaneous electrical nerve stimulation (TENS) and acupuncture-like transcutaneous electrical nerve stimulation (ALTENS) in the treatment of patients with chronic low back pain. In: Bombardier C, Nachemson A, Deyo R, de Bie R, Bouter L, Shekelle P *et al.* ed. *CMSG Back Module of the Cochrane Database of Systematic Reviews* [updated 5 december 1996]. Oxford: The Cochrane Collaboration, 1997.

Gam AN, Thorsen H, Lonnberg F. The effect of low-level laser therapy on musculoskeletal pain: a meta-analysis. *Pain* 1993; **52**:63–6.

Garzillo MJ, Garzillo TA. Does obesity cause low back pain? *Journal of Manipulative and Physiological Therapy* 1994; **17**:601–4.

Gebhardt WA. Effectiveness of training to prevent job-related back pain: a meta-analysis. *British Journal of Clinical Psychology* 1994; **33**:571–4.

Gebthardt WA. Effectiveness of training to prevent job-related back pain: a meta-analysis. *British Journal of Clinical Psychology* 1994; **33**:571–4.

Geis GS. Overall safety of Arthrotec. *Scandinavian Journal of Rheumatology* 1992; (suppl.)**96**:33–6.

Genuis ML. The use of hypnosis in helping cancer patients control anxiety, pain, and emesis: a review of recent empirical studies. *American Journal of Clinical Hypnosis* 1995; **37**:316–25.

Ghent WR, Eskin BA, Low DA, Hill LP. Iodine replacement in fibrocystic disease of the breast [see comments]. *Canadian Journal of Surgery* 1993; **36**:453–60.

Glazer S, Portenoy RK. Systemic local anesthetics in pain control. *Journal of Pain and Symptom Management* 1991; **6**:30–9.

Good M. Effect of relaxation and music on postoperative pain: a review. *Journal of Advanced Nursing* 1996; **24**:905–14.

Goodkin K, Vrancken MAE, Feaster D. On the putative efficacy of the antidepressants in chronic, benign pain syndromes. An update. *Pain Forum* 1995; **4**:237–47.

Goodnick PJ, Sandoval R. Psychotropic treatment of chronic fatigue syndrome and related disorders. *Journal of Clinical Psychiatry* 1993; **54**:13–20.

Gøtzsche PC. Meta analysis of grip strength: most common, but superfluous variable in comparative NSAID trials. *Danish Medical Bulletin* 1989; **36**:493–5.

Gøtzsche PC. Meta-analysis of NSAIDs: contribution of drugs, doses, trial designs, and meta-analytic techniques. *Scandinavian Journal of Rheumatology* 1993; **22**:255–60.

Gøtzsche PC. Methodology and overt and hidden bias in reports of 196 double blind trials of nonsteroidal antiinflammatory drugs in rheumatoid arthritis. *Controlled Clinical Trials* 1989; **10**:31–56.

Gøzsche PC. Patients' preference in indomethacin trials: an overview. *Lancet* 1989; **1**:88–91.

Gøtzsche PC. Review of dose response studies of NSAIDs in rheumatoid arthritis. *Danish Medical Bulletin* 1989; **36**:395–9.

Gøtzsche PC. Sensitivity of effect variables in rheumatoid arthritis: a meta analysis of 130 placebo controlled NSAID trials. *Journal of Clinical Epidemiology* 1990; **43**:1313–18.

Gøtzschc PC, Pødenphant J, Olesen M, Halberg P. Meta-analysis of second-line antirheumatic drugs: sample bias and uncertain benefit. *Journal of Clinical Epidemiology* 1992; **45**:587–94.

Grant A. The choice of suture materials and techniques for repair of perineal trauma: an overview of the evidence from controlled trials. *British Journal of Obstetrics and Gynaecology* 1989; **96**:1281–9.

Grant A, Sleep J. Relief of perineal pain and discomfort after childbirth In: *Effective care in pregnancy and childbirth*. Chalmers I,

Enkin M, Keirse MJNC, ed. Oxford University Press, 1989:1347–58.

Haase W, Fischer M. [Statistical meta-analysis of multicenter clinical studies of ibuprofen with regard to cohort size] Statistische metaanalyse von multizentrischen klinischen studien mit ibuprofen im hinblick auf die kohortengrosse. *Zeitschrift Rheumatolie* 1991; **50**:77–83.

Halpern S, Preston R. Postdural puncture headache and spinal needle design. Metaanalyses. *Anesthesiology* 1994; **81**:1376–83.

Hanks GW. Controlled release morphine (MST Contin) in advanced cancer. The European experience. *Cancer* 1989; **63**:2378–82.

Harrison DL, Slack MK. Meta-analytic review of the effect of subcutaneous sumatriptan in migraine headache. *Journal of Pharmacy Technology* 1996; **12**:109–14.

Haselkorn JK, Turner JA, Diehr PK, Ciol MA, Deyo RA. Meta-analysis. A useful tool for the spine researcher. *Spine* 1994; **19**:S2076–82.

Hathaway D. Effect of preoperative instruction on postoperative outcomes: a meta-analysis. *Nursing Research* 1986; **35**:269–75.

Heller CA, Ingelfinger JA, Goldman P. Nonsteroidal antiinflammatory drugs and aspirin–analyzing the scores. *Pharmacotherapy* 1985; **5**:30–8.

Hersh EV, Cooper SA, Betts N, Wedell D, MacAfee K, Quinn P et al. Single dose and multidose analgesic study of ibuprofen and meclofenamate sodium after third molar surgery. *Oral Surgery, Oral Medicine and Oral Pathology* 1993; **76**:680–7.

Hill AG. Review of flufenamic acid in rheumatoid arthritis. *Annals of Physical Medicine* 1967; Supplement 87–92.

Hoeveel voegt codeine toe aan paracetamol bij eenmalig postoperatief [How much does codeine add to paracetamol in single postoperative application?]. *Geneesmid delenbulletin* 1996; **30**:136.

Hoffman RM, Kent DL, Deyo RA. Diagnostic accuracy and clinical utility of thermography for lumbar radiculopathy. A meta-analysis [see comments]. *Spine* 1991; **16**:623–8.

Holmes B, Brogden RN, Heel RC, Speight TM, Avery GS. Flunarizine. A review of its pharmacodynamic and pharmacokinetic properties and therapeutic use. *Drugs* 1984; **27**:6–44.

Holroyd KA, Athens OH, Penzien DB, Jackson MS, Rokicki La, Cordingley GE. Flunarizine vs propranolol: a meta-analysis of clinical trials. *Headache* 1992; **32**:256.

Holroyd KA, Penzien DB. Client variables and the behavioral treatment of recurrent tension headache: a meta analytic review. *Journal of Behavioral Medicine* 1986; **9**:515–36.

Holroyd KA, Penzien DB. Meta-analysis minus the analysis: a prescription for confusion. *Pain* 1989; **39**:359–61.

Holroyd KA, Penzien DB. Pharmacological versus non pharmacological prophylaxis of recurrent migraine headache: a meta analytic review of clinical trials. *Pain* 1990; **42**:1–13.

Holroyd KA, Penzien DB, Cordingley GE. Propranolol in the management of recurrent migraine: a meta-analytic review. *Headache* 1991; **31**:333–40.

Howell C, Chalmers I. A review of prospectively controlled comparisons of epidural with non-epidural forms of pain relief during labour. *International Journal of Obstetrics and Anesthesiology* 1991; **2**:1–17.

Hurwitz EL, Aker PD, Adams AH, Meeker WC, Shekelle PG, Barr J.S.J. Manipulation and mobilization of the cervical spine: A systematic review of the literature. *Spine* 1996; **21**:1746–60.

Hyman RB, Feldman HR, Harris RB, Levin RF, Malloy GB. The effects of relaxation training on clinical symptoms: a meta analysis. *Nursing Research* 1989; **38**:216–20.

Jadad AR. Meta-analysis in pain relief: a valuable but easily misused tool. *Current Opinion in Anaesthesiology* 1996; **9**:426–9.

Jadad AR, Carroll D, Glynn CJ, McQuay HJ. Intravenous regional sympathetic blockade for pain relief in reflex sympathetic dystrophy: a systematic review and a randomized, double-blind crossover study. *Journal of Pain and Symptom Management* 1995; **10**:13–20.

Jadad AR, McQuay HJ. Meta-analyses to evaluate analgesic interventions: a systematic qualitative review of their methodology. *Journal of Clinical Epidemiology* 1996; **49**:235–43.

Jadad AR, Moore RA, Carroll D, Jenkinson C, Reynolds DJM, Gavaghan DJ et al. Assessing the quality of reports of randomized clinical trials: is blinding necessary? *Controlled Clinical Trials* 1996; **17**:1–12.

Johanson JF, Rimm A. Optimal nonsurgical treatment of hemorrhoids: a comparative analysis of infrared coagulation, rubber band ligation and injection sclerotherapy. *American Journal of Gastroenterology* 1992; **87**:1601–6.

Kaiko RF, Grandy RP, Oshlack B, Pav J, Horodniak J, Thomas G et al. The United States experience with oral controlled release morphine (MS Contin tablets). Parts I and II. Review of nine dose titration studies and clinical pharmacology of 15 mg, 30 mg, 60 mg, and 100 mg tablet strengths in normal subjects. *Cancer* 1989; **63**:2348–54.

Kalso E, Tramer M, Carroll D, McQuay H, Moore RA. Pain relief from intra-articular morphine after knee surgery: A qualitative systematic review. *Pain* 1997; **71**:642–51.

Kellihan MJ, Mangino PD. Pamidronate. *Annals of Pharmacotherapeutics* 1992; **26**:1262–9.

Kerns RD. A call for improved clinical trials of the efficacy of antidepressants in the management of chronic, nonmalignant pain. *Pain Forum* 1995; **4**:256–8.

Kinnison M, Powe N, Steinberg E. Results of randomized controlled trials of low versus high osmolaity contrast media. *Radiology* 1989; **170**:381–9.

Koes BW, Assendelft WJ, van der Heijden G, Bouter LM, Knipschild PG. Spinal manipulation and mobilisation for back and neck pain: a blinded review. *British Medical Journal* 1991; **303**:1298–303.

Koes BW, Bouter LM, van der Heijden G. Methodological quality of randomized clinical trials on treatment efficacy in low back pain. *Spine* 1995; **20**:228–35.

Koes BW, Bouter LM, Beckerman H, van der Heijden G, Knipschild PG. Physiotherapy exercises and back pain: a blinded review. *British Medical Journal* 1991; **302**:1572–6.

Koes BW, Scholten RPM, Mens JMA, Bouter LM. Efficacy of epidural steroid injections for low-back pain and sciatica: a systematic review of randomized clinical trials. *Pain* 1995; **63**:279–88.

Koes BW, van Tulder MW, van der Windt WM, Bouter LM. The efficacy of back schools: a review of randomized clinical trials. *Journal of Clinical Epidemiology* 1994; **47**:851–62.

Kubiena G. [Considerations of the placebo problem in acupuncture. Reflections on usefulness, ethical justification, standardization and differentiated use of placebos in acupuncture]. *Wien Klinische Wochenschrift* 1989; **101**:362–7.

Labrecque M, Dostaler LP, Rousselle R, Nguyen T, Poirier S. Efficacy of nonsteroidal anti-inflammatory drugs in the treatment of acute renal colic. A meta-analysis. *Archives of Internal Medicine* 1994; **154**:1381–7.

Ladas SD, Raptis SA. Conservative treatment of acute pancreatitis: the use of somatostatin. *Hepatogastroenterology* 1992; **39**:466–9.

Lahad A, Malter AD, Berg AO, Deyo RA. The effectiveness of four interventions for the prevention of low back pain. *Journal of American Medical Association* 1994; **272**:1286–91.

Lancaster T, Silagy C, Gray S. Primary care management of acute herpes zoster: systematic review of evidence from randomized controlled trials. *British Journal of General Practice* 1995; **45**:39–45.

Laska EM, Sunshine A, Mueller F, Elvers WB, Siegel C, Rubin A. Caffeine as an analgesic adjuvant. *Journal of the American Medical Association* 1984; **251**:1711–18.

Laska EM, Sunshine A, Zighelbolm I, Roure C, Marrero I, Wanderling J *et al.* Effect of caffeine on acetaminophen analgesia. *Clinical Pharmacology and Therapeutics* 1983; **33**:498–509.

Lataste X, Taylor P, Notter M. DHE nasal spray in the acute management of migraine attacks. *Cephalalgia* 1989; **9**:342–3.

Laurent MR, Buchanan WW, Bellamy N. Methods of assessment used in ankylosing spondylitis clinical trials: a review [see comments]. *British Journal of Rheumatology* 1991; **30**:326–9.

Letzel H, Schoop W. [Gingko biloba extract EGb 761 and pentoxifylline in intermittent claudication. Secondary analysis of the clinical effectiveness] Gingko-biloba-Extrakt EGb 761 und Pentoxifyllin bei Claudicatio intermittens. Sekundaranalyse zur klinischen Wirksamkeit. *Vasa* 1992; **21**:403–10.

Lipton RB, Stewart WF. The epidemiology of migraine. *European Neurology* 1994; **34**(suppl. 2):6–11.

Loosemore TM, Chalmers TC, Dormandy JA. A meta-analysis of randomized placebo control trials in Fontaine stages III and IV peripheral occlusive arterial disease. *International Journal of Angiology* 1994; **13**:133–42.

Lycka BA. Postherpetic neuralgia and systemic corticosteroid therapy. Efficacy and safety. *International Journal of Dermatology* 1990; **29**:523–7.

Macarthur C, Saunders N, Feldman W. Helicobacter pylori, gastroduodenal disease, and recurrent abdominal pain in children. *Journal of American Medical Association* 1995; **273**:729–34.

Magni G. The use of antidepressants in the treatment of chronic pain. A review of the current evidence. *Drugs* 1991; **42**:730–48.

Mahon WA, De Gregorio M. Benzydamine: a critical review of clinical data. *International Journal of Tissue Reaction* 1985; **7**:229–35.

Major P. [Should non-steroidal anti-inflammatory agents be used in acute soft tissue injuries?] Bor ikke-steroide antiinflammatoriske midler brukes ved akutte blotdelsskader? *Tidsskrift for den Norske Laegeforening* 1992; **112**:1614–15.

Malone MD, Strube MJ. Meta-analysis of non-medical treatments for chronic pain. *Pain* 1988; **34**:231–44.

Malone MD, Strube MJ, Scogin FR. Reply to Holroyd and Penzien. *Pain* 1989; **39**:362–3.

Max MB. Thirteen consecutive well-designed randomized trials show that antidepressants reduce pain in diabetic neuropathy and postherpetic neuralgia. *Pain Forum* 1995; **4**:248–253.

McGee J, Alexander M. Phenothiazine analgesia fact or fantasy? *American Journal of Hospital Pharmacology* 1979; **36**:633–40.

McQuay HJ. Pre-emptive analgesia: a systematic review of clinical studies. *Annals of Medicine* 1995; **27**:249–56.

McQuay H, Carroll D, Jadad AR, Wiffen P, Moore A. Anticonvulsant drugs for management of pain: a systematic review. *British Medical Journal* 1995; **311**:1047–52.

McQuay HJ, Carroll D, Moore RA. Injected morphine in postoperative pain; a quantitative systematic review. submitted.

McQuay HJ, Carroll D, Moore RA. Radiotherapy for painful bony metastases: a systematic review. *Clinical Oncology* 1997; **9**:150–4.

McQuay H, Carroll D, Moore A. Variation in the placebo effect in randomised controlled trials of analgesics: All is as blind as it seems. *Pain* 1996; **64**:331–5.

McQuay H, Moore RA. Epidural steroids (letter). *Anaesthesia and Intensive Care* 1996; **24**:284–6.

McQuay HJ, Tramer M, Nye BA, Carroll D, Wiffen PJ, Moore RA. A systematic review of antidepressants in neuropathic pain. *Pain* 1996; **68**:217–27.

Mendelson G. Acupuncture analgesia. I. Review of clinical studies. *Australian and New Zealand Medical Journal* 1977; **7**:642–8.

Mizraji M. Clinical response to etodolac in the management of pain. *European Journal of Rheumatology and Inflammation* 1990; **10**:35–43.

Montastruc JL, Senard JM. [Calcium channel blockers and prevention of migraine] Medicaments anticalciques et prophylaxie de la migraine. *Pathologie Biologie* 1992; **40**:381–8.

Moore A, Collins S, Carroll D, McQuay H. Paracetamol with and without codeine in acute pain: a quantitative systematic review. *Pain* 1997; **70**:193–201.

Moore A, McQuay H, Gavaghan D. Deriving dichotomous outcome measures from continuous data in randomised controlled trials of analgesics. *Pain* 1996; **66**:229–37.

Moore RA, Collins S, McQuay HJ. Variation in the placebo effect; the impact on individual trials and consequences for meta-analysis. In: Jensen TS, Hammond DL, Jensen TS, ed. *Proceedings of the 8th World Congress on Pain. Progress in pain research and management*, Vol. 2. Seattle: IASP Press, 1997: 469–76.

Moore RA, McQuay HJ. Single-patient data meta-analysis of 3453 postoperative patients: Oral tramadol versus placebo, codeine and combination analgesics. *Pain* 1997; **69**:287–94.

Moore RA, Nye BA, Carroll D, Wiffen PJ, Tramèr M, McQuay HJ. A systematic review of topically-applied non-steroidal anti-inflammatory drugs. *British Medical Journal*. in press.

Moote CA. Ibuprofen arginine in the management of pain. A review. *Clinical Drug Investigation* 1996; **11**:1–7.

Morton SC, Williams MS, Keeler EB, Gambone JC, Kahn KL. Effect of epidural analgesia for labor on the cesarean delivery rate. *Obstetrics and Gynecology* 1994; **83**:1045–52.

Mullen PD, Laville EA, Biddle AK, Lorig K. Efficacy of psychoeducational interventions on pain, depression, and disability in people with arthritis: a meta analysis. *Journal of Rheumatology* 1987; **14** (suppl.):33–9.

Murphy NG, Zurier RB. Treatment of rheumatoid arthritis. *Current Opinion in Rheumatology* 1991; **3**:441–8.

Naldi L, Zucchi A, Brevi A, Cavalieri D'Oro L, Cainelli T. Corticosteroids and post-herpetic neuralgia. *Lancet* 1990; **336**:947.

Nicholas JJ. Physical modalities in rheumatological rehabilitation. *Archives of Physical and Medical Rehabilitation* 1994; **75**:994–1001.

NIH Technology Assessment Panel on Integration of Behavioural and Relaxation Approaches into the Treatment of Chronic Pain and Insomnia. Integration of behavioural and relaxation approaches into the treatment of chronic pain and insomnia. *Journal of American Medical Association* 1996; **276**:313–18.

Olesen J. Role of calcium entry blockers in the prophylaxis of migraine. *European Neurology* 1986; **25** (suppl.):72–9.

Onghena P, Van Houdenhove B. Antidepressant-induced analgesia in chronic non-malignant pain: a meta-analysis of 39 placebo-controlled studies. *Pain* 1992; **49**:205–19.

Ottenbacher K, DiFabio RP. Efficacy of spinal manipulation/mobilization therapy. A meta analysis. *Spine* 1985; **10**:833–7.

Pace NL. The best prophylaxis for succinylcholine myalgias: extension of a previous meta-analysis [letter]. *Anesthesia and Analgesia* 1993; **77**:1080–1.

Pace NL. Prevention of succinylcholine myalgias: a meta-analysis. *Anesthesia and Analgesia* 1990; **70**:477–83.

Patel M, Gutzwiller F, Paccaud F, Marazzi A. A meta-analysis of acupuncture for chronic pain. *International Journal of Epidemiology* 1989; **18**:900–6.

Penzien DB, Holroyd KA, Hursey KG, Holm JE, Wittchen H. *The behavioral treatment of migraine headache: a meta-analytic review of the literature.* Based on doctoral dissertation by Penzien, D.B. 1987:1–67.

Penzien DB, Holroyd KA. The behavioral treatment of migraine headache: a meta-analytic review of the literature. *Dissertation Abstracts International* 1987; 47:Order No. DA8629941.

Penzien DB, Rains JC, Holroyd KA. A review of alternative behavioral treatments for headache. *Mis Psychology* 1992; **17**:8–9.

Philipp M, Fickinger M. Psychotropic drugs in the management of chronic pain syndromes. *Pharmacopsychiatry* 1993; **26**:221–34.

Plantema F. Worldwide studies comparing piroxicam and naproxen. *Acta Obstetrica Gynecologica Scandinavica* 1986; (suppl.):138.

Pope JE, Anderson JJ, Felson DT. A meta-analysis of the effects of nonsteroidal anti-inflammatory drugs on blood pressure. *Archives of Internal Medicine* 1993; **153**:477–84.

Porzio F. Meta-analysis of three double-blind comparative trials with sustained-release etodolac in the treatment of osteoarthritis of the knee. *Rheumatology International* 1993; **13**:S19–24.

Porzio F. Sublingual piroxicam FDDF in the management of pain associated with rheumatic and nonrheumatic conditions: The Italian experience. *European Journal of Rheumatology and Inflammation* 1995; **15**:11–17.

Post B, Philbrick J. Do corticosteroids prevent postherpetic neuralgia? A review of the evidence. *Journal of the American Academy of Dermatology* 1988; **18**:605–10.

Powell FC, Hanigan WC, Olivero WC. A risk/benefit analysis of spinal manipulation therapy for relief of lumbar or cervical pain. *Neurosurgery* 1993; **33**:73–8; discussion 78–9.

Poynard T, Naveau S, Mory B, Chaput JC. Meta-analysis of smooth muscle relaxants in the treatment of irritable bowel syndrome. *Alimentation Pharmacology Therapeutics* 1994; **8**:499–510.

Poynard T, Valterio C. Meta-analysis of hydroxyethylrutosides in the treatment of chronic venous insufficiency. *Vasa* 1994; **23**:244–50.

Pradalier A, Vincent D. [Migraine and non-steroidal anti-inflammatory agents] Migraine et anti-inflammatoires non-steroidiens. *Pathologie Biologie* 1992; **40**:397–405.

Puett DW, Griffin MR. Published trials of nonmedicinal and noninvasive therapies for hip and knee osteoarthritis. *Annals of Internal Medicine* 1994; **121**:133–40.

Pustaver MR. Mechanical low back pain: etiology and conservative management. *Journal of Manipulative and Physiological Therapeutics* 1994; **17**:376–84.

Quan M. Pelvic inflammatory disease: diagnosis and management. *Journal of the American Board of Family Practitioners* 1994; **7**:110–23.

Radack K, Deck C. Beta-adrenergic blocker therapy does not worsen intermittent claudication in subjects with peripheral arterial disease. A meta-analysis of randomized controlled trials. *Archives of Internal Medicine* 1991; **151**:1769–76.

Radack K, Deck C. Do nonsteroidal anti inflammatory drugs interfere with blood pressure control in hypertensive patients? *Journal of General Internal Medicine* 1987; **2**:108–12.

Radack K, Wyderski RJ. Conservative management of intermittent claudication. *Annals of Internal Medicine* 1990; **113**:135–46.

Rahimtoola S. A perspective on the three large multicenter randomized clinical trials of coronary bypass surgery for chronic stable angina. *Circulation* 1985; **72**:V123–35.

Reeve J, Menon D, Corabian P. Transcutaneous electrical nerve stimulation (TENS): a technology assessment. *International Journal of Technology Assessment in Health Care* 1996; **12**:299–324.

Richardson PH, Williams AC. Meta-analysis of antidepressant-induced analgesia in chronic pain: comment. *Pain* 1993; **52**:247–9.

Riedemann PJ, Bersinic S, Cuddy LJ, Torrance GW, Tugwell PX. A study to determine the efficacy of safety and tenoxicam versus piroxicam, diclofenac and indomethacin in patients with osteoarthritis: a meta-analysis. *Journal of Rheumatology* 1993; **20**:2095–103.

Riethmüller-Winzen H. Flupirtine in the treatment of postoperative pain. *Postgraduate Medical Journal* 1987; **63**:61–5.

Robinson M, Mills RJ, Euler AR. Ranitidine prevents duodenal ulcers associated with non-steroidal anti-inflammatory drug therapy. *Alimentation Pharmacology and Therapeutics* 1991; **5**:143–50.

Robinson RG, Preston DF, Schiefelbein M, Baxter KG. Strontium 89 therapy for the palliation of pain due to osseous metastases. *Journal of American Medical Association* 1995; **274**:420–4.

Roderick PJ, Wilkes HC, Meade TW. The gastrointestinal toxicity of aspirin: an overview of randomised controlled trials. *British Journal of Clinical Pharmacology* 1993; **35**:219–26.

Rosch W. Efficacy of cisapride in the treatment of epigastric pain and concomitant symptoms in non ulcer dyspepsia. *Scandinavian Journal of Gastroenterology* 1989; (suppl.); 165.

Saag KG, Criswell LA, Sems KM, Nettleman MD, Kolluri S. Low-dose corticosteroids in rheumatoid arthritis: A meta-analysis of their moderate-term effectiveness. *Arthritis and Rheumatism* 1996; **39**:1818–25.

Sacks HS, Ancona-Berk VA, Berrier J, Nagalingam R, Chalmers TC. Dipyridamole in the treatment of angina pectoris: a meta-analysis. *Clinical Pharmacology and Therapeutics* 1988; **43**:610–15.

Sand T. Which factors affect reported headache incidences after lumbar myelography? A statistical analysis of publications in the literature. *Neuroradiology* 1989; **31**:55–9.

Schiassi M, Bianchini C, Restelli A, Zoni G. Tolerability profile of the antiinflammatory compound imidazole salicylate: a met-analysis of safety data in 1408 patients. *International Journal of Tissue Research* 1989; **11**:321–6.

Schmader K, Studenski S. Are current therapies useful for the prevention of postherpetic neuralgia? A critical analysis of the literature. *Journal of General Internal Medicine* 1989; **4**:83–9.

Schuhfried O, Fialka-Moser V. [Iontophoresis in the treatment of pain]. *Wien Medizinischi Wochenschrift* 1995; **145**:4–8.

Schulz KF, Grimes DA, Altman DG, Hayes RJ. Blinding and exclusions after allocation in randomised controlled trials: survey of published parallel group trials in obstetrics and gynaecology. *British Medical Journal* 1996; **312**:742–4.

Shekelle PG, Adams AH, Chassin MR, Hurwitz EL, Brook RH. Spinal manipulation for low-back pain [see comments]. *Annals of Internal Medicine* 1992; **117**:590–8.

Siminoski K, Josse RG, Bowyer M. Calcitonin in the treatment of osteoporosis. *Canadian Medical Association Journal* 1996; **155**:962–5.

Simkin P. Non-pharmacological methods of pain relief during labour. In: *Effective care in pregnancy and childbirth.* Chalmers I, Enkin M, Keirse MJNC, ed. Oxford University Press. 1989; 893–911.

Simmons J, Stavinoha W, Knodel L. Update and review of chemonucleolysis. *Clinical Orthopaedics* 1984; March:51–60.

Sindhu F. Are non-pharmacological nursing interventions for the management of pain effective?–A meta-analysis. *Journal of Advanced Nursing* 1996; **24**:1152–1159.

Smith MC, Holcombe JK, Stullenbarger E. A meta-analysis of intervention effectiveness for symptom management in oncology nursing research. *Oncology Nursing Forum* 1994; **21**:1201–9; discussion 1209–10.

Solomon GD. Verapamil in migraine prophylaxis–a five year review. *Headache* 1989; **29**:425–7.

Spierings EL, Messinger HB. Flunarizine vs. pizotifen in migraine prophylaxis: a review of comparative studies. *Cephalalgia* 1988; 8(suppl.):27–30.

Stalnikowicz R, Rachmilewitz D. NSAID-induced gastroduodenal damage: is prevention needed? A review and metaanalysis. *Journal of Clinical Gastroenterology* 1993; 17:238–43.

Stewart WF, Simon D, Shechter A, Lipton RB. Population variation in migraine prevalence: a meta-analysis. *Journal of Clinical Epidemiology* 1995; 48:269–80.

Stulberg B, Bauer T, Belhobek G. Making core decompression work. *Clinical Orthopaedics* 1990; Dec:186–95.

Suls J, Fletcher B. The relative efficacy of avoidant and nonavoidant coping strategies: a meta analysis. *Health and Psychology* 1985; 4:249–88.

Suls J, Wan CK. Effects of sensory and procedural information on coping with stressful medical procedures and pain: a meta-analysis. *Journal of Consulting and Clinical Psychology* 1989; 57:372–9.

Sutters KA, Miaskowski C. The problem of pain in children with cancer: a research review. *Oncology Nursing Forum* 1992; 19:465–71.

Teasell RW, Harth M. Functional restoration: Returning patients with chronic low back pain. *Spine* 1996; 21:844–847.

ter Riet G, Kleijnen J, Knipschild P. Acupuncture and chronic pain: a criteria-based meta-analysis. *Journal of Epidemiology* 1990; 43:1191–9.

Tfelt-Hansen P. Efficacy of beta blockers in migraine. A critical review. *Cephalalgia* 1986; 6(suppl.):15–24.

Tfelt-Hansen P. Sumatriptan for the treatment of migraine attacks-a review of controlled clinical studies. *Cephalalgia* 1993; 13:238–44.

Thomas D, Williams RA, Smith DS. The Frozen Shoulder: A Review of Manipulative Treatment. *Rheumatology and Rehabilitation* 1980; 19:173–9.

Thomson AM, Hillier VF. A re-evaluation of the effect of pethidine on the length of labour. *Journal of Advanced Nursing* 1994; 19:448–56.

Trabant H, Widdra W, De LS. Efficacy and safety of intranasal buserelin acetate in the treatment of endometriosis: a review of six clinical trials and comparison with danazol. *Progress in Clinical and Biological Research* 1990; 323:357–82.

Tramèr M, Williams J, Carroll D, Wiffen PJ, McQuay HJ, Moore RA. Systematic review of direct comparisons of non-steroidal anti-inflammatory drugs given by different routes for acute pain. *Acta Anaesthesiologica Scandinavica*. in press.

Turner JA. Efficacy of antidepressant medication for chronic pain problems. *Pain Forum* 1995; 4:254–5.

Turner JA, Denny MC. Do antidepressant medications relieve chronic low back pain?. *Journal of Family Practice* 1993; 37:545–53.

Turner JA, Deyo RA, Loeser JD, Von Korff M, Fordyce WE. The importance of placebo effects in pain treatment and research. *Journal of American Medical Association* 1994; 271:1609–14.

Turner JA, Ersek M, Herron L, Deyo R. Surgery for lumbar spinal stenosis. Attempted meta-analysis of the literature. *Spine* 1992; 17:1–8.

Turner JA, Loeser JD, Bell KG. Spinal cord stimulation for chronic low back pain; a systematic literature synthesis. *Neurosurgery* 1995; 37:1088–96.

Vaiani G, Grossi E. Meta-analysis of italian clinical trials of nabumetone. *Drugs* 1990; 40:48–9.

van den Hoogen HM, Koes BW, van Eijk JT, Bouter LM. On the accuracy of history, physical examination, and erythrocyte sedimentation rate in diagnosing low back pain in general practice. A criteria-based review of the literature. *Spine* 1995; 20:318–27.

van der Heijden CJM, van der Windt DAW, Kleijnen J, Koes BW, Bouter LM. Steroid injections for shoulder disorders: a systematic review of randomized clinical trials. *British Journal of General Practice* 1996; 46:309–16.

van der Heijden GJ, Beurskens AJ, Koes BW, Assendelft WJ, de Vet HC, Bouter LM. The efficacy of traction for back and neck pain: a systematic, blinded review of randomized clinical trial methods. *Physical Therapy* 1995; 75:93–104.

Vischer T. Efficacy and tolerability of tenoxicam an overview. *European Journal of Rheumatology and Inflammation* 1987; 9:51–7.

Vischer T. Efficacy and tolerability of tenoxicam an overview. *Scandinavian Journal of Rheumatology* 1987; 65:(suppl.):107–12.

Volmink J, Lancaster T, Gray S, Silagy C. Treatments for postherpetic neuralgia: A systematic review of randomized controlled trials. *Family Practice* 1996; 13:84–91.

Watts RW, Silagy CA. A meta-analysis on the efficacy of epidural corticosteroids in the treatment of sciatica. *Anaesthesia and Intensive Care* 1995; 23:564–9.

White KP, Harth M. An analytical review of 24 controlled clinical trials for fibromyalgia syndrome (FMS). *Pain* 1996; 64:211–19.

Wilkie DJ, Savedra MC, Holzemer WL, Tesler MD, Paul SM. Use of the McGill Pain Questionnaire to measure pain: a meta-analysis. *Nursing Research* 1990; 39:36–41.

Windle M, Booker L, Rayburn W. Postpartum pain after vaginal delivery. A review of comparative analgesic trials. *Journal of Reproductive Medicine* 1989; 34:891–5.

Wood MJ. How to measure and reduce the burden of zoster-associated pain. *Scandinavian Journal of Infectious Diseases* 1996; (suppl.):55–8.

Wood MJ, Kay R, Dworkin RH, Soong SJ, Whitley RJ. Oral acyclovir therapy accelerates pain resolution in patients with herpes zoster: A meta-analysis of placebo-controlled trials. *Clinical Infectious Diseases* 1996; 22:341–7.

Wright JM. Review of the syptomatic treatment of diabetic neuropathy. *Pharmacotherapy* 1994; 14:689–97.

Yee LY, Lopez JR. Transdermal fentanyl [see comments]. *Annals of Pharmacotherapeutics* 1992; 26:1393–9.

Zhang WY, Li Wan Po A. Analgesic efficacy of paracetamol and its combination with codeine and caffeine in surgical pain–A meta-analysis. *Journal of Clinical Pharmacology and Therapeutics* 1996; 21:261–82.

Zhang WY, Li Wan Po A. The effectiveness of topically applied capsaicin. A meta-analysis. *European Journal of Clinical Pharmacology* 1994; 46:517–22.

Part II

ACUTE PAIN

8

Acute pain: introduction

Summary

Systematic reviews of randomized controlled trials provide the highest level of evidence for treatments. There is now good evidence from systematic reviews about the relative efficacy of oral analgesics in moderate and severe postoperative pain. Using this knowledge carefully should improve postoperative care after acute pain.

Introduction

It should be unnecessary for patients with acute pain to have to endure severe pain in hospital, to have to stay in hospital because of poor pain relief, or to have to contact health care professionals because of continuing pain after they have left hospital.

It is hard to be precise about how many patients with acute pain endure severe pain in hospital, but Table 3 in Chapter 1 showed that 87% of over 3000 patients surveyed had pain of severe or moderate intensity, and that for a third of them pain was present all or most of the time. Equally, it is hard to be precise about the effect poorly controlled pain has on the incidence of patients having to stay in hospital, or on the incidence of consultations after leaving hospital. Ideal targets seem to be that less than 1% should have to stay, and less than 1% should have to consult [1]. Audits of day surgery show that poor pain control can certainly produce higher rates than 1% for both categories [2], and that providing better pain control produced a worthwhile reduction in both types of problem.

We have to pick our way through the evidence to achieve best outcome. There is a complicated relationship between evidence, guidelines, research and legal considerations, and the patients' outcomes assessed by audit (Fig. 1).

The rational approach to acute pain management is to use the highest quality evidence available. In the context of acute pain management, this comes from systematic reviews of valid randomized trials. We still have to adapt to the circumstance of the individual, but our policies will be more discerning.

This book focuses on treatments that are simple, clinically appropriate, and evidence-based. We are fortunate that there is now steady supply of systematic reviews in the pain world (Chapter 7), and an updated listing is maintained on the Internet at <http://www.jr2.ox.ac.uk/Bandolier/painres/MApain.html>. In the acute pain chapters we have therefore concentrated on developing a league table, or rank ordering, for which pain-killer or analgesic works best by mouth after surgery. There are surprises in this ranking, because the 'standard' take-home analgesic package often contains anal-

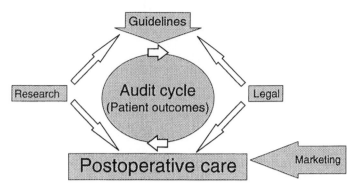

Fig. 1 Influences on postoperative care.

gesic that do poorly on the ranking. We have also looked at how well the oral pain-killers work compared with injections of morphine or of non-steroidal anti-inflammatory drugs (NSAIDs). We have thrown the net quite wide, and also include information on transcutaneous electrical nerve stimulations (TENS), injections of morphine into the knee joint and other peripheral sites, and on whether the timing of the analgesic (before or after surgery) makes any clinical difference.

Background and key questions

Background

Acute pain management is more than a collection of interventions. It is a package of care that needs to be examined as a whole as well as in its parts. Publications that analyse the process of acute pain provision are rare, perhaps because they attract few academic plaudits. There is good evidence that the risk of adverse events is increased when high-tech approaches are used for drug administration [3].

Acute pain is not confined to postoperative wards, but is a problem in many clinical settings (Table 1).

After surgery, pain is predictable, but in other settings its onset is unexpected, due to sudden illness or accident. Our procedures need to be effective for both the predictable and the unexpected.

The tools

The tools for treating pain are common to all types of acute pain although particular clinical circumstances may require different management strategies (Fig. 2).

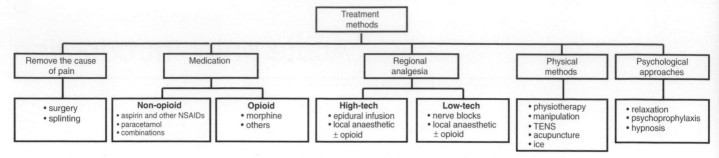

Fig. 2   Acute pain: interventions

Table 1   Acute pain settings

Postoperative
- inpatient
- day surgery
- wound dressings

Medical illness
- myocardial infarction
- sickle-cell crisis
- renal colic

Musculoskeletal
- acute low back pain
- rheumatoid arthritis
- acute on chronic

Cancer

Trauma

Burns

Childbirth

Medication

The majority of acute pain is managed solely with medication. In England during 1995 there were 32 million primary care prescriptions for non-opioids (mainly paracetamol and its combinations), 17 million for non-steroidal anti-inflammatory drugs, and 4 million for opioids [4].

Pain charts

Pain charts used as part of normal practice will improve quality of care [5, 6]. The fact of a chart is more important than its form, with pain measurements recorded at the same time as sedation, respiratory frequency, and nausea, and part of on-going audit. An example is the Burford chart [7]. There are special scales for children [8]. The chart we give to patients to use at home is shown in Fig. 3.

Acute pain services

One remedy for poor management is the provision of an acute pain service [9]. The dispute about what should be provided ranges from a full 'menu' including all the high-tech

options [10] to a service limited to supervision of good practice guidelines for low-tech approaches and staff education [5, 6]. Training and education should be the main tasks of an acute pain service, making sure that the focus is on the effective or most effective measures.

Key questions

Several key questions for pain relief are obvious:

- If patients can swallow then should the oral route be preferred?
- Should we use prophylaxis rather than treat-as-necessary—are the arguments for prophylaxis convincing?
- When is speed of effect a primary factor, so that injected routes are preferable to oral?
- When should we use injected opioid?
- When are injections of local anaesthetic with or without opioids useful in the acute pain setting?

For the future we need to know why some patients' acute pain turns into chronic pain.

Can the patient swallow?

Most postoperative pain is managed solely with medication. Perhaps because anaesthetists work with injected drugs there is a natural belief that drugs which are injected are more powerful than drugs taken by mouth.

Some questions:

- Which classes of drugs are the most effective postoperative analgesics? (or which are least effective)
- Within a class of drugs does the same dose work better when injected than when taken orally?

It is important to know which oral analgesics to recommend to patients because so much care is now given in the home. We are biased to think of patients after major surgery, but they too need oral analgesics when they can swallow. The evidence from trials which compare drugs with placebo may be used to build a ranking of relative efficacy.

For the acute pain part of this book all the trials of a particular drug compared with placebo in postoperative pain were obtained. The drug's performance in the trials was then converted into a common currency, the proportion of patients with moderate or severe postoperative pain who

Name ....   Treatment week ....

Please fill in this chart each evening before going to bed. Record your pain intensity and the amount of pain relief. If you have had any side-effects please note them in the side-effects box.

	Date							
Pain intensity How bad has your pain been today?	Severe							
	Moderate							
	Mild							
	None							
Pain relief How much pain relief have the tablets given today?	Complete							
	Good							
	Moderate							
	Slight							
	None							
Side-effects Has the treatment upset you in any way?								

How effective was the treatment this week? *poor fair good very good excellent* Please circle your choice

Fig. 3   The Oxford pain chart.

achieve at least 50% pain relief compared with placebo over 6 hours.

The most effective drugs have a low number-needed-to-treat (NNT) of about 2, meaning that for every two patients who receive the drug one will achieve at least 50% relief because of the treatment (the other patient may obtain relief but it does not reach the 50% level). The NNT is *treatment-specific*, which is useful for comparison of relative efficacy. But because these NNT comparisons are against placebo, the best NNT of 2 means that while 50 of 100 patients will get at least 50% relief because of the treatment, another 20 will have a placebo response which gives them at least 50% relief, so that with ibuprofen 70 of 100 will have effective pain relief.

For paracetamol 1 g the NNT is 4. Combination of paracetamol with codeine 60 mg improves the NNT to 3. Ibuprofen is better at 2. The clear message is that of the oral analgesics, NSAIDs perform best, and that paracetamol alone or in combinations is also effective. The strongest oral analgesic regimen would be oral NSAIDs supplemented as necessary with a paracetamol opioid combination. As pain wanes then the prescription should be paracetamol-based, supplemented if necessary by NSAIDs. When used in acute pain, a regimen like this resulted in high quality pain relief without recourse to general practitioner visits [2].

Even if patients can swallow is it best to give drugs by injection or suppository?

There is no evidence that NSAIDs given rectally or by injection perform better than the same drug at the same dose given by mouth (Chapter 11); two randomized, double-blind placebo-controlled comparisons of oral ibuprofen arginine (400 mg) failed to distinguish any difference from intramuscular ketorolac 30 mg [11, 12]. These other non-oral routes become appropriate when patients cannot swallow.

The patient cannot swallow analgesics

We only have preliminary information on the relative efficacy of injected opioids or NSAIDs (Chapter 13), that is how does the league table of oral analgesic efficacy relate to a league table of injected analgesic efficacy, or indeed to regional anaesthetic techniques. Some statements can be made, however:

- Injecting morphine at a dose of 10 mg provides similar analgesia to oral NSAID [13].
- Injecting morphine at doses of 10–20 mg provides similar analgesia to injected NSAID [14].
- Injecting NSAID provides similar analgesia to oral NSAID [11, 12].

- Injecting 20 mg of morphine provides greater analgesia then injecting 10 mg, and greater analgesia than the best performers on the oral league table [14].

Other techniques

Transcutaneous electrical nerve stimulation (TENS)

There is some disarray in professional opinion about the use of TENS in acute postoperative pain. Although the Agency for Health Care Policy and Research [15] recommends TENS for acute pain management, the earlier report of the UK College of Anaesthetists' working party on pain after surgery [9] does not. Chapter 20 deals with this difficult topic, and Chapter 21 examines the evidence underpinning the substantial use of TENS in labour pain.

Psychological methods

There is evidence that psychological approaches are beneficial [16]. Cognitive-behavioural methods can reduce pain and distress in burn patients. Preparation before surgery can reduce postoperative analgesic consumption. The evidence for the use of relaxation and music on postoperative pain is confounded by the poor quality of trials [17].

Pain which persists: prophylaxis or wait until it happens?

The intriguing problems in acute pain are:

- Is there a link between bad 'acute' pain and perseveration of this pain into a chronic status?
- Can we do anything to prevent this?

What remains unexplained is why some patients end up with chronic pain after acute pain when others do not. A simplistic explanation is that those with chronic pain have nerve damage at surgery. An alternative explanation is that it is the patients with severe acute pain who develop the chronic pain. The easy linkage is then to propose that if the acute pain was better controlled the chronic pain would not develop [18, 19].

Pre-emptive analgesia

The evidence for clinical advantage of giving an intervention before pain as opposed to giving the same intervention after pain still unconvincing [20]. Certainly, by far the majority of trials of pre-pain versus post-pain dosing has failed to show any clinically meaningful benefit.

Peripheral opioids

At least for intra-articular peripheral opioids the story becomes a little clearer. A systematic review of valid trials of intra-articular morphine in knee surgery has shown mor-

phine in the knee joint can indeed provide analgesia (Chapter 17, [21]). This analgesia can continue for up to 24 hours, although there is no dose-response. It is the long duration of action which suggests this technique might have practical application beyond its research interest [22].

Conclusion

The availability of high quality evidence gives a firm foundation for building better postoperative care. We can make informed decisions about drugs and route of administration for individual patients and services, both for pain and for nausea and vomiting. Bringing this together into an efficient and effective service will be the challenge, so that audit or controlled trials can demonstrate the effectiveness of our postoperative care.

References

1. Millar JM, Rudkin GE, Hitchcock M. *Practical anaesthesia and analgesia for day surgery.* Oxford: Bios, 1997.
2. Haynes TK, Evans DEN, Roberts D. Pain relief after day surgery: quality improvement by audit. *Journal of One-day Surgery* 1995; Summer: 12–15.
3. Bates DW, Cullen DJ, Laird N, Petersen LA, Small SD, Servi D *et al.* Incidence of adverse drug events and potential adverse drug events. *Journal of American Medical Association* 1995; **274**:29–34.
4. Government Statistical Service. *Prescription cost analysis for England 1995.* London: Department of Health, 1996.
5. Gould TH, Crosby DL, Harmer M, Lloyd SM, Lunn JN, Rees GAD *et al.* Policy for controlling pain after surgery: effect of sequential changes in management. *British Medical Journal* 1992; **305**:1187–93.
6. Rawal N, Berggren L. Organization of acute pain services: a low-cost model. *Pain* 1994; **57**:117–23.
7. Burford Nursing Development Unit. Nurses and pain. *Nursing Times* 1984; **18**:94.
8. McGrath PJ, Ritchie JA, Unruh AM. Paediatric pain. In: Carroll D, Bowsher D, Eds. *Pain management and nursing care.* Oxford: Butterworth Heinemann, 1993:100–23.
9. Royal College of Surgeons of England, the College of Anaesthetists. *Report of the working party on pain after surgery.* London: Royal College of Surgeons, 1990.
10. Ready LB, Oden R, Chadwick HS, Benedetti C, Rooke GA, Caplan R *et al.* Development of an anaesthesiology based postoperative pain management service. *Anesthesiology* 1988; **68**:100–6.
11. Laveneziana D, Riva A, Bonazzi M, Cipolla M, Migliavacca S. Comparative efficacy of oral ibuprofen arginine and intramuscular ketorolac in patients with postoperative pain. *Clinical Drug Investigation* 1996; **11**:8–14.
12. Pagnoni B, Vignali M, Colella S, Monopoli R, Tiengo N. Comparative efficacy of oral ibuprofen arginine and intramuscular ketorolac in patients with postcaesarean section pain. *Clinical Drug Investigation* 1996; **11**:15–21.
13. Mansfield M, Firth F, Glynn C, Kinsella J. A comparison of ibuprofen arginine with morphine sulphate for pain relief after orthopaedic surgery. *European Journal of Anaesthesiology* 1996; **13**:492–7.

14. Norholt S, SindetPedersen S, Larsen U, Bang U, Ingerslev J, Nielsen O *et al*. Pain control after dental surgery: A double-blind, randomised trial of lornoxicam versus morphine. *Pain* 1996; 67:335–43.

15. Acute Pain Management Guideline Panel. *Acute pain management: operative or medical procedures and trauma*. Clinical Practice Guideline No. 1. Agency for Health Care Policy and Research, U.S. Department of Health and Human Services. AHCPR Publication No. 92-0032. Rockville, MD: Public Health Service, 1992:24–5.

16. Justins DM, Richardson PH. Clinical management of acute pain. *British Medical Bulletin* 1991; 47:561–83.

17. Good M. Effect of relaxation and music on postoperative pain: a review. *Journal of Advanced Nursing* 1996; 24:905–14.

18. Eija K, Tiina T, Pertti NJ. Amitriptyline effectively relieves neuropathic pain following treatment of breast cancer. *Pain* 1996; 64:293–302.

19. Katz J, Jackson M, Kavanagh B, Sandler A. Acute pain after thoracic surgery predicts long-term post-thoracotomy pain. *Clinical Journal of Pain* 1996; 12:50–5.

20. McQuay HJ. Pre-emptive analgesia: a systematic review of clinical studies. *Annals of Medicine* 1995; 27:249–56.

21. Kalso E, Tramer M, Carroll D, McQuay H, Moore RA. Pain relief from intra-articular morphine after knee surgery: A qualitative systematic review. *Pain* 1997; 71:642–51.

22. Kanbak NM, Akpolat N, Öcal T, Doral NM, Ercan M, Erdem K. Intraarticular morphine administration provides pain relief after knee arthroscopy. *European Journal of Anaesthesiology* 1997; 14:153–6.

9

Paracetamol with and without codeine in acute pain

Summary

This is a systematic review of randomized controlled trials (RCTs) to assess the analgesia obtained from single oral doses of paracetamol alone and in combination with codeine in postoperative pain.

We found 39 trials of paracetamol against placebo with 4124 patients, 21 trials of paracetamol plus codeine against placebo with 1450 patients and 12 trials of paracetamol plus codeine against the same dose of paracetamol with 794 patients. Pain relief information was extracted, and converted into dichotomous information—number of patients with at least 50% pain relief. Wide variations in responses to placebo (0–72%) and active (5–89%) were observed.

In postoperative pain states paracetamol 1000 mg alone against placebo had a number-needed-to-treat (NNT) of 4.6 (3.9–5.4) and paracetamol 600/650 mg alone an NNT of 5.3 (4.1–7.2). Paracetamol 600/650 mg plus codeine 60 mg verses placebo had a better NNT of 3.1 (2.6–3.9), with no overlap of 95% confidence intervals with paracetamol 600/650 mg alone. In direct comparisons the additional analgesic effect of 60 mg of codeine added to paracetamol was 11 extra patients in every 100 achieving at least 50% pain relief. In indirect comparisons of each with placebo it was 14 extra patients per 100. This was an NNT for adding codeine 60 mg of 7.7 (5.1–20).

The results confirm that paracetamol is an effective analgesic, and that codeine 60 mg added to paracetamol produces worthwhile additional pain relief even in single oral doses.

Introduction

Paracetamol is an important non-opioid analgesic, commonly prescribed, as well as being available without prescription. In England in 1995, paracetamol alone for adults accounted for over 5 million prescriptions (16% of total non-opioid analgesic prescriptions), with 4.5 million prescriptions of paediatric suspensions [2]. In combination with codeine, paracetamol accounted for a further 6.4 million prescriptions (20% of total non-opioid analgesics). Paracetamol alone and in combination with a variety of opioids accounted for 93% of prescriptions in this British National Formulary (BNF) classification.

Policy decisions and guidelines are increasingly being made on the basis of hard evidence. Trying to judge the relative efficacy of analgesics against one another is not easy because there are few such direct comparisons. Only five direct comparisons were found of paracetamol 1000 mg and ibuprofen 400 mg in acute pain [3].

Relative efficacy can also be determined indirectly, from comparisons of each analgesic with placebo, using a common descriptor of efficacy, and then comparing the results for various analgesic interventions, both pharmacological and non-pharmacological. In this review of paracetamol we compare its analgesic efficacy with information about other drugs again determined by similar quantitative systematic reviews.

Methods

Randomized controlled trials of paracetamol in postoperative pain (post-dental extraction, post-surgical, or postpartum pain) were sought. A number of different search strategies were used to identify eligible reports in MEDLINE (1966–May 1996), EMBASE (1980–96), the Cochrane Library (March 1996), and the Oxford Pain Relief Database (1950–94) [4]. The words: 'paracetamol', 'acetaminophen', and 'trial' were used in a free text search, including combinations of these words, and without restriction to language. Additional reports were identified from reference lists of retrieved reports, review articles (including a recent systematic review of paracetamol plus codeine [5], and textbooks.

Inclusion criteria for paracetamol

Neither pharmaceutical companies nor authors of papers were contacted for unpublished reports. Abstracts and review articles were not considered. The inclusion criteria used were: randomized allocation to treatment groups which compared either paracetamol or a paracetamol and codeine combination with placebo or a paracetamol and codeine combination with the same dose of paracetamol alone, full journal publication, established postoperative pain with the pain outcome measured using a five-point pain relief scale with standard wording (none, slight, moderate, good, complete), or a four-point pain intensity scale (none, mild, moderate, severe), or a

---

The topic discussed in this chapter is also published in part in Moore *et al.* 1997 [1].

visual analogue scale (VAS) for pain relief or pain intensity, TOTPAR or SPID (at 4, 5, or 6 hours) as a derived pain relief outcome (or sufficient data provided to allow their calculation), postoperative oral administration, adult patients, baseline pain of moderate to severe intensity, (for VAS this equates to > 30 mm [6]), and double-blind design. We excluded reports for the relief of other pain conditions, paracetamol used in combination with drugs other than codeine, and trials where the number of patients per treatment group was less than ten [7]. In postpartum pain trials were included if the pain investigated was due to episiotomy or caesarean section combined with uterine cramps, but trials investigating uterine cramps alone were excluded.

Data extraction and analysis

From each report we took: the numbers of patients treated, the mean TOTPAR, SPID, VAS-TOTPAR, or VAS-SPID, study duration and the dose given. Information on adverse events was also extracted. For each report, the mean TOTPAR, SPID, VAS-TOTPAR, or VAS-SPID values for active and placebo were converted to %maxTOTPAR or %maxSPID by division into the calculated maximum value [8]. The proportion of patients in each treatment group who achieved at least 50%maxTOTPAR was calculated using verified equations [9–11]. These proportions were then converted into the number of patients achieving at least 50%max TOTPAR by multiplying by the total number of patients in the treatment group. Information on the number of patients with at least 50%maxTOTPAR for active and placebo was then used to calculate relative benefit (RB) and NNT.

Relative benefit (RB) estimates were calculated with 95% confidence intervals (CI) using a random effects model [12]; the random effects model was chosen because this produces the most conservative estimate (homogeneity was assumed when $P > 0.1$). NNT and 95% confidence intervals were calculated by the method of Cook and Sackett [13]. A statistically significant difference from control was assumed when the 95% confidence interval of the relative benefit did not include 1.

Results

Paracetamol vs. placebo

The searches found 37 reports of 39 trials that fulfilled the inclusion criteria; 2530 patients were given paracetamol and 1594 placebo. Details of the trials are in Appendix 1. Twenty-one trials investigated oral surgery pain (post-dental pain, predominantly third molar extraction with bone removal), 8 post-surgical (elective general, gynecological, and orthopaedic surgery) and 10 postpartum (episiotomy and post-Caesarean section). Doses of paracetamol were 500 mg in 6 trials, 600 mg in 6, 650 mg in 11 and 1000 mg in 20; for analysis, data from paracetamol 600 mg and 650 mg

were combined. One report on episiotomy provided dichotomous information on the overall patient global rating of pain relief [14]. This report was included. The proportion of patients with good or excellent pain relief was used.

The variation in placebo response rates (i.e. the proportion of patients with at least 50% pain relief) was from 0% to 72% of patients with at least 50%maxTOTPAR (Fig. 1). The placebo response rate ranged from 0% to 72% in post-dental pain, 11% to 48% in post-surgical pain, and 0% to 34% in postpartum pain. The variation in response rates with all doses of paracetamol was 5% to 83% (Fig. 1). The mean response rate for paracetamol 600/650 mg was 42%, and that for placebo was 23%.

Combining data across conditions, the pooled relative benefits for all doses of paracetamol versus placebo were significant (Table 1). At a dose of 600/650 mg paracetamol had an NNT for at least 50% pain relief compared with placebo in single dose administration of 5.3 (4.1–7.2) and at 1000 mg the NNT was 4.6 (3.9–5.4), with overlap between the confidence intervals (CIs).

Drug-related study withdrawals occurred rarely. One study [15] had three withdrawals, one on placebo and two on paracetamol. Another [16] had two patients who withdrew on paracetamol. These studies reported a variable incidence of adverse events which were mild and transient, with no difference in incidence between paracetamol and placebo.

Paracetamol plus codeine vs. placebo

We found 20 reports of 20 trials that fulfilled the inclusion criteria; 721 patients were given paracetamol and 664 placebo. Details of the trials are given in Appendix 2. Doses were paracetamol 300 mg plus codeine 30 mg in five trials, paracetamol 600 plus codeine 60 mg in eight, paracetamol 650 mg plus codeine 60 mg in five, and paracetamol 1000 mg plus

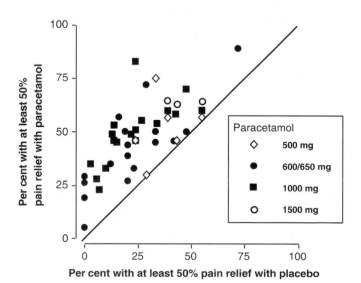

Fig. 1 Single dose studies of paracetamol vs. placebo.

Table 1   Summary relative benefit and number-needed-to-treat (NNT) for trials of paracetamol vs. placebo

No. of trials	Paracetamol dose (mg)	At least 50%maxTOTPAR on paracetamol	At least 50%maxTOTPAR on placebo	Relative benefit (95% CI)	NNT (95% CI)
6	500	194/353	109/296	1.4 (1.1–1.9)	5.6 (3.9–9.5)
17	600/650	243/594	125/573	1.7 (1.3–2.2)	5.3 (4.1–7.2)
20	1000	620/1376	207/907	2.3 (1.7–2.9)	4.6 (3.9–5.4)
3	1500	133/207	63/141	1.4 (1.2–1.9)	5.0 (3.3–11)

codeine 60 mg in two. One report on episiotomy provided dichotomous information on the overall patient global rating of pain relief [17]. This report was included. The proportion of patients with good or excellent pain relief was used. Pain relief was measured over four to six hours in 19 of the reports; one had observations for just three hours.

The variation in placebo response rates was from 0% to 72% of patients with at least 50%maxTOTPAR. The variation in response rates to all doses of paracetamol plus codeine was 20% to 83% (Fig. 2). The mean response rate for paracetamol 600/650 mg plus codeine 60 mg was 51%, and that for placebo was 21%.

Combining data across conditions, paracetamol 300 mg plus codeine 30 mg had an NNT for at least 50% pain relief compared with placebo in single dose administration of 5.3 (3.8–8.0), paracetamol 600/650 mg plus codeine 60 mg an NNT of 3.1 (2.6–3.8) and paracetamol 1000 mg plus codeine 60 mg an NNT of 1.9 (1.5–2.6), although in only two trials (Table 2).

There were no serious adverse events which necessitated withdrawal from any study.

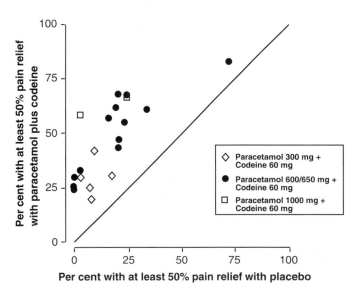

Fig. 2   Single dose studies of paracetamol plus codeine vs. placebo.

Paracetamol plus codeine vs. paracetamol alone

We found 12 reports of 12 trials that fulfilled the inclusion criteria; 395 patients were given paracetamol and 399 placebo. Four reports were identified that fulfilled inclusion criteria except that they had pain outcomes other than five-point categorical pain relief scores. Details of the trials are given in Appendix 3. Ten trials were in oral surgery and three in post-surgical pain. Doses were paracetamol 600 mg plus codeine 60 mg in seven trials, paracetamol 650 mg plus codeine 60 mg in four, and paracetamol 1000 mg plus codeine 60 mg in two. Pain relief was measured over four to six hours in twelve reports; one measured pain relief over three hours.

The variation in response rates for paracetamol alone was from 5% to 89% of patients with at least 50%maxTOTPAR. The variation in response rates to all doses of paracetamol plus codeine was 24% to 83%.

Only one of the reports had a lower 95% confidence interval of the relative benefit that did not include 1 (Fig. 3). The combined relative benefit for this homogeneous data set was 1.25 (1.09–1.43). Combining data across conditions, the NNT for addition of codeine 60 mg to all doses of paracetamol for at least 50% pain relief in single dose administration was 7.7 (5.1–17).

There were no serious adverse events which necessitated withdrawal from any study.

Comment

Paracetamol 1000 mg alone had an overall NNT of 4.6 for at least 50% pain relief compared with placebo in single dose administration. This means that one of every five patients with pain of moderate to severe intensity will get at least 50% pain relief, who would not have done had they been given a placebo. The equivalent NNT at 600/650 mg was 5.3, indicating lower efficacy, although the dose-response was not significant.

Paracetamol 600/650 mg plus codeine 60 mg had an NNT of 3.1 for at least 50% pain relief compared with placebo in single dose administration, meaning that one of every three patients with pain of moderate to severe intensity will get at least 50% pain relief, who would not have done had they been given a placebo (Table 2). There was no overlap

Table 2 Summary relative benefit and number-needed-to-treat (NNT) for trials of paracetamol and codeine vs. placebo and paracetamol alone

No. of trials	Drug dose (mg) paracetamol + codeine	At least 50%maxTOTPAR on paracetamol + codeine	At least 50%maxTOTPAR on placebo	At least 50%maxTOTPAR on paracetamol alone	Relative benefit (95% CI)	NNT (95% CI)
Paracetamol + codeine vs. placebo						
5	300 + 30	69/246	17/196		3.0 (1.8–5.0)	5.3 (3.8–8.0)
13	600/650 + 60	200/398	80/418		2.6 (1.7–4.0)	3.1 (2.6–3.9)
2	1000 + 60	48/77	5/50		6.2 (0.8–47)	1.9 (1.5–2.6)
Paracetamol + codeine vs. same dose of paracetamol alone						
10	600/650 + 60	165/309		129/313	1.3 (1.0–1.6)	8.3 (5.0 -23)
2	1000 + 60	57/86		44/86	1.3 (1.1–1.5)	6.7 (3.4–174)
12	All doses + 60	222/395		173/399	1.2 (1.1–1.5)	7.7 (5.1–17)

Doses of paracetamol are given first. Studies were predominantly in oral surgery (14 trials for paracetamol plus codeine vs. placebo and 10 trials for paracetamol plus codeine vs. paracetamol alone).

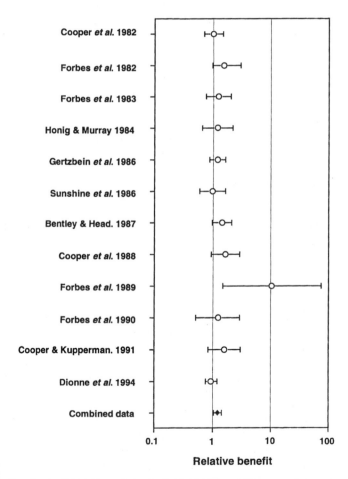

Fig. 3 Relative benefit for individual trials of 60 mg codeine plus paracetamol compared with the same dose of paracetamol alone. (See Appendix 3 for the references.)

between the 95% confidence interval of the NNT for paracetamol 600/650 mg plus codeine 60 mg in 13 trials (2.6–3.9) and that of paracetamol 600/650 mg alone in 17 trials (4.1–7.2). This indicates that addition of codeine 60 mg provides a substantial increase in analgesia in single dose administration. This is demonstrated clearly in Fig. 4, where wide confidence intervals accompany point estimates of the NNT where there were small numbers of patients. Despite this, paracetamol combined with 60 mg of codeine is clearly a powerful analgesic.

The extra analgesic effect of adding codeine 60 mg to paracetamol can be estimated in two ways. Since both paracetamol alone and paracetamol plus codeine were each compared with placebo, then any increased response rate (proportion of patients with at least 50% pain relief) may be ascribed to the addition of codeine. For paracetamol 600/650 mg alone against placebo, the difference between active (42%) and control (23%) response rates was 19%. For paracetamol 600/650 mg plus codeine 60 mg the difference between active (51%) and control (21%) was 33%. Therefore the extra 11% response was due to adding codeine 60 mg.

There were also direct comparisons of paracetamol (all doses) plus codeine 60 mg with the same dose of paracetamol alone. Here again, any increased response rate can be ascribed to the addition of codeine. For paracetamol plus codeine 60 mg versus the same dose of paracetamol the difference between active (55%) and control (41%) was 14%. This agreement between direct and indirect measures helps to justify the meta-analytical methods. The extra 14% response for codeine 60 mg corresponds to an NNT for at least 50% pain relief in single dose administration of 7.7 (5.1–17) (Table 2). This means that for every eight patients given paracetamol 600/650 mg plus codeine 60 mg, one extra will achieve at least 50% pain relief who would not have done had they received paracetamol 600/650 mg alone.

The variation in placebo and active response rates was large, but this degree of variation is common in pain studies [18], as well as in studies with more objective outcomes like postoperative vomiting [19], and in the response of infants to

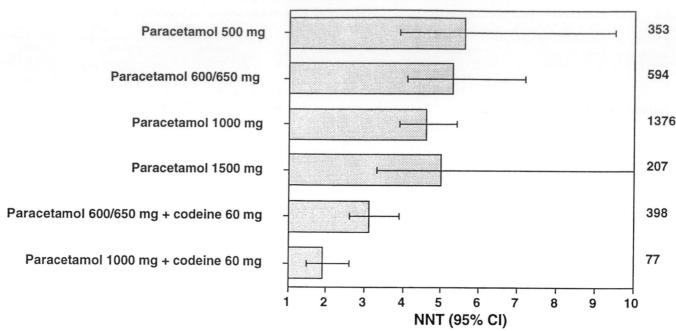

Fig. 4 Relative effectiveness of paracetamol doses and paracetamol plus codeine combinations. Number of Patients given active on right axis.

pulmonary surfactant [20]. The variability in both the placebo and active response rates (Fig. 1 and 2) underpins the use of standard methods in pain research, where sensitivity of the model is demonstrated by separation of standard analgesic from placebo. This variability also emphasises both the need to include placebo groups in analgesic trials, and the need to understand better those factors that contribute to the variability in placebo responses in pain.

The power of the systematic review method is demonstrated here in several ways. The analgesic effect of paracetamol at two doses has been determined with confidence from all the available published data. The rather slight effects of codeine added to paracetamol (which are difficult to measure in single trials with limited numbers of patients) has been confirmed in direct and indirect comparison.

References

1. Moore A, Collins S, Carroll D, McQuay H. Paracetamol with and without codeine in acute pain: a quantitative systematic review. *Pain* 1997; **70**:193–201.
2. Government Statistical Service. *Prescription cost analysis for England 1995*. London: Department of Health, 1996.
3. Jadad AR. Meta-analysis of randomised clinical trials in pain relief. University of Oxford: D.Phil.thesis, 1994.
4. Jadad AR, Carroll D, Moore A, McQuay H. Developing a database of published reports of randomised clinical trials in pain research. *Pain* 1996; **66**:239–46.
5. de Craen AJM, Di Giulio G, LampeSchoenmaeckers AJE, Kessels AGH, Kleijnen J. Analgesic efficacy and safety of paracetamol-codeine combinations versus paracetamol alone: A systematic review. *British Medical Journal* 1996; **313**:321–5.
6. Collins SL, Moore RA, McQuay HJ. The visual analogue pain intensity scale: what is moderate pain in millimeters? *Pain* 1997; **72**:95–7.
7. L'Abbé KA, Detsky AS, O'Rourke K. Meta-analysis in clinical research. *Annals of Internal Medicine* 1987; **107**:224–33.
8. Cooper SA. Single-dose analgesic studies: the upside and downside of assay sensitivity. In: Max MB, Portenoy RK, Laska EM, ed. *The design of analgesic clinical trials (Advances in pain research and therapy*, Vol. 18). New York: Raven Press, 1991:117–24.
9. Moore A, McQuay H, Gavaghan D. Deriving dichotomous outcome measures from continuous data in randomised controlled trials of analgesics. *Pain* 1996; **66**:229–37.
10. Moore A, McQuay H, Gavaghan D. Deriving dichotomous outcome measures from continuous data in randomised controlled trials of analgesics: Verification from independent data. *Pain* 1997; **69**:127–30.
11. Moore A, Moore O, McQuay H, Gavaghan D. Deriving dichotomous outcome measures from continuous data in randomised controlled trials of analgesics: Use of pain intensity and visual analogue scales. *Pain* 1997; **69**:311–15.
12. DerSimonian R, Laird N. Meta-analysis of clinical trials. *Controlled Clinical Trials* 1986; **7**:177–88.
13. Cook RJ, Sackett DL. The number needed to treat: a clinically useful measure of treatment effect. *British Medical Journal* 1995; **310**:452–4.
14. Berry FN, Miller JM, Levin HM, Bare WW, Hopkinson JH3, Feldman AJ. Relief of severe pain with acetaminophen in a new dose formulation versus propoxyphene hydrochloride 65 mg. and placebo: a comparative double blind study. *Current Therapeutic Research* 1975; **17**:361–8.
15. Dolci G, Ripari M, Pacifici L, Umile A. Evaluation of piroxicam-beta-cyclodextrin, piroxicam, paracetamol and placebo in post-operative oral surgery pain. *International Journal of Clinical Pharmacology Research* 1994; **14**:185–91.

16. Kiersch TA, Halladay SC, Hormel PC. A single-dose, double-blind comparison of naproxen sodium, acetaminophen, and placebo in postoperative dental pain. *Clinical Therapeutics* 1994; **16**:394–404.

17. Turek M, Baird W. Double blind parallel comparison of ketoprofen (Orudis), acetaminophen plus codeine, and placebo in postoperative pain. *Journal of Clinical Pharmacology* 1988; **28**:S23–8.

18. McQuay HJ, Tramer M, Nye BA, Carroll D, Wiffen PJ, Moore RA. A systematic review of antidepressants in neuropathic pain. *Pain* 1996; **68**:217–27.

19. Tramer M, Moore A, McQuay H. Prevention of vomiting after paediatric strabismus surgery: a systematic review using the numbers-needed-to-treat method. *British Journal of Anaesthesiology* 1995; **75**:556–61.

20. Soll JC, McQueen MC. Respiratory distress syndrome. In: Sinclair JC, Bracken ME, ed. *Effective care of the newborn infant*. Oxford University Press, 1992: Chapter 15, p. 333.

21. Moore RA, McQuay HJ. Single-patient data meta-analysis of 3453 postoperative patients: Oral tramadol versus placebo, codeine and combination analgesics. *Pain* 1997; **69**:287–94.

Appendix 1
Paracetamol vs. placebo: trial details

Ref.	Condition & no. of patients	Design, study duration & follow-up	Outcome measures	Dose regimen	Analgesic outcome results	Remedication	Withdrawals & exclusions	Adverse effects	Quality score
[Beaver & McMillan 1980]	Episiotomy & uterine cramp (Vaginal delivery <48 h) n = 108 Age?	RCT, DB, single oral dose, 5 parallel groups. 3 h washout prior to start & med given >30 min before or >2 h after patients meal. Evaluated in hospital by nurse observer at 0 then hourly for 6 h or until pain returned to premed level.	PI (4-pt scale) PR (5-pt scale) 50% PR (y/n) Global rating (5-pt scale) NB episiotomy pain was assessed as 'right now' & uterine cramp pain as 'during the last h'	Placebo n = 22 Paracetamol (1000 mg) n = 22	Paracetamol was significantly superior to placebo (P<0.05–0.01) for all measures except those based on change in PI.	Patients were allowed to remed after 2 h if pain returned to pre-med levels. After remed PR = 0 for all further timepoints.	108 analysed 'There were no drop-outs'.	NSD between groups. All AE were mild & subjective. Total no. of patients reporting AE: Placebo 7/22 with 8 AE Paracetamol 11/22 with 13 AE.	4
[Bentley & Head 1987]	3rd molar bony impacted n = 128 Age, mean mid 20s	RCT, DB, single oral dose, 4 parallel groups. No info on anaes except 'no sedative or narcotic agents were used before, during or after surgery'. Self-assessed at home at 0, 1, 2, 3, 4, 5 h, then posted reports to investigator.	PI (10-pt scale) PR (5-pt scale)	Placebo n = 17 Paracetamol (1000 mg) n = 41	Paracetamol showed significant superiority for all measures of efficacy.	Rescue analgesic—Tylenol No. 3. Patients who remed <5 h, last PI & PR scores carried on for all further timepoints.	120 analysed. Exclusions: 3 did not take the med, 1 took only a portion, 1 took no med until the day after surgery, 1 remed after 30 min, 1 vomited within 30 min of taking the med & 1 patient did not return the forms.	53 had 1 or more AE, 86 were reported in total, majority were dizziness, drowsiness, nausea & vomiting. There was NSD between treatment groups. No. patients with AE; paracetamol 21/42 with 31 AE Placebo 9/19 with 16 AE.	3
[Berry et al. 1975]	Episiotomy n = 225 Age: 15+	RCT, DB, single oral dose, 3 parallel groups, 12 h washout prior to start. Assessed by observer(s) in hospital at 0, 0.5, 1, 2, 3, 4 h.	PI (5-pt scale) PR (5-pt scale): (NB non-standard scale) Gastric discomfort (4-pt scale) Global rating (5 word scale)	Placebo n = 76 Paracetamol (1000 mg) n = 76	Total pain scores & total relief from pain scores showed paracetamol to be significantly superior to placebo. Global rating > good Placebo 18/76 Paracetamol 43/76.	After a reasonable period rescue analgesia could be prescribed at the investigator's discretion & the patient regarded as a treatment failure (no info on how data handled). Placebo 23/76 Paracetamol 2/76.	No details.	'None of the patients experienced adverse drug reactions'. No. patients reporting Gastric discomfort; Paracetamol (slight) 2/76. Placebo (mod) 2/76	3
[Bjune et al. 1996]	Caesarean section n = 125 Age: 27–37	RCT, DB, single oral dose, 3 parallel groups, 4 h washout prior to start. Baseline pain >40 mm = moderate, >60 mm = severe. Evaluated in hospital at 0, 0.5, 1 h then hourly for 6 h.	VAS-PI ('no pain' to 'unbearable pain') PR (5-pt scale)	Placebo n = 21 (9 moderate, 12 severe baseline pain) Paracetamol (1000 mg) n = 43 (17 moderate, 26 severe baseline pain)	For the patients with moderate pain there were no differences between the groups for any measures of efficacy. For patients with severe pain the active groups were significantly superior to placebo for most measures of efficacy (P<0.005).	Remed after 1st h (PI = 0 & PR last score used for all further timepoints).	108 analysed. Exclusions: 6 patients did not adhere to 4 h washout, 5 had PI <40 mm & 5 were excluded for other minor protocol violations.	No. of patients with AE: Placebo 1/25 with 1 AE. Paracetamol 10/50 with 14 AE.	3
[Cooper et al. 1980]	Impacted 3rd molar n = 298 Age: mean early 20s	RCT, DB, single oral dose, 6 parallel groups. No info on anaes. Self-assessed at home at 0, 1, 2, 3, 4 h (questionnaire)—majority collected 1 week later by observer, few returned by mail (patients telephoned if problems encountered).	PI (4-pt scale) PR (5-pt scale) Global rating (5-pt scale) 50% relief of baseline pain (y/n) Time to remed	Placebo n = 38 Paracetamol (500 mg) n = 37	Paracetamol showed significant analgesic efficacy for all measures.	t >1 h before remed (unclear how data handled). Remed <4 h Placebo 26/38. Paracetamol 25/3.	247 analysed. Exclusions: 21 were lost to follow-up, 10 dropped out before ingesting med. (no details), 20 ingested med but were excluded for protocol violations (no details).	No. of patients with AE: Placebo 6/38 with 7 AE. Paracetamol 3/37 with 6 AE.	4
[Cooper et al. 1981]	Impacted 3rd molar n = 248 Age, mean early 20s	RCT, DB, single oral dose, 5 parallel grps. Either GA or LA. Self-assessed at home at 0, 1, 2, 3, 4 h (questionnaire).	PI (4-pt scale) PR (5-pt scale) Global rating (5-pt scale) 50% relief of baseline pain (y/n) Time to remed	Placebo n = 37 Paracetamol (650 mg) n = 37	All active treatments were significantly superior to placebo for all measures. (Mean values for SPID, peak PID, TOTPAR etc, in Table 2).	Remed after 1st h if needed (last score used for all further timepoints) Remed <4 h Placebo 20/37 Paracetamol 2/37.	200 analysed. Exclusions: 17 did not ingest med, 31 ingested med but violated protocol (remed before 1st h obs, constant deviation of more than 15 min from evaluation times, not returning questionnaire & lost to follow-up).	No serious AE was reported. No. of patients with AE: Placebo 4/37 with 5 AE. Paracetamol 12/37 with 15 AE.	4

Ref.	Condition & no. of patients	Design, study duration & follow-up	Outcome measures	Dose regimen	Analgesic outcome results	Remedication	Withdrawals & exclusions	Adverse effects	Quality score
[Cooper *et al.* 1986]	Oral surgery (involving bone removal) n = 112 Age: 16+	RCT, DB, single oral dose, 3 parallel grps, single centre & 1 surgeon. No info on anaes. Self-assessed at home at 0, 1, 2, 3, 4, 5, 6 h (diary).	PI (4-pt scale) PR (5-pt scale) Pain half gone? (y/n) Global rating (5 pt) Time to remed	Placebo n = 22 Paracetamol (1000 mg) n = 38	For all measures paracetamol was significantly superior to placebo (P<0.05). (Table 2 for mean values SPID, TOTPAR, 50% red, etc).	Remed after 1st h if needed (last score used for all further timepoint).	99 analysed. Exclusions: 6 did not require analgesia, 3 fell asleep, & the other 4 were 'various protocol violations'.	No serious AE was reported. Over half reported were drowsiness & there were 2 reports of nausea. No. of AE reported: Paracetamol 12 Placebo 0.	3
[Cooper *et al.* 1988]	Impacted 3rd molar n = 165 Age: 18–57	RCT, DB, single oral dose, 3 parallel grps, single centre & 1 surgeon. LA with sed &/or nitrous oxide. 4 h washout prior to start. Self-assessed at home at 0, 0.5, 1, 2, 3, 4, 5, 6 h (diary).	PI (4-pt scale) PR (5pt-scale) Pain half gone? (y/n) Global rating (5 pt) Time to remed	Placebo n = 40 Paracetamol (600 mg) n = 36	Paracetamol appeared clinically more effective than placebo but it was not significantly superior.	Remed after 1st h (last or baseline score used for all further timepoints).	143 analysed. Exclusions: 11 were lost to follow-up, 8 did not require med. & 3 for 'various protocol violations'.	No serious AE were reported, No. of AE reported: Placebo 3 Paracetamol 8.	4
[Cooper *et al.* 1989]	Removal of impacted teeth n = 194 Age: 16+	RCT, DB, single oral dose, 3 parallel grps. LA with IV sed., atropine &/or nitrous oxide. 4 h washout prior to start. Self-assessed at home at 0, 0.5, 1, 2, 3, 4, 5, 6 h (diary).	PI (4-pt scale) PR (5-pt scale) Pain half gone? (y/n) Global rating (5 pt) Time to remed.	Placebo n = 64 Paracetamol (1000 mg) n = 59	Paracetamol was significantly superior to the placebo (P<0.05 to P<0.001) for all measures.(Table 2 for mean values, SPID, TOTPAR, etc.).	Remed after 1st h (last or baseline score used for all further timepoints) Approx 50% paracetamol & 36% placebo completed least 4 h before remed. Sig longer mean time to remed for paracetamol (P<05) than for placebo.	184 analysed. Exclusions: 4 slept through more than 2 observations, 2 were lost to follow-up, 2 did not need to medicate, 1 had inadequate baseline PI & 1 failed to complete the evaluations at the set times.	190 were evaluated for AE (all who ingested the med). No serious AE were reported—drowsiness was the most common. No. of patients with AE: Placebo 7/64 with 7 AE Paracetamol 11/63 with 13 AE.	5
[Cooper & Kuppeman 1991]	Removal of 1 or more impacted teeth n = 247 Age: 'young adults'	RCT, DB, single oral dose, 6 parallel groups. LA (lidocaine + epinephrine) with IV diazepam & methohexital—on occasion nitrous oxide was also used. Self-assessed at home at 0, 0.5 h then hourly for 6 h (diaries).	PI (4-pt scale) (PR (5-pt scale) Global Rating (5-pt scale) Time to remed.	Placebo n = 44 Paracetamol (650 mg) n = 37	Paracetamol was the only active drug not to be significantly superior to placebo for any measure.	t >1 h before remed, data included & baseline or last score (most severe) used for all further timepoints.	226 analysed. Exclusions; 13 did not require med., 3 were lost to follow-up, 2 remed, with slight pain before the 2nd h obs., 2 remed before the 1st h obs,. 1 fell asleep for over 2 h.	All AE mild. No. patients with AE: Placebo 7/44 with 9 AE, Paracetamol 6/37 with 7 AE.	3
[Dionne *et al.* 1994]	Impacted 3rd molar n = 135 Age: 16+	RCT, DB, single oral dose, 5 parallel groups. GA & LA. 4 h washout prior to start. Self-assessed at clinic for at least the first 2 h then at home hourly for 6 h .	PI (4-pt scale) PR (5-pt scale) Global rating (5-pt scale) Time to remed	Placebo n = 25 Paracetamol (650 mg) n = 27	Paracetamol did not show a significant difference to placebo for any measure of analgesia.	t ≥ 2 h before remed, data included & baseline used for all further timepoints.	124 analysed. Exclusions: 4 previously enrolled in the study, 3 remed before t = 2 h, 2 were lost to follow-up, 1 was ineligible because of codeine sensitivity.	All AE mild. No. of patients with AE: Placebo 5/25 with 5 AE. Paracetamol 7/27 with 9AE.	3
[Dolci *et al.* 1994]	Removal of single impacted 3rd molar n = 336 Age: 18+	RCT, DB, single oral dose, 4 parallel groups. Multicentre (11). No info on anaes. 24 h washout prior to start. Evaluations made at 0, 0.5, 1, 1.5, 2 h in the clinic then at 3 & 4 h at home (diary).	PI (4-pt scale) PR (5-pt scale) Global rating (5-pt scale)	Placebo n = 76 Paracetamol (500 mg) n = 72	PID/PR: Paracetamol was significantly superior to Placebo P<0.01) at t = 30 min & (P<0.01) from t = 1 to t = 4 h. SPID/TOTPAR: Paracetamol was significantly superior from t = 1 to t = 4. Dichot. data avail. for global rating—see Table V p. 190.	Rescue analgesia was permitted after 90 min, no further eval. made post remed. No. remed at t >1.5 h: Placebo 46/76 Paracetamol 15/72.	298 analysed. Exclusions: 15 were lost to follow-up, 6 remed before 1.5 h 3 experienced an AE & did not complete the assessments & 14 did not experience > moderate baseline pain.	4 withdrew from the study due to AE: Paracetamol, 1 for nausea, & 1 for swelling Placebo, 1 for fever nausea, & diarrhoea. Total no. of patients with AE: Paracetamol 7/80 with 7 AE Placebo 8/82 with 12 AE.	4
[Fassolt & Stocker 1983]	Postoperative ('simple surgery'—15+ surgical techniques named) n = 146 Age: 18+	RCT, DB, single oral dose, 5 parallel groups. GA used. 4 h washout prior to start. Evaluations made at 0, 30 min then hourly for 6 h by the same trained observer in hospital.	PI (5-pt scale & VAS) PR (5-pt scale) Global rating (5-pt scale) Time to remed	Placebo n = 28 Paracetamol (650 mg) n = 29	All active drugs were significantly superior for all measures of efficacy (except Suprofen 200 which showed NSD in the global rating).	Remed allowed after 2 h (last score used for all further timepoints) No. of patients not remed 6 h: Placebo 9/28 Paracetamol 25/29.	No info given	No serious AE reported—no further details given.	2
[Forbes *et al.* 1982]	Impacted 3rd molar (1 or more) n = 177 Age: 15+	DB, single oral dose, 5 parallel groups. No info on anaes. Self-assessed at home at 0, 1 then hourly for 12 h.	PI (4-pt scale) PR (5-pt scale) 50% PR (y/n) Global rating (5-pt scale) Time to remed	Placebo n = 30 Paracetamol (600 mg) n = 34	At 4 h paracetamol was significantly superior to placebo for PR, Peak PR, & 50% PR (P<0.01).	If remed <2 h excluded. If >2 h <12 h PR = 0 & PI baseline or last. % patients remed >2 h but <12h. Placebo 93% Paracetamol 85%.	159 analysed. Exclusions: 4 lost to follow-up, 3 did not take med. 7 took remed <2 h with mild pain & 3 did not complete the forms properly.	None of the active treatments produced more AE than the placebo. None were serious.	3

Ref.	Condition & no. of patients	Design, study duration & follow-up	Outcome measures	Dose regimen	Analgesic outcome results	Remedication	Withdrawals & exclusions	Adverse effects	Quality score
[Forbes et al. 1983]	Postoperative (general, gynae, or othopaedic surgery) n = 132 Age: 18+	RCT, DB, single oral dose, 5 parallel groups. GA, given on request 1st day able to take oral analgesia. Self-assessed in hospital at 0, 0.5, 1, 1.5, 2 then hourly for 12 h . Single nurse observer present for 1st 6 h, 2nd 6 h monitored by ward staff.	PI (4-pt scale) PR (5-pt scale) Pain half gone? (y/n) Global rating (5-pt scale) Time to remed	Placebo n = 26 Paracetamol (600 mg) n = 26	For 6-h data Paracetamol was significantly superior for all measures & for 12-h data all except SPID	Patients were remed on demand if <2 h excluded. If remed <12 h PR = 0, PI = baseline or last score for remaining timepoints.	132 analysed. There were no exclusions	No serious AE reported. Most common were drowsiness, dizziness & dry mouth. No. of patients with AE: Placebo 4/26 with 5 AE. Paracetamol 11/26 with 11 AE.	5
[Forbes et al. 1984]	Postoperative (general, gynae, or othopaedic surgery) n = 132 Age: 18+	RCT, DB, single oral dose, 5 parallel groups. GA, trial drug given on request 1st day after surgery. Assessed in hospital by single nurse-observer at 0, 15 min, 30 min, then hourly for 6 h.	PI (4-pt scale) PR (5-pt scale) Pain half gone? (y/n) Acceptability (5-pt scale, each h) Time to remed	Placebo n = 33 Paracetamol (650 mg) n = 31	Paracetamol was significantly superior for all measures of efficacy from t = 1 h to t = 4. But only marginally sig. for peal PID & peak PR.	If remed <6 h PR = 0, PI = baseline or last for all remaining timepoints	129 analysed. Exclusions: 2 remed <2 h & 1 received an interfering med.	No serious AE recorded. Sedation accounted for 2/3 of the AEs. No. of patients with AE: Placebo 8/33 with 9 AE. Paracetamol 9/33 with 10 AE.	4
[Forbes et al. 1984]	Impacted 3rd molar (1 or more) n = 191 Age: 15+	RCT, DB, single oral dose, 4 parallel groups. GA/LA—unclear. Self-assess at home at 0, 1 then hourly for 6 h, returned 5 days later for review & debrief.	PI (4-pt scale) PR (5-pt scale) Pain half gone? (y/n) Global rating (5-pt scale) Time to remed	Placebo n = 36 Paracetamol (650 mg) n = 39	Paracetamol significantly superior for all measures of total & peak analgesia	Patients could remed after 2 h but were asked to complete the next evaluation before doing so (PI last or baseline score, PR = 0 for all further timepoints). % remed by h 6: Paracetamol 74% Placebo 97%.	148 analysed. Exclusions: 1 did not return results, 1 was lost to follow-up, 26 did not req. med, 8 did not follow the instructions & 7 remed <2 h.	NSD in AE between treatments, none were serious. Most freq was drowsiness. No. of patients with AE: Placebo 2/40 with 2 AE. Paracetamol 1/43 with 2 AE.	5
[Forbes et al. 1989]	Impacted 3rd molar (1 or more) n = 107 Age:15+	RCT, DB, single oral dose, 4 parallel groups at 2 centres. GA & LA—unclear. Patients self-assessed at home at 0, 1, 2 then hourly for 12 h or until remed (diary) returned 5 days later for review & debrief.	PI (4-pt scale) PR (5pt scale) Global rating (5pt scale) Time to Remed	Placebo n = 23 Paracetamol (600 mg) n = 22	For 12 hr: Paracetamol was not significantly superior for any measure. For 4 hr: Paracetamol was significantly superior for SPID, TOTPAR & h of 50% rel.	Patients could remed after 2 h but were asked to complete the next evaluation before doing so (PI last or baseline score, PR = 0 for all further timepoints). % remed by h 12; Paracetamol 95% Placebo 91%	88 analysed. Exclusions: 9 did not take the med., 2 remedicated before the 2 h point, 1 remedicated with slight pain, 4 did not complete their evaluation, 1 took only part of the med. & 2 remedicated despite of having some relief from the study med.	No serious AE reported. No. of patients with AE: Placebo 2/26 with 2 AE. Paracetamol 3/26 with 3 AE. NB includes AE reported post remed.	5
[Forbes et al. 1990]	Impacted 3rd molar (1 or more) n = 269 Age: 15+	RCT, DB, single then multiple oral dose, 6 parallel groups. GA/LA—unclear. Self-assess at home at 0, 1 then hourly for 6 h—returned 5 days later for review & debrief.	PI (4-pt scale) PR (5-pt scale) Pain half gone? (y/n) Global rating (5pt scale) Time to remed	Placebo n = 34 Paracetamol (600 mg) n = 36	All active medications were significantly superior for all measures of total & peak analgesia.	Remed allowed after 2 h but asked to complete the next eval (PI last or baseline score, PR = 0 used for all remaining timepoints). % remed by h 6; Placebo 33% Paracetamol 29%.	206 analysed. Exclusions; 3 lost to follow-up, 1 lost report card, 22 did not req med. 8 remed despite having relief from study med, 6 remed with only slight pain, 13 remed <2 h. 7 failed to follow instructions, 3 did not complete the forms.	No AE was serious. No. of patients reporting AE; Placebo 0/38 Paracetamol 5/41 with 5 AE.	5
[Honig & Murray 1984]	Postope (elective surgery —abdominal, orthopaedic, rectal, thoracic & vascular) n = 116 Age 19–87	RCT, single oral dose, 4 parallel groups. No info on anaes, 4 h washout prior to start. Interviewed in hospital by nurse observer at 1, 0.5, 1 h then hourly for 6 h.	PI (4-pt scale) PR (5-pt scale) 50% PR (y/n) Global rating (5pt scale)	Placebo n = 30 Paracetamol (600 mg) n = 28	TOTPAR & global rating; Paracetamol was significantly superior to Placebo (P <0.05).	If remed last score was used for all further timepoints. No. of patients who did not remed in 6 h; Placebo n = 14/30 Paracetamol n = 16/28	No details given.	None severe except 1 severe dry mouth. Reported in all groups & were primarily CNS & gastrointestinal effects.	3
[Jain et al. 1986]	Postope (general, gynae, or orthopaedic surgery) n = 128 Age: 18–70	RCT, DB, single oral dose, 4 parallel groups. GA, trial drug given within 72 h of surgery on request for analgesia. 4 h washout prior to start. Assessed in hospital by nurse-observer at 0, 15 min, 30 min then hourly for 6 h.	PI (4-pt scale) PR (5pt scale)	Placebo n = 32 Paracetamol (650 mg) n = 30	Paracetamol was only significantly superior for Maxrel (P <0.05)	Remed <2 h data excluded. If >2 h last measure used for all remaining timepoints. Total no. of remed; Placebo 11/32 Paracetamol 10/30 Nalbu 9/34 Combo 5/32	122 analysed. Exclusions: 2 had improperly blinded drugs, 2 remed <2 h & 2 received interfering med.	No serious AE reported. NSD in occurrence between groups. Total no. of patients with AE: Placebo 6/32 with 8 AE. Paracetamol 9/30 with 9 AE.	4

Ref.	Condition & no. of patients	Design, study duration & follow-up	Outcome measures	Dose regimen	Analgesic outcome results	Remedication	Withdrawals & exclusions	Adverse effects	Quality score
[Kiersch et al. 1994]	Impacted 3rd molar (3 or 4) n = 232 Age: 14+	RCT, DB, single oral dose, 3 parallel groups. LA, 48 h washout prior to start. Self-assessed in clinic for first 2 h then at home. Assessed at 0, 20 min, 30 min, 40 min, 1 h then hourly for 12 h.	PI (4-pt scale) PR (5-pt scale) Pain half gone? (y/n) Global rating (5-pt scale) Time to remed PI VAS (100 mm)	Placebo n = 30 Paracetamol (1000 mg) n = 30	Paracetamol was significantly superior to Placebo for most efficacy measures in the first 6 h.	'Patients were asked to allow 2 h.....before taking alternate med'. Time to remed (median); Placebo 2.0 h Paracetamol 3.1 h	226 analysed. Exclusions: 1 experienced nausea & vomiting so did not ingest the treatment, 2 did not require analgesia, 1 failed to follow the instructions & 2 vomited within 10 min of taking the trial drug.	None serious. No. of patients reporting AE; Placebo 13/45 with 18 AE. Paracetamol 31/92 with 35 AE.	4
[Laska et al. 1983] **Study 1**	Postpartum (post episiotomy & post-surgical inc uterine cramping) n = 480 Age: did not say	RCT, DB, single oral dose, 7 parallel groups. 4 h washout prior to start. Evaluated by same nurse observer in hospital at 0, 0.5, 1 h then hourly for 4 h.	PI (4-pt scale) PR (5-pt scale)— NB non-standard scale (% pain relief)	Placebo n = 40 Paracetamol (500 mg) n = 54 Paracetamol (1000 mg) n = 50 Paracetamol (1500 mg) n = 60	Paracetamol 500 mg was not significantly superior to placebo for any measure. The 1000 mg & 1500 mg doses were significantly superior to placebo for both SPID & TOTPAR (P<0.01) but only the 1500 mg dose was significantly superior to placebo for %SPID.	Remed after 1st h (PI = 0 & PR last score used for all further timepoints).	373 analysed. Exclusions: 26 for protocol violations, 12 had missing caffeine forms & 69 used caffeine during the study.	No. of patients with AE; Placebo 1/40 with 1 AE (vomited). Paracetamol (500 mg) No AE reported. Paracetamol 1000 mg 1/50 with 1 AE (vomited). Paracetamol (1500 mg) No AE reported.	4
[Laska et al. 1983] **Study 2**	Postpartum (post episiotomy & post-surgical inc uterine cramping) n = 577 Age: did not say	RCT, DB, single oral dose, 7 parallel groups. 4 h washout prior to start. Evaluated by same nurse observer in hospital at 0, 0.5, 1 h then hourly for 4 hr.	PI (4-pt scale) PR (5-pt scale)— NB non-standard scale (% pain relief)	Placebo n = 44 Paracetamol (500 mg) n = 68 Paracetamol (1000 mg) n = 68 Paracetamol (1500 mg) n = 66	None of the doses of paracetamol were significantly superior to placebo for any measure of analgesia.	Remed after 1st h (PI = 0 & PR last score used for all further timepoints).	434 analysed. Exclusions: 4 for protocol violations & 139 used caffeine during the study.	No AE were reported.	4
[Laska et al. 1983] **Study 3**	Postpartum (post-episiotomy & post-surgical) n = 552 Age: did not say	RCT, DB, single oral dose, 7 parallel groups. 4 h washout prior to start. Evaluated by same nurse observer in hospital at 0, 0.5, 1 h then hourly for 4 h.	PI (4-pt scale) PR (5-pt scale)— NB non-standard scale (% pain relief)	Placebo n = 57 Paracetamol (500 mg) n = 81 Paracetamol (1000 mg) n = 81 Paracetamol (1500 mg) n = 81	All doses of paracetamol were significantly superior to placebo for SPID, TOTPAR, % SPID & ONSET (P<0.05).	Remed after 1st h (PI = 0 & PR last score used for all further timepoints).	358 analysed. Exclusions: 14 for protocol violations.	No AE were reported.	4
[Lehnert et al. 1990]	3rd molar n = 150 Age: did not say	RCT, DB, single oral dose, 3 parallel groups. 4 h washout prior to start. Self assessed at 0, 0.5, 1h then hourly for 6 h.	PI (4-pt scale) PR (5-pt scale) Global rating (4-pt scale)	Placebo n = 40 Paracetamol (1000 mg) n = 49	Paracetamol was significantly superior to Placebo for all measures of efficacy.	If remed <6 h patient was considered a dropout; no data on how data was handled.	133 analysed. Exclusions; 11 did not take the med, 3 were lost to follow-up & 3 for various protocol violations.	No. of patients reporting AE; Placebo 4/40 with ? AE. Paracetamol 5/49 with ? AE.	5
[McQuay et al. 1988]	Postop (elective orthopaedic surgery) n = 158 Age: 18–70	RCT, DB, single oral dose, 5 parallel groups. GA, trial drug given 1/2 days after surgery. 3 h washout prior to start. Assessed in hospital by nurse-observer at 0, 0.5, 1 & 1.5 then hourly for 6 h.	PI (4-pt scale, VAS & 8 word verbal rating) PR (5-pt scale & VAS) Pain half gone? (y/n) Global rating (5-pt scale—both patient & observer) Time to remed Vital Signs	Placebo n = 30 Paracetamol (1000 mg) n = 30 (NB these are the numbers after exclusions)	Paracetamol was significantly superior to Placebo for all integrated measures of efficacy.	If remed after 1 h PI scored at baseline & PR = 0. For no. of pat. remed <6 h; all active treatments were ss (P<0.01) to placebo.	150 analysed. Exclusions: 2 were discharged before the end, 3 received drugs prohibited by protocol, 1 vomited intact med within 15 min & 2 patients pain assessments were not adequately completed.	None serious & NSD between groups No. of patients reporting AE: Placebo 6/30 with 8 AE. Paracetamol 6/30 with 10 AE.	4
[Mehlisch & Frakes, 1984]	Oral surgery (involving bone removal) n = 174 AGE: 16+	RCT, DB, single oral dose, 3 parallel groups. No info on anaes except no long acting IM or IV anaes used, 4 h washout period prior to start. Assessed in clinic nurse-observer at 30 min then hourly for 6 h.	PI (4-pt scale) PR (5-pt scale) Pain half gone? (y/n) Global rating (5-pt scale) Time to remed	Placebo n = 55 Paracetamol (1000 mg) n = 58	Paracetamol was significantly superior (P<0.05) to Placebo for all measures. Paracetamol was also ss to Aspirin for maxSPID (P<0.05), maxTOTPAR (P<0.03) & global (P<0.02)	Remed if req after 1 h—If remed patient considered treatment failure (no details on how data was handled) Full Dichot data on times of med Table IV. No. of patients not remed before t >6 h; Paracetamol 13/58 Placebo 3/55	162 analysed. Exclusions: 9 failed to comply with protocol & 3 were lost to follow-up.	NSD between No. of AE for paracetamol & placebo—no other details given.	4

Ref.	Condition & no. of patients	Design, study duration & follow-up	Outcome measures	Dose regimen	Analgesic outcome results	Remediation	Withdrawals & exclusions	Adverse effects	Quality score
[Mehlisch *et al.* 1990]	Oral surgery (various procedures) $n = 706$ Age 17–64	RCT, DB, single oral dose, 3 parallel groups. LA, 6 h washout prior to start. Self-assessed at 0, 0.5, 1 h then hourly for 6 h. Multi-centre (7 investigators)	PI (4-pt scale) PR (5-pt scale)	Placebo $n = 85$ Paracetamol (1000 mg) $n = 309$	Both active treatments were significantly superior to placebo.	If remedicated PI = baseline & PR = 0.	697 analysed. Exclusions: 4 lost to follow-up, 4 entered in trial twice & 1 failed to meet inclusion criteria.	No. of patients reporting AE; Placebo 12/85 with ? AE. Paracetamol 32/307 with ? AE.	4
[Mehlisch *et al.* 1995]	3rd molar (at least 1 embedded) $n = 706$ Age 15+	RCT, DB, single oral dose, 3 parallel groups. LA, 12 h washout prior to start. Self-assessed at 0, 15 min, 45 min, 1 h & 90 min then hourly for 6 h.	PI (4-pt scale) PR (5-pt scale) Global rating (5-pt scale)	Placebo $n = 40$ Paracetamol (1000 mg) $n = 101$	Paracetamol was significantly superior to Placebo for all measures of efficacy.	If remed before 1 h, data was excluded from the analysis. A value of 0 was assigned for PID & PR at all time-points after remed. Proportion of Patients remed: Placebo 88% Paracetamol 52%	399 analysed. Exclusions: 1 patient failed to complete the diary.	None serious. No. of patients reporting AE; Placebo 4/40 with ? AE. Paracetamol 17/101 with ? AE	3.
[Rubin & Winter, 1984]	Episiotomy (Post uncomplicated delivery) $n = 500$ Age 13–40	RCT, DB, single oral dose, 4 parallel groups, 6 h washout prior to start. Evaluated at 0, 0.5, 1 then hourly for 4 h by the same observer.	PI (4-pt scale)	Placebo $n = 125$ Paracetamol (1000 mg) $n = 125$	All 3 active groups produced significantly superior pain relief to placebo from t = 0.5 h to the end of the study.	If remed <2 h excluded. If remed >2 h PI last or baseline was allocated for remaining timepoints.	476 analysed. Exclusions: 5 withdrew without taking the med & 19 remedicated before 2 h.	None serious. No. of patients reporting AE; Placebo 6/109 with 6 AE Paracetamol 6/123 with 6 AE	4
[Schachtel *et al.* 1989]	Episiotomy uncomplicated delivery) $n = 115$ Age 16–37	RCT, DB, single oral dose, 3 parallel groups. 4 h washout prior to start. Assessed (where & by who not clear) at 0, 0.5, 1 then hrly for 4 h.	PI (4-pt scale) PR (5-pt scale) Global rating (5-pt scale)	Placebo $n = 38$ Paracetamol (1000 mg) $n = 37$	Paracetamol was significantly superior ($P < 0.05$) to placebo for TOTPAR, global & no. remed.	Remed after 1 h—if did considered treatment failures, last/baseline PI & PR = 0 scored for the remaining timepoints. Remed <6 h; Paracetamol 13/37 Placebo 22/38	111 analysed. Exclusions: 4 patients remed but did not record at what time.	No AE were reported. Placebo 0/37 Paracetamol 0/37.	4
[Seymour *et al.* 1996]	3rd molar extraction $n = 206$ Age: Adults	RCT, DB, single oral dose, 5 parallel groups. 12 h washout prior to start. Evaluated at 0, 0.25, 0.5, 0.75, 1, 1.5, 2 h then hrly for 6 h. Baseline pain >30 mm.	PI VAS ('no pain' to 'unbearable pain') Global rating (5 pt by patient)	Placebo $n = 41$ Paracetamol (500 mg) $n = 41$ Paracetamol (1000 mg) $n = 41$	All active treatments resulted in significantly less pain than placebo ($P < 0.01$)	If remed <1 h excluded. If >1 h last PI value was allocated for all remaining timepoints.	200 analysed. Exclusions: 6 for remed in the first h.	No patients reported any AEs.	4
[Sunshine *et al.* 1986]	Impacted 3rd molar $n = 182$ Age 16+	RCT, DB, single oral dose, 6 parallel groups. LA (lidocaine/epinephrine). 4 h washout prior to start. Evaluations at 0, 0.5, 1, 2 & 3 h in clinic by single observer. At 4, 5 & 6 h self-assessed. 1 week later met with observer & reviewed the forms.	PI (4-pt scale) PR (5-pt scale) Global rating (4-pt scale) Overall improvement (7pt scale) Time to remed	Placebo $n = 30$ Paracetamol (650 mg) $n = 30$	Paracetamol was significantly superior ($P < 0.05$) to Placebo for; PID 1–3 h, PR at 4 h, PR at 2 h & t to Peak effect (See Table II).	If <1 h excluded. If >1 h use last PI or baseline & PR = 0. Full dichot data in table III. No. of patients remed; Placebo 13/30 Paracetamol 14/30	182 analysed. No exclusions	No serious AE, NSD between groups. No. of patients reporting AE; Placebo 1/30. Paracetamol 1/30.	5
[Sunshine *et al.* 1989]	Episiotomy (multiparous inpatients) $n = 200$ Age: 18+	RCT, DB, single oral dose, 3 parallel groups. Only inc patients with severe pain. 4 h washout prior to start. Evaluations in hospital by nurse observer at 0, 0.5, 1 then hrly for 6 h (if asleep—woken). Interviewed in patients 1st language (Spanish).	PI (4-pt scale) PR (5-pt scale) Global rating (4-pt scale) Overall improvement (7-pt scale) Time to remed	Placebo $n = 50$ Paracetamol (650 mg) $n = 75$	Paracetamol was significantly superior ($P < 0.05$) to placebo for all measures of efficacy.	If remed <2 h excluded. If remed >2 h PI last or baseline & PR = 0 for remaining timepoints. No remeds <2 h. Remed >2 h: Placebo 8/50 Paracetamol 2/75.	200 analysed. No exclusions	Only 2 patients with AE neither were in the Paracetamol nor Placebo groups. AE were mild dizziness, sleepiness & sweating.	4
[Sunshine *et al.* 1993]	Postop (Caesarean Section) $n = 240$ Age: 18+	RCT, DB, single oral dose then multi-dose, 5 parallel groups. Only inc. patients with severe pain, 4 h washout prior to start. Eval carried out by same nurse observer at 0, 0.5, 1 then hourly for 8 h. Interviewed in patients 1st language (Spanish).	PI (4-pt scale) PR (5-pt scale) Global rating (5-pt scale) Time to meaningful relief	Placebo $n = 48$ Paracetamol (650 mg) $n = 48$	Paracetamol was not significantly superior ($P < 0.05$) to placebo for any measure.	If remed <1 h after 1st dose, dropped & replaced. If remed >1 h after 1st dose eligible for the repeat dose phase. No. of patients remed <8 h: Placebo 35/48 Paracetamol 42/48.	All 240 enrolled were analysed	No details for single dose phase.	4

Ref.	Condition & no. of patients	Design, study duration & follow-up	Outcome measures	Dose regimen	Analgesic outcome results	Remedication	Withdrawals & exclusions	Adverse effects	Quality score
[Winnem *et al.* 1981]	Post orthopaedic surgery *n* = 80 Age 17–9 = 63	RCT, DB, single oral dose, 4 parallel groups, 4 h washout period prior to start. Evaluated by nurse observer at 0, 0.5, 1 h then hourly for 6 h.	PI (4-pt scale) PI VAS ('no pain' to 'unbearable pain')	Placebo *n* = 20 Paracetamol (1000 mg) *n* = 20	Paracetamol was significantly superior to placebo for all measures of pain relief (*P* <0.05).	If remed after 2 h withdrawn & all subsequent scores were assumed to be baseline.	79 analysed: Exclusions: 1 for vomiting med	No AE were observed.	4
[Winter *et al.* 1983]	Oral Surgery (various procedures) *n* = 168 Age 16–75	RCT, DB, single oral dose, 4 parallel groups. 4 h washout period prior to start. GA & or LA. Self-assessed at 0, 0.5, 1, 2, 3 & 4 h.	PI (4-pt scale) PR (5-pt scale) 50% PR Global Rating (5-pt scale)	Placebo *n* = 41 Paracetamol (1000 mg) *n* = 41	Paracetamol was significantly superior to placebo for all measures of analgesic efficacy. Both produced sig analgesia as early as t = 0.5h.	Remed was allowed after 2 h or if pain returned to premed levels. 2 patients remed ≥ 2 h (1 placebo + 1 paracetamol).	164 analysed Exclusions: 3 Protocol violations & 1 did not received study drug	No serious AE were reported. No. Patients with AE; Placebo 1/41 (severe headache). Paracetamol 0/41.	4
[Young *et al.* 1979]	Postop (various elective procedures) *n* = 120 Age 12–83	RCT, DB, single oral dose, 4 parallel groups. GA—Halothane/Nit Ox/OX, 4 h washout prior to start. Evaluated in hospital by single observer at 0, 0.5, 1, 2, 3 & 4 h.	PI (4-pt scale) PR (5-pt scale) 2 Global Ratings (5-pt scale)—Both Pat & obs opinion	Study 1: Placebo *n* = 29 Paracetamol (650 mg) *n* = 30	Paracetamol was only significantly superior (*P* <0.05) to placebo at t = 2 h PR score.	'Any concomitant or additional med given was duly noted'. No details given on this data or how it was handled.	119 analysed. Exclusion: 1 patient had received analgesia within 2 h of the study.	No serious AE reported. No. of patients reporting AE; Placebo 1/30 (sedation). Paracetamol 3/30 (nausea).	4

AE, adverse effect; DB, double-blind; GA, general anaesthesia; LA, local anaesthesia; NSD, no significant difference; PI, pain intensity; PR, pain relief; SPID, summed pain intensity differences; TOTPAR, total pain relief; VAS, visual analogue scale. References to Tables and Figures are from the original reports.

Appendix 1 references

Beaver WT, McMillan D. Methodological considerations in the evaluation of analgesic combinations: acetami-5215 nophen (paracetamol) and hydrocodone in postpartum pain. *British Journal of Clinical Pharmacology* 1980; **10 10**: (Suppl.) S215–23.

Bentley KC, Head TW. The additive analgesic efficacy of acetaminophen, 1000 mg, and codeine, 60 mg, in dental pain. *Clinical Pharmacology and Therapeutics* 1987; **42**:634–40.

Berry FN, Miller JM, Levin HM, Bare WW, Hopkinson JH3, Feldman AJ. Relief of severe pain with acetaminophen in a new dose formulation versus propoxyphene hydrochloride 65 mg. and placebo: a comparative double blind study. *Current Therapeutic Research* 1975; **17**:361–8.

Bjune K, Stubhaug A, Dodgson MS, Breivik H. Additive analgesic effect of codeine and paracetamol can be detected in strong, but not moderate, pain after Caesarean section. Baseline pain-intensity is a determinant of assay-sensitivity in a postoperative analgesic trial. *Acta Anaesthesiologica Scandinavica* 1996; **40**:399–07.

Cooper SA, Breen JF, Giuliani RL. The relative efficacy of indoprofen compared with opioid analgesic combinations. *Journal of Oral Surgery* 1981; **39**:21–5.

Cooper SA, Erlichman MC, Mardirossian G. Double blind comparison of an acetaminophen codeine caffeine combination in oral surgery pain. *Anesthesia Progress* 1986; **33**:139–42.

Cooper SA, Firestein A, Cohn P. Double blind comparison of meclofenamate sodium with acetaminophen, acetaminophen with codeine and placebo for relief of postsurgical dental pain. *Journal of Clinical Dentistry* 1988; **1**:31–4.

Cooper SA, Kupperman A. The analgesic efficacy of flurbiprofen compared to acetaminophen with codeine. *Journal of Clinical Dentistry* 1991; **2**:70–4.

Cooper SA, Precheur H, Rauch D, Rosenheck A, Ladov M, Engel J. Evaluation of oxycodone and acetaminophen in treatment of postoperative dental pain. *Oral Surgery, Oral Medicine, Oral Pathology* 1980; **50**:496–501.

Cooper SA, Schachtel BP, Goldman E, Gelb S, Cohn P. Ibuprofen and acetaminophen in the relief of acute pain: a randomized, double blind, placebo controlled study. *Journal of Clinical Pharmacology* 1989; **29**:1026–30.

Dionne RA, Snyder J, Hargreaves KM. Analgesic efficacy of flurbiprofen in comparison with acetaminophen, acetaminophen plus codeine, and placebo after impacted third molar removal. *Journal of Oral and Maxillofacial Surgery* 1994; **52**:919–24; discussion 25–6.

Dolci G, Ripari M, Pacifici L, Umile A. Evaluation of piroxicam-beta-cyclodextrin, piroxicam, paracetamol and placebo in postoperative oral surgery pain. *International Journal of Clinical and Pharmacology Research* 1994; **14**:185–91.

Fassolt A, Stocker H. [Treatment of postoperative wound pain with suprofen] Behandlung des postoperative Wundschmerzes mit Suprofen. *Arzneimittelforschung* 1983; **33**:1327–30.

Forbes JA, Barkaszi BA, Ragland RN, Hankle JJ. Analgesic effect of acetaminophen, phenyltoloxamine and their combination in postoperative oral surgery pain. *Pharmacotherapy* 1984; **4**:221–6.

Forbes JA, Beaver WT, White EH, White RW, Neilson GB, Shackleford RW. Diflunisal. A new oral analgesic with an unusually long duration of action. *Journal of American Medical Association* 1982; **248**:2139–42.

Forbes JA, Butterworth GA, Burchfield WH, Yorio CC, Selinger LR, Rosenmertz SK *et al.* Evaluation of flurbiprofen, acetaminophen, an acetaminophen-codeine combination, and placebo in postoperative oral surgery pain. *Pharmacotherapy* 1989; **9**:322–30.

Forbes JA, Kehm CJ, Grodin CD, Beaver WT. Evaluation of ketorolac, ibuprofen, acetaminophen, and an acetaminophen codeine combination in postoperative oral surgery pain. *Pharmacotherapy* 1990; **10**:94S–105S.

Forbes JA, Kolodny AL, Beaver WT, Shackleford RW, Scarlett VR. A 12 hour evaluation of the analgesic efficacy of diflunisal, acetaminophen, and acetaminophen codeine combination, and placebo in postoperative pain. *Pharmacotherapy* 1983; **3**:47S–54.

Forbes JA, Kolodny AL, Chachich BM, Beaver WT. Nalbuphine, acetaminophen, and their combination in postoperative pain. *Clinical Pharmacology and Therapeutics* 1984; **35**:843–51.

Honig S, Murray KA. An appraisal of codeine as an analgesic: single dose analysis. *Journal of Clinical Pharmacology* 1984; **24**:96–102.

Jain AK, Ryan JR, McMahon FG, Smith G. Comparison of oral nalbuphine, acetaminophen, and their combination in postoperative pain. *Clinical Pharmacology and Therapeutics* 1986; **39**:295–9.

Kiersch TA, Halladay SC, Hormel PC. A single-dose, double-blind comparison of naproxen sodium, acetaminophen, and placebo in postoperative dental pain. *Clinical Therapeutics* 1994; **16**:394–404.

Laska EM, Sunshine A, Zighelboim I, Roure C, Marrero I, Wanderling J *et al*. Effect of Caffeine on Acetaminophen Analgesia. *Clinical Pharmacology and Therapeutics* 1983; **33**:498–509.

Lehnert S, Reuther J, Wahl G, Barthel K. [The efficacy of paracetamol (Tylenol) and acetyl salicylic acid (Aspirin) in treating postoperative pain] Wirksamkeit von Paracetamol (Tylenol) und Acetylsalizylsaure (Aspirin) bei postoperativen Schmerzen. *Deutsche Zahnarztl Zeitschrift* 1990; **45**:23–6.

McQuay HJ, Carroll D, Frankland T, Harvey M, Moore A. Bromfenac, acetaminophen, and placebo in orthopedic postoperative pain. *Clinical Pharmacology and Therapeutics* 1990; **47**:760–6.

Mehlisch DR, Frakes LA. A controlled comparative evaluation of acetaminophen and aspirin in the treatment of postoperative pain. *Clinical Therapeutics* 1984; **7**:89–97.

Mehlisch DR, Jasper RD, Brown P, Korn SH, McCarroll K, Murakami AA. Comparative study of ibuprofen lysine and acetaminophen in patients with postoperative dental pain. *Clinical Therapeutics* 1995; **17**:852–60.

Mehlisch DR, Sollecito WA, Helfrick JF, Leibold DG, Markowitz R, Schow CEJ *et al*. Multicenter clinical trial of ibuprofen and acetaminophen in the treatment of postoperative dental pain. *Journal of the American Dental Association* 1990; **121**:257–63.

Rubin A, Winter LJ. A double blind randomized study of an aspirin/caffeine combination versus acetaminophen/aspirin combination versus acetaminophen versus placebo in patients with moderate to severe post partum pain. *Journal of International Medical Research* 1984; **12**:338–45.

Schachtel B, Thoden W, Baybutt R. Ibuprofen and acetaminophen in the relief of postpartum episiotomy pain. *Journal of Clinical Pharmacology* 1989; **29**:550–3.

Seymour RA, Kelly PJ, Hawkesford JE. The efficacy of ketoprofen and paracetamol (acetaminophen) in postoperative pain after third molar surgery. *British Journal of Clinical Pharmacology* 1996; **41**:581–5.

Sunshine A, Marrero I, Olson N, McCormick N, Laska EM. Comparative study of flurbiprofen, zomepirac sodium, acetaminophen plus codeine, and acetaminophen for the relief of postsurgical dental pain. *American Journal of Medicine* 1986; **80**:50–4.

Sunshine A, Olson NZ, Zighelboim I, De Castro A. Ketoprofen, acetaminophen plus oxycodone, and acetaminophen in the relief of postoperative pain. *Clinical Pharmacology and Therapeutics* 1993; **54**:546–55.

Sunshine A, Zighelboim I, De Castro A, Sorrentino JV, Smith DS, Bartizek RD *et al*. Augmentation of acetaminophen analgesia by the antihistamine phenyltoloxamine. *Journal of Clinical Pharmacology* 1989; **29**:660–4.

Winnem B, Samstad B, Breivik H. Paracetamol, tiaramide and placebo for pain relief after orthopedic surgery. *Acta Anaesthesiologica Scandinavica* 1981; **25**:209–14.

Winter LJ, Appleby F, Ciccone PE, Pigeon JG. A comparative study of an acetaminophen analgesic combination and aspirin in the treatment of post-operative oral surgery pain. *Current Therapeutic Research* 1983; **33**:115–22.

Young RE, Quigley JJ, Archambault WAJ, Gordon LL. Butorphanol/acetaminophen double blind study in postoperative pain. *Journal of Medicine* 1979; **10**:239–56.

Appendix 2
Paracetamol plus codeine vs. placebo: trial details

Ref.	Condition & no. of patients	Design, study duration & follow-up	Outcome measures	Dose regimen	Analgesic outcome results	Remediation	Withdrawals & exclusions	Adverse effects	Quality score
[Bentley & Head 1987]	3rd molar bony impacted n = 128 Age: mean mid 20s	RCT, DB, single oral dose, 4 parallel groups. No info on anaes except 'no sedative or narcotic agents were used before, during or after surgery'. Self-assessed at home at 0, 1, 2, 3, 4, 5 h then posted reports to investigator.	PI (10-pt scale) PR (5-pt scale)	Placebo n = 17 Paracetamol (1000 mg) + codeine (60 mg) n = 41	The combination was significantly superior to placebo for all measures of efficacy, but was not significantly different to paracetamol for any measure.	Rescue analgesic: Tylenol No. 3. Patients who remed <5 h, last PI & PR scores carried on for all further timepoints.	120 analysed. Exclusions: 3 did not take the med, 1 took only a portion, 1 took no med until the day after surgery, 1 remed after 30 min, 1 vomited within 30 min of taking the med & 1 patient did not return the forms.	53 had 1 or more AE, 86 were reported in total, majority were dizziness, drowsiness, nausea & vomiting. There was NSD between treatment groups. No. of patients with AE; Placebo 9/19 with 16 AE Paracetamol + codeine 15/42 with 24 AE	3
[Bjune et al. 1996]	Caesarean section n = 125 Age: 27–37	RCT, DB, single oral dose, 3 parallel groups, 4 h washout prior to start. Baseline pain >40 mm = moderate, >60 mm = severe. Evaluated in hospital at 0, 0.5, 1 h then hourly for 6 h.	PI/VAS ('no pain' to 'unbearable pain') PR (5-pt scale)	Placebo n = 21 (9 moderate, 12 severe baseline pain) Paracetamol (800 mg) + codeine (60 mg) n = 44 (23 moderate, 21 severe baseline pain)	For the patients with moderate pain there were no diff between the groups for any measures of efficacy. For patients with severe pain the active groups were significantly superior to placebo for most measures of efficacy (P < 0.005)	Remed after 1st h (PI = 0 & PR last score used for all further timepoints).	108 analysed. Exclusions: 6 patients did not adhere to 4 h washout, 5 had PI <40 mm & 5 were excluded for other minor protocol violations.	No. of patients with AE; Placebo 1/25 with 1 AE Paracetamol + codeine 10/50 with 11 AE	3
[Cooper et al 1981]	Impacted 3rd molar n = 248 Age: mean early 20s	RCT, DB, single oral dose, 5 parallel groups. Either GA or LA. Self assessed at home at 0, 1, 2, 3, 4 h (questionnaire).	PI (4-pt scale) PR (5-pt scale) Global rating (5-pt scale) 50% relief of baseline pain (y/n) Time to remed	Placebo n = 37 Paracetamol (650 mg) + codeine (60 mg) n = 42	All active treatments were significantly superior to Placebo for all measures. The combination was slightly more effective than the Paracetamol alone but the diff was not significant.	Remed after 1st h if needed (last score used for all further timepoints). Remed <4 h; Placebo 20/37 Paracetamol 2/37	200 analysed. Exclusions: 17 did not ingest med, 31 ingested med but violated protocol (remed before 1st h obs, constant deviation of more than 15 min from evaluation times, not returning questionnaire & lost to follow-up)	No serious AE was reported. No. of patients with AE; Placebo 4/37 with 5 AE Paracetamol + codeine 10/42 with 10 AE	4
[Cooper et al. 1988]	Impacted 3rd molar n = 165 Age: 18–57	RCT, DB, single oral dose, 3 parallel groups, single centre & 1 surgeon. LA with sed &/or Nitrous oxide. 4 h washout prior to start. Self assessed at home at 0, 0.5, 1, 2, 3, 4, 5, 6 h (diary)	PI (4-pt scale) PR (5-pt scale) Pain half gone? (y/n) Global rating (5-pt) Time to remed	Placebo n = 40 Paracetamol (600 mg) + codeine (60 mg) n = 31	The combination was significantly superior to Placebo for every measure & to Paracetamol for TOTPAR. (P < 0.05)	Remed after 1st h (last or baseline score used for all further timepoints).	143 analysed. Exclusions: 11 were lost to follow-up, 8 did not require med. & 3 for 'various protocol violations'.	No serious AE were reported. No. of AE reported; Placebo 3 Paracetamol + codeine 4	4
[Cooper & Kupperman 1991]	Removal of 1 or more impacted teeth n = 247 Age: 'young adults'	RCT, DB, single oral dose, 6 parallel Groups. LA (lidocaine + epinephrine) with IV diazepam & methohexital—on occasion nitrous oxide was also used. Self-assessed at home at 0, 0.5 h then hourly till 6 h (diaries).	PI (4-pt scale) PR (5-pt scale) Global rating (5-pt scale) Time to remed	Placebo n = 44 Paracetamol (650 mg) + codeine (60 mg) n = 39	The combination was significantly superior to placebo for most measures & to Paracetamol or TOTPAR & the global rating.	t >1 h before remed, data included & baseline or last score (most severe) used for all further timepoints.	226 analysed. Exclusions; 13 did not require med. 3 were lost to follow-up, 2 remed with slight pain before the 2nd h obs., 2 remed before the 1st h obs. 1 fell asleep for over 2 h	All AE mild. No. of patients with AE; Placebo 7/44 with 9 AE Paracetamol + codeine 8/39 with 11 AE	3
[Dionne et al. 1994]	Impacted 3rd molar n = 135 Age 16+	RCT, DB, single oral dose, 5 parallel groups. GA & LA. 4 h washout prior to start. Self-assessed at clinic for at least the first 2 h then at home hourly till 6 h.	PI (4-pt scale) PR (5-pt scale) Global rating (5-pt scale) Time to remed	Placebo n = 25 Paracetamol (650 mg) + codeine (60 mg) n = 24	Neither Paracetamol nor the combination showed a significant diff to placebo for any measure of analgesia.	t ≥ 2 h before remed, data included & baseline used for all further timepoints.	124 analysed. Exclusions: 4 previously enrolled in the study, 3 remed before t = 2 h, 2 were lost to follow-up, 1 with ineligible because of codeine sensitivity	All AE mild. No. of patients with AE; Placebo 5/25 with 5 AE Paracetamol + codeine 9/24 with 10 AE	3
[Forbes et al. 1982]	Impacted 3rd molar (1 or more) n = 177 Age: 15+	DB, single oral dose, 5 parallel groups. No info on anaes. Self-assessed at home at 0, 1 then hourly till 12 h.	PI (4-pt scale) PR (5-pt scale) 50% PR (y/n) Global rating (5-pt scale) Time to remed	Placebo n = 30 Paracetamol (600 mg) + codeine (60 mg) n = 31	The combination was significantly superior to Placebo for all measures.	If remed <2 h excluded. If >2 h <12 h PR = 0 & PI baseline or last. % patients remed >2 h but <12 h. Placebo 93% Paracetamol 85%	159 analysed. Exclusions: 4 lost to follow-up, 3 did not take med, 7 took remed <2 h, 1 med with mild pain & 3 did not complete the forms properly.	None of the active treatments produced more AE than the Placebo. None were serious.	3

Ref.	Condition & no. of patients	Design, study duration & follow-up	Outcome measures	Dose regimen	Analgesic outcome results	Remediation	Withdrawals & exclusions	Adverse effects	Quality score
[Forbes et al. 1983]	Postop (general, gynae, or orthopaedic surgery) $n = 132$ Age: 18+	RCT, DB, single oral dose, 5 parallel groups. GA, given on request 1st day able to take oral analgesia. Self-assessed in hospital at 0, 0.5, 1, 1.5, 2 then hourly till 12 h Single nurse observer present for 1st 6 h, 2nd 6 h monitored by ward staff.	PI (4-pt scale) PR (5-pt scale) Pain half gone? (y/n) Global rating (5-pt scale) Time to remed	Placebo $n = 26$ Paracetamol (600 mg) + codeine (60 mg) $n = 26$	Until 6 h data the combination was significantly superior to placebo & until 12 h data, all except SPID.	Patients with remed on demand if <2 h excluded. If remed <12 h PR = 0, PI = baseline or last score for remaining timepoints.	132 analysed. There were no exclusions.	No serious AE reported. Most common were drowsiness, dizziness & dry mouth. No. of patients with AE; Placebo 4/26 with 5 AE Paracetamol + codeine 11/26 with AE	5
[Forbes et al. 1989]	Impacted 3rd molar (1 or more) $n = 107$ Age 15+	RCT, DB, single oral dose, 4 parallel groups at 2 centres. GA & LA—unclear. Patients self-assessed at home at 0, 1, 2 then hourly till 12 h or until remed (diary)—returned 5 days later for review & debrief.	PI (4-pt scale) PR (5-pt scale) Global rating (5-pt scale) Time to remed	Placebo $n = 23$ Paracetamol (600 mg) + codeine (60 mg) $n = 17$	At 4 h: The combination was significantly superior to Placebo & to Paracetamol for TOTPAR. ($P <0.05$)	Patients could remed after 2 h but were asked to completed the next evaluation before doing so (PI last or baseline score, PR = 0 for all further timepoints). % remed by hr 12; Paracetamol 95% Placebo 91%	88 analysed Exclusions: 9 did not take the med, 2 remed before the 2 h point, 1 remed with slight pain, 4 did not complete their evaluation, 1 took only part of the med & 2 remed despite of having some relief from the study med.	No serious AE reported No. of patients with AE; Placebo 2/26 with 2 AE Paracetamol + codeine 1/17 with 1 AE (NB includes AE reported postremed)	5
[Forbes et al. 1990] b	Impacted 3rd molar (1 or more) $n = 269$ Age: 15+	RCT, DB, single then multiple oral dose, 6 parallel groups. GA/LA—unclear. Self-assess at home at 0, 1 then hourly till 6 h—returned 5 days later for review & debrief.	PI (4-pt scale) PR (5-pt scale) Pain half gone? (y/n) Global rating (5-pt scale) Time to remed	Placebo $n = 34$ Paracetamol (600 mg) + codeine (60 mg) $n = 38$	All active medications were significantly superior for all measures of total & peak analgesia.	Remed allowed after 2 h but asked to complete the next eval (PI last or baseline score, PR = 0 used for all remaining timepoints). % remed by hour 6; Placebo 33% Paracetamol 29%	206 analysed. Exclusions; 3 lost to follow-up, 1 lost report card, 22 did not req med, 8 remed despite having relief from study med, 6 remed with only slight pain, 13 remed < 2 h, 7 failed to follow instructions, 3 did not complete the forms.	No AE was serious No. of patients reporting AE; Placebo 0/38 Paracetamol + codeine 8/40 with 9 AE	5
[Honig & Murray 1984]	Postop (elective surgery— abdominal, orthopaedic, rectal, thoracic & vascular) $n = 116$ Age: 19–87	RCT, DB, single oral dose, 4 parallel groups. No info on anaes, 4 h washout prior to start. Interviewed in hospital by nurse observer at 0, 0.5, 1 h then hourly till 6 h.	PI (4-pt scale) PR (5-pt scale) 50% PR (y/n) Global rating (5-pt scale)	Placebo $n = 30$ Paracetamol (600 mg) + codeine (60 mg) $n = 30$	The combination was significantly superior to placebo for all measures of efficacy	If remed last score was used for all further timepoints. No. of patients who did not remed in 6 h; Placebo $n = 14/30$ Paracetamol $n = 16/28$	No details given	None severe except 1 severe dry mouth. Reported in all groups & were primarily CNS & gastrointestinal effects.	3
[Pande et al. 1996]	3rd molar extraction $n = 100$ Age—did not say	RCT, DB, single oral dose, 4 Parallel groups. Self-assessed at home at 0, 0.5, 1 h then hourly till 6 h .	PI (4-pt scale) PR (5-pt scale) Global rating by patient	Placebo $n = 26$ Paracetamol (600m g) + codeine (60 mg) $n = 23$	The combination was significantly superior to placebo ($P < 0.001$).	If t ≥1 h before remed, data included but no information on how it was handled.	100 analysed, no exclusions.	No serious AE was reported. No. of patients with AE; Placebo ?/26 with 3 AE Paracetamol + codeine ?/23 with AE	4
[Stubhaug et al. 1995]	Post-orthopaedic surgery $n = 144$ Age: Adults	RCT, DB, single oral dose, 4 parallel groups, 4 h washout prior to start. Evaluated at 0, 0.5, 1 h then hourly till 6 h by observer. Baseline pain was >60 mm on VAS scale.	PI VAS ('no pain') to 'unbearable pain') Global rating by patient & observer	Placebo $n = 33$ Paracetamol (1000 mg) + codeine (60 mg) $n = 36$	The combination was significantly superior to placebo for all measures of efficacy.	If the patient remed the PI score was assumed to be the last for all further timepoints.	137 analysed. Exclusions: 3 vomited med, 3 received other analgesics & 1 experienced complications during the study.	No serious AE was reported. No. of patients with AE; Placebo 15/36 with 16 AE Paracetamol + codeine 10/37 with 17 AE	4
[Sunshine et al. 1986]	Impacted 3rd molar $n = 182$ Age: 16+	RCT, DB, single oral dose, 6 parallel groups. LA (lidocaine/epineph-rine). 4 h washout prior to start. Evaluations at 0, 0.5, 1, 2 & 3 h in clinic by single observer. at 4, 5 & 6 h self-assessed. 1 wk later met with observer & reviewed the forms.	PI (4-pt scale) PR (5-pt scale) Global rating (4-pt scale) Overall improvement (7-pt scale) Time to remed	Placebo $n = 30$ Paracetamol (650 mg) + codeine (60 mg) $n = 31$	The combination was significantly superior to placebo for most measures of efficacy. ($P < 0.05$)	If <1 h excluded. If >1 h use last PI or baseline & PR = 0. Full dichot data in table III. No. of patients remed; Placebo 13/30 Paracetamol 14/30	182 analysed. No exclusions.	No serious AE, NSD between groups. No. of patients reporting AE; Placebo 1/30 Paracetamol + codeine 3/31	5
[Desjardins et al. 1986]	Oral surgery $n = 137$ Age 18+	RCT, DB, single oral dose, 3 parallel groups, LA. 4 h washout prior to start. Self-assessed at home at 0, 0.5 then hourly till 6 h.	PI (4-pt scale) PR (5-pt scale) 50% PR (y/n) Global rating (5-pt scale) Anxiety (4-pt scale) Relaxation (4-pt scale)	Placebo $n = 41$ Paracetamol (300 mg) + codeine (30 mg) $n = 39$	The combination was only significantly superior to Placebo for global rating & total anxiety. ($P < 0.05$)	If t ≥1 h before remed, data included & last score for PI & PR used for all further timepoints.	123 analysed. Exclusions: 14 did not med or were lost to follow-up or provided uninterpretable results	No serious AE reported. No. of patients with AE; Placebo 4/41 with 4 AE Paracetamol + codeine 2/39 with 3 AE	4

Ref.	Condition & no. of patients	Design, study duration & follow-up	Outcome measures	Dose regimen	Analgesic outcome results	Remediation	Withdrawals & exclusions	Adverse effects	Quality score
[Forbes et al. 1986]	Impacted 3rd molar (1 or more) n = 146 Age: 15+	RCT, DB, single oral dose, 3 parallel groups, LA. Patients self-assessed at home at 0, 1 then hourly till 6h (diary)—returned 5 days later for review & debrief.	PI (4-pt scale) PR (5-pt scale) 50% PR (y/n) Global rating (5-pt scale) Anxiety (4-pt scale) Relaxation (4-pt scale)	Placebo n = 38 Paracetamol (300 mg) + codeine (30 mg) n = 43	The combination was significantly superior to the placebo for all measures of efficacy.	If remed <2 h excluded. If >2 h <6 h PR = 0 & PI baseline or last which ever was greater.	122 analysed. Exclusions: 1 did not return the form, 6 did not need analgesia & 17 had invalid data.	No serious AE reported. No. of patients with AE; Placebo 9/46 with 11 AE. Paracetamol + codeine 6/46 with 8 AE.	5
[Forbes et al. 1990] a	Impacted 3rd molar (1 or more) n = 162 Age: 15+	RCT, DB, single oral dose, 4 parallel groups. LA. Patients self-assessed at home at 0, 1 then hourly till 6 h (diary)—returned 5 days later for review & debrief.	PI (4-pt scale) PR (5-pt scale) Pain half gone? (y/n) Global rating (5-pt scale) Time to remed	Placebo n = 32 Paracetamol (600 mg) + codeine (60 mg) n = 27	The combination was significantly superior to the placebo for all measures of efficacy.	If remed <2 h excluded. If >2 h <6 h PR = 0 & PI baseline or last which ever was greater. No. of remed before t = 6 h; Placebo 27 Combination 23	128 analysed. Exclusions: 1 failed to return the form, 19 did not require analgesia & 14 had invalid data	No serious AE reported. No. of patients with AE; Placebo 5/34 with 6 AE. Paracetamol + codeine 9/31 with 12 AE.	5
[Forbes et al. 1994]	Impacted 3rd molar (1 or more) n = 324 Age: 15+	RCT, DB, single oral dose, 3 parallel groups. LA. Patients self-assessed at home at 0, 0.5, 1 then hourly till 6 h (diary)—returned 5 days later for review & debrief.	PI (4-pt scale) PR (5-pt scale) Pain half gone? (y/n) Global rating (5-pt scale) Time to remed	Placebo n = 45 Paracetamol (300 mg) + codeine (30 mg) n = 93	The combination was significantly superior to the placebo for all measures of mean & peak analgesia.	If remed <2 h excluded. If >2 h <6 h PR = 0 & PI baseline or last which ever was greater.	232 analysed. Exclusions: 1 lost to follow-up, 32 did not require analgesia & 51 had invalid data	No serious AE reported. No. of patients with AE; Placebo 10/65 with 12 AE. Paracetamol + codeine 18/107 with 21 AE.	5
[Heidrich et al. 1985]	Orthopaedic surgery n = 120 Age: 18–65	RCT, DB, single oral dose, 3 parallel groups. No info on anaes, 3 h washout prior to start. Interviewed in hospital by nurse observer at 0, 0.5, 1 h then hourly till 6 h	PI (4-pt scale) PR (5-pt scale) Global rating (5-pt scale) PI & PR VAS McGill Questionnaire Mood Questionnaire & VAS	Placebo n = 40 Paracetamol (300 mg) + codeine (30 mg) n = 40	Orthogonal analyses of variance showed the Combination gave greater relief from pain than Placebo	No info on remed	No info on withdrawals or exclusions	There were no diff among ant of the treatments in terms of side effects. No patient withdrew because of AE.	2
[Petti 1985]	Orthopaedic or general surgery n = 141 Age: 18–80	RCT, SB, single oral dose, 4 parallel groups. No info on anaes, 4 h washout prior to start. Interviewed in hospital by observer at 0, 0.5 1 h then hourly till 6 h. NB all patients had a baseline PI of 2 (moderate).	PI (4-pt scale) PR (5-pt scale) Global rating (5-pt scale) Severity of AE (5-pt scale)	Placebo n = 32 Paracetamol (300 mg) + codeine (30 mg) n = 31	Does not say anything directly about the Combination	Remed allowed after 2 h. If remed scores of PR = 0 & PI = 2 were allocated & the patient was excluded from further evaluations	129 analysed. Exclusions: 12 were excluded for protocol violations	No serious AE reported. Only 1 AE was reported which was dry mouth in the Paracetamol + codeine group.	2
[Turek & Baird 1988]	Elective surgery n = 161 Age: 18+	RCT, DB, single oral dose, 4 parallel groups. No info on anaes, 3 h washout prior to start. Interviewed in hospital by nurse observer at 0, 0.5, 1 h then hourly till 6 h.	PI (4-pt scale) PR (5-pt scale) Global rating (5-pt scale) Subjective Assessment of improvement (7-pt scale)	Placebo n = 41 Paracetamol (650 mg) + codeine (60 mg) n = 39	The combination was significantly superior to placebo for most measures of efficacy.	If remed <1 h excluded. If >1 h <6 h PR = 0 & PI = baseline was allocated for all further timepoints.	160 analysed. Exclusions: 1 from placebo for taking concomitant med	No serious AE reported. No. of patients with AE; Placebo 4/41 with 6 AE. Paracetamol + codeine 11/39 with 20 AE.	3

See Appendix 1 for key to abbreviations.

Appendix 2 references

Bentley KC, Head TW. The additive analgesic efficacy of aceta-minophen, 1000 mg, and codeine, 60 mg, in dental pain. *Clinical Pharmacology and Therapeutics* 1987; **42**:634–40.

Bjune K, Stubhaug A, Dodgson MS, Breivik H. Additive analgesic effect of codeine and paracetamol can be detected in strong, but not moderate, pain after Caesarean section. Baseline pain-intensity is a determinant of assay-sensitivity in a postoperative analgesic trial. *Acta Anesthesiologica Scandinavica* 1996; **40**:399–407.

Cooper SA, Breen JF, Giuliani RL. The relative efficacy of indopro-fen compared with opioid analgesic combinations. *Journal of Oral Surgery* 1981; **39**:21–5.

Cooper SA, Firestein A, Cohn P. Double blind comparison of meclofenamate sodium with acetaminophen, aceta-minophen with codeine and placebo for relief of postsurgical dental pain. *Journal of Clinical Dentistry* 1988; **1**:31–4.

Cooper SA, Kupperman A. The analgesic efficacy of flurbiprofen compared to acetaminophen with codeine. *Journal of Clinical Dentistry* 1991; **2**:70–4.

Desjardins PJ, Cooper SA, Finizio T. Efficacy of low dose combination analgesics: acetaminophen/codeine, aspirin/butalbital/caffeine/codeine, and placebo in oral surgery pain. *Anesthesia Progress* 1986; **33**:143–6.

Dionne RA, Snyder J, Hargreaves KM. Analgesic efficacy of flurbiprofen in comparison with acetaminophen, acetaminophen plus codeine, and placebo after impacted third molar removal. *Journal of Oral and Maxillofacial Surgery* 1994; **52**:919–24; discussion 25–6.

Forbes JA, Bates JA, Edquist IA, Burchfield WH, Smith FG, Schwartz MK *et al.* Evaluation of two opioid-acetaminophen combinations and placebo in postoperative oral surgery pain. *Pharmacotherapy* 1994; **14**:139–46.

Forbes JA, Beaver WT, White EH, White RW, Neilson GB, Shackleford RW. Diflunisal. A new oral analgesic with an unusually long duration of action. *Journal of American Medical Association* 1982; **248**:2139–42.

Forbes JA, Butterworth GA, Burchfield WH, Yorio CC, Selinger LR, Rosenmertz SK *et al.* Evaluation of flurbiprofen, acetaminophen, an acetaminophen-codeine combination, and placebo in postoperative oral surgery pain. *Pharmacotherapy* 1989; **9**:322–30.

Forbes JA, Butterworth GA, Burchfield WH, Beaver WT. Evaluation of ketorolac, aspirin, and an acetaminophen-codeine combination in postoperative oral surgery pain. *Pharmacotherapy* 1990a; **10**:S77–93.

Forbes JA, Jones KF, Smith WK, Gongloff CM. Analgesic effect of an aspirin codeine butalbital caffeine combination and an acetaminophen codeine combination in postoperative oral surgery pain. *Pharmacotherapy* 1986; **6**:240–7.

Forbes JA, Kehm CJ, Grodin CD, Beaver WT. Evaluation of ketorolac, ibuprofen, acetaminophen, and an acetaminophen codeine combination in postoperative oral surgery pain. *Pharmacotherapy* 1990b; **10**:S94–105.

Forbes JA, Kolodny AL, Beaver WT, Shackleford RW, Scarlett VR. A 12 hour evaluation of the analgesic efficacy of diflunisal, acetaminophen, and acetaminophen codeine combination, and placebo in postoperative pain. *Pharmacotherapy* 1983; **3**:47S–54S.

Heidrich G, Slavic Svircev V, Kaiko RF. Efficacy and quality of ibuprofen and acetaminophen plus codeine analgesia. *Pain* 1985; **22**:385–97.

Honig S, Murray KA. An appraisal of codeine as an analgesic: single dose analysis. *Journal of Clinical Pharmacology* 1984; **24**:96–102.

Pande AC, Pyke RE, Greiner M, Cooper SA, Benjamin R, Pierce MW. Analgesic efficacy of the kappa-receptor agonist, enadoline, in dental surgery pain. *Clinical Neuropharmacology* 1996; **19**:92–7.

Petti A. Postoperative pain relief with pentazocine and acetaminophen: comparison with other analgesic combinations and placebo. *Clinical Therapeutics* 1985; **8**:126–33.

Stubhaug A, Grimstad J, Breivik H. Lack of analgesic effect of 50 and 100 mg oral tramadol after orthopaedic surgery: a randomized, double-blind, placebo and standard active drug comparison. *Pain* 1995; **62**:111–18.

Sunshine A, Marrero I, Olson N, McCormick N, Laska EM. Comparative study of flurbiprofen, zomepirac sodium, acetaminophen plus codeine, and acetaminophen for the relief of postsurgical dental pain. *American Journal of Medicine* 1986; **80**:50–4.

Turek M, Baird W. Double blind parallel comparison of ketoprofen (Orudis), acetaminophen plus codeine, and placebo in postoperative pain. *Journal of Clinical Pharmacology* 1988; **28**:S23–8.

Appendix 3
Paracetamol plus codeine vs. paracetamol: trial details

Ref.	Condition & no. of patients	Design, study duration & follow-up	Outcome measures	Dose regimen	Analgesic outcome results	Remedication	Withdrawals & exclusions	Adverse effects	Quality score
[Bentley & Head 1987]	3rd molar bony impacted n = 128 Age: mean mid 20s	RCT, DB, single oral dose, 4 parallel groups. No info on anaes except 'no sedative or narcotic agents were used before, during or after surgery'. Self-assessed at home at 0, 1, 2, 3, 4, 5 h then posted reports to investigator.	PI (10-pt scale) PR (5-pt scale)	Paracetamol (1000 mg) + codeine (60 mg) n = 41 Paracetamol (1000 mg) n = 41	Both paracetamol & the combination were significantly superior to placebo for all measures of efficacy, but the combination was not significantly different to paracetamol for any measure.	Rescue analgesic—Tylenol No. 3. Patients who remed <5 h, last PI & PR scores carried on for all further timepoints.	120 analysed. Exclusions: 3 did not take the med, 1 took only a portion, 1 took no med until the day after surgery, 1 remed after 30 min, 1 vomitted within 30 min of taking the med & 1 patient did not return the forms.	53 had 1 or more AE, 86 were reported in total, majority were dizziness, drowsiness, nausea & vomiting. There was NSD between treatment groups. No. of patients with AE; Paracetamol + codeine 15/42 with 24 AE. Paracetamol 21/42 with 31 AE.	3
[Cooper et al. 1981]	Impacted 3rd molar n = 248 Age: mean early 20s	RCT, DB, single oral dose, 5 parallel groups. Either GA or LA. Self assessed at home at 0, 1, 2, 3, 4 h (questionnaire).	PI (4-pt scale) PR (5-pt scale) Global rating (5-pt scale) 50% relief of baseline pain (y/n) Time to remed	Paracetamol (650 mg) + codeine (60 mg) n = 42 Paracetamol (650 mg) n = 37	All active treatments were significantly superior to placebo for all measures. The combination was slightly more effective than the Paracetamol alone but the diff was not significant.	Remed after 1st h if needed (last score used for all further timepoints). Remed <4 h; Placebo 20/37 Paracetamol 2/37	200 analysed. Exclusions: 17 did not ingest med, 31 ingested med but violated protocol (remed before 1st h obs, constant deviation of more than 15 min from evaluation times, not returning questionnaire & lost to follow-up)	No serious AE was reported. No. of patients with AE; Paracetamol + codeine 10/42 with 10 AE Paracetamol 12/37 with 15 AE.	4
[Cooper et al. 1988]	Impacted 3rd molar n = 165 Age: 18–57	RCT, DB, single oral dose, 3 parallel groups, single centre & 1 surgeon. LA with sed &/or Nitrous oxide. 4 h washout prior to start. Self-assessed at home at 0, 0.5, 1, 2, 3, 4, 5 6 h (diary).	PI (4-pt scale) PR (5-pt scale) Pain half gone? (y/n) Global rating (5-pt) Time to remed	Paracetamol (650 mg) + codeine (60 mg) n = 31 Paracetamol (600 mg) n = 36	The combination was significantly superior to placebo for every measure & to Paracetamol for TOTPAR. Paracetamol appeared clinically more effective than Placebo but it was not significant. (P <0.05)	Remed after 1st h (last or baseline score used for all further timepoints).	143 analysed. Exclusions: 11 were lost to follow-up, 8 did not require med. & 3 for 'various protocol violations'.	No serious AE were reported. No. of AE reported; Paracetamol + codeine 4. Paracetamol 8.	4
[Cooper & Kupperman 1991]	Removal of 1 or more impacted teeth n = 247 Age: 'young adults'	RCT, DB, single oral dose, 6 parallel groups. LA (lidocaine + epinephrine) with IV diazepam & methohexital—on occasion nitrous oxide was also used. Self-assessed at home at 0, 0.5 h then hourly till 6 h (diaries).	PI (4-pt scale) PR (5-pt scale) Global rating (5-pt scale) Time to remed	Paracetamol (650 mg) + codeine (60 mg) n = 39 Paracetamol (650 mg) n = 37	Paracetamol was the only active drug not to be significantly superior to Placebo for any measure. The combination was significantly superior to placebo for most measures & to Paracetamol for TOTPAR & the global rating.	t >1 h before remed, data included & baseline or last score (most severe) used for all further timepoints).	226 analysed. Exclusions; 13 did not require med. 3 were lost to follow-up, 2 remed, with slight pain before the 2nd h obs, 2 remed before the 1st h obs, 1 fell asleep for over 2 h	All AE mild. No. of patients with AE; Paracetamol + codeine 8/39 with 11 AE. Paracetamol 6/37 with 7AE.	3
[Dionne et al. 1994]	Impacted 3rd molar n = 135 Age: 16+	RCT, DB, single oral dose, 5 parallel groups. GA & LA. 4 h washout prior to start. Self assessed at clinic for at least the first 2 h then at home hourly for 6 h.	PI (4-pt scale) PR (5-pt scale) Global rating (5-pt scale) Time to remed	Paracetamol (650 mg) + codeine (60 mg) n = 24 Paracetamol (650 mg) n = 27	Neither Paracetamol nor the combination showed a significant diff to placebo for any measure of analgesia.	t ≥2 h before remed, data included & baseline used for all further timepoints.	124 analysed. Exclusions: 4 previously enrolled in the study, 3 remed before t = 2 h, 2 were lost to follow-up, 1 with ineligible because of codeine sensitivity	All AE mild. No. of patients with AE; Paracetamol + codeine 9/24 with 10 AE Paracetamol 7/27 with 9 AE.	3
[Forbes et al. 1982]	Impacted 3rd molar (1 or more) n = 177 Age: 15+	DB, single oral dose, 5 parallel groups. No info on anaes. Self-assessed at home at 0, 1 then hourly for 12 h.	PI (4-pt scale) PR (5-pt scale) 50% PR (y/n) Global rating (5-pt scale) Time to remed	Paracetamol (600 mg) + codeine (60 mg) n = 31 Paracetamol (600 mg) n = 34	At 4 h Paracetamol was significantly superior to Placebo for PR, Peak PR & 50% PR (P <0.01). The combination was significantly superior to Placebo for all measures.	If remed <2 h excluded. If >2 h <12 h PR = baseline or last. % patients remed >2 h but <12 h; Placebo 93% Paracetamol 85%	159 analysed. Exclusions: 4 lost to follow-up, 3 did not take med, 7 took remed <2 h, 1 med with mild pain & 3 did not complete the forms properly.	None of the active treatments produced more AE than the Placebo. None were serious.	3
[Forbes et al. 1983]	Postop (general, gynae, or orthopaedic surgery) n = 132 Age: 18+	RCT, DB, single oral dose, 5 parallel groups. GA, given on request 1st day able to take oral analgesia. Self-assessed in hospital at 0, 0.5, 1, 1.5, 2 then hourly for 12 h Single nurse observer present for 1st 6 h, 2nd 6 h monitored by ward staff.	PI (4-pt scale) PR (5-pt scale) Pain half gone? (y/n) Global rating (5-pt scale) Time to remed	Paracetamol (600 mg) + Placebo (60 mg) n = 26 Paracetamol (600 mg) n = 26	For 6 h data both Paracetamol & the combination were significantly superior to Placebo for all measures & for 12-h data, all except SPID.	Patients were remed on demand if <2 h excluded. If remed <2 h PR = 0, PI = baseline or last score for remaining timepoints.	132 analysed. There were no exclusions.	No serious AE reported. Most common were drowsiness, dizziness & dry mouth. No. of patients with AE; Paracetamol + codeine 11/26 with 16 AE. Paracetamol 11/26 with 11 AE.	5

Ref.	Condition & no. of patients	Design, study duration & follow-up	Outcome measures	Dose regimen	Analgesic outcome results	Remediation	Withdrawals & exclusions	Adverse effects	Quality score
[Forbes et al. 1989]	Impacted 3rd molar (1 or more) n = 107 Age: 15+	RCT, DB, single oral dose, 4 parallel groups at 2 centres. GA & LA—unclear. Patients self-assessed at home at 0, 1, 2 then hourly for 12 h or until remed (diary)—returned 5 days later for review & debrief.	PI (4-pt scale) PR (5-pt scale) Global rating (5-pt scale) Time to Remed	Paracetamol (600 mg) + codeine (60 mg) n = 17 Paracetamol (600 mg) n = 22	At 4 h: Paracetamol & the combination were significantly superior to Placebo. The combination was also significantly superior to Paracetamol for TOTPAR. (P <0.05)	Patients could remed after 2 h but were asked to complete the next evaluation before doing so (PI last or baseline score, PR = 0 for all further timepoints). % remed by h 12; Paracetamol 95% Placebo 91%	88 analysed. Exclusions: 9 did not take the med, 2 remed before the 2 h point, 1 remed with slight pain, 4 did not complete their evaluation, 1 took only part of the med & 2 remed despite of having some relief from the study med.	No serious AE reported. No. of patients with AE; Paracetamol + codeine 1/17 with 1 AE Paracetamol 3/36 with 3 AE (NB includes AE reported post remed).	5
[Forbes et al. 1990]	Impacted 3rd molar (1 or more) n = 269 Age: 15+	RCT, DB, single then multiple oral dose, 6 parallel groups. GA/LA—unclear. Self-assess at home at 0, 1 then hourly for 6 h—returned 5 days later for review & debrief.	PI (4-pt scale) PR (5-pt scale) Pain half gone? (y/n) Global rating (5-pt scale) Time to remed	Paracetamol (600 mg) + codeine (60 mg) n = 38 Paracetamol (600 mg) n = 36)	All active med were significantly superior for all measures of total & peak analgesia.	Remed allowed after 2 h but asked to complete the next eval (PI last or baseline score, PR = 0 used for all remaining timepoints). % remed by hour 6; Placebo 33% Paracetamol 29%	206 analysed. Exclusions: 3 lost to follow-up, 1 lost report card, 22 did not req med, 8 remed despite having relief from study med, 6 remed with only slight pain, 13 remed <2 h, 7 failed to follow instructions, 3 did not complete the forms.	No AE was serious. No. of patients reporting AE; Paracetamol + codeine 8/40 with 9 AE Paracetamol 5/41 with 5 AE.	5
[Gertzbein et al. 1986]	Postop (elective surgery— orthopaedic or general) n = 116 Age: 16–65	RCT, single oral dose, 3 parallel groups. No info on anaes, 1st oral analgesic given. Interviewed in hospital by nurse observer at 0, 0.5, 1 h then hourly for 5 h	PI (5-pt scale) PR (5-pt scale) 50% PR (y/n) Global rating (4-pt scale)—patient & observer PI VAS ('No pain' to 'Worst pain I can imagine')	Paracetamol (1000 mg) + codeine (60 mg) n = 45 Paracetamol (1000 mg) n = 45	The combination was seen to give higher efficacy results than paracetamol alone but was not significantly superior for any measure.	Remed allowed after 1 h (PI = last score & PR = 0 used for all remaining timepoints). Mean time to remed; Combination 230 min Paracetamol 214 min	113 analysed. Exclusions:1 refused to comply with instructions, 1 vomited within 1 h of taking the study med & 1 took concomitant analgesia.	No serious AE reported. No. of patients with AE: Paracetamol + codeine 13/47 with 13 AE Paracetamol 13/46 with 15 AE.	4
[Honig & Murray 1984]	Postop (elective surgery— abdominal, orthopaedic, rectal, thoracic & vascular) n = 116 Age: 19–87	RCT, DB, single oral dose, 4 parallel groups. No info on anaes, 4 h washout prior to start. Interviewed in hospital by nurse observer at 0, 0.5, 1 h then hourly for 6 h	PI (4-pt scale) PR (5-pt scale) 50% PR (y/n) Global rating (5-pt scale)	Paracetamol (600 mg) + codeine (60 mg) n = 30 Paracetamol (600 mg) n = 28	TOTPAR & Global rating; Both paracetamol & the combination were significantly superior to Placebo (P <0.05). The combination was also significantly superior for SPID & no. remed before 6 h.	If remed last score was used for all further timepoints. No. of patients who did not remed in 6 h; Placebo n = 14/30 Paracetamol n = 16/28	No details given.	None severe except 1 severe dry mouth. Reported in all groups & were primarily CNS & gastrointestinal effects.	3
[Sunshine et al. 1986]	Impacted 3rd molar n = 182 Age: 16+	RCT, DB, single oral dose, 6 parallel groups. LA (lidocaine/ epinephrine) 4 h washout prior to start. Evaluations at 0, 0.5, 1, 2 & 3 h in clinic by single observer. At 4, 5 & 6 h self-assessed. 1 wk later met with observer & reviewed the forms.	PI (4-pt scale) PR (5-pt scale) Global rating (4-pt scale) Overall improvement (7-pt scale) Time to remed	Paracetamol (650 mg) + codeine (60 mg) n = 31 Paracetamol (650 mg) n = 30	Both Paracetamol & the combination were significantly superior (P <0.05) to Placebo for; PID 1–3 h, SUMPID at 4 h, PR at 2 h & t to Peak effect. The combination was also significantly superior to TOTPAR.	If <1 h excluded. If >1 h use last PI or baseline & PR = 0. Full dichot data in table III. No. of patients remed; Placebo 13/30 Paracetamol 14/30.	182 analysed. No exclusions.	No serious AE, NSD between groups. No. of patients reporting AE; Paracetamol + codeine 3/31 Paracetamol 1/30.	5

See Appendix 1 for key to abbreviations.

Appendix 3 references

Bentley KC, Head TW. The additive analgesic efficacy of aceta-minophen, 1000 mg, and codeine, 60 mg, in dental pain. *Clinical Pharmacology and Therapeutics* 1987; **42**:634–40.

Cooper SA, Breen JF, Giuliani RL. The relative efficacy of indopro-fen compared with opioid analgesic combinations. *Journal of Oral Surgery* 1981; **39**:21–5.

Cooper SA, Firestein A, Cohn P. Double blind comparison of meclofenamate sodium with acetaminophen, acetaminophen with codeine and placebo for relief of postsurgical dental pain. *Journal of Clinical Dentistry* 1988; **1**:31–4.

Cooper SA, Kupperman A. The analgesic efficacy of flurbiprofen compared to acetaminophen with codeine. *Journal of Clinical Dentistry* 1991; **2**:70–4.

Dionne RA, Snyder J, Hargreaves KM. Analgesic efficacy of flur-biprofen in comparison with acetaminophen, acetaminophen plus codeine, and placebo after impacted third molar removal. *Journal of Oral and Maxillofacial Surgery* 1994; **52**:919–24; discussion 25–6.

Forbes JA, Beaver WT, White EH, White RW, Neilson GB, Shackleford RW. Diflunisal. A new oral analgesic with an un-usually long duration of action. *Journal of American Medical Association* 1982; **248**:2139–42.

Forbes JA, Butterworth GA, Burchfield WH, Yorio CC, Selinger LR, Rosenmertz SK *et al.* Evaluation of flurbiprofen, aceta-minophen, an acetaminophen-codeine combination, and placebo in postoperative oral surgery pain. *Pharmacotherapy* 1989; **9**:322–30.

Forbes JA, Kehm CJ, Grodin CD, Beaver WT. Evaluation of ketoro-lac, ibuprofen, acetaminophen, and an acetaminophen codeine combination in postoperative oral surgery pain. *Pharmacotherapy* 1990; **10**:94S–105S.

Forbes JA, Kolodny AL, Beaver WT, Shackleford RW, Scarlett VR. A 12 hour evaluation of the analgesic efficacy of diflunisal, acetaminophen, and acetaminophen codeine combination, and placebo in postoperative pain. *Pharmacotherapy* 1983; **3**:S47–54.

Gertzbein SD, Tile M, McMurty RY, Kellam JF, Hunter GA, Keith RG *et al*. Analysis of the analgesic efficacy of acetaminophen 1000 mg, codeine phosphate 60 mg, and the combination of acetaminophen 1000 mg and codeine phosphate 60 mg in the relief of postoperative pain. *Pharmacotherapy* 1986; **6**:104–7.

Honig S, Murray KA. An appraisal of codeine as an analgesic: single dose analysis. *Journal of Clinical Pharmacology* 1984; **24**:96–102.

Sunshine A, Marrero I, Olson N, McCormick N, Laska EM. Comparative study of flurbiprofen, zomepirac sodium, acetaminophen plus codeine, and acetaminophen for the relief of postsurgical dental pain. *American Journal of Medicine* 1986; **80**:50–4.

10

Oral ibuprofen and diclofenac in postoperative pain

Summary

The aim was to compare ibuprofen and diclofenac in postoperative pain. Studies were identified by searching MEDLINE (1966–December 1996), EMBASE (1980–January 1997), the Cochrane Library (August 1996), Biological Abstracts (January 1985–December 1996), and the Oxford Pain Relief Database (1950–94). Additional reports were identified from the reference lists of reports, review articles, and textbooks.

We sought randomized, controlled, single dose comparisons of ibuprofen or diclofenac against placebo. Summed pain relief or pain intensity difference over four to six hours was extracted, and converted into dichotomous information yielding the number of patients with at least 50% pain relief. This was then used to calculate the relative benefit and the number-needed-to-treat (NNT) for one patient to achieve at least 50% pain relief.

Thirty-four reports compared ibuprofen and placebo (3591 patients), six compared diclofenac with placebo (840 patients), and there were two direct comparisons of diclofenac 50 mg and ibuprofen 400 mg (130 patients). In postoperative pain, ibuprofen 200 mg had an NNT of 3.3 (95% confidence interval 2.8–4.0) compared with placebo, ibuprofen 400 mg had an NNT of 2.7 (2.5–3.0), and ibuprofen 600 mg had an NNT of 2.4 (1.9–3.3). Diclofenac 50 mg had an NNT of 2.3 (2.0–2.7) compared with placebo in established postoperative pain and diclofenac 100 mg had an NNT of 1.8 (1.5–2.1).

When diclofenac 50 mg was compared directly with ibuprofen 400 mg, there was no significant difference between the two treatments. Ibuprofen showed a clear dose response with similar relative efficacy to diclofenac. Both drugs work well. Choosing between them is an issue of dose, safety, and cost.

Introduction

Ibuprofen and diclofenac are two of the most widely used non-steroidal anti-inflammatory (NSAID) analgesics, with ibuprofen commonly available without prescription. In England in 1996, ibuprofen accounted for nearly 5.5 million prescriptions (31% of total NSAID prescriptions) and diclofenac for nearly 6 million prescriptions (34%), although it is not known how much of this was for acute pain conditions [2].

The topic discussed in this chapter is also published in part in Collins *et al.* [1].

With an increasing amount of surgery being performed as day cases it is important to know which drug should be recommended for postoperative pain relief. We sought to compare the relative efficacy of the two drugs to allow a balanced decision to be made based on efficacy, safety, and cost.

Methods

Single dose, randomized controlled trials of ibuprofen and diclofenac in postoperative pain (post-dental extraction, post-surgical, or postpartum pain) were sought. Different search strategies were used to identify eligible reports from MEDLINE (1966–December 1996), EMBASE (1980–January 1997), the Cochrane Library (August 1996), Biological Abstracts (January 1985–December 1996), and the Oxford Pain Relief Database (1950–94) [3]. A search was undertaken for each drug using the words: 'clinical trial', 'trial', 'study', 'random*', 'double blind', 'analgesi*', and 'pain*', along with 'ibuprofen', 'Brufen', 'propionic acid', and 'isobutylphenyl propionic acid', for the ibuprofen search and, for the diclofenac search, 'diclofenac', and 76 brand names [4]. Each was a broad free text search, including various combinations of the words, and without restriction to language. Additional reports were identified from the reference lists of retrieved reports, review articles, and textbooks.

Excluded reports

We excluded reports of ibuprofen or diclofenac for the relief of other pain conditions, controlled release formulations, ibuprofen or diclofenac used in combination with other drugs, trials which reported data from a cross-over design as a single data set, trials where the number of patients per treatment group was less than ten [6], and trials which included pain relief data collected after additional analgesia was given.

Included reports

Neither pharmaceutical companies nor authors of papers were contacted for unpublished reports. Abstracts and review articles were not considered. The inclusion criteria used were: randomized allocation to treatment groups which included ibuprofen or diclofenac and placebo, full journal publication, established postoperative pain with the pain outcome measured using a five-point pain relief scale with standard wording (none, slight, moderate, good, complete) or a four-point pain intensity scale (none, mild, moderate, or severe) or a visual analogue scale (VAS) for pain relief or pain intensity, TOTPAR or SPID (at four, five or six hours) as a derived pain relief outcome (or sufficient data provided to allow their calculation), postoperative oral administration for ibuprofen and postoperative oral, rectal, intravenous, or intramuscular administration for diclofenac, adult patients, baseline pain of moderate to severe intensity (for VAS this equates to > 30 mm [5]) and double-blind design.

Data extraction and analysis

From each report we took: the numbers of patients treated, the mean TOTPAR, SPID, VAS-TOTPAR, or VAS-SPID, study-duration, and the dose given. Information on adverse events was also extracted. For each report, the mean TOTPAR, SPID, VAS-TOTPAR or VAS-SPID values for active and placebo were converted to %maxTOTPAR or %maxSPID by division into the calculated maximum value [7]. The proportion of patients in each treatment group who achieved at least 50%maxTOTPAR was calculated using verified equations [8–10]. These proportions were then converted into the number of patients achieving at least 50%maxTOTPAR by multiplying by the total number of patients in the treatment group. Information on the number of patients with at least 50%maxTOTPAR for active and placebo was then used to calculate relative benefit (RB) and NNT.

Relative benefit (RB) estimates were calculated with 95% confidence intervals (CIs) using a random effects model [11]; the random effects model was chosen because this produces the most conservative estimate (homogeneity was assumed when $P > 0.1$). NNT and 95% confidence intervals were calculated by the method of Cook and Sackett [12]. A statistically significant difference from control was assumed when the 95% confidence interval of the relative benefit did not include 1.

The number of patients experiencing at least 50% pain relief with placebo (the control event rate, CER) can vary greatly with the relatively small sample sizes typically used in analgesic trials affecting the apparent efficacy of an analgesic [13]. To allow for this variation the RB and NNT for each dose of ibuprofen and diclofenac were also calculated using a fixed CER of 19%. This CER was obtained from data for 4378 patients given placebo, pooled from 124 single dose analgesic trials meeting identical inclusion criteria included in this and similar systematic reviews [14–17] (843/4378 patients experienced at least 50% pain relief).

Results

Ibuprofen vs. placebo

Thirty-four reports of 35 trials fulfilled our inclusion criteria; 2214 patients were given ibuprofen and 1377 placebo.

Citations to the 34 included reports are given in Appendix 1, together with details of the studies. One author was contacted and kindly provided information on the number of patients in each treatment arm [18].

Twenty-five trials investigated oral surgery pain (predominantly third molar extraction with bone removal), five trials investigated postpartum pain (predominantly episiotomy and Caesarean section), and four trials investigated postoperative pain (one tonsillectomy, one inguinal hernia, one orthopaedic surgery, and one general surgery). Doses of ibuprofen were 50 mg in one trial, 100 mg in two, 200 mg in eight, 400 mg in thirty, 600 mg in three, and 800 mg in one.

The control event rate (the proportion of patients given placebo experiencing at least 50% pain relief, CER) ranged from 0% to 67% (median 12%) (Fig. 1). The experimental response rate (the proportion of patients given ibuprofen experiencing at least 50% pain relief, EER) for the single trial of ibuprofen 50 mg was 28%. The two trials of ibuprofen 100 mg gave EER values of 27% and 8%. The EER for ibuprofen 200 mg varied between 6% and 57% (median 39%) and for ibuprofen 400 mg varied between 13% and 100% (median 60%). The EER for the single trial of ibuprofen 800 mg was 100%. The 100 mg and 200 mg data sets were homogeneous but the 400 mg and 600 mg data sets were not.

One trial [19] used a syrup formulation of ibuprofen, two trials [20, 21] used soluble ibuprofen and liquid in gelatin capsules, two trials [22, 23] used ibuprofen lysine, and two trials [24, 25] used soluble ibuprofen arginine. When these more readily absorbed formulations were pooled and the

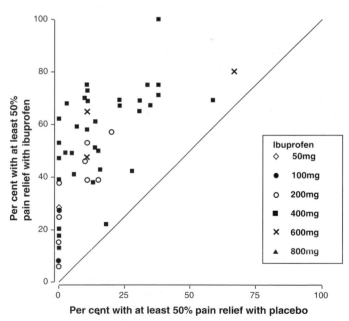

Fig. 1   Ibuprofen vs. placebo. Each point represents one trial with the proportion of patients achieving at least 50% pain relief on the study drug plotted on the y-axis, and the proportion of patients achieving the same endpoint with placebo on the x-axis.

results compared with those of the standard tablet formulation, no difference was found in the relative benefit or NNTs. The NNT for a single dose of ibuprofen 400 mg standard formulation tablets (1356 patients) compared with placebo was 2.8 (2.5–3.1) and for ibuprofen 400 mg soluble formulations (250 patients) the NNT was 2.5 (2.1–3.1). All formulations were therefore pooled for the overall analysis.

The single data set for ibuprofen 50 mg showed no significant difference from placebo. The pooled relative benefits for ibuprofen 100 mg, 200 mg, 400 mg, and 600 mg were significantly different from placebo, as was the single data set for ibuprofen 800 mg (Table 1). At a dose of 50 mg ibuprofen had an NNT of 3.6 (2.5–6.1) for at least 50% pain relief over 4 to 6 hours compared with placebo in pain of moderate to severe intensity, at 100 mg the NNT was 5.6 (3.8–9.9), at 200 mg the NNT was 3.3 (2.8–4.0), at 400 mg the NNT was 2.7 (2.5–3.0), at 600 mg the NNT was 2.4 (1.9–3.3), and at 800 mg the NNT was 1.6 (1.3–2.2). The dose-response for ibuprofen is shown in Fig. 2.

When a fixed CER of 19% was applied there was a clear dose-response with no overlap in the confidence intervals except for the 600 mg and 800 mg doses (Table 1, Fig. 5).

Drug-related study withdrawals occurred rarely. One study [26] had one withdrawal on ibuprofen for vomiting which the authors did not attribute to the medication. One study [21] had three withdrawals on ibuprofen and one on placebo for vomiting soon after ingestion of study drug. Another study [19] had one patient who withdrew on placebo. The studies reported a variable incidence of minor adverse events which were all mild and transient, with no difference in incidence between ibuprofen and placebo.

Diclofenac vs. placebo

Although the search identified nearly 2000 trials the majority were in chronic pain or the drug was administered before the patient experienced pain. Over 500 reports were found of trials involving rectal, intravenous, and intramuscular diclofenac. Predominantly, the reports were not in established postoperative pain, were not placebo-controlled or did not use standard pain outcome measures. Only six trials fulfilled our inclusion criteria; all were for oral diclofenac (528 patients were given diclofenac and 312 placebo). Five reports

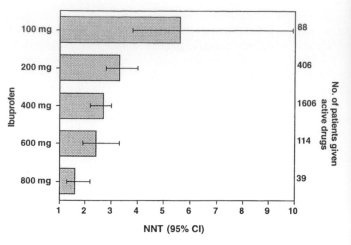

Fig. 2   Dose-response for ibuprofen trials.

identified by the search could not be obtained despite attempts to contact the authors, ordering through the British Library and help from the librarians at Novartis and Knoll pharmaceuticals [27–31]. Citations to the six included reports are given in Appendix 2, together with details of the studies. One author was contacted for information on the number of patients in each treatment arm [32]; they were unable to provide this information and so an equal split of 50 patients per group was assumed.

Five trials investigated oral surgery pain (third molar extraction with bone removal) and one pain following gynaecological surgery. Doses of diclofenac were 25 mg in one trial, 50 mg in six, and 100 mg in three. Three trials used the immediate release diclofenac potassium formulation [32–34] and two used dispersible diclofenac [35, 36]. One trial used both the immediate release and enteric coated formulations [37]. To ensure comparability only the data from the immediate release formulation were included.

The CER ranged from 8% to 38% (median 10%) (Fig. 3). The EER for the single trial of diclofenac 25 mg was 46%. The EER for diclofenac 50 mg varied between 53% and 75% (median 58%) and for diclofenac 100 mg varied between 56% and 72% (median 67%). The 100 mg data set was homogeneous but the 50 mg data set was not.

Table 1   Summary of relative benefit (RB) and number-needed-to-treat (NNT) for trials of ibuprofen vs. placebo

No. of trials	Ibuprofen dose (mg)	No. of patients with >50% pain relief: ibuprofen	No. of patients with >50% pain relief: placebo	RB (random-effects model) (95% CI)	NNT (95% CI)	NNT with 19% CER (95% CI)
1	50	16/57	0/51	144 (0.3–>1000)	3.6 (2.5–6.1)	12.5 (4.1–∞)
2	100	16/88	0/98	72 (16–318)	5.6 (3.8–9.9)	−100 (10–∞)
8	200	151/406	22/320	3.5 (2.3–5.3)	3.3 (2.8–4.0)	5.6 (4.1–8.5)
30	400	858/1606	214/1292	3.3 (2.5–4.3)	2.7 (2.5–3.0)	2.9 (2.7–3.2)
3	600	90/114	40/108	2.5 (1.2–5.5)	2.4 (1.9–3.3)	1.7 (1.4–2)
1	800	39/39	14/37	2.6 (1.8–4)	1.6 (1.3–2.2)	1.2 (1.1–1.5)

CER, control event rate.

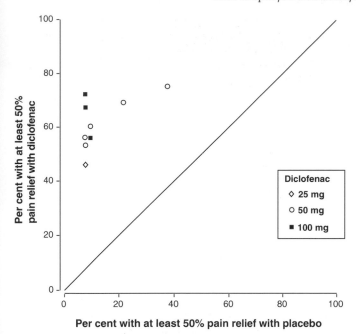

Fig. 3 Diclofenac vs. placebo.

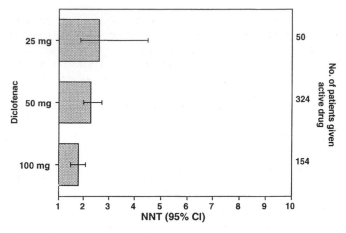

Fig. 4 Dose-response for diclofenac trials.

The pooled relative benefits for all doses of diclofenac versus placebo were significant (Table 2). At a dose of 25 mg diclofenac had an NNT of 2.6 (1.9–4.5) for at least 50% pain relief over 4 to 6 hours compared with placebo in pain of moderate to severe intensity. At 50 mg the NNT was 2.3 (2.0–2.7) and at 100 mg the NNT was 1.8 (1.5–2.1), with overlapping confidence intervals. The dose response for diclofenac is shown in Fig. 4.

With a fixed CER of 19% the NNT for diclofenac 25 mg was 3.9 (2.3–12), for 50 mg it was 2.3 (2.0–2.7) and for 100 mg it was 2.2 (1.8–2.8), with overlapping confidence intervals (Table 1; Fig. 5).

Drug-related study withdrawals occurred rarely. One study [33] had one withdrawal on diclofenac 100 mg for nausea and vomiting. The studies reported a variable incidence of minor adverse events none of which were serious and with no difference in incidence between diclofenac and placebo.

Diclofenac vs. ibuprofen

There were two direct comparisons of diclofenac 50 mg and ibuprofen 400 [35, 36]. Both trials were in dental pain (third

molar removal); 118 patients received diclofenac and 112 ibuprofen. There was no significant difference between diclofenac 50 mg and ibuprofen 400 mg (relative benefit 1.0 (0.9–1.2)).

Comment

A single dose of ibuprofen 400 mg had an NNT of 2.7 for at least 50% pain relief compared with placebo. This means that one out of every three patients with pain of moderate to severe intensity will experience at least 50% pain relief with ibuprofen which they would not have had with placebo. The equivalent NNT of a single dose of ibuprofen 600 mg was 2.4 and for ibuprofen 200 mg was 3.3, showing a dose-response, although the confidence intervals overlapped (Table 1). When a fixed CER was used to smooth out the variation in the CERs of the individual trials the confidence intervals for the NNTs did not overlap, supporting the dose response finding (Fig. 5). Moreover, the use of a fixed (population) CER had little effect on the NNT in circumstances where there were either large numbers of patients or where there were large effects (Tables 1 and 2). Only in small trials with limited analgesic efficacy (low doses) did the use of the fixed CER alter the NNT significantly.

A single dose of diclofenac 50 mg had an NNT of 2.3 for at least 50% pain relief compared with placebo. The equivalent NNT for diclofenac 100 mg was 1.8 and for diclofenac 25 mg was 2.6, indicating a dose-response although the confidence intervals overlapped (Table 2). With a fixed CER

Table 2 Summary of relative benefit (RB) and number-needed-to-treat (NNT) for trials of diclofenac vs. placebo

No. of trials	Diclofenac dose (mg)	No. of patients with >50% pain relief: diclofenac	No. of patients with >50% pain relief: placebo	RB (random-effects model) (95% CI)	NNT (95% CI)	NNT with 19% CER (95% CI)
1	25	23/50	4/50	5.8 (2.1–15.4)	2.6 (1.9–4.5)	3.9 (2.3–12.1)
6	50	203/324	57/312	4.3 (2.4–7.8)	2.3 (2–2.7)	2.3 (2–2.7)
3	100	100/154	13/154	7.2 (5.5–9.4)	1.8 (1.5–2.1)	2.2 (1.8–2.8)

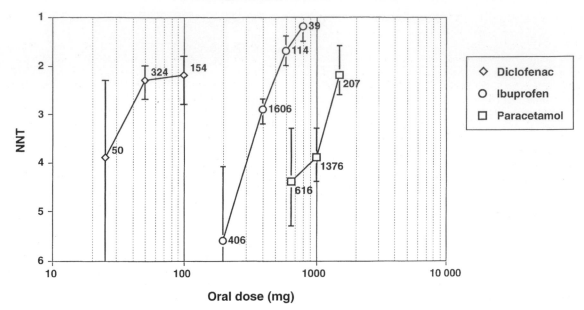

Fig. 5   Dose-response for diclofenac, ibuprofen, and paracetamol using a fixed 19% placebo response rate. Numbers indicate patients given active treatment. (The value next to the symbol indicates the number of patients receiving that dose of study drug. The data for paracetamol comes from Chapter 9.)

of 19% the confidence intervals of the two higher doses overlapped completely (Table 2, Fig. 5).

Diclofenac is widely regarded as a more effective NSAID than ibuprofen. Our results do not support this. When diclofenac 50 mg and ibuprofen 400 mg were compared directly there was no significant difference between them. When compared with placebo, diclofenac 50 mg and ibuprofen 600 mg had very similar NNTs with complete overlap of the confidence intervals. Single trials of NSAIDs have often reported flat dose-response curves typified by diclofenac in Fig. 5. With the advantage of the much larger numbers of patients in this meta-analysis the 'true' dose-response for ibuprofen is shown (Fig. 5), with the interesting finding that higher doses (> 1 g) of paracetamol also follow traditional dose-response curve contours.

The issue of the relative efficacy of the two drugs therefore comes down to dose (Figs 2, 4, and 5). An ibuprofen dose of 400 mg is one-sixth of the maximum daily dose. Diclofenac 50 mg is one-third of the maximum daily dose. This may explain prescriber confusion.

References

1. Collins SL, Moore A, McQuay HJ, Wiffen PJ. Oral ibuprofen and diclofenac in postoperative pain: a quantitative systematic review. submitted
2. Government Statistical Service. *Prescription cost analysis for England 1996*. London: Department of Health, 1997.
3. Jadad AR, Carroll D, Moore A, McQuay H. Developing a database of published reports of randomised clinical trials in pain research. *Pain* 1996; 66:239–46.
4. Reynolds JEF. *Martindale: the extra pharmacopoeia*, (30th edn). London: Pharmaceutical Press, 1993:292–314.
5. Collins SL, Moore RA, McQuay HJ. The visual analogue pain intensity scale: what is moderate pain in millimetres? *Pain* 1997; **72**:95–7.
6. L'Abbé KA, Detsky AS, O'Rourke K. Meta-analysis in clinical research *Annals of Internal Medicine* 1987; **107**:224–33.
7. Cooper SA. Single-dose analgesic studies: the upside and downside of assay sensitivity. In: Max MB, Portenoy RK, Laska EM, ed. *The design of analgesic clinical trials (Advances in pain research and therapy*, Vol. 18). New York: Raven Press, 1991:117–24.
8. Moore A, McQuay H, Gavaghan D. Deriving dichotomous outcome measures from continuous data in randomised controlled trials of analgesics. *Pain* 1996; 66:229–37.
9. Moore A, McQuay H, Gavaghan D. Deriving dichotomous outcome measures from continuous data in randomised controlled trials of analgesics: Verification from independent data. *Pain* 1997; 69:127–30.
10. Moore A, Moore O, McQuay H, Gavaghan D. Deriving dichotomous outcome measures from continuous data in randomised controlled trials of analgesics: Use of pain intensity and visual analogue scales. *Pain* 1997; 69:311–15.
11. DerSimonian R, Laird N. Meta-analysis of clinical trials. *Controlled Clinical Trials* 1986; **7**:177–88.
12. Cook RJ, Sackett DL. The number needed to treat: a clinically useful measure of treatment effect. *British Medical Journal* 1995; **310**:452–4.
13. Moore RA, Collins S, McQuay HJ. Variation in the placebo effect; the impact on individual trials and consequences for meta-analysis. In: Jensen TS, Hammond DL, Jensen TS, ed. Proceedings of the 8th World Congress on Pain. *Progress in pain research and management*, Vol. 2. Seattle: IASP Press, 1997: 469–76.

14. Moore A, Collins S, Carroll D, McQuay H. Paracetamol with and without codeine in acute pain: a quantitative systematic review. *Pain* 1997; 70:193–201.
15. Moore RA, McQuay HJ. Single-patient data meta-analysis of 3453 postoperative patients: Oral tramadol versus placebo, codeine and combination analgesics. *Pain* 1997; 69:287–94.
16. Collins SL, Edwards J, Moore A, McQuay HJ. Oral dextropropoxyphene in postoperative pain: a quantitative systematic review. *European Journal of Clinical Pharmacology*. in press.
17. Edwards JE, McQuay HJ, Moore RA. Systematic review: dihydrocodeine in postoperative pain. submitted.
18. Laska EM, Sunshine A, Marrero I, Olson N, Siegel C, McCormick N. The correlation between blood levels of ibuprofen and clinical analgesic response. *Clinical Pharmacology and Therapeutics* 1986; 40:1–7.
19. Parker D, Gibbin K, Noyelle R. Syrup formulations for post tonsillectomy analgesia: a double blind study comparing ibuprofen, aspirin and placebo. *Journal of Laryngology and Otology* 1986; 100:1055–60.
20. Seymour RA, Hawkesford JE, Weldon M, Brewster D. An evaluation of different ibuprofen preparations in the control of postoperative pain after third molar surgery. *British Journal of Clinical Pharmacology* 1991; 31:83–7.
21. Seymour R, WardBooth P, Kelly P. Evaluation of different doses of soluble ibuprofen and ibuprofen tablets in postoperative dental pain. *British Journal of Oral and Maxillofacial Surgery* 1996; 34:110–14.
22. Mehlisch DR, Jasper RD, Brown P, Korn SH, McCarroll K, Murakami AA. Comparative study of ibuprofen lysine and acetaminophen in patients with postoperative dental pain. *Clinical Therapeutics* 1995; 17:852–60.
23. Nelson SL, brahim JS, Korn SH, Greene SS, Suchower LJ. Comparison of single-dose ibuprofen lysine, acetyl-salicylic acid, and placebo for moderate-to-severe postoperative dental pain. *Clinical Therapeutics* 1994; 16:458–65.
24. Laveneziana D, Riva A, Bonazzi M, Cipolla M, Migliavacca S. Comparative efficacy of oral ibuprofen arginine and intramuscular ketorolac in patients with postoperative pain. *Clinical Drug Investigation* 1996; 11:8–14.
25. Pagnoni B, Ravanelli A, Degradi L, Rossi R, Tiengo M. Clinical efficacy of ibuprofen arginine in the management of postoperative pain associated with suction termination of pregnancy. A double-blind placebo-controlled study. *Clinical Drug Investigation* 1996; 11:27–32.
26. Fricke J, Halladay S, Francisco C. Efficacy and safety of naproxen sodium and ibuprofen for pain relief after oral surgery. *Current Therapeutic Research: Clinical and Experimental* 1993; 54:619–27.
27. Carlos D. Comparative study of the efficacy of diclofenac NA, meperidine HCL and nalbuphine HCL in post-operative

analgesia. *Philippine Journal of Internal Medicine* 1984; 22:51–5.
28. Frezza R, Bolognesi P, Bernardi F. [Comparison of the action of 3 non-steroidal anti-inflammatory agents in the control of post-operative pain. Effectiveness of NSAID against pain] Confronto sull'azione di tre antinfiammatori non steroidei nel controllo de dolore odontoiatrico post-chirurgico. Efficaaci i FANS contro il dolore. *Attual Dent* 1985; 1:40–2.
29. Iqbal K, Biswas G, Mondo S, Afzalunnessa B. Assessment of post operative analgesia: A comparative study of pethidine and diclofenac sodium. *Journal of the Bangladesh College of Physicians and Surgeons* 1986; 4:1–7.
30. Joubert JJ. An assesment of the efficacy and tolerability of Voltaren in the treatment of inflammation after extraction of teeth. *Journal of the Dental Association of South Africa* 1977; 32:581–3.
31. Vigneron JR, Thys R. [Study of the anti-inflammatory and analgesic actions of diclofenac in traumatology and orthopedic surgery] Etude de l'action anti-inflammatoire et antalgique du diclofenac en traumatologie et chriurgie orthopedique. *Revue Médicale Liège* 1977; 32:10–14.
32. Nelson S, Brahim J. An evaluation of the analgesic efficacy of diclofenac potassium, aspirin, and placebo in postoperative dental pain. *Today's Therapeutic Trends* 1994; 12:3–14.
33. Hebertson R, Storey N. The comparative efficacy of diclofenac potassium, aspirin, and placebo in the treatment of patients with pain following gynecologic surgery. *Today's Therapeutic Trends* 1994; 12:33–45.
34. Mehlisch D, Brown P. Single-dose therapy with diclofenac potassium, aspirin, or placebo following dental impaction surgery. *Today's Therapeutic Trends* 1994; 12:15–31.
35. Ahlström U, Bakshi R, Nilsson P, Wahlander L. The analgesic efficacy of diclofenac dispersible and ibuprofen in postoperative pain after dental extraction. *European Journal of Clinical Pharmacology* 1993; 44:587–8.
36. Bakshi R, Frenkel G, Dietlein G, Meurer Witt B, Schneider B, Sinterhauf U. A placebo-controlled comparative evaluation of diclofenac dispersible versus ibuprofen in postoperative pain after third molar surgery. *Journal of Clinical Pharmacology* 1994; 34:225–30.
37. Bakshi R, Jacobs L, Lehnert S, Picha B, Reuther J. A double-blind, placebo-controlled trial comparing the analgesic efficacy of two formulations of diclofenac in postoperative dental pain. *Current Therapeutic Research: Clinical and Experimental* 1992; 52:435–42.
38. Henry D, Lim LL, Rodriguez LAG, Gutthann SP, Carson JL, Griffin M *et al.* Variability in risk of gastrointestinal complications with individual non-steroidal anti-inflammatory drugs: results of a collabo-rative meta-analysis. *British Medical Journal* 1996; 312:1563–6.

Appendix 1
Ibuprofen vs. placebo: trial details

Ref.	Condition & no. of patients	Design, study duration & follow-up	Outcome measures	Dose regimen	Analgesic outcome results	Remediation	Withdrawals & exclusions	Adverse effects
[Ahlstrom *et al.* 1993]	3rd molar extraction n = 127 Age: 18–40	RCT, DB, single oral dose, parallel groups. 4 h washout before start. Evaluated at 0, 20, 40 min 1 h then hourly intervals for 6 h. Med taken when baseline pain was at least moderate intensity (>30 mm)	PI (VAS scale) 'No pain at all'. Agonizing pain. Global rating by patient	Ibuprofen (400 mg) n = 32 Placebo n = 30	Ibuprofen was significantly superior to placebo by 40 min (P = 0.01) this continued for 6 h. TOTPI & SPID; Ibuprofen was significantly superior to placebo (P < 0.0001) 6-h SPID: ibuprofen 188 mm Placebo 32 mm.	Patients were allowed to remed after 1 h. After remed PI = last score was carried forward for all further timepoints.	97 analysed. Exclusions: 30 for various protocol violations.	No serious AE were reported & no patient withdrew as a result of AE. No. of patients reporting AE; Ibuprofen 3/32 with ? AE Placebo 2/30 with ? AE.
[Arnold *et al.* 1990]	General surgery (inc. gynae & orthopaedic) n = 59 Age: 22–70	RCT, DB, single oral dose, parallel groups. Assessed by single nurse observer at 0. 0.5 1 h then hourly intervals for 6 h. Med taken when baseline pain was of moderate to severe intensity.	PI (4-pt scale): standard PR (5-pt scale): standard Time to meaningful relief Global rating (5-pt scale) by patient	Ibuprofen (400 mg) n = 15 Placebo n = 14	Ibuprofen was not significantly superior to placebo for either SPID or TOTPAR. 6 h TOTPAR: Ibuprofen 4.2 Placebo 1.5.	After remed PR = 0 & PI = baseline score for all further timepoints	No info given on any exclusions.	The diff in occurrence of AE. was not significant between groups. No patient withdrew from either the ibuprofen or placebo group as a result of AE.
[Bakshi *et al.* 1994]	3rd molar extraction n = 257 Age: Adults up to 65	RCT, DB, single oral dose, parallel groups. LA. Self-assessed at 0, 20 min, 40 min, 1 h, 1.5 h, 2 h then hourly intervals for 6 h. Med taken when baseline pain was of at least severe intensity.	PI (VAS scale)—'no pain – pain could not be worse' PR (5-pt scale) – (none,poor, mod., sufficient. total) Global rating (5-pt scale) by patient & by observer	Ibuprofen (400 mg) n = 80 Placebo n = 82	Ibuprofen was significantly superior to placebo for TOTPAR & both global ratings (P < 0.01). 6 h TOTPAR: Ibuprofen 14.9 Placebo 8.85.	Patients were allowed to remed after 1 h. If they remed before then their data was excluded from the efficacy analysis. After remed PR = 0 & PI = last score for all further timepoints.	245 analysed. Exclusions: 9 did not experience severe pain, 2 remed before 1 h, 1 completed the diaries incorrectly.	No serious AE were reported & no patient withdrew as a result of AE. No. of patients reporting AE; Ibuprofen 6/80 with ? AE Placebo 5/82 with ? AE.
[Cooper *et al.* 1977]	3rd molar extraction n = 245 Age: ?	RCT, DB, single oral dose, parallel groups. LA. Self-assessed at home at 0 then hourly intervals for 4 h. Med taken when baseline pain was of moderate to severe intensity.	PI (4-pt scale): standard PR (5-pt scale): standard 50% PR (y/n) Global rating (5-pt scale) by patient	Ibuprofen (400 mg) n = 40 Ibuprofen (200 mg) n = 38 Placebo n = 40	Ibuprofen at both doses was significantly superior to placebo for all measures of efficacy (P < 0.05) 4-h TOTPAR: Ibuprofen 400 mg 7.32 Ibuprofen 400 mg 6.27 Placebo 3.32.	Patients were allowed to remed after 2 h. If they remed before then their data was excluded from the efficacy analysis. After remed PR = 0 & PI = baseline score for all further timepoints.	192 analysed. Exclusions: 17 provided uninterpretable data, 12 took confounding med, 10 were lost to follow-up, 9 did not need med, 5 fell asleep.	No serious AE. were reported & no patient withdrew as a result of AE. No individual data was provided but there was no significant diff in occurrence between groups.
[Cooper *et al.* 1982]	3rd molar extraction n = 316 Age: 16–65	RCT, DB, single oral dose, parallel groups. Mostly LA. Self-assessed at home at 0 then hourly intervals for 4 h. Med taken when baseline pain was of moderate to severe intensity.	PI (4-pt scale): standard PR (5-pt scale): standard 50% PR (y/n) Global rating (5-pt scale) by patient	Ibuprofen (400 mg) n = 38 Placebo n = 46 Ibuprofen (400 mg) + Codeine n = 41 Codeine (60 mg) n = 41	All active treatments were significantly superior to placebo for SPID & TOTPAR (no P value given). 4 h TOTPAR: Ibuprofen 8.39 Placebo 2.65 Ibuprofen + codeine 9.39 Codeine 4.12.	Patients were allowed to remed after 1 h. If they remed before then their data was excluded from the efficacy analysis. After remed PR = 0 & PI = baseline score for all further timepoints.	249 analysed. Exclusions: 30 were lost to follow-up, 15 did not req. med, 11 remed before 1 h, 6 missed more the 1 evaluation, 3 medicated with slight pain, 1 did not take all the med, 1 medicated over 24 h after surgery.	No serious AE. were reported & no patient withdrew as a result of AE. No. of patients reporting AE; Ibuprofen 11/38 with 12 AE. Placebo 5/46 with 6 AE Ibuprofen + codeine 18/41 with 20 AE Codeine 11/41 with 11 AE.
[Cooper *et al.* 1988]	3rd molar extraction n = 201 Age: Adults	RCT, DB, single oral dose, parallel groups. LA + sedative. Self-assessed at home at 0 then hourly intervals for 6 h. Med taken when baseline pain was of moderate to severe intensity.	PI (4-pt scale): standard PR (5-pt scale): standard 50% PR (y/n) Global rating (5-pt scale) by patient	Ibuprofen (400 mg) n = 37 Placebo n = 43	Ibuprofen was significantly superior to placebo for all measures of efficacy (P < 0.01). 6 h TOTPAR: Ibuprofen 11.32 Placebo 4.67.	Patients were allowed to remed after 1 h. If they remed before then their data was excluded from the efficacy analysis. After remed PR = 0 & PI = baseline score for all further timepoints.	161 analysed. Exclusions: 20 did not req. med, 13 were lost to follow-up, 7 for various protocol violations.	No serious AE. were reported & no patient withdrew as a result of AE. No. of patients reporting AE; Ibuprofen 10/40 with 14 AE Placebo 7/45 with 7 AE.

Ref.	Condition & no. of patients	Design, study duration & follow-up	Outcome measures	Dose regimen	Analgesic outcome results	Remedication	Withdrawals & exclusions	Adverse effects
[Cooper *et al.* 1989]	3rd molar extraction *n* = 194 Age: 16+	RCT, DB, single oral dose, parallel groups LA. Self-assessed at home at 0, 0.5, 1 h then hourly intervals for 6 h. Med taken when baseline pain was of moderate to severe intensity.	PI (4-pt scale): standard PR (5-pt scale): standard 50% PR (y/n) Global rating (5-pt scale) by patient	Ibuprofen (400 mg) *n* = 61 Placebo *n* = 64	Ibuprofen was significantly superior to placebo for all measures of efficacy (*P* < 0.001) 6 h TOTPAR: Ibuprofen 11.32 Placebo 4.67	Patients were allowed to remed before 1 h. If they remed before then their data was excluded from the efficacy analysis. No details on how the data was handled for remed.	184 analysed. Exclusions: 2 were lost to follow-up, 2 did not req. med, 4 missed more than 1 evaluation, 1 had insufficient baseline pain, 1 failed to complete the diary of the appropriate time	No AE were reported & no patient withdrew as a result of AE. No. of patients reporting AE; Ibuprofen 5/63 with 6 AE Placebo 7/64 with 7 AE.
[Forbes *et al.* 1984]	3rd molar extraction *n* = 136 Age: 15+	RCT, DB, single oral dose, parallel groups GA. Self-assessed at home at 0 then hourly intervals for 12 h. Med taken when baseline pain was of moderate to severe intensity. Follow-up 5 days post surgery with the research nurse.	PI (4-pt scale): standard PR (5-pt scale): standard 50% PR (y/n) Global rating (5-pt scale) by patient	Ibuprofen (400 mg) *n* = 28 Placebo *n* = 28	Ibuprofen was significantly superior to placebo for all measures of efficacy (*P* < 0.01) 6 h TOTPAR: Ibuprofen 15.79 Placebo 3.79 4 h TOTPAR: Ibuprofen 10.75 Placebo 2.79	Patients were allowed to remed after 1 h. If they remed before then their data was excluded from the efficacy analysis. After remed PR = 0 & PI = baseline or last score (whichever was greater) for all further timepoints.	109 analysed. Exclusions: 21 did not req. med, 2 took rescue med instead of the trial med, 2 remed despite having some relief, 2 remed before 2 h.	No serious AE were reported & no patient withdrew as a result of AE. No. of patients reporting AE; Ibuprofen 5/28 with 6 AE Placebo 3/28 with 3 AE
[Forbes *et al.* 1990]	3rd molar extraction *n* = 269 Age: 15+	RCT, DB, single then multiple oral dose parallel groups. GA/ LA–unclear. Self-assessed at home at 0,1 then hourly for 6 h. Med taken when baseline pain was of moderate to severe intensity. Follow-up 5 days post surgery.	PI (4-pt scale): standard PR (5-pt scale): standard 50% PR (y/n) Global rating (5-pt scale) by patient	Ibuprofen (400 mg) *n* = 32 Placebo *n* = 34	Ibuprofen was significantly superior to placebo for all measures of analgesia (*P* < 0.05 at least) 6 h TOTPAR: Ibuprofen 10.47 Placebo 1.88	Patients were allowed to remed after 2 h. If they remed before then their data was excluded from the efficacy analysis. After remed PR = 0 & PI = baseline or last score (whichever was greater) for all further timepoints.	206 analysed. Exclusions: 3 lost to follow-up, 1 lost report card, 22 did not req. med, 8 remed despite having relief from study med, 6 remed with only slight pain, 13 remed <2 h, 7 failed to follow instructions, 3 did not complete the forms.	No serious AE were reported & no patient withdrew as a result of AE. No. of patients reporting AE; Ibuprofen 8/43 with 9 AE Placebo 0/38 with 0 AE
[Forbes *et al.* 1991]	3rd molar extraction *n* = 395 Age: 15+	RCT, DB, single oral dose, parallel groups. LA. 4 h caffeine washout prior to start. Self-assessed at 0, 0.5, 1 h then hourly intervals for 8 h. Med taken when baseline pain was mod-severe. Follow-up 5 days post surgery. Multi-centre (2 sites).	PI (4-pt scale) standard PR (5-pt scale): standard 50% PR (y/n) Global rating (5-pt scale) by patient	Ibuprofen (50 mg) *n* = 57 Ibuprofen (100 mg) *n* = 49 Ibuprofen (200 mg) *n* = 48 Placebo *n* = 51 Ibuprofen (100 mg) + caffeine (100 mg) *n* = 49 Ibuprofen (200 mg) + caffeine (100 mg) *n* = 44	All Ibuprofen treatments were sig superior to placebo for all measures (*P* < 0.05 at least) 8 h TOTPAR: Ibu 50 8.82 Ibu 100 8.46 Ibu 200 10.00 Placebo 2.58 100 combo 11.29 200 combo 15.58 {6 h TOTPAR calculated from the mean hourly scores}	Patients were allowed to remed after 2 h. If they remed before then their data was excluded from the efficacy analysis. After remed PR = 0 & PI = baseline or last score (whichever was greater) for all further timepoints.	298 analysed. Exclusions: 33 did not req. med, 14 remed <2 h, 1 ate caffeine containing food, 2 med for a headache, 1 rated only one side of mouth, 1 form completed by relative, 3 lacked consistency, 22 evaluated at incorrect time, 3 incomplete forms.	No serious AE were reported & no patient withdrew as a result of AE. Ibuprofen 50 10/63 with 15 AE Ibuprofen 100 5/62 with 6 AE Ibuprofen 200 6/60 with 6 AE Placebo 8/61 with 8 AE 100 mg Caffeine Combo 12/58 with 15 AE 200 mg Caffeine Combo 8/58 with 9 AE
[Forbes *et al.* 1991]	3rd molar extraction *n* = 288 Age: 15+	RCT, DB, single oral dose, parallel groups. LA. Self-assessed at home at 0, 1 then hourly for 8 h. Med taken when baseline pain was of moderate to severe intensity. Follow-up 5 days post surgery	PI (4-pt scale): standard PR (5-pt scale) : standard 50% PR (y/n) Global rating (5-pt scale) by patient	Ibuprofen (400 mg) *n* = 37 Placebo *n* = 39	Ibuprofen was significantly superior to placebo for all measures of efficacy (*P* < 0.05 at least) 8 h TOTPAR: Ibuprofen 14.30 Placebo 2.59 6 h TOTPAR calculated from the mean hourly scores Ibuprofen 10.97 Placebo 2.49	Patients were allowed to remed after 2 h. If they remed before then their data was excluded from the efficacy analysis. After remed PR = 0 & PI = baseline or last score (whichever was greater) for all further timepoints.	241 analysed. Exclusions: 7 were lost to follow-up, 12 did not req. med., 4 remed with some relief, 1 remed with slight pain, 19 remed before 2 h, 2 lacked consistency, 1 did not complete the form, 1 took only part of the med.	No serious AE were reported & no patient withdrew as a result of AE. No. of patients reporting AE; Ibuprofen 7/43 with 8 AE Placebo 3/47 with 3 AE
[Forbes *et al.* 1992]	3rd molar extraction *n* = 338 Age: 15+	RCT, DB, single oral dose, parallel groups. LA. Self-assessed at home at 0, 1 then hourly for 8 h. Med taken when baseline pain was of moderate to severe intensity. Follow-up 5 days post surgery.	PI (4-pt scale) : standard PR (5-pt scale) : standard 50% PR (y/n) Global rating (5-pt scale) by patient	Ibuprofen (400 mg) *n* = 38 Placebo *n* = 38	Ibuprofen was significantly superior to placebo for all measures of efficacy (*P* < 0.01) 8 h TOTPAR: Ibuprofen 14.82 Placebo 2.34 6 h TOTPAR calculated from the mean hourly scores Ibuprofen 11.79 Placebo 2.06	Patients were allowed to remed after 2 h. If they remed before then their data was excluded from the efficacy analysis. After remed PR = 0 & PI = baseline or last score (whichever was greater) for all further timepoints.	280 analysed. Exclusions: 3 did not return form, 14 did not req. med, 4 remed despite some relief, 6 remed with slight pain, 18 remed before 2 h, 2 lacked consistency, 2 did not complete form, 2 took only part of med, 5 took back up med.	No serious AE were reported & no patient withdrew as a result of AE. No. of patients reporting AE; Ibuprofen 4/45 with 8 AE Placebo 2/46 with 5 AE

Ref.	Condition & no. of patients	Design, study duration & follow-up	Outcome measures	Dose regimen	Analgesic outcome results	Remediation	Withdrawals & exclusions	Adverse effects
[Frame *et al.* 1989]	3rd molar extraction *n* = 148 Age: 16+	RCT, DB, single oral dose, parallel groups LA. Self-assessed at home at 0, 0.5, 1 then hourly for 5 h. Med taken when baseline pain was of at least moderate intensity.	PI (9-pt scale): non-standard PR (5-pt scale): standard 50% PR (y/N)	Ibuprofen (400 mg) *n* = 42 Placebo *n* = 38	At 2 & 3 h ibuprofen was significantly superior to placebo. 5-h TOTPAR calculated from the graph Ibuprofen 12.85 Placebo 7.95	Patients were allowed to remed after 2 h. No info provided on how data was handled for patients who remed	123 analysed. Exclusions: 9 did not take the med, 7 were lost to follow-up, 1 was asleep so did not complete the forms, 1 had complications so did not complete the form, 7 had slight pain.	No serious AE were reported & no patient withdrew as a result of AE. No. of patients reporting AE; Ibuprofen 2/42 with 2 AE Placebo 1/38 with 3 AE
[Fricke *et al.* 1993]	3rd molar extraction *n* = 207 Age: 15+	RCT, DB, single oral dose, parallel groups. 72 h washout prior to start. LA. Self-assessed at home at 0, 20, 30, 40, 60 min then hourly for 12 h. Med taken when baseline pain was of moderate intensity. Review 1/2 days after the trial.	PI (4-pt scale): standard PR (5-pt scale): standard 50% PR (y/n) Global rating (5-pt scale) by patient 50% PR (y/n) PI (VAS): no pain to worst pain imaginable	Ibuprofen (400 mg) *n* = 81 Placebo *n* = 39	Ibuprofen was significantly superior to placebo for all measures after 30 min. 6 h TOTPAR Ibuprofen 10.9 Placebo 2.9	Patients were allowed to remed after 2 h. After remed PR = 0 & PI = baseline or last score (whichever was greater) for all further timepoints.	201 analysed. Exclusions: 1 took the med twice, 5 had insufficient pain.	No serious AE were reported & 1 patient in the ibuprofen group withdrew as a result of vomiting which the investigators did not attribute to the med. No. of patients reporting AE; Ibuprofen 8/81 with 13 AE Placebo 1/39 with 1 AE
[Gay *et al.* 1996]	3rd molar extraction *n* = 206 Age: 18–60	RCT, DB, single oral dose, parallel groups. 12 h washout prior to start LA, Self-assessed at 'regular intervals' for 6 h. Med taken when baseline pain was of moderate to severe intensity.	PI (4-pt scale): standard PR (5-pt scale): standard 50% PR (y/n) Global rating (5-pt scale) by patient PI (VAS): no pain to worst pain imaginable	Ibuprofen (400 mg) *n* = 41 Placebo *n* = 39	Ibuprofen was significantly superior to placebo for all summary measures of analgesia (*P* < 0.05). 6 h TOTPAR Ibuprofen 13.6 Placebo 5.2	Patients were allowed to remed after 1 h. If they remed before then their data was excluded from the efficacy analysis. After remed PR = 0 & PI = baseline of last score (whichever was greater) for all further timepoints.	194 analysed. Exclusions: 2 remed before 1 h, 10 failed to complete the assessments within 15 min of the scheduled time.	No serious AE were reported & no patient withdrew as a result of AE. No. of patients reporting AE; Ibuprofen 3/41 with 3 AE Placebo 4/41 with 7 AE
[Heidrich *et al.* 1985]	Orthopaedic surgery *n* = 120 Age: 18–65	RCT, DB, single oral dose, parallel groups. 4 h washout prior to start. Assessed by trained nurse observer at 0, 0.5, 1 then hourly intervals for 6 h. Med taken when baseline pain was of moderate to severe intensity.	PI (4-pt scale) PR (5-pt scale) PI-VAS 'no relief' —'complete relief' PI (VAS): 'no pain'. —'worst pain imaginable' McGill pain questionnaire	Ibuprofen (400 mg) *n* = 40 Placebo *n* = 40	Orthogonal analyses of variance showed ibuprofen produced greater relief from pain than placebo. 6 h VAS-TOTPAR Ibuprofen 234 Placebo 104	No info was given on patients who remed	No info given on any exclusions.	'There were no diff among treatments in terms of side effects. No patient withdrew because of AE'.
[Hersch *et al.* 1993]	3rd molar extraction *n* = 254 Age: 16+	RCT, DB, single oral dose, parallel groups. 4 h washout prior to start. LA. Self-assessed at 0, 0.5, 1 then hourly for 8 h (for the first 2 h this was in the clinic). Med taken when baseline pain was of moderate to severe intensity.	PI (4-pt scale): standard PR (5-pt scale): standard Global rating (5-pt scale) by patient	Ibuprofen (400 mg) *n* = 49 Ibuprofen (200 mg) *n* = 51 Placebo *n* = 51	Ibuprofen at both doses was significantly superior to placebo for all measures of analgesia (*P* < 0.05). 6 h TOTPAR calculated from the graph Ibuprofen 400 mg 9.1 Ibuprofen 200 mg 6.68 Placebo 1.18	Patients were allowed to remed after 1 h. If they remed before then their data was excluded from the efficacy analysis. After remed PR = 0 & PI = baseline or last score (whichever was greater) for all further timepoints.	254 analysed No exclusions.	No serious AE were reported & no patient withdrew as a result of AE. No. of patients reporting AE; Ibuprofen 400 mg 6/49 with 7 AE Ibuprofen 200 mg 4/51 with 4 AE Placebo 9/51 with 9 AE
[Hersch *et al.* 1993]	3rd molar extraction *n* = 114 Age: Did not say	RCT, DB, pre-surgery placebo then single oral dose, parallel groups. LA. Self-assessed at 0, 0.5, 1 then hourly for 6 h. Med taken when baseline pain was of moderate to severe intensity.	PI (4-pt scale): standard PR (5-pt scale): standard 50% PR (y/n) Global rating (5-pt scale) by patient	Placebo then Ibuprofen (400 mg) *n* = 12 Placebo then Placebo *n* = 16	Ibuprofen was significantly superior to placebo for all summary measures of analgesia. 6 h TOTPAR Ibuprofen 15.67 Placebo 9.00	Patients were allowed to remed after 1 h. After remed PR = 0 & PI = baseline or last score (whichever was greater) for all further timepoints.	81 analysed. Exclusions: 19 lost to follow-up, 11 did not req. med, 3 excluded for various protocol violations.	No info was given on AE.

Ref.	Condition & no. of patients	Design, study duration & follow-up	Outcome measures	Dose regimen	Analgesic outcome results	Remediation	Withdrawals & exclusions	Adverse effects
[Jain *et al.* 1986]	3rd molar extraction n = 260 Age: 18–65	RCT, DB, single oral dose, parallel groups. Self-assessed at home at 0, 1 then hourly for 6 h. Med taken when baseline pain was of moderate to severe intensity.	PI (4-pt scale): standard wording but scale 1–4 PR (5-pt scale): non-standard Global rating (5-pt scale) by patient PI (VAS): 'no pain' – 'worst ever pain'	Ibuprofen (400 mg) n = 49 Ibuprofen (200 mg) n = 47 Ibuprofen (100 mg) n = 39 Placebo n = 47	All doses of ibuprofen were significantly superior to placebo ($P < 0.001$). 6-h SPID Ibuprofen 400 mg 3.0 Ibuprofen 200 mg 2.26 Ibuprofen 100 mg 1.54 Placebo 1.73.	Patients were allowed to remed after 1 h. If they remed before then their data was excluded from the efficacy analysis. After remed PR = 0 & PI = last score for all further timepoints.	227 analysed. Exclusions: 10 remed before 1 h, 19 did not take the med or were lost to follow-up, 2 had mild baseline pain, 1 missed >2 evaluations & 1 used confounding drugs.	No serious AE were reported & no patient withdrew as a result of AE. No. of patients reporting AE: Ibuprofen 400 mg 10/? with 12 AE Ibuprofen 200 mg 6/? with 8 AE Ibuprofen 100 mg 13/? with 15 AE Placebo 12/? with 15 AE.
[Jain *et al.* 1988]	Episiotomy n = 161 Age: 18+	RCT, DB, single oral dose, parallel groups. 4 h washout prior to start. Assessed by trained nurse observer at 0, 0.5, 1 then hourly for 6 h. Med taken when baseline pain was of moderate to severe intensity	PI (4-pt scale): standard PR (5-pt scale): standard Time to meaningful relief Global rating (5-pt scale) by patient Overall improvement (7-pt scale) by patient	Ibuprofen (400 mg) n = 49 Placebo n = 48	Ibuprofen was significantly superior to placebo for most summary measures of analgesia ($P < 0.01$). 6 h TOTPAR Ibuprofen 14.4 Placebo 8.61.	Patients were allowed to remed after 2 h. If they remed before then their data was excluded from the efficacy analysis. After remed PR = baseline or last score (whichever was greater) for all further timepoints.	147 analysed. Exclusions: 11 remed before 2 h, 2 received confounding agents, 1 was under 18 yrs old.	No serious AE were reported & no patient withdrew as a result of AE. No. of patients reporting AE; Ibuprofen 2/49 with 2 AE Placebo 1/48 with 1 AE
[Kiersch *et al.* 1993]	3rd molar extraction n = 205 Age: 15+	RCT, DB, single oral dose, parallel groups. 72 h washout prior to start. Self-assessed at home at 0, 20, 30, 40, 60 min then hourly for 12 h. Med taken when baseline pain was of at least moderate intensity. Review 1/2 days after the trial.	PI (4-pt scale): standard PR (5-pt scale): standard 50% PR (y/n) Global rating (5-pt scale) by patient PI (VAS): no pain to worst pain imaginable	Ibuprofen (200 mg) n = 81 Placebo n = 42	Ibuprofen was significantly superior to placebo for all summary measures of analgesia ($P < 0.001$). 6 h TOTPAR Ibuprofen 10.3 Placebo 3.7	Patients were allowed to remed after 2 h. No info was given on how the data was then handled.	203 analysed. Exclusions: 2 for protocol violations.	No serious AE were reported & no patient withdrew as a result of AE. No. of patients reporting AE; Ibuprofen 16/81 with 20 AE Placebo 5/43 with 5 AE
[Laska *et al.* 1986]	3rd molar extraction n = 200 Age: 16+	RCT, DB, single oral dose, parallel groups. 4 h washout prior to start. Self-assessed at 0, 0.5, 1 then hourly for 6 h. Med taken when baseline pain was of moderate to severe intensity.	PI (4-pt scale): standard PR (5-pt scale) Global rating by patient Blood serum levels	Ibuprofen (400 mg) n = ? Ibuprofen (600 mg) n = ? Ibuprofen (800 mg) n = ? Placebo n = ? assumed an equal distribution of 40 patients per group	All three doses of ibuprofen were significantly superior to placebo for %SPID. 6 h SPID calculated from the PID graph Ibuprofen 400 mg 13.4 Ibuprofen 600 mg 14.1 Ibuprofen 800 mg 13.9 Placebo 5.3.	Patients were allowed to remed after 1 h. If they remed before then their data was excluded from the efficacy analysis. After remed PR = 0 & PI = baseline or last score (whichever was greater) for all further timepoints.	195 analysed. Exclusions: 4 remed before 1 h & 1 vomited within 5 min of taking the study med.	No patient withdrew as a result of AE. No. of patients reporting AE; Ibuprofen 400 mg 1/? with 1 AE Placebo 3/? with 3 AE.
[Lavenziana *et al.* 1996]	Postop (inguinal hernia) n = 125 Age: 18–75	RCT, DB, single oral dose, parallel groups. 6 h washout prior to start. Assessed in hospital at 0, 15, 30, 45, 60, 90 min, 2 h then hourly for up to 6 h. Med taken when baseline pain was of moderate to severe intensity.	PI (VAS): 'no pain' 'unbearable pain' Global rating (5-pt scale) by patient	Ibuprofen arginine soluble (400 mg) n = 42 Placebo n = 41	Patients with 61–80 mm baseline pain—were significantly superior to placebo ($P < 0.05$). Patients with >81 mm baseline pain—no significant diff. VAS-SPID from graph Ibuprofen 250 Placebo 215.	Patients were allowed to remed after 1 h. Patients were asked to wait until their pain returned to baseline Intensity before remed but no info was given on how the data was then handled.	124 analysed. Exclusions: 1 patient for insufficient pain.	No AE were reported.

Ref.	Condition & no. of patients	Design, study duration & follow-up	Outcome measures	Dose regimen	Analgesic outcome results	Remedication	Withdrawals & exclusions	Adverse effects
[McQuay et al. 1996]	3rd molar extraction n = 218 Age: 16–53	RCT, DB, single oral dose, parallel groups. 12 h washout prior to start. LA. Self-assessed for 6 h (did not say at what points). Med taken if baseline pain was of moderate to severe intensity within 2 h of surgery.	PI (4-pt scale): standard PR (5-pt scale): standard Global rating (5-pt scale) by patient PI (VAS): no pain to worst pain imaginable PR (VAS): no relief to complete relief Random 8 word scale Mood (VAS) Stopwatch to meaningful relief	Ibuprofen (400 mg) n = 30 Ibuprofen (200 mg) n = 31 Placebo n = 11	Ibuprofen at both doses was significantly superior to placebo for all measures of analgesia. 6 h TOTPAR calculated from the graph Ibuprofen 400 mg 9.1 Ibuprofen 200 mg 6.68 Placebo 1.18.	Patients were allowed to remed after 45 min. If they remed before then their data was excluded from the efficacy analysis. After remed PR = 0 & PI = baseline for all further timepoints.	161 analysed. Exclusions: 15 no pain, 10 concurrent illness, 7 analgesics within 48 h, 4 withdrew before study began, 4 did not attend, 3 previous NSAID allergy, 1 possible pregnancy, 1 migraine after surgery, 1 surgery cancelled, 3 remed before 45 min.	No serious AE were reported & no patient withdrew as a result of AE. No. of patients reporting AE; Ibuprofen 400 mg 2/30 with 3 AE Ibuprofen 200 mg 4/31 with 4 AE Placebo 1/11 with 1 AE.
[Mehlisch et al. 1990]	Various oral surgery procedures n = 706 Age: 18–64	RCT, DB, single oral dose, parallel groups. 6 h washout prior to start. Self-assessed at 0, 0.5, 1 h then hourly for up to 6 h. Med taken when baseline pain was of moderate to severe intensity.	PI (4-pt scale): standard wording scale 1–4 PR (4-pt scale): non-standard	Ibuprofen (400 mg) n = 306 Placebo n = 85	Ibuprofen was significantly superior for most summary measures of efficacy. 6-h SPID Ibuprofen 5.84 Placebo 0.99	Patients were allowed to remed. After remed PR = 0 & PI = baseline score for all further timepoints.	697 analysed. Exclusions: 4 were lost to follow-up, 4 were entered in the trial twice (1st entry only was analysed for efficacy but both were included in safety analysis) & 1 was excluded for failing to meet inclusion criteria.	No serious AE were reported & no patient withdrew as a result of AE. No. of patients reporting AE; Ibuprofen 31/310 with ? AE. Placebo 12/85 with ? AE.
[Mehlisch et al. 1995]	3rd molar extraction n = 205 Age: 15+	RCT, DB, single oral dose, parallel groups. 12 h washout prior to start. LA. Self-assessed at 0, 15, 30, 45, 90 min, 2 h then hourly for 6 h. Med taken when baseline pain was of moderate to severe intensity.	PI (4-pt scale): standard PR (5-pt scale): standard Global rating (5-pt scale) by patient	Ibuprofen (400 mg) n = 98 Placebo n = 40	Ibuprofen was significantly superior to placebo for all measures of analgesia (P < 0.05). 6 h TOTPAR Ibuprofen 14.39 Placebo 2.62	Patients were allowed to remed after 1 h (but were encouraged to wait for 4 h). If they remed before then their data was excluded from the efficacy analysis. After remed PR & PID = 0 for all further timepoints.	239 analysed. Exclusion: 1 patient only had 1 molar removed & failed to complete the diary.	No serious AE were reported & no patient withdrew as a result of AE. No. of patients reporting AE; Ibuprofen 12/98 with ? AE. Placebo 4/40 with ? AE
[Nelson et al. 1994]	3rd molar extraction n = 183 Age: 15+	RCT, DB, single oral dose, parallel groups. 12 h washout prior to start. LA. Self-assessed at 0, 15, 30, 45, 60, 90 min, 2 h then hourly for 6 h. Med taken when baseline pain was of moderate to severe intensity.	PI (4-pt scale): standard PR (5-pt scale): standard 50% PR (y/n) Global rating (5-pt scale) by patient	Ibuprofen (200 mg) n = 75 Placebo n = 40	Ibuprofen was significantly superior to placebo for PR & PID from 30 min to the end. 6 h TOTPAR Ibuprofen 12.31 Placebo 5.56	Patients were allowed to remed after 1 h. If they remed before then their data was excluded from the efficacy analysis. After remed PR = 0 & PI = 0 for all further timepoints.	180 analysed. Exclusions: 2 remed before 1 h, 1 did not record baseline pain intensity.	No serious AE were reported & no patient withdrew as a result of AE. No. of patients reporting AE; Ibuprofen 16/77 with ? AE Placebo 11/41 with ? AE.
[Pagnoni et al. 1996]	Caesarean section n = 92 Age: 18+	RCT, DB, single oral dose, parallel groups. 6 h washout prior to start. GA. Assessed in hospital at 0, 15, 30, 45, 60, 90 min, 2 h then hourly for 6 h. Med taken when baseline pain was >55 mm.	PI (VAS): 'no pain' —'unbearable pain' Global rating (5-pt scale) by patient	Ibuprofen arginine soluble (400 mg) n = 30 Placebo n = 32	The sum of PID & the mean AUC showed ibuprofen to be significantly superior to placebo (P < 0.001) the mean peak PID value was also significantly superior to placebo (P < 0.05). 6 h VAS-SPID from graph Ibuprofen 181 mm Placebo 65 mm	Patients were allowed to remed after 1 h. If they remed before then their data was excluded from the efficacy analysis. After remed PI = last recorded value for all further timepoints.	92 analysed. Exclusions: none	No AE reported.
[Parker et al. 1986]	Tonsillectomy n = 139 Age: 16–66	RCT, DB, single oral dose then multiple doses, parallel groups. GA. Assessed in hospital at 0, 0.5, 1 then hourly for 4 h. Med taken when baseline pain was of moderate to severe intensity.	PI (9-pt scale): non-standard PR (5-pt scale): standard 50% PR (y/n) Observer noted their impression of the patients progress	Ibuprofen syrup (600 mg) n = 44 Placebo n = 33	Ibuprofen was significantly superior to placebo at 30 min & 1 h. 4 h TOTPAR Ibuprofen 10.92 Placebo 9.37	No info was given on patients who remed	110 analysed. No info was given on the 29 exclusions.	No details were given on the AE occurring during the single dose. For the multiple doses 1 patient in the placebo group withdrew as a result of AE. The number of AE reported was similar for both groups.

Ref.	Condition & no. of patients	Design, study duration & follow-up	Outcome measures	Dose regimen	Analgesic outcome results	Remediation	Withdrawals & exclusions	Adverse effects
[Schachtel et al. 1989]	Episiotomy $n = 115$ Age: 16–37	RCT, DB, single oral dose then multiple doses, parallel groups. 4 h washout prior to start. Assessed in hospital at 0, 0.5, 1 then hourly for 4 h. Med taken when baseline pain was of moderate to severe intensity.	PI (4-pt scale): standard PR (5-pt scale): standard Global rating (5-pt scale) by patient	Ibuprofen (400 mg) $n = 36$ Placebo $n = 38$	Ibuprofen was significantly superior to placebo for all measures of analgesia ($P < 0.05$) at least. 4 h TOTPAR Ibuprofen 10.4 Placebo 5.5	Patients were allowed to remed after 1 h. If they remed before then their data was excluded from the efficacy analysis. After remed PR = 0 & PI = last or baseline (which ever was greater) for all further timepoints.	111 analysed. Exclusions: 4 remed before 1 h.	No AE reported.
[Seymour et al. 1991]	3rd molar extraction $n = 205$ Age: Adults	RCT, DB, single oral dose, parallel groups. GA. Assessed in hospital by the same observer at 0, 10, 20, 30, 45, 60, 90 min, 2 h then hourly for 6 h. Med taken when baseline pain was >30 mm.	PI (VAS): 'no pair' – 'unbearable pain' Global rating (5-pt scale) by patient	Study 1 Ibuprofen (400 mg) tablets $n = 31$ Ibuprofen (400 mg) liquid in gelatin capsules $n = 32$ Placebo $n = 32$ Study 2 Ibuprofen (400 mg) tablets $n = 30$ Ibuprofen (400 mg) soluble $n = 32$ Placebo $n = 30$	1: Both Ibuprofen were sig superior to placebo; NSD between the 2 active groups. 2: Sol Ibuprofen was sig superior to placebo from 20 min; tablets from 30 min 6 h VAS-SPID Gel 233 mm Tablets 243 Placebo 120 Sol 228 mm Tablets 214 Placebo 86	Patients were allowed to remed. After remed PI = last score for all further timepoints.	187 analysed but claimed to have enrolled only 180?	No serious AE were reported & no patient withdrew as a result of AE. Only 1 patient reported an AE, they were in the placebo groups of study 1.
[Seymour et al. 1966]	3rd molar extraction $n = 148$ Age: Adults	RCT, DB, single oral dose, parallel groups. GA. Assessed in hospital by nurse observer at 0, 10, 20, 30, 45, 60, 75, 90, 120, 150 min, 3 h then hourly for 6 h. Med taken when baseline pain was >30 mm.	PI (VAS): 'no pain' – 'unbearable pain' Global rating (5-pt scale) by patient	Ibuprofen (600 mg) tablets $n = 17$ Ibuprofen (600 mg) soluble $n = 17$ Ibuprofen (400 mg) tablets $n = 15$ Ibuprofen (400 mg) soluble $n = 16$ Ibuprofen (200 mg) tablets $n = 18$ Ibuprofen (200 mg) soluble $n = 17$ Placebo $n = 19$	All ibuprofen treatments except ibuprofen 200 mg resulted in significantly less pain than placebo for all efficacy measures ($P < 0.05$). 6 h VAS-SPID Ibuprofen 600 T 230 Ibuprofen 600 S 148 Ibuprofen 400 T 258 Ibuprofen 400 S 238 Ibuprofen 200 T 140 Ibuprofen 200 S 198 Placebo 44	Patients were allowed to remed. After remed PI = last score for all further timepoints.	199 analysed. Exclusions: 4 were excluded for 'unwanted effects' & 25 failed to reach a sufficient baseline pain intensity.	4 patients reported AE, 3 had received ibuprofen (did not clarify which dose) & 1 had taken placebo.
[Sunshine et al. 1983]	Episiotomy $n = 115$ Age: 18+	RCT, DB, single oral dose, parallel groups. 4 h washout prior to start. Assessed in hospital by the same observer at 0, 0.5, 1 h then hourly for 4 h. Med taken when baseline pain was of moderate to severe intensity.	PI (4-pt scale): standard PR (5-pt scale): non-standard (percentages not descriptive wording) Global rating of med (4-pt scale) by patient Global rating of personal improvement (7-pt scale) by patient	Ibuprofen (400 mg) $n = 30$ Placebo $n = 30$	Ibuprofen was significantly superior to placebo for all measures of analgesia from 1 h onwards. 4 h SPID Ibuprofen 6.47 Placebo 1.12	Patients were allowed to remed after 1 h. If they remed before then their data was excluded from the efficacy analysis. After remed PR = 0 & PI = last for all further timepoints.	120 analysed. Exclusions: none	No patient reported any AE.

Ref.	Condition & no. of patients	Design, study duration & follow-up	Outcome measures	Dose regimen	Analgesic outcome results	Remedication	Withdrawals & exclusions	Adverse effects
[Sunshine *et al.* 1987]	Episiotomy, Caesarean section or gynae surgery n = 200 Age: ?	RCT, DB, single oral dose, parallel groups. 4 h washout prior to start. Assessed in hospital by the same observer at 0, 0.5, 1 h then hourly for 4 h. Med taken when baseline pain was of moderate to severe intensity.	PI (4-pt scale): standard PR (5-pt scale): non-standard (percentages not descriptive wording) Global rating of med (4-pt scale) by patient Global rating of personal improvement (7-pt scale) by patient	Ibuprofen (400 mg) n = 38 Placebo n = 40	All active treatments were significantly superior to placebo for TOTPAR & all except codeine for SPID. 4 h SPID Ibuprofen 8.1 Placebo 5.2	Patients were allowed to remed after 1 h. If they remed before then their data was excluded from the efficacy analysis. After remed PR = 0 & PI = last for all further timepoints.	195 analysed. Exclusions: 1 had not complied with the washout period & 4 did not complete the evaluations.	No AE were reported in either the placebo or ibuprofen groups.

AE, adverse effect; DB, double-blind; GA, general anaesthesia; LA, local anaesthesia; NSD, no significant difference; PI, pain intensity; PR, pain relief; SPID, summed pain intensity differences; TOTPAR, total pain relief; VAS, visual analogue scale.

Appendix 2
Diclofenac vs. placebo: trial details

Ref.	Condition & no. of patients	Design, study duration & follow-up	Outcome measures	Dose regimen	Analgesic outcome results	Remedication	Withdrawals & exclusions	Adverse effects
[Ahlstrom *et al.* 1993]	3rd molar extraction n = 127 Age: 18–40	RCT, DB, single oral dose, parallel groups. 4 h washout prior to start. Evaluated at 0, 20, 40 min 1 h then hourly intervals for 6 h. Med taken when baseline pain was at least moderate intensity (>30 mm).	PI (VAS): 'no pain at all' – 'agonizing pain' Global rating by patient	Diclofenac (50 mg) drinkable n = 35 Placebo n = 30	Diclofenac was significantly superior to Placebo by 40 min (*P* = 0.001) this continued for 6 h. TOTPI & SPID; Diclofenac was significantly superior to placebo (*P* < 0.0001). 6-h SPID: Diclofenac 173 mm Placebo 32 mm	Patients were allowed to remed after 1 h. After remed PI = last score was carried forward for all further timepoints.	97 analysed. Exclusions: 30 for various protocol violations.	No serious AE were reported & no patient withdrew as a result of AE. No. of patients reporting AE; Diclofenac 6/35 with ? AE Placebo 2/30 with ? AE.
[Bakshi *et al.* 1992]	3rd molar extraction n = 180 Age: Adults	RCT, DB, single oral dose, parallel groups. 4 h washout prior to start. Self-assessed at 0, 15, 30 min, 1 h then hourly intervals for 6 h. Med taken when baseline pain was of at least moderate intensity.	PI (4-pt scale): standard PR (4-pt scale): non-standard 50% PR (y/n) Global rating (4-pt scale) by patient	Diclofenac potassium (50 mg)— sugar coated n = 51 Diclofenac sodium (50 mg)— enteric coated n = 54 Placebo n = 46	Diclofenac K was significantly superior to placebo for SPID, TOTPAR, MAXPID & MAXPAR (*P* < 0.001). Diclofenac Na was significantly superior to placebo for SPID (*P* = 0.023) & MAXPID (*P* = 0.018) 6-h SPID: Diclofenac K 7.8 Diclofenac Na 5.3 Placebo 2.6	Patients were allowed to remed after 1 h. If they remed before then their data was excluded from the efficacy analysis. After remed PR = 0 & PI = last score or baseline (whichever was greater) for all further timepoints.	151 analysed. Exclusions: 26 did not require med & 3 were lost to follow-up.	No serious AE were reported & no patient withdrew as a result of AE. No. of patients reporting AE; Diclofenac K 3/51 with 5 AE Diclofenac Na 1/54 with 1 AE Placebo 3/46 with 3 AE.
[Bakshi *et al.* 1994]	3rd molar extraction n = 257 Age: Adults–65	RCT, DB, single oral dose, parallel groups. LA. Self-assessed at 0, 20 min, 40 min, 1 h, 1.5 h, 2 h then hourly intervals for 6 h. Med taken when baseline pain was of at least severe intensity.	PI (VAS): 'no pain – pain could not be worse' PR (5-pt scale): (none, poor, mod, sufficient, total) Global rating (5-pt scale) by patient & by observer—non standard	Diclofenac (50 mg) dispersible n = 83 Placebo n = 82	Diclofenac was significantly superior to placebo for TOTPAR & both global ratings (*P* < 0.01). 6-h TOTPAR: Diclofenac 15.45 Placebo 8.85	Patients were allowed to remed after 1 h. If they remed before then their data was excluded from the efficacy analysis. After remed PR = 0 & PI = last score for all further timepoints.	245 analysed. Exclusions: 9 did not experience severe pain, 2 remed before 1 h, 1 completed the diaries incorrectly.	No serious AE were reported & no patient withdrew as a result of AE. No. of patients reporting AE; Diclofenac 4/83 with ? AE Placebo 5/82 with ? AE.
[Hebertson *et al.* 1994]	Gynae surgery n = 217 Age: 16+	RCT, DB, single oral dose, parallel groups. 4 h washout prior to start. Assessed by observer at 0, 0.5, 1 h then hourly intervals for 8 h. Med taken when baseline pain was of moderate to severe intensity & groups stratified by baseline PI.	PI (4-pt scale): standard PR (5-pt scale): standard Global rating (5-pt scale) by patient	Diclofenac (50 mg) n = 52 Diclofenac (100 mg) n = 52 Placebo n = 52	Both diclofenac doses were significantly superior to placebo for pain relief at each timepoint from 1 h onwards. 6-h TOTPAR from graph: Diclofenac 50 mg 12.1 Diclofenac 100 mg 12.2 Placebo 3.7	Patients were allowed to remed after 1 h. If they remed before their data was excluded from the efficacy analysis. After remed the patients were discontinued but no info was given on how their data was then handled.	209 analysed for at least 1 efficacy analysis. 194 analysed for 8 h SPID & TOTPAR. No info given on any exclusions.	All AE were gastrointestinal except 1 in the placebo group (not defined), 1 withdrew from Diclofenac 100 mg for nausea & vomiting. No. of patients reporting AE; Diclofenac 50 mg 3/54 with ? AE Diclofenac 100 mg 2/55 with ? AE Placebo 2/54 with ? AE
[Mehlisch *et al.* 1994]	3rd molar extraction n = 208 Age: 16–70	RCT, DB, single oral dose, parallel groups. LA. 4 h washout prior to start. Self-assessed at 0, 0.5, 1 h then hourly for up to 8 h. Med taken when baseline pain was of moderate to severe intensity.	PI (4-pt scale): standard PR (5-pt scale): standard Global rating (5-pt scale) by patient	Diclofenac (50 mg) n = 53 Diclofenac (100 mg) n = 52 Placebo n = 52	Both Diclofenac groups were significantly superior to placebo for all timepoints with regard to pain relief. 6-h TOTPAR from graph: Diclofenac 50 mg 11.6 Diclofenac 100 mg 14.3 Placebo 3.3	Patients were allowed to remed after 2 h. After remed PR = 0 & PI = last score for all further timepoints.	There were no exclusions.	No serious AE were reported & no patient withdrew as a result of AE. No. of patients reporting AE; Diclofenac 50 mg 2/53 with ? AE Diclofenac 100 mg 2/52 with ? AE Placebo 2/52 with ? AE

Ref.	Condition & no. of patients	Design, study duration & follow-up	Outcome measures	Dose regimen	Analgesic outcome results	Remediation	Withdrawals & exclusions	Adverse effects
[Nelson *et al.* 1994]	3rd molar extraction n = 255 Age: 16–70	RCT, DB, single oral close, parallel groups. LA. 4 h washout prior to start. Self-assessed at 0, 0.5, 1 h then hourly for up to 8 h. Med taken when baseline pain was of moderate to severe intensity.	PI (4-pt scale): standard PR (5-pt scale): standard	Diclofenac (25 mg) n = ? Diclofenac (50 mg) n = ? Diclofenac (100 mg) n = ? Placebo n = ? NB assumed an equal distribution 51 per group (inc ASA group)	All diclofenac groups were significantly superior to placebo for pain relief from 1 h onwards. 6-h TOTPAR from graph: Diclofenac 25 mg 10.5 Diclofenac 50 mg 12.2 Diclofenac 100 mg 14.8 Placebo 3.6	Patients were allowed to remed at 1 h, no info was given as to how their data was then handled.	252 analysed for at least 1 efficacy analysis. No exclusions other than remed were given.	No serious AE were reported & no patient withdrew as a result of AE. No. of patients reporting AE; Diclofenac 25 mg 5 with ? AE Diclofenac 50 mg 4 with ? AE Diclofenac 100 mg 4 with ? AE Placebo 6 with ? AE

See Appendix 1 for key to abbreviations.

Appendices 1 and 2 references

Ahlström U, Bakshi R, Nilsson P, Wåhlander L. The analgesic efficacy of diclofenac dispersible and ibuprofen in postoperative pain after dental extraction. *European Journal of Clinical Pharmacology* 1993; **44**:587–8.

Arnold JD. Ketoprofen, ibuprofen, and placebo in the relief of postoperative pain. *Advances in Therapeutics* 1990; **7**:264–275.

Bakshi R, Frenkel G, Dietlein G, Meurer With B, Schneider B, Sinterhauf U. A placebo-controlled comparative evaluation of diclofenac dispersible versus ibuprofen in postoperative pain after third molar surgery. *Journal of Clinical Pharmacology* 1994; **34**:225–30.

Bakshi R, Jacobs LD, Lehnert S, Picha B, Reuther J. A double-blind, placebo-controlled trial comparing the analgesic efficacy of two formulations of diclofenac in postoperative dental pain. *Current Therapeutic Research* 1992; **52**:435–42.

Cooper SA, Berrie R, Cohn P. Comparison of ketoprofen, ibuprofen and placebo in a dental surgery pain model. *Advances in Therapeutics* 1988; **5**:43–53.

Cooper SA, Engel J, Ladov M, Precheur H, Rosenheck A, Rauch D. Analgesic efficacy of an ibuprofen codeine combination. *Pharmacotherapy* 1982; **2**:162–7.

Cooper SA, Needle SE, Kruger GO Comparative analgesic potency of aspirin and ibuprofen. *Journal of Oral Surgery* 1977; **35**:898–903.

Cooper SA, Schachtel BP, Goldman E, Gelb S, Cohn P. Ibuprofen and acetaminophen in the relief of acute pain: a randomized, double blind, placebo controlled study. *Journal of Clinical Pharmacology* 1989; **29**:1026–30.

Forbes JA, Barkaszi BA, Ragland RN Hankle JJ. Analgesic effect of fendosal, ibuprofen and aspirin in postoperative oral surgery pain. *Pharmacotherapy* 1984; **4**:385–91.

Forbes JA, Beaver WT, Jones KF, Edquist IA, *et al.* Gongloff CM, Smith WK et al. Analgesic efficacy of bromfenac, ibuprofen, and aspirin in postoperative oral surgery pain. *Clinical Pharmacology and Therapeutics* 1992; **51**:343–52.

Forbes JA, Beaver WT, Jones KF, Kehm CJ, Smith WK *et al.* Effect of caffeine on ibuprofen analgesia in postoperative oral surgery pain. *Clinical Pharmacology and Therapentics* 1991; **49**:674–84.

Forbes JA, Edquist IA, Smith FG, Schwartz MK, Beaver WT. Evaluation of bromfenac, aspirin, and ibuprofen in postoperative oral surgery pain. *Pharmacotherapy* 1991; **11**:64–70.

Forbes JA, Kehm CJ, Grodin CD, Beaver WT. Evaluation of ketorolac, ibuprofen, acetaminophen, and an acetaminophen codeine combination in postoperative oral surgery pain. *Pharmacotherapy* 1990; **10**:S94–105.

Frame JW, Evans CR, Flaum GR, Langford R, Rout PG. A comparison of ibuprofen and dihydrocodeine in relieving pain following wisdom teeth removal. *British Dental Journal* 1989; **166**:121–4.

Fricke JR, Halladay SC, Francisco CA. Efficacy and safety of naproxen sodium and ibuprofen for pain relief after oral surgery. *Current Therapeutic Research* 1993; **54**:619–27.

Gay C, Planas E, Donado M, Martinez JM, Artigas R, Torres F *et al.* Analgesic efficacy of low doses of dexketoprofen in the dental pain model: A randomised, double-blind, placebo-controlled study. *Clinical Drug Investigation* 1996; **11**:320–30.

Hebertson RM, Storey N. The comparative efficacy of diclofenac potassium, aspirin, and placebo in the treatment of patients with pain following gynecologic surgery. *Today's Therapeutics Trends* 1994; **12**:33–45.

Heidrich G, Slavic Svircev V, Kaiko RF. Efficacy and quality of ibuprofen and acetaminophen plus codeine analgesia. *Pain* 1985; **22**:385–97.

Hersh EV, Cooper S, Betts N, Wedell D, MacAfee K, Quinn P *et al.* Single dose and multidose analgesic study of ibuprofen and meclofenamate sodium after third molar surgery. *Oral Surgery, Oral Medicine Oral Pathology* 1993; **76**:680–7.

Hersh EV, Ocns H, Quinn P, MacAfee K, Cooper SA. Narcotic receptor blockade and its effect on the analgesic response to placebo and ibuprofen after oral surgery. *Oral Surgery, Oral Medicine Oral Pathology* 1993; **75**:539–46.

Jain AK, Ryan JR, McMahon FG, Kuebel JO, Walters PJ, Noveck C. Analgesic efficacy of low dose ibuprofen in dental extraction pain. *Pharmacotherapy* 1986; **6**:318–22.

Jain AK, Mcmahon FG, Ryan JR, Narcisse C. A double-blind study of ibuprofen 200 mg in combination with caffeine 100 mg, ibuprofen 400 mg, and placebo in episiotomy pain. *Current Therapeutic Research* 1988; **43**:762–79.

Kiersch TA, Halladay SC, Koschik M. A double-blind, randomized study of naproxen sodium, ibuprofen, and placebo in postoperative dental pain. *Clinical Therapeutics* 1993; **15**:845–54.

Laska EM, Sunshine A, Marrero I, Olson N, Siegel C, McCormick N. The corelation between blood levels of ibuprofen and clinical analgesic response. *Clinical Pharmacology and Therapeutics* 1986; **40**:1–7.

Laveneziana D, Riva A, Bonazzi M, Cipolla M, Migliavacca S. Comparative efficacy of oral ibuprofen arginine and intramuscular ketorolac in patients with postoperative pain, *Clinical Drug Investigations* 1996; **11**:8–14.

McQuay HJ, Angell K, Carroll D, Moore RA, Juniper RP. Ibuprofen compared with ibuprofen plus caffeine after third molar surgery. *Pain* 1996; **66**:247–51.

Mehlisch DR, Brown P. Single-dose therapy with diclofenac potassium, aspirin, or placebo following dental impaction surgery. *Today's Therapeutic Trends* 1994; **12**:15–31.

Mehlisch DR, Jasper RD, Brown P, Korn SH, McCarroll K, Murakami AA. Comparative study of ibuprofen lysine and acetaminophen in patients with postoperative dental pain. *Clinical Therapeutics* 1995; **17**:852–60.

Mehlisch DR, Sollecito WA, Helfrick JF, Leibold DG, Markowitz R, Schow CE Jr *et al.* Multicenter clinical trial of ibuprofen and acetaminophen in the treatment of postoperative dental pain. *Journal of the American Dental Association* 1990; **121**:257–63.

Nelson S, Brahim J. An evaluation of the analgesic efficacy of diclofenac potassium, aspirin, and placebo in postoperative dental pain. *Today's Therapeutic Trends* 1994; **12**:3–14.

Nelson SL, Brahim JS, Korn SH, Greene SS, Suchower LJ. Comparison of single-dose ibuprofen lysine, acetylsalicylic acid, and placebo for moderate-to-severe postoperative dental pain. *Clinical Therapeutics* 1994; **16**:458–65.

Pagnoni B, Ravanelli A, Degradi L, Rossi R, Tiengo M. Clinical efficacy of ibuprofen arginine in the management of postoperative pain associated with suction termination of pregnancy. A double-blind placebo-controlled study. *Clinical Drug Investigations* 1996; **11**:27–32.

Parker DA, Gibbin KP, Noyelle RM. Syrup formulations for post tonsillectomy analgesia: a double blind study comparing ibuprofen, aspirin and placebo. *Journal of Laryngology and Otology* 1986; **100**:1055–60.

Schachtel BP, Thoden WR, Baybutt RI. Ibuprofen and acetaminophen in the relief of postpartum episiotomy pain. *Journal of Clinical Pharmacology* 1989; **29**:550–3.

Seymour RA, Hawkesford JE, Weldon M, Brewster D. An evaluation of different ibuprofen preparations in the control of postoperative pain after third molar surgery. *British Journal of Clinical Pharmacology* 1991; **31**:83–7.

Seymour RA, WardBooth P, Kelly PJ. Evaluation of different doses of soluble ibuprofen and ibuprofen tablets in postoperative dental pain. *British Journal of Oral and Maxillofacial Surgery* 1996; **34**:110–114.

Sunshine A, Olson NZ, Laska EM, Zighelboim I, De Castro A, De Sarrazin C. Ibuprofen, zomepirac, aspirin, and placebo in the relief of postepisiotomy pain. *Clinical Pharmacology and Therapeutics* 1983; **34**:254–8.

Sunshine A, Roure C, Olson N, Laska EM, Zorrilla C, Rivera J. Analgesic efficacy of two ibuprofen codeine combinations for the treatment of postepisiotomy and postoperative pain. *Clinical Pharmacology and Therapeutics* 1987; **42**:374–380.

11

Comparing analgesic efficacy of non-steroidal anti-inflammatory drugs given by different routes in acute and chronic pain

Summary

The aim of this systematic review was to test the evidence for a difference in analgesic efficacy and adverse effects of non-steroidal anti-inflammatory drugs (NSAIDs) given by different routes. Relevant published randomized controlled trials were comparisons of the same drug given by different routes. Presence of internal sensitivity was sought as a validity criteria. Analgesic and adverse effect outcomes were summarized, and synthesized qualitatively.

In 26 trials (2225 analysed patients) eight different NSAIDs were tested in 58 comparisons. Fifteen trials (58%) compared the same drug by different routes. Drugs were given by intravenous, intramuscular, intrawound, rectal, and oral route in postoperative pain (14 trials), renal colic (4), acute musculoskeletal pain (1), dysmenorrhoea (1), and rheumatoid arthritis (6). Five of the 15 direct comparisons were invalid because they reported no difference between routes but without evidence of internal sensitivity.

In all three direct comparisons in renal colic intravenous NSAIDs had a faster onset of action than intramuscular or rectal. In one direct comparison in dysmenorrhoea, oral NSAID was better than rectal. In the five direct comparisons in postoperative pain results were inconsistent. In one direct comparison in rheumatoid arthritis intramuscular NSAID was better than oral. Injected and rectal administration had some specific adverse effects.

In renal colic there is evidence that NSAIDs act quickest when given intravenously. This may be clinically relevant. In all other pain conditions there is a lack of evidence of any difference between routes. In pain conditions other than renal colic, there is, therefore, a strong argument to give NSAIDs orally rather than by injection.

Introduction

Oral non-steroidal anti-inflammatory drugs (NSAIDs) are an important component of simple 'low-tech' pharmacological control of both acute and chronic pain. Oral NSAIDs can be surprisingly effective in patients with moderate to severe postoperative pain. Compared with placebo, oral ibuprofen 400 mg will result in one in every three patients getting at least 50% relief of pain over six hours [2]. This is a high standard of effectiveness, and it is one against which more complicated methods of delivering adequate analgesia have to be judged. Invasive procedures like continuous extradural opioid infusion, or patient-controlled analgesia, carry recognized risks [3] and may not be available or appropriate for the majority of acute or chronic pain patients.

Although oral NSAIDs can be effective, the advent of rectal and injectable formulations of NSAIDs has led to a fashion for using these routes. This is reflected in the United States Agency for Health Care and Policy Research Acute Pain Guidelines, where the options for postoperative pain include systemic administration of NSAIDs with no mention of the oral route [4]. There are clinical circumstances where use of the oral route is not possible, such as patients who cannot swallow, who are unconscious, nauseated, or who have an ileus. If NSAIDs are indicated for such patients then rectal or injectable formulations are the only options. In the much commoner circumstance of a preoperative premedication, conscious day case patients who can swallow, or other acute and chronic pain conditions, is there any reason to use rectal or injected formulations rather than oral? Those reasons could be greater efficacy, or similar efficacy with fewer adverse effects. The evidence for any such advantage over oral use is unclear, and this review assesses the existing evidence from published reports of direct comparisons of NSAIDs given by different routes in acute and chronic pain.

Methods

Full reports of published randomized controlled trials of direct comparisons of NSAIDs, given by different routes of administration, and tested in acute or chronic pain with pain outcomes, were sought. A number of different search strategies [5] were used to identify eligible reports in MEDLINE (Knowledge Server, Silver Platter, 1966–96), EMBASE (1986–96), and the Oxford Pain Relief Database (1950–93). The words: NSAID, 'non-steroidal anti-inflammatory,' and individual drug names were used with the words: 'postoperative pain', 'renal colic', '*colic', 'intravenous', 'intramuscular', and 'rectal' in searching, including combinations of these words, and without restriction to language. Additional reports were

The topic discussed in this chapter is also published in full in Tramèr et al. [1].

identified from the reference lists of retrieved reports, review articles and textbooks, manual searching locally available anaesthetic journals, and by contacting pharmaceutical companies with licensed parenteral or rectal NSAID preparations.

Excluded reports

Abstracts, letters, review articles, and use of topical formulations (skin, mucous membranes, eye) or intra-articular use were not considered. Unpublished reports were not sought. Reports where the numbers of patients per treatment group were fewer than 10 were excluded. Authors were not contacted.

Included reports

Each report which could possibly meet the inclusion criteria was read by at least two authors independently and scored for inclusion and methodological quality using a validated three-item, five-point scale [6]. Authors met to agree scores. Reports which were described as 'randomized' were given one point, and a further point if the method of randomization was described and adequate (such as a table of random numbers). There was a *pre-hoc* agreement that trials without concealment of treatment allocation (allocation according to patient's date of birth, for instance) would be excluded from further analysis because of the well-documented risk of overestimation of treatment effects in such trials [7, 8]. One point was given when the trial was described as 'double-blind'. When the method of double-blinding was described and adequate (double-dummy method, for instance), a further point was given. Finally, reports which described the number and reasons for withdrawals were given one point. Thus, the maximum score of an included randomized controlled trial was 5 and the minimum score was 1.

Data extraction and analysis

These trials compared drug efficacy across different routes of administration. Therefore, our primary focus was trials that compared the same drug given by different routes. Only such direct comparisons were regarded as relevant to this review. Comparisons of different drugs across routes were regarded as irrelevant and were not analysed. Comparisons between NSAID and non-NSAID controls (opioid, placebo) were not considered.

Each trial was checked for specific design details with potential impact on trial validity. These details were first, whether or not the design included internal sensitivity measures, either a negative control (placebo or no treatment) or at least two dose levels of an active. There was a prior agreement that trials that reported equivalence (i.e. no difference) between routes but which had no index of internal sensitivity would be regarded as invalid and would not be considered for data synthesis. Second, the extent to which blinding was protected by using a double-dummy design was checked.

Finally, we recorded baseline pain intensity in trials where pain was treated (chronic pain settings, for instance), and pain intensity without analgesic intervention in prophylaxis trials (postoperative setting, for instance).

Information about the clinical setting, inclusion criteria, number of patients, study design, and drugs, route, and doses used was extracted from the reports, together with information on analgesic measurements and results, and adverse effects. Analgesic efficacy was estimated by extracting data of significant difference ($P < 0.05$, as reported in the original trials) between NSAID arms. Relevant outcomes were pain intensity at rest or on movement, and additional analgesic consumption. Quantitative analysis of combined data was proposed. There was a prior hypothesis that there was no clinically relevant difference between routes of administration with NSAIDs, and, specifically, that the oral route would be no different from the other routes of administration.

Results

Twenty-six randomized controlled trials (2225 analysed patients), published between 1970 and 1996, were considered eligible for the review (Table 1).

Fourteen trials were in postoperative pain (1268 patients) [9–22], four in renal colic (647 patients) [23–26], one in acute musculoskeletal pain (77 patients) [27], one in dysmenorrhoea (32 patients) [28], and six in rheumatoid arthritis (201 patients) [29–34]. Different doses of eight different NSAIDs (diclofenac, ibuprofen, indomethacin, ketoprofen, ketorolac, naproxen, piroxicam, tenoxicam), given by intravenous, intramuscular, intrawound, rectal, and oral route, were tested in 58 single dose or multiple dose comparisons.

The median quality score of all trials was 3 (range 1–5). Quantitative analysis was not considered appropriate because of the variety of clinical settings, drugs, doses, routes, and pain outcomes reported. Instead, any statistically significant difference between treatments was extracted from the original reports and documented in table format as done previously for other qualitative systematic reviews [35, 36]. We then decided on a 'vote-counting' procedure, giving positive or negative votes, if there was evidence of presence or absence respectively of a significant difference between routes.

Fifteen trials (58% of all analysed trials) were relevant to this review because they compared the same drug by different routes [9–14, 23–25, 28–33]. In nine of them (35% of all trials) the same drug was compared at the same dose [9, 11, 12, 23, 28–32].

Five of the 15 relevant trials reported equivalence between routes but had no index of internal sensitivity [14, 30–33]. These trials were not, therefore, analysed further.

Of the 10 relevant trials which reported a significant difference between routes, or which reported equivalence but had an index of internal sensitivity (i.e. which were valid), five were in postoperative pain [9–13], three were in renal colic [23–25], one was in dysmenorrhoea [28], and one was in rheumatoid arthritis [29]. Six of them used a double-dummy design [9, 10, 23, 24, 28, 29].

Postoperative pain

Of 14 trials in postoperative pain, five were valid direct comparisons. They compared diclofenac or ketorolac across routes.

In one trial, diclofenac 1 mg/kg injected intravenously at induction of anaesthesia led to significantly lower pain intensity scores 30 minutes after surgery than the same dose given intramuscularly at induction [12]. In two other trials no difference was found between ketorolac 30 mg given either intravenously or intramuscularly at induction [9, 11]. In one of these trials inguinal hernia repair was done under local anaesthesia with very low pain scores during the postoperative observation period whether or not an NSAID or no treatment was given [11]. In the same trial both intramuscular and intravenous ketorolac 30 mg at induction led to significantly lower pain scores and less rescue analgesics at 90 minutes after surgery than the same dose taken orally, but one hour before surgery [11]. Group sizes in this trial were small (i.e. 14 patients per group) and no double-dummy design was used.

Another trial with larger groups (50 patients per group), but again without a double-dummy design, reported less pain and rescue analgesics at discharge with diclofenac 75 mg intramuscularly compared with the same drug given orally but at a lower dose (50 mg) [13]. Yet another trial compared diclofenac 150 mg taken orally with 50 mg intramuscularly plus 100 mg orally [10]. The drugs were given as a premedication using a double-dummy design, and group sizes were large (50 patients per group). No difference was found between the two forms of administration.

Renal colic

Of four trials in renal colic, there were three valid direct comparisons [23–25]. They compared dipyrone, diclofenac, and indomethacin given by different routes. Two used a double-dummy design [23, 24]. In one, baseline pain before treatment was started (at least 50 mm on a 100 mm visual analogue scale) was defined [23]. Group sizes in these three trials were between 22 and 76 patients.

In one trial, pain relief was tested with dipyrone 1 g or 2 g, and diclofenac 75 mg, given intramuscularly compared with intravenously [23]. At 10 and 20 minutes after administration of the drugs the proportion of patients with at least 50% improvement was significantly in favour of the intravenous route with each drug and dose.

In the two other trials intravenous indomethacin 50 mg was compared with the same drug given rectally but double the dose [24, 25]. Despite there being only half the intravenous dose both trials reported significant improvement (less pain intensity, less rescue analgesics) with the intravenous route compared with the rectal. Again these differences were apparent only at 10 or 20 minutes.

Dysmenorrhoea

We found only one trial in dysmenorrhoea [28]. This crossover trial in 38 patients compared oral with rectal naproxen, both 500 mg six-hourly, using a double-dummy design. Relief of spasmodic pain was significantly better with the oral route.

Chronic pain

Six trials in rheumatoid arthritis were retrieved. Five of them were direct comparisons, but only one small trial using a double-dummy design with 20 patients per group was valid [29]. Patients with defined baseline pain (at least 40 mm on a 100 mm scale) receiving ketoprofen 100 mg intramuscularly reported a significantly shorter delay until the lowest pain intensity score was achieved than in patients receiving the same dose of the same drug orally.

Other pain conditions

No direct comparisons from other pain conditions were found.

Adverse effects

Commonly reported adverse effects independent of the route of administration were nausea, vomiting, dizziness, drowsiness, sedation, anxiety, dyspepsia, indigestion, and dry mouth (Table 1). Two studies reported bleeding time changes [12, 21]. In 12 patients with rheumatoid arthritis treated with indomethacin 100–150 mg orally and rectally, respectively, in a cross-over design for two weeks, endoscopically diagnosed gastric mucosal damage was independent of the route of administration [31].

Adverse effects related to the route of administration were most often reported for intramuscular and rectal regimens (Table 1). Discomfort at the site of injection [19, 20] was the most frequent complaint in relation to intramuscular injections. After rectal administration, diarrhoea [14, 30], rectal irritation [28, 31, 34], and non-retention of suppositories [24] were reported.

Comment

Many doctors use injected or rectal NSAIDs when the oral route could be used. This is despite advice to use the least invasive route possible, with the statement that no study has specifically compared the analgesic efficacy of alternative routes of the same drug [37]. Reasons for choosing injected or rectal formulations rather than oral, when the oral route could be used, might be for greater efficacy or faster onset of pain relief. The safety argument would be that these efficacy benefits were achieved at no greater (or acceptably greater) level of adverse effects. Patients may prefer oral to rectal dosing [38]. There are also legal ramifications, because of the obligation for consent if drugs are given rectally while the patient is asleep [39].

We wanted to compare, using evidence from systematically searched published reports of randomized controlled trials

Table 1   Details of randomized controlled trials

Ref.	Regimen: drug, dose, route (no. of patients)ª	No.	Setting	Pain outcomes	Internal sensitivityᵇ		Double-dummy	Overall efficacyᶜ	Adverse effects	Quality score
					Index	Given				
Postoperative										
[9]	**Ketorolac 30 mg IV + saline IM treatment (38)** / **Ketorolac 30 mg IM + saline IV treatment (38)** / Saline IM + IV treatment (37)	113	Major orthopaedic (moderate or severe pain)	Time to onset of analgesia: not sig. Time to first subsequent analgesic: ketorolic IV = IM >placebo. Number of patients achieving a 1-point decrease of pain scale within 30': ketorolac IM = placebo; IV >placebo. Patients achieving...	Placebo	yes	yes	IV = IM	No serious AEs.	5
[10]	**Diclofenac 50 mg po rapid + 100 mg po retard PM (20) (51)** / **Diclofenac 50 mg IM + 100 mg po retard PM (20) (51)** / Placebo (49)	151	3rd molar	IV >placebo. Patients' rating: ketorolac IV >placebo. Pain relief 0-8 h (VAS mean): diclofenac po & IM sig better than placebo. Rescue analgesics: sig less needed in diclofenac groups. Dipyrone at 90': IM 2/14; IW 3/14; IV 1/14, po 7/14 (sig); control 10/14.	Placebo	yes	yes	po + po = po + IM	Diclofenac po 17/51; diclofenac in 16/51; placebo 16/49.	2
[11]	**Ketorolac 30 mg IM ind (14)** / **Ketorolac 30 mg IW ind (14)** / **Ketorolac 30 mg IV ind (14)** / **Ketorolac 30 mg po PM (1 h) (14)** / no treatment (14)	90	Inguinal hernia repair (LA)	Buprenorphine at 90': IM, IW, IV, po 0/14, control 5/14. VAS-PI supine/sitting (90'): IM, IW, & IV sig better than po & control.	No treatment control	yes	no	IM = IV = IW >po	Statec: as none.	2
[12]	**Diclofenac 1 mg/kg IV ind (40)** / **Diclofenac 1 mg/kg IM ind (40)** / Fentanyl 1 µg/kg IV ind (40) / Saline IM ind (40)	160	3rd molar	Analgesic needs 'nil': diclofenac IV 14/40, diclofenac IM 12/40, fentany 3/40, saline 5/40. VAS-PI (mean) at 30' postop (60' postinjection): diclofenac IV sig better than all other groups.	Placebo	yes	no	IV >IM	Bleeding time infra (30' postinjection): sig increased with IM diclofenac. No other AEs reported.	1
[13]	**Diclofenac 75 mg IM PM (10-20') (50)** / **Diclofenac 50 mg po PM (10-20') (50)** / Ketorolac 30 mg IM PM (10-20') (50) / Saline IM PM (10-20') (50)	200	Minor gynae	No pain (discharge): diclofenac IM 43/50 & po 34/50; ketorolac IM 44/50; placebo 34/50 (IM NSAID vs. po or placebo sig diff). No analgesics (discharge): diclofenac IM 37/50 & po 27/50; ketorolac IM 38/50, placebo 27/50.	Plaebo	yes	no	IM >po	Emesis: no diff. Anxiety: sig less in IM groups. No other AE reported.	2
[14]	**Diclofenac 75 mg IM post + 75 mg/12 h: total 300 mg/48 h (16)** / **Diclofenac 10 mg po post + 100 mg/12 h: total 500 mg/48 h (16)**	32	Thoracotomy	Pain intensity (VAS mean): NSD IM vs. pr. Analgesic consumption (mean mg papaveretum): NSD. Pain after 24 h (mild or mild): ketorolac IV 11/20, diclofenac pr 14/20.	no	no	no	IM = pr	IM 1/16, pr 5/16 (2 diarrhoea).	1
[15]	Diclofenac 10 mg pr PM (1 h) (20) / Ketorolac 10 mg IV ind (20)	40	Knee arthroscopy	Activity restriction (none or mild): ketorolac IV 12/20, diclofenac pr 16/20.	no	no	yes	IV = pr	No AEs reported.	3
[16]	Ketorolac 60 mg IM PM (30') (29) / Piroxicam 40 mg po PM (90') (28) / Fentanyl 100 µg IV ind + 2 × 25 µg IV intra (27)	84	Gynae laparoscopy	Pain intensity (mild at discharge): ketorolac IM 90%, piroxicam po 97%, fentanyl 63%. Morphine required in postanaesthetic care unit: ketorolac IM 16/29, piroxicam po 25/28; fentanyl 20/27. VAS-PI at 5h: ketorolac IV sig better than piroxicam & ibuprofen.	no	yes	yes	IM >po	Ketorolac IM 7/29, piroxicam po 18/28; fentany 8/27.	4
[17]	Paracetamol 650 mg po post (30') (20) / Ibuprofen 600 mg po post (30') (20) / Ketorolac 60 mg IV end (20)	60	Strabismus (adults)	Additional analgesia at 5h: paracetamol 4/20; ibuprofen po 0/20, ketorolac IV 13/20.	no	yes	no	IV >po	Nausea: ketorolac IV 0/20; paracetamol 2/20, ibuprofen 2/20. No other AEs mentioned.	3
[18]	Ketorolac 30 mg IM ind (31) / Indomethacin 100 mg pr ind (31) / Placebo IM & pr (25)	87	Gynae or breast	VAS-PI: sig lower with NSAID at 15' & 90', but not at 60' (pr = IM). No additional analgesics: both NSAIDs sig. better than placebo.	Placebo	yes	yes	pr = IM	Ketorolac IM 7/31; indomethacin pr 9/31; placebo 8/25.	3
[19]	Indomethacin 100 mg pr + saline IM ind (38) / Ketorolac 30 mg IM + placebo pr ind (51) / Placebo pr & IM ind (48)	137	Gynae laparoscopy	Analgesic use up to 180' (fentanyl, paracetamol/codeine): not sig. VAS-PI: no diff at 30' & 60'. Post-hoc sig diff between ketorolac & placebo at 180'.	Placebo	no	yes	pr–IM	No diff in the frequency of complaints of pain at injection site.	2
[20]	Tenoxicam 20 mg IV intra + 20 mg po post (12) / Diclofenac 75 mg IM intra + 50 mg po post (13)	25	3rd molar	VAS-PI: sig lower with diclofenac at 1 h, 2 h & 3 h. 'Objective pain score' (BP, crying, agitation, movement verbal report).	no	yes	no	(IM + po) >(IV + po)	Discomfort due to IM injection: 13/13 with diclofenac.	1
[21]	Ketorolac 1 mg/kg IV ind (25) / Paracetamol 35 mg/kg pr ind (25)	50	Tonsillectomy (children)	Ketorolac > paracetamol at 2 h. No diff at 30', 1 h & 3 h. Additional analgesics up to 3 h: morphine & codeine: no diff; paracetamol: sig less with ketorolac.	no	yes	no	IV = pr	Extra 'omeostatic measurements: sig more with ketorolac (not related to route).	2
[22]	Diclofenac 100 mg pr PM (1 h) + placebo po (19) / Piroxicam 40 mg po PM (1 h) + placebo pr (20)	39	3rd molar	Median time to rescue analgesic: diclofenac 350' piroxicam 305' (P >0.05). No analgesic after 18 h: diclofenac 2/19, piroxicam 6/20. VAS-PI similar at any time.	no	no	yes	po = pr	Vomiting piroxicam 3/20, diclofenac 0/19. Nausea: piroxicam 2/20, diclofenac 1/19.	4
Renal colic										
[23]	**Dipyrone 1 g IM + placebo IV (71)** / **Dipyrone 1 g IV + placebo IM (30)** / **Dipyrone 2 g IV + placebo IM (76)** / **Dipyrone 2 g IM + placebo IV (71)** / **Diclofenac 75 mg IM + placebo IV (32)** / **Diclofenac 75 mg IV + placebo IM (22)**	302	Renal colic (VAS-PI >50)	Proportion of patients with more than 50% improvement: sig diff dipyrone 2 g IV >1 g IV at 10'; dipyrone 75 mg IV >IM at 20'; dipyrone 2 g IV >2 g IM at 10' & 20'; dipyrone 1 g IV >1 g IM at 20'.	Dose-response	yes	yes	IV >IM / IV >IM / IV >IM	IV: vomiting 1 × (diclofenac). IM: drowsiness 3 × (1 dipyrone 1 g, 1 dipyrone 2 g, 1 diclofenac); drowsiness 1 × (diclofenac).	4
[24]	**Indomethacin 100 mg pr (47)** / **Indomethacin 50 mg IV (37)**	84	Renal colic	VAS-PI at 10': IV sig lower than pr; at 30' no diff. Supplementary analgesics: pr 16/47, IV 8/37.	no	yes	yes	IV = pr	30/84 non-drug related withdrawals (non-retention of suppositories & others). Drug-related pr 8/47; IV 18/37.	1
[25]	Indomethacin 100 mg pr (63) / Indomethacin 50 mg IV (53) / Indomethacin 50 mg IV (44)	116	Renal colic	VAS-PI at 10' & 20': IV sig lower than pr; at 30' no diff. Supplementary analgesics: pr 17/63; IV 5/53 (P = 0.03).	no	no	no	IV >pr	IV 44/53, pr 29/63 (P = 0.03).	3
[26]	Diclofenac 50 mg IM (47) / Avafortan (dipyrone plus antispasmodic) IV (5–)	145	Renal colic	Pain relief ('complete') after 1st dose at 30': indomethacin IV 37/44, diclofenac IM 31/47, avafortan 45/54. Pain relief ('complete') after 1st dose at 30': indomethacin IV 37/44, diclofenac IM 31/47. NSAID IV sig better than IM.	no	yes	no	IV >IM	Indomethacin IV 5/44, diclofenac IM 3/44, avafortan 0/54.	2

Table 1   *continued*

Ref.	Regimen: drug, dose, route (no. of patients)[a]	No.	Setting	Pain outcomes	Internal sensitivity[b]		Double-dummy	Overall efficacy	Adverse effects	Quality score
					Index	Given				
Acute musculoskeletal pain										
[27]	Ketorolac 60 mg IM + placebo po (40) Ibuprofen 800 mg po + placebo IM (37)	77	Acute musculo-skeletal pain (treatment)	VAS-PI 0–120': no sig diff between keto IM & ibu po.	no	no	yes	IM = po	Dyspepsia: ketorolac 1/40; ibuprofen 2/37. Sedation: ketorolac 1/40; ibuprofen 0/37. Dry mouth: ketorolac 0/40; ibuprofen 1/37.	5
Dysmenorrhoea										
[28]	Cross-over (n = 32) **Naproxen 500 mg po 6-hourly + placebo pr** **Naproxen 500 mg pr 6-hourly + placebo po**	32	Primary dysmenorrhoea	No diff in number of additional analgesics taken. Spasmodic pain relief (score): sig better with po route. All other symptoms (score): no diff. Patients' overall assessment no diff.	no	no	**yes**	**po >pr**	pr irritation after naproxen suppositories: 2/32.	4
Rheumatoid arthritis										
[29]	**Ketoprofen 2 × 50 mg po + placebo IM (20)** **Ketoprofen 100 mg IM + placebo po (20)**	40	Rheumatoid arthritis (VAS-PI >40)	Decrease in VAS-PI, patients' global judgement, maximum decrease in VAS-PI after treatment: po better than IM (not sig). Delay until lowest pain intensity: IM shorter than po ($P < 0.05$). Articular index, grip strength, pain score (analogue 0–9), morning stiffness.	no	**yes**	**yes**	**IM>po**	Active po (6/20): 3 nausea, 1 vomiting, 1 indigestion, 1 diarrhoea, 1 headache, 2 vertigo, 1 dyspnea. Active IM (5/20): 1 headache, 2 somnolence, 1 pruritus, 1 vertigo. po: 17/13, pr: 11/13.	3
[30]	Cross-over (n = 13): placebo pr + placebo po for 1 wk. then **Indomethacin 100 mg pr + placebo po for 1 wk** **Indomethacin 100 mg po + placebo pr for 1 wk**	13 cross-over	Rheumatoid arthritis	digital joint size, rescue analgesics (paracetamol). & patient's preference: no diff between po & pr.	no	no	yes	po = pr	Diarrhoea: 4/13 pr. Indigestion: 5/13 po, 2/13, pr.	4
[31]	Cross-over (n = 12): placebo pr + placebo po for 2 wk. then **Indomethacin 100–150 mg po + placebo pr for 2 wk** **Indomethacin 100–150 mg pr + placebo po for 2 wk**	12 cross-over	Rheumatoid arthritis	Morning stiffness & pain (pain intensity on 50 mm VAS): no diff between pr & po.	no	no	yes	po = pr	Endoscopy: equal amount of gastric mucosal damage, pr discomfort with suppositories: 8 po active + pr placebo, 7 pr active + po placebo, 7 po & pr placebo.	3
[32]	Cross-over (n = 20): **Indomethacin 100 mg pr + placebo po for day 1 & 3** **Indomethacin 100 mg po + placebo pr for day 2 & 4**	20 cross-over	Rheumatoid arthritis	Patients' preference: po sig better than pr. No diff: pain, morning stiffness, duration of stiffness. Day- & night pain (4-pt scale), morning stiffness (min): no diff.	no	no	yes	po = pr	Nausea, anorexia, epigastric discomfort: po 2/20, pr 2/20. po (5): headache, dizziness, 'loose bowel motions', stomach pain. pr (8): headache, 'loose bowel motions'.	3
[33]	Cross-over (n = 22): **Indomethacin SR 75 mg po + placebo pr for 2 wk** **Indomethacin 100 mg pr + placebo po for 2 wk**	22 cross-over	Rheumatoid arthritis	Conventional grip strength: pr sig better than po (6 mm). Morning stiffness (duration): po sig better than pr. Awakenings during the night: pr sig better than po. No diff: pain on awakening (VAS), articular index, patients' & doctors' assessment (7-step scale), rescue analgesics.	no	no	yes	po = pr		4
[34]	Cross-over (n = 94) Ketoprofen CR 200 mg po + placebo pr for 3 wk Indomethacin 10 mg pr + placebo po for 3 wk	94	Rheumatoid arthritis		no	no	yes	po = pr	pr irritation: indomethacin 7/94. GI problems: ketoprofen 40/94, indomethacin 28/94.	4
Sum		**2158**								

', minutes; >, better than; <, worse than; =, similar; AEs, adverse effects; end, end of surgery; GA, general anaesthesia; GI, gastrointestinal; IM, intramuscular; ind, induction; intra, intraoperative; IV, intravenous; IW, intrawound; LA, local anaesthesia; NSD, no significant difference; PI, pain intensity; po, oral; pr, rectal; VAS, visual analogue scale; VAS-PI, visual analogue scale of pain intensity; CR, controlled release.

a **Bold** type indicates relevant trials & same drug across route.
b **Bold** type indicates fulfilled validity criteria in relevant trials.

with direct comparisons, the benefit and risk of NSAIDs given by different routes in acute and chronic pain. Systematic reviews are powerful instruments to gain more insight into treatment efficacy and harm. Ideally, dichotomous outcomes would be extracted from original reports and combined using biostatistical methods. In some circumstances dichotomous data may be extracted from measurements which were originally not binary outcomes [40].

However, such quantitative analysis was not possible here because of the variety of clinical settings, drugs, doses, routes, and pain outcomes reported. Systematic reviewers may then have to rely on statistically significant results as reported in the original reports and apply a vote-counting procedure [35]. It is obvious that such a qualitative approach is vulnerable to bias. Vote counting take no account of the size of the trial or of the size of any difference in effect. In such analyses pre-set validity criteria become especially important to minimize the risk of bias [36].

These trials highlighted different methodological problems affecting the validity of the trials.

First, if the null hypothesis was that there was no difference between the routes one might expect comparisons of the same drug given by different routes. One might even wish to concentrate only on comparisons of the same drugs at the same dose. However, only about half of these trials compared the same NSAID across routes, and, therefore, addressed what we regarded as the clinically relevant question. Only one-third of all trials would have satisfied stricter validity rules (i.e. direct comparison of the same drug at the same dose).

Second, the classical approach to design of analgesic trials is to build in an index of internal sensitivity, either by using a placebo (or no treatment) control, or by including a high and a low dose of a standard analgesic to establish a dose-response relationship. What such designs seek to achieve is a defence against equivalence of treatments. Lack of internal sensitivity is a key issue in equivalence trials [41]. This has been shown in systematic reviews of analgesic trials [36]. Without such controls equivalence in a comparison of two or more drugs may mean that the methods of measuring pain or its relief failed in that study, rather than that this was a true negative result of no difference between the analgesic effect of the drugs. Power calculations cannot be a defence against method failure. Only a positive result (significant difference) despite the lack of negative controls is an adequate vindication of such methods.

Eight (31%) of the 26 trials built in a method ensuring internal sensitivity in the form of a placebo control [9, 10, 12, 13, 18, 19], a no-treatment control [11], or two dose levels of the same drug given by the same route [23]. Five direct comparisons reported equivalence between routes but had no index of internal sensitivity. These trials, therefore, were invalid and were excluded from further analysis.

Third, although all these trials were by definition comparisons of NSAIDs given by different routes, only 17 (65%) used a double-dummy design. The blinding of the other trials must be questioned. In trials with deficient blinding the therapeutic effect may be exaggerated [7]. While all trials in rheumatoid arthritis used a double-dummy technique, this

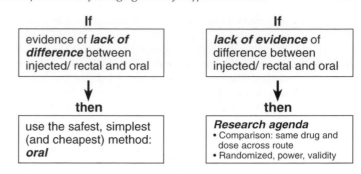

was true for only half of the surgical trials. An extreme example was the comparison of an oral drug given one hour before surgery with the same drug given by injection at induction [11]. This trial did not use a double-dummy method and reported better analgesic efficacy with the parenteral route compared with the oral.

Finally, a *pre-hoc* defined pain intensity, sufficient to provide measurable change after study treatment, was reported in only a minority of trials measuring pain relief [9, 23, 29]. Very low pain intensity scores independent of the treatment were reported in some trials where pain was meant to be prevented, such as in the surgical setting. If there is no pain, analgesia cannot be measured. A pain trial without an adequate baseline pain intensity is not a valid assay [36].

Applying our rules of validity to these 26 trials reveals the following. Only 15 (58%) of all systematically searched trials were relevant to this review (i.e. investigated the same drug given by different routes). Five of them had to be excluded because their result could not be interpreted (i.e. they reported equivalence but had no index of internal sensitivity). This meant that actually only 10 trials (38% of all trials) could be analysed. Only six of them used a double-dummy design. In renal colic there was evidence from three valid direct comparisons that the intravenous route acted significantly faster than rectal or intramuscular. Although this difference was only evident during the first 10 to 20 minutes, the faster onset of action is likely to be of clinical relevance in this specific setting. In the only trial in dysmenorrhoea one outcome measurement indicated that oral NSAIDs may be better than rectal. In one trial in rheumatoid arthritis one isolated endpoint suggested that intramuscular ketoprofen may be superior to oral. The clinical utility of this is unclear. Finally, in the surgical setting results were far from being conclusive.

Reporting of adverse effects was generally poor and mostly not related to route of administration. Rectal and intramuscular routes were most likely to have specific local adverse effects. These have to be taken into account when advantages of one route over the other are discussed.

With the exception of the renal colic setting these trials constitute a lack of evidence for any difference rather than evidence of lack of difference between NSAIDs given by different routes. This is not just semantics, because if there is adequate evidence of a lack of difference then practice should change, reverting to the safest and simplest option, the oral route. If there is a lack of evidence (rather than evidence of a lack of difference) then a research agenda is set, to determine whether or not there is any clinical advantage of one route over another. It could be argued that patients should again receive the safest and simplest option unless they agree to participate in a randomized comparison of different routes of administration. The research agenda should be to design simple comparisons of the same drug at the same dose across route, with validity, and ideally with standardized outcome measures in the various studies to make combined quantitative analysis possible.

It does not seem right that over 2200 patients have already participated in trials over the past 26 years, and still for the majority of clinical settings we cannot answer the simple question: 'Is it better to give NSAIDs by injection or suppository, than to take them orally?'

References

1. Tramèr M, Williams J, Carroll D, Wiffen PJ, McQuay HJ, Moore RA. Systematic review of direct comparisons of non-steroidal anti-inflammatory drugs given by different routes for acute pain. *Acta Anaesthesiologica Scandinavica*. in press.
2. Collins SL, Moore A, McQuay HJ, Wiffen PJ. Oral ibuprofen and diclofenac in postoperative pain: a quantitative systematic review. submitted 1997.
3. Bates DW, Cullen DJ, Laird N, Petersen LA, Small SD, Servi D et al. Incidence of adverse drug events and potential adverse drug events. *Journal of American Medical Association* 1995; **274**:29–34.
4. Acute Pain Management Guideline Panel. *Acute pain management: operative or medical procedures and trauma.* Clinical Practice Guideline No. 1. Agency for Health Care Policy and Research, U.S. Department of Health and Human Services. AHCPR Publication No. 92-0032. Rockville, MD: Public Health Service, 1992:24–5.
5. Jadad AR, McQuay HJ. A high-yield strategy to identify randomized controlled trials for systematic reviews. *Online Journal of Current Clinical Trials* [serial online] 1993; Doc No 33:3973 words; 39 paragraphs. 5 tables.
6. Jadad AR, Moore RA, Carroll D, Jenkinson C, Reynolds DJM, Gavaghan DJ et al. Assessing the quality of reports of randomized clinical trials: is blinding necessary? *Controlled Clinical Trials* 1996; **17**:1–12.
7. Schulz KF, Chalmers I, Hayes RJ, Altman DG. Empirical evidence of bias: dimensions of methodological quality associated with estimates of treatment effects in controlled trials. *Journal of the American Medical Association* 1995; **273**:408–12.
8. Carroll D, Tramer M, McQuay H, Nye B, Moore A. Randomization is important in studies with pain outcomes: Systematic review of transcutaneous electrical nerve stimulation in acute postoperative pain. *British Journal of Anaesthesia* 1996; **77**:798–803.
9. Parke TJ, Millett S, Old S, Goodwin APL, Rice ASC. Ketorolac for early postoperative analgesia. *Journal of Clinical Anesthesia* 1995; **7**:465–9.
10. Hyrkas T, Ylipaavalniemi P, Oikarinen VJ, Hampf G. Postoperative pain prevention by a single-dose formulation of diclofenac producing a steady plasma concentration. *Journal of Oral Maxillofacial Surgery* 1992; **50**:124–7.
11. Ben-David B, Baune-Goldstein U, Goldik Z, Gaitini L. Is preoperative ketorolac a useful adjunct to regional anesthesia for inguinal herniorrhaphy? *Acta Anaesthesiologica Scandinavica* 1996; **40**:358–63.
12. Campbell WI, Kendrick R, Patterson C. Intravenous diclofenac sodium. Does its administration before operation suppress postoperative pain? *Anaesthesia* 1990; **45**:763–6.
13. Jakobsson J, Rane K, Davidson S. Intramuscular NSAIDs reduce post-operative pain after minor outpatient anaesthesia. *European Journal of Anaesthesiology* 1996; **13**:67–71.
14. Moore AP, Thorpe JA, Mulley BA, Cruise M. Which diclofenac form is best? Post-thoracotamy pain: intramuscular v. rectal administration of diclofenac. *Hospital Pharmacy Practice* 1993; September:431–2, 435.
15. Dennis AR, Leeson-Payne CG, Hobbs GJ. A comparison of diclofenac with ketorolac for pain relief after knee arthroscopy. *Anaesthesia* 1995; **50**:904–6.
16. Lysak SZ, Anderson PT, Carithers RA, DeVane GG, Smith ML, Bates GW. Postoperative effects of fentanyl, ketorolac, and piroxicam as analgesics for outpatient laparoscopic procedures. *Obstetrics and Gynecology* 1994; **83**:270–5.
17. Morrison NA, Repka MX. Ketorolac versus acetaminophen or ibuprofen in controlling postoperative pain in patients with strabismus. *Ophthalmology* 1994; **101**:915–18.
18. Morley-Forster P, Newton PT, Cook M. Ketorolac and indomethacin are equally efficacious for the relief of minor postoperative pain. *Canadian Journal of Anaesthesia* 1993; **40**:1126–30.
19. Murrell GC, Leake T, Hughes PJ. A comparison of the efficacy of ketorolac and indomethacin for postoperative analgesia following laparoscopic surgery in day patients. *Anaesthesia and Intensive Care* 1996; **24**:237–40.
20. Roelofse JA, van der Bijl P, Joubert JJ. An open comparative study of the analgesic effects of tenoxicam and diclofenac sodium after third molar surgery. *Anesthesia and Pain Control in Dentistry* 1993; **2**:217–22.
21. Rusy LM, Houck CS, Sullivan LJ, Ohlms LA, Jones DT, McGill TJ et al. A double-blind evaluation of ketorolac tromethamine versus acetaminophen in pediatric tonsillectomy: analgesia and bleeding. *Anesthesia and Analgesia* 1995; **80**:226–9.
22. Wakeling HG, Barry PC, Butler PJ. Postoperative analgesia in dental day case surgery. A comparison between Feldene 'Melt' (piroxicam) and diclofenac suppositories. *Anaesthesia* 1996; **51**:784–6.
23. Muriel-Villoria X, Muriel-Villoria C, Zungri-Telo E, Diaz-Curiel M, Fernandez-Guerrero M, Moreno J et al. Comparison of the onset and duration of the analgesic effect of dipyrone, 1 or 2 g, by the intramuscular or intravenous route, in acute renal colic. *European Journal of Clinical Pharmacology* 1995; **48**:103–7.
24. Nelson CE, Nylander C, Olsson AM, Olsson R, Pettersson BA, Wallstrom I. Rectal v. intravenous administration of indomethacin in the treatment of renal colic. *Acta Chirurgica Scandinavica* 1988; **154**:253–5.
25. Nissen I, Birke H, Olsen J, Wurtz E, Lorentzen K, Salomon H et al. Treatment of ureteric colic. Intravenous versus rectal administration of indomethacin. *British Journal of Urology* 1990; **65**:576–9.
26. El-Sherif A, Foda R, Norlen L, Yahia H. Treatment of renal colic by prostaglandin synthetase inhibitors and avafortan (analgesic antispasmodic). *British Journal of Urology* 1990; **66**:602–5.
27. Turturro MA, Paris PM, Seaberg DC. Intramuscular ketorolac versus oral ibuprofen in acute musculoskeletal pain. *Annals of Emergency Medicine* 1995; **26**:117–20.

28. Ylikorkala O, Puolakka J, Kauppila A. Comparison between naproxen tablets and suppositories in primary dysmenorrhea. *Prostaglandins* 1980; **20**:463–8.

29. Dougados M, Listrat V, Duchesne L, Amor B. [Comparative efficacy of ketoprofen related to the route of administration (intramuscular or per os). A doubleblind study versus placebo in rheumatoid arthritis] Efficacite comparee du ketoprofene en fonction de sa voie d'administration (intra-musculaire ou per os). Une etude en double aveugle contre placebo au cours de la polyarthrite rhumatoide. *Revue du Rhumatisme et de Maladies Osteo-articulaire* 1992; **59**:769–73.

30. Baber N, Sibeon R, Laws E, Halliday L, Orme M, Littler T. Indomethacin in rheumatoid arthritis: comparison of oral and rectal dosing. *British Journal of Clinical Pharmacology* 1980; **10**:387–92.

31. Hansen TM, Matzen P, Madsen P. Endoscopic evaluation of the effect of indomethacin capsules and suppositories on the gastric mucosa in rheumatic patients. *Journal of Rheumatology* 1984; **11**:484–7.

32. Huskisson EC, Taylor RT, Burston D, Chuter PJ, Hart FD. Evening indomethacin in the treatment of rheumatoid arthritis. *Annals of Rheumatic Disease* 1970; **29**:393–6.

33. Iversen O, Fowles M, Vlieg M, Smidt N, Wigley R. Sustained release indomethacin: a double blind comparison with indomethacin suppositories. *New Zealand Medical Journal* 1981; **93**:261–2.

34. Uddenfeldt P, Leden I, Rubin B. A double-blind comparison of oral ketoprofen 'controlled release' and indomethacin suppository in the treatment of rheumatoid arthritis with special regard to morning stiffness and pain on awakening. *Current Medical Research Opinion* 1993; **13**:127–32.

35. Carroll D, Tramer M, McQuay H, Nye B, Moore A. Transcutaneous electrical nerve stimulation in labour pain: A systematic review. *British Journal of Obstetrics and Gynaecology* 1997; **104**:169–75.

36. Kalso E, Tramer M, Carroll D, McQuay H, Moore RA. Pain relief from intra-articular morphine after knee surgery: A qualitative systematic review. *Pain* 1997; **71**:642–51.

37. Cashman J, McAnulty G. Nonsteroidal anti-inflammatory drugs in perisurgical pain management. Mechanisms of action and rationale for optimum use. *Drugs* 1995; **49**:51–70.

38. Vyvyan HAL, Hanafiah Z. Patients' attitudes to rectal drug administration. *Anaesthesia* 1995; **50**:983–4.

39. Mitchell J. A fundamental problem of consent. *British Medical Journal* 1995; **310**:43–8.

40. McQuay HJ, Moore RA. Using numerical results from systematic reviews in clinical practice. *Annals of Internal Medicine* 1997; **126**:712–20.

41. Jones B, Jarvis P, Lewis JA, Ebbutt AF. Trials to assess equivalence: the importance of rigorous methods. *British Medical Journal* 1996; **313**:36–9.

12
Topically applied non-steroidal anti-inflammatory drugs

Summary

This systematic review assessed the effectiveness and safety of topical non-steroidal anti-inflammatory drugs (NSAIDs) in acute (soft tissue trauma, strains and sprains) and chronic pain conditions (osteoarthritis, tendinitis). Eighty-six, randomized controlled trials involving 10 160 patients were found. Measures approximating at least half pain relief, local, and systemic adverse effects were extracted. Analysis was done at one week for acute and two weeks for chronic conditions using relative benefit and number-needed-to-treat (NNT)

In acute pain conditions placebo controlled trials had a relative benefit of 1.7 (1.5–1.9) and NNT of 3.9 (3.4–4.4). Analysing by drug (at least three trials), ketoprofen (NNT 2.6), felbinac (3.0), ibuprofen (3.5), and piroxicam (4.2) had significant efficacy. Benzydamine and indomethacin were not distinguished from placebo.

In chronic pain conditions placebo controlled trials had a relative benefit of 2.0 (1.5–2.7) and NNT of 3.1 (2.7–3.8). Small trials (< 40 treated patients) exaggerated effectiveness of topical non-steroidals in acute conditions only (by 24%). There was no relationship between trial quality and treatment effect.

In both acute and chronic pain, local and systemic adverse events and drug-related study withdrawal had a low incidence, and were no different from placebo. Topical NSAIDs drugs are effective in relieving pain in acute and chronic conditions.

Introduction

Some topical NSAIDs are available without prescription and are widely advertised for acute and chronic painful conditions. In the United Kingdom, some 20–24 million (predominantly oral) NSAID prescriptions are written each year, 5% of the National Health Service total prescriptions, with many more available without prescription. The attributable risk of going to hospital with gastrointestinal problems is 1.3% to 1.6% annually for regular users or oral non-steroidals [1]. This raises the question whether using oral NSAIDs is worse than the disease for some patients [2]. Despite licensed status there is scepticism that topical NSAIDs have any action other than as rubefacients [2, 3]. This systematic review was undertaken to examine the evidence that topical NSAIDs are effective and safe, and to determine whether there is evidence for differences between topical preparations.

Methods

Reports were sought of randomized controlled trials of topical NSAIDs which pain was an outcome. Reports were included which compared topical NSAID(s) with placebo, with another topical non-steroidal, or with an oral non-steroidal. A number of different search strategies in MEDLINE (1966–September 1996), EMBASE (1981–September 1996), and the Oxford Pain Relief Database (1950–94) [4] were used to locate reports, using individual drug name (generic and proprietary), together with the words: 'administration, topical', 'gel', 'ointment', 'aerosol', 'cream', and combinations of these, without restriction to English language. Additional reports were identified from reference lists of retrieved reports and review articles. Librarians and medical directors of the 12 pharmaceutical companies in the United Kingdom identified as marketing topical NSAIDs were asked for reports of randomized controlled trials of their products, including any unpublished reports. Abstracts were not sought. Authors were not contacted.

Randomized controlled trials of NSAIDs with pain as an outcome in acute conditions (strains, sprains, sports injuries) or chronic conditions (arthritic, rheumatic) were included. Those in vaginitis, oral, or buccal conditions, thrombophlebitis or experimental pain settings were not.

Two of the authors screened reports to eliminate those without pain outcomes, which were not randomized, or were abstracts or reviews. Each report which could possibly be described as a randomized controlled trial (RCT) was read independently by each of the authors and scored using a three-item, 1–5 score, quality scale [5]. Consensus was then achieved. The maximum score of an included RCT was 5 and the minimum score was 1.

Information about treatment(s) and control(s), condition studied, number of patients randomized and analysed, study design, observation periods, outcome measures used for pain or global evaluation, analgesic outcome results, local skin irritation, systemic adverse effects, and study withdrawal due to adverse effects was taken from each report by authors meeting to concur.

We defined a clinically relevant outcome as at least 50% pain relief. Only information that was available in dichotomous form was used for analysis. A hierarchy of measures was used for extraction which approximated, in this order of preference:

1. Patient global judgement (excellent/good).
2. Pain on movement (no pain/slight pain).
3. Spontaneous pain or pain at rest (no pain/slight pain).
4. Physician global judgement (excellent/good) if defined against a stated scale.

The denominator was taken as the number of patients randomized (i.e. an intention to treat analysis). For acute conditions we took the effectiveness measure nearest to one week after start of treatment, and for chronic conditions two weeks. Our prior hypotheses were that topical NSAIDs were no better than placebo and that there was no difference between them.

The scatter of success rates with topical NSAIDs versus success rate with placebo [6] was used as a graphical means of exploring the consistency of efficacy and the homogeneity of the data. On such plots a scatter lying predominantly between the line of equality and the axis of the active intervention (topical non-steroidal) would suggest consistent efficacy with the intervention, and relative homogeneity.

Relative risk or benefit with 95% confidence interval was calculated for pain data using a random effects model [7] because the results were heterogeneous. Heterogeneity was assumed when $P > 0.1$. This was done pooling all data, pooling data for an individual drug where there were at least three trials, and for sensitivity analysis by quality score and treatment group size. We used a fixed-effects model [8] for the (homogeneous) adverse effect data. A statistically significant improvement over control was assumed when the lower limit of the 95% confidence interval of the relative benefit was > 1. Number-needed-to-treat (NNT) and 95% confidence interval (CI) was calculated for effect data [9, 10]. The NNT indicated how many patients with acute or chronic pain have to be treated with topical NSAIDs for one of them to achieve at least 50% pain relief who would not have done with placebo. A significant difference between NNTs was assumed when confidence intervals did not overlap.

Results

Searches found 86 reports (10 160 patients) that fulfilled inclusion criteria, 76 of which had dichotomous pain out-comes, including three unpublished reports with 1695 patients from a pharmaceutical company. The number of reports, patients, and the distribution of quality scores is divided by acute or chronic, both placebo and active controlled, are shown in Table 1. Over 75% of placebo controlled trials had quality scores of 3 or more. Conversely, 60% of active controlled trials had scores of 2 or less. Full details of trial design, outcome measures, and results are in the Appendices.

Acute conditions

Thirty-seven reports of 40 placebo controlled trials of topical NSAID drugs were found (details in Appendix 1). The mean size of the group treated with topical drugs was 47 patients (median 32). Studies were conducted in recent soft tissue injury, sprains, strains, or trauma. Dichotomous pain out-comes were available from 1747 patients with active treatment and 1492 on placebo. An additional 24 reports of 24 trials compared different topical NSAIDs, or formulations, or route of administration in 4171 patients. In three studies, topical was compared with oral non-steroidal, one of which also had a placebo control.

Relative benefit and 95% confidence intervals are shown for each placebo controlled trial in Fig. 1. Twenty-seven of the 37 comparisons showed statistical superiority of topical non-steroidal over placebo. The scatter of the proportion of patients with at least 50% pain relief with topical non-steroidal or placebo is shown in Fig. 2. Thirty-six of the 37 comparisons were in the segment favouring treatment over placebo. The three trials that did not have dichotomous out-comes also reported statistical benefit of topical non-steroidal over placebo.

Pooled relative benefit for all 37 comparisons was 1.7 (1.5–1.9) and the NNT was 3.9 (3.4–4.3) (Table 2). Pooling data just from trials with a quality score of at least 3 produced the same results. Sensitivity analysis by treatment group size showed that trials with a group size of at least 40 treated patients produced higher (worse) estimates for NNT of 4.8 (4.0–5.7) than all trials together. Trials with fewer than 40 treated patients produced a significantly lower (better) NNT of 2.6 (2.3–3.1) than either bigger trials or all trials.

Pooling data for each drug studied in three or more trials showed ketoprofen, felbinac, ibuprofen, and piroxicam to be

Table 1 Number of reports, patients, and the distribution of quality scores

Trials	No. of reports	No. of patients	Quality score (1–5)				
			1	2	3	4	5
Acute pain placebo controlled	37	3556	1	6	10	13	7
Acute pain active controlled	24	4171	4	11	4	5	0
Chronic pain placebo controlled	13	1161	0	3	5	5	0
Chronic pain active controlled	12	1272	2	5	3	2	0

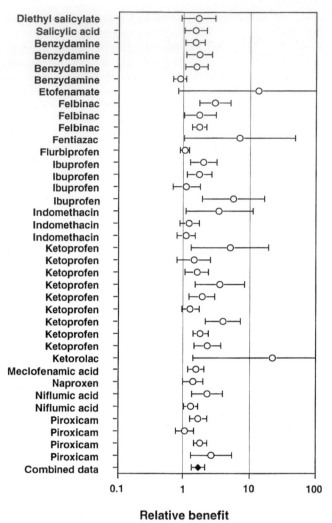

Fig. 1 Placebo controlled trials of topical NSAIDs: one-week outcome in acute painful conditions.

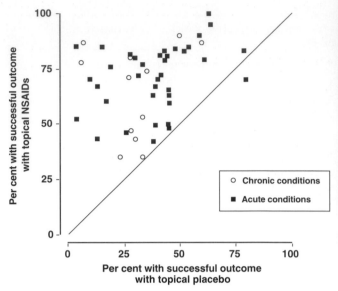

Fig. 2 Placebo controlled trials of topical NSAIDs in acute and chronic conditions.

statistically superior to placebo with NNT of 2.6–4.2. Indomethacin and benzydamine were no better than placebo (Table 2).

The percentage of patients achieving at least 50% pain relief with active treatment or placebo in all studies in all trials (placebo and active controlled) in acute conditions is shown in Fig. 3 (lower panel). The range with placebo was 0% to 80%. With topical non-steroidal it was 30% to 100%. There was no significant difference in the (low) frequency of local or systemic adverse effects, or drug-related withdrawal (Table 2).

Chronic conditions

The 13 placebo controlled trials (Appendix 2) were predominantly in single joint arthritis and rheumatological disorders, with dichotomous outcomes from 547 patients on active treatment and 550 on placebo in 12 trials. Twelve other

trials (Appendix 2) compared different topical NSAIDs in 1272 patients. In two of these, topical was compared with oral NSAIDs.

Relative benefit and 95% confidence intervals for each drug compared with placebo are shown in Fig. 4. Seven of the 12 studies showed statistical superiority of topical NSAIDs over placebo. The scatter of the proportion of patients with at least 50% pain relief with topical or placebo is shown in Fig. 2. All 12 comparisons were in the segment favouring treatment over placebo. The one trial which did not have dichotomous outcomes also reported statistical benefit of topical NSAIDs over placebo.

Pooled relative benefit for all 12 comparisons was 2.0 (1.5–2.7) and the NNT was 3.1 (2.7–3.8) (Table 2). Sensitivity analysis by quality score or treatment group size produced no significant change in these estimates. No single topical NSAID was tested in as many as three placebo controlled studies and combined estimates could not therefore be calculated for any single drug.

The percentage of patients achieving at least 50% pain relief with active treatment or placebo in all studies in all trials (placebo and active controlled) in chronic conditions is shown in Fig. 3 (upper panel). The range with placebo was 5% to 60%. With topical NSAIDs it was 30% to 95%. There was no significant difference in the (low) frequency of local or systemic adverse effects, or drug-related withdrawal (Table 2).

Comparison with oral NSAIDs

Five studies compared topical with oral NSAIDs, three in acute conditions [11, 13] and two in chronic [14, 15]. None showed statistical benefit of oral over topical NSAIDs.

Table 2 Combined results and sensitivity analysis for topical NSAIDs in acute and chronic painful conditions

Drug	No. of trials	No. of patients	Average no. of treated patients	CER	EER	RR	NNT (95% CI)
Acute painful conditions							
Combined efficacy data	37	3329	47	39	71	1.7 (1.5–1.9)	3.9 (3.4–4.4)
Local AE				3	2.6	1.2 (0.8–1.7)	
Systemic AE				0.7	0.8	1.0 (0.6–1.8)	
Withdrawal due to AE				0.4	0.6	0.8 (0.4–1.4)	
Trials of quality score 3–5	30	2834	52	38	72	1.7 (1.5–1.9)	3.9 (3.4–4.4)
Trials with treatment groups of <40 patients	20	933	24	35	76	1.9 (1.6–2.2)	2.6 (2.3–3.1)
Trials with treatment groups of 40–80 patients	8	810	51	44	66	1.6 (1.1–2.2)	5.0 (3.7–7.4)
Trials with treatment groups of >80 patients	7	1496	123	41	67	1.6 (1.3–1.9)	4.6 (3.7–5.9)
Ketoprofen	9	724	43	36	74	2.0 (1.5–2.6)	2.6 (2.3–3.2)
Felbinac	3	413	70	32	66	2.0 (1.5–2.7)	3.0 (2.4–4.1)
Ibuprofen	4	284	36	34	70	1.9 (1.2–3.0)	3.5 (2.5–5.6)
Piroxicam	4	589	74	39	69	1.6 (1.2–2.2)	4.2 (3.1–6.1)
Benzydamine	4	245	31	62	84	1.4 (0.9–2.0)	6.7 (3.8–23)
Indomethacin	3	394	66	32	47	1.3 (0.9–1.8)	10 (5.0–∞)
Chronic painful conditions							
Combined efficacy data	12	1097		30	65	2.0 (1.5–2.7)	3.1 (2.7–3.8)
Local AE				5.3	5.9	0.9 (0.4–1.7)	
Systemic AE				1.3	1.1	1.1 (0.5–2.3)	
Withdrawal due to AE				0.7	0.7	1.0 (0.4–2.4)	
Trials of quality score 3–5 only	9	987	55	27	62	2.2 (1.5–3.1)	3.1 (2.6–3.8)
Trials with treatment groups of <40 patients	6	261	22	31	69	2.2 (1.5–3.1)	2.6 (2.0–3.6)
Trials with treatment groups at >40 patients	6	836	70	29	61	2.0 (1.7–2.4)	3.3 (2.8–4.3)

CER, control event rate; CI, confidence intervals; EER, experimental event rate; RR, relative benefit or risk.
Response is either proportion of patients with successful outcome or percentage of patients with an AE. An infinite NNT confidence interval indicates that there may be no benefit of the treatment over placebo.

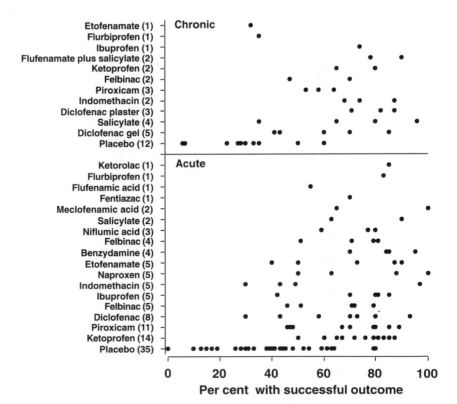

Fig. 3 Successful outcome for treatment arms from placebo and active controlled trials in chronic and acute painful conditions: drug and number of trials

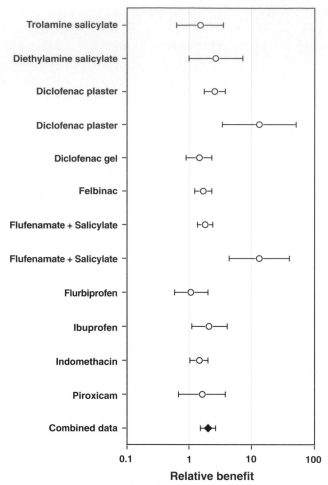

Fig. 4 Placebo controlled trials of topical NSAIDs: two-week outcome in chronic painful conditions.

Comment

Topical NSAIDs were significantly more effective than placebo. This is not just due to rubbing. Placebo preparations were also rubbed onto the affected parts. The significant difference was therefore additional to any effect of rubbing. Topical preparations produced NNTs in the range of 3 to 5 (Table 2). At least one patient in about three using a topical non-steroidal will achieve at least 50% pain relief who would not have done had they used a placebo.

Although this result may surprise some, it is not because the trials were poor. Placebo controlled studies in both acute and chronic conditions had quality scores of 3 or more on a scale of 1 to 5 in over 75% of reports (Table 1). This is important, since trials of lower methodological quality (2 or less using the same validated scale as here) have been shown to have a more favourable outcome [16].

We judged it sensible to pool data for individual drugs only when there were at least three randomized trials. In acute conditions there was enough information to make comparisons (Table 2). The average response for placebo was similar for

individual drugs apart from benzydamine. Ketoprofen, felbinac, ibuprofen, and piroxicam were all statistically superior to placebo, in contrast to indomethacin and benzydamine which were not. Confidence intervals for the NNT for ketoprofen did not overlap with those of benzydamine or indomethacin. There is no clear message as to which of ketoprofen, felbinac, ibuprofen, or piroxicam was best, or indeed whether there was any difference in efficacy. They all work.

Local skin reactions were rare (3.6%), and systemic effects were rarer (less than 0.5%). Local or systemic adverse effects of sufficient severity to cause withdrawal from the study were also rare (0.5%). Adverse effects were no more common than with placebo.

Topical NSAIDs are not associated with the gastrointestinal adverse effects seen with the same drugs taken orally [17]. The low incidence of systemic adverse effects for topical NSAIDs probably results from the much lower plasma concentrations from similar doses applied topically to those administered orally [13, 18]. Topical application of ibuprofen resulted in significant tissue concentrations in deep tissue compartments, more than enough to inhibit inflammatory enzymes [18, 19].

These positive results for topical non-steroidals could be argued as being skewed by publication restricted to positive findings. It is next to impossible to rebut this argument. We made strenuous efforts to unearth unpublished data. Ironically, one pharmaceutical company withheld results they claimed to be positive and favourable to their product. Rosenthal's file drawer argument [20] says we would need many negative results (more than 692 for acute, 37 for chronic) to overturn these positive results.

More important is the empirical evidence that small trials (arbitrarily set at fewer than 40 patients per group as being between the mean and median sizes of 47 and 32 patients per treated group) produced exaggerated estimates of clinical efficacy by 24% (4.8 minus 3.9/3.9, Table 2) with confidence intervals that did not overlap. By contrast, trial quality made no difference despite evidence to the contrary from other settings [16]. Size of treatment group may be an important issue for credibility of estimates of clinical efficacy in treatments, just like randomization [21, 22] and double-blinding [21]. Just as it may be hazardous to change practice on the basis of a single small trial, similarly, beware meta-analysis restricted to multiple small trials [23].

The important research agenda is to identify those patients with chronic disease, particularly elderly patients, who may benefit from using topical rather than oral NSAIDs. We need to compare the pain relief and mobility, harm, and cost for these alternatives. The few studies we identified comparing oral with topical non-steroidals had inadequate design and power to answer these important questions. In the meantime, the message is that topical NSAIDs are effective and safe.

REFERENCES

1. Wynne HA, Campbell M. Pharmacoeconomics of nonsteroidal anti-inflammatory drugs (NSAIDs). *PharmacoEconomics* 1993; 3:107–23.

2. Bateman DN, Kennedy JG. Non-steroidal anti-inflammatory drugs and elderly patients. The medicine may be worse than the disease. *British Medical Journal* 1995; **310**:817–8.

3. Anonymous. Rational use of NSAIDs for musculoskeletal disorders. *Drug and Therapeutics Bulletin* 1994; **32**:91–5.

4. Jadad AR, Carroll D, Moore A, McQuay H. Developing a database of published reports of randomised clinical trials in pain research. *Pain* 1996; **66**:239–46.

5. Jadad AR, Moore RA, Carroll D, Jenkinson C, Reynolds DJM, Gavaghan DJ *et al*. Assessing the quality of reports of randomized clinical trials: is blinding necessary? *Controlled Clinical Trials* 1996; **17**:1–12.

6. L'Abbé KA, Detsky AS, O'Rourke K. Meta-analysis in clinical research. *Annals of Internal Medicine* 1987; **107**:224–33.

7. DerSimonian R, Laird N. Meta-analysis of clinical trials. *Controlled Clinical Trials* 1986; **7**:177–88.

8. Yusuf S, Peto R, Lewis J, Collins R, Sleight P. Betablockade during and after myocardial infarction: an overview of the randomized trials. *Progress in Cardiovascular Disease* 1985; **27**:335–71.

9. Laupacis A, Sackett DL, Roberts RS. An assessment of clinically useful measures of the consequences of treatment. *New England Journal of Medicine* 1988; **318**:1728–33.

10. Cook RJ, Sackett DL. The number needed to treat: a clinically useful measure of treatment effect. *British Medical Journal* 1995; **310**:452–4.

11. Åkermark C, Forsskåhl B. Topical indomethacin in overuse injuries in athletes. A randomized double blind study comparing Elmetacin® with oral indomethacin and placebo. *International Journal of Sports Medicine* 1990; **11**:393–6.

12. Hosie GAC. The topical NSAID, felbinac, versus oral ibuprofen: a comparison of efficacy in the treatment of acute lower back injury. *British Journal of Clinical Research* 1993; **4**:5–17.

13. Vanderstraeten G, Schuermans P. Study on the effect of etofenamate 10% cream in comparison with an oral NSAID in strains and sprains due to sports injuries. *Acta Belgica Medica Physica* 1990; **13**:139–41.

14. Browning RC, Johson K. Reducing the dose of oral NSAIDs by use of feldene gel: an open study in elderly patients with osteoarthritis. *Advances in Therapeutic Research* 1994; **11**:198–206.

15. Golden EL. A double-blind comparison of orally ingested aspirin and a topically applied salicylate cream in the relief of rheumatic pain. *Current Therapeutic Research* 1978; **24**:524–9.

16. Khan KS, Daya S, Jadad AR. The importance of quality of primary studies in producing unbiased systematic reviews. *Archives of Internal Medicine* 1996; **156**:661–6.

17. Evans JMM, McMahon A, McGilchrist M, White G, Murray F, McDevitt D *et al*. Topical non-steroidal antiinflammatory drugs and admission to hospital for upper gastrointestinal bleeding and perforation: a record linkage case-control study. *British Medical Journal* 1995; **311**:22–6.

18. Berner G, Engels B, Vögtle-Junkert U. Percutaneous ibuprofen therapy with Trauma-Dolgit gel: bioequivalence studies. *Drugs Under Experimental and Clinical Research* 1989; **15**:559–64.

19. Treffel P, Gabard B. Feasibility of measuring the biavailability of topical ibuprofen in commercial formulations using drug content in epidermis and a methyl nicotinate skin inflammation assay. *Skin Pharmacology* 1993; **6**:268–75.

20. Rosenthal R. The 'File Drawer Problem' and Tolerance for null results. *Psychology Bulletin* 1979; **86**:638–41.

21. Schulz KF, Chalmers I, Hayes RJ, Altman DG. Empirical evidence of bias: dimensions of methodological quality associated with estimates of treatment effects in controlled trials. *Journal of the American Medical Association* 1995; **273**:408–12.

22. Carroll D, Tramer M, McQuay H, Nye B, Moore A. Randomization is important in studies with pain outcomes: Systematic review of transcutaneous electrical nerve stimulation in acute postoperative pain. *British Journal of Anaesthesia* 1996; **77**:798–803.

23. Egger M, Smith GD. Misleading meta-analysis. Lessons from 'an effective, safe, simple' intervention that wasn't. *British Medical Journal* 1995; **310**:752–4.

Appendix 1A
Details of trial design, outcome measures, and results in placebo controlled trials in acute painful conditions

Ref.	Condition	Drug	No., study design & follow-up	Outcome measures	Dose regimen	Analgesic outcome results	Skin irritation	Withdrawals & adverse effects	Quality score
[Airaksinen et al. 1993]	Acute soft tissue injuries <1 wk	Ketoprofen 2.5% gel, placebo gel	n = 56 parallel group 0, 3, 7 days	1. VAS-PT on rest & movement 2. Patient & investigator global rating.	5 g twice daily	1. Overall sig reduction in pain at rest with ketoprofen (NSD for placebo). 2. Sig diff (P <0.05) in no. of patients improved (pt global): 24/29 ketoprofen, 4/27 placebo.	5/29 ketoprofen, 14/27 placebo.	Withdrawals: 0/29 ketoprofen, 0/27 placebo AE; 129 placebo.	2
[Akermark et al. 1990]	Repetitive sports injuries	Indomethacin 1% spray, indomethacin oral, placebo spray/oral	n = 70 parallel group double dummy 3, 7, 14 days	1. Improvement visual analogue. 2. Physician global 5-pt scale. 3. Pain on movement, palpation, activity 4-pt scale	Indomethacin spray 0.5–1.5 ml 3–5 times a day indomethacin 3 × 25 mg tablets	1. Indomethacin spray showed sig improvement (P <0.05) day 3 & 7. 2. Marked improvement or symptom-free at 1 wk 10/22 indomethacin spray, 5/23 indomethacin oral, 3/24 placebo. 3. Marked improvement or symptom-free at 2 wk, 16/22 indomethacin.	4/23 Indomethacin spray, 0/23 Indomethacin oral, 0/24 placebo.	Withdrawals: 1/23 indomethacin spray, 1/23 indomethacin oral 0/24 placebo, AE; 4/23 indomethacin spray, 10/23 indomethacin oral, 0/24 placebo.	5
[Aoki et al. 1984]	Acute orthopaedic trauma	Piroxicam 0.5% gel, indomethacin 1% gel, placebo gel	n = 252 multicentre parallel group 0, 3, 7 days	Multiple outcomes 1. Overall improvement patient. 2. Pain intensity—movement, spontaneous.	1 g 3–4 times a day	1. Sig diff in overall improvement (P<0.05) piroxicam best. 2. Improvement day 7 piroxicam sig > placebo (P<0.01). 3. No. of patients better or much better: 56/84 piroxicam, 41/84 indomethacin, 33/84 placebo.	1/84 piroxicam, 2/84 indomethacin 2/84 placebo.	Withdrawals & AE: 0/84 piroxicam, 0/84 indomethacin, 0/84 placebo.	4
[Auclair et al. 1989]	Achilles heel, tendinitis of recent origin	Niflumic acid 2.5% gel, placebo gel	n = 243 parallel group 7, 21 days	1. Pain (VAS) on palpation. 2. Pain intensity at dorsiflexion 3. Global patient.	5 gm gel 3 times daily	1. Sig more pain reduction than placebo. 2. Pain on dorsiflexion disappeared or improved, 75/117 niflumic acid, 69/110 on placebo. 3. Global very good/good, 69/117, 54/109.	5/123 niflumic acid, 6/116 placebo.	AE withdrawal 1/123 niflumic acid, 0/116 placebo.	3
[Baracchi et al. 1982]	Acute soft tissue trauma	Ibyorifeb 10% cream, placebo cream	n = 40 parallel group 3, 5, 7, 10, 12, 14 days	1. Cat spontaneous pain, pain on movement, & pressure 2. Investigator global.	Twice daily	1. Ibuprofen sig > placebo (for spontaneous pain P = 0.001). 2. Global (good or excellent response): 17/20 ibuprofen, 3/20 placebo.	No. rep of local effects	Well tolerated.	4
[Campbell & Dunn 1994]	Acute ankle sprain <24 h	Ibuprofen 5% cream, placebo cream	n = 100 parallel group 2 wk diaries	VAS on rest & movement.	4 inches, 4 times a day	1. Ibuprofen > placebo on days 2 & 3. 2. No. of patients with improved walking ability at 7 day: 21/50 ibuprofen, 19/50 placebo.	Not rep	Withdrawals: 0/50 ibuprofen 0/50 placebo AE: 1/50 ibuprofen, 0/50 placebo, 55/100 returned diaries.	4
[Candela et al. 1986]	Traumatic sport injuries	Ketoprofen placebo gel	n = 30 parallel group 5, 10, 15 days	Cat scales, pain on pressure, on movement, functional limitation.	Twice daily	1. Ketoprofen > placebo. 2. No. of patients better/much better at day 10: 10/15 ketoprofen, 2/15 placebo.	Not rep	Not rep	1
[Chaterjee 1977]	Soft tissue injuries	Benzydamine 3% cream, placebo cream	n = 51 parallel group 6 days	Verbal rating pain: spontaneous, pressure, movement.	3 times a day	1. Benzydamine > placebo at 6 days spontaneous pain, pressure, movement. 2. On day 6 no. of patients none or slight pain on movement: 21/25 benzydamine, 12/25 placebo.	Not rep	Withdrawals & AE: 0/25 benzydamine, 0/25 placebo.	4
[Diebschlag 1986]	Ankle sprains	Diclofenac gel, placebo gel	n = 20 cross-over 2 × 1 wk	1. Ankle joint volume measurement 2. VAS-PI.	ad libitum	1. Reduced swelling & less pain with diclofenac.	Not rep	Withdrawals & AE: 0/20 diclofenac, 0/20 placebo.	3
[Diebschlag et al. 1990]	Acute ankle sprain	Ketorolac 2% gel, etofenamate 5% gel, placebo gel	n = 37 parallel group 2, 3, 4, 8, 14 days	1. Ankle joint volume measurement 2. VAS-PI	3 g 3 times a day	1. Ketorolac > placebo & etofenamate 2. No. improved day 3, 0/12 placebo, 11/13 ketorolac, 6/12 etofenamate.	1/13 ketorolac, 1/12 etofenamate, 0/12 placebo.	Withdrawals & AE: 0/12 placebo, 0/13 ketorolac, 0/12 etofenamate	4
[Diebschlag & Knocker 1987]	Ankle sprain <48 h	Salicylic acid ointment, placebo ointment	n = 80 parallel group 2, 3, 4, 8, 15 days	1. Ankle joint volume measurement. 2. VAS pain on rest & movement	10–15 cm ointment twice daily	Salicylic acid > placebo for all measures.	Not rep	Withdrawals & AE: 0/40 salicylic acid, 0/40 placebo.	5

Ref.	Condition	Drug	No., study design & follow-up	Outcome measures	Dose regimen	Analgesic outcome results	Skin irritation	Withdrawals & adverse effects	Quality score
[Dreiser 1988]	Acute tendinitis <1 month	Ibuprofen 5% cream, placebo cream	n = 64 parallel group 7 days	VAS pain on rest, pressure, movement.	4 cm 3 times a day	1. Ibuprofen > placebo (P <0.01). 2. Global improvement: 26/32 ibuprofen, 13/28 placebo	0/32 ibuprofen, 0/32 placebo.	Withdrawals & AE: 0/32 ibuprofen, 0/32 placebo.	3
[Dreiser 1988]	Simple sprains	Ketoprofen 5% gel, placebo gel	n = 60 parallel group 7 days	VAS-PI, on rest, movement. patient global	5 cm twice daily	Global improvement: 18/30 ketoprofen 5/30 placebo.	0/30 ketoprofen, 1/30 placebo.	Withdrawals & AE: 0/30 ketoprofen, 0/30 placebo.	5
[Dreiser et al. 1990]	Uncomplicated ankle sprains	Niflumic acid 2.5% gel, placebo gel	n = 60 parallel group 7 days	VAS-PI, investigator pain intensity, patient & investigator global.	5 g gel 3 times a day	Patient global (improved or healed) 23/30 niflumic acid, 10/30 placebo.	3/30 niflumic acid, 1/30 placebo.	Withdrawals & AE: 0/30 niflumic acid, 0/30 placebo.	5
[Dreiser et al. 1994]	Ankle joint pain after post-traumatic strain	Furbiprofen patch 40 mg, placebo patch	n = 131 parallel group 7 days	VAS spontaneous pain by patient.	2 patches a day	Mean VAS sig lower with furbiprofen pain better than moderate at day 7: 53/64 furbiprofen, 52/66 placebo.	Not rep	Withdrawals: 0/64 furbiprofen, 0/66 placebo.	4
[Fantato & De Gregorio 1971]	Oedema & post-traumatic pain	Benzydamine 3% cream, placebo cream	n = 52 parallel group 6 days	1. 4-pt verbal rating. 2. Investigator global with cat scale.	3 times a day	1. Benzydamine > placebo. 2. ≥50% fall in symptom score, 22/26 benzydamine, 14/26 placebo.	Not rep	Not rep	5
[Frahm 1993]	Acute knee or ankle sprains	Salicylic acid cream, 2% placebo cream	n = 156 parallel group 9 days	1. VAS-PI on movement & at rest.	10 cm cream twice daily	VAS-PI sig less on day 9 for salicylic acid cream.	0/78 salicylic acid, 0/78 placebo.	Withdrawals: 0/78 salicylic acid, 0/78 placebo AE: 0/78 salicylic acid, 1/78 placebo.	5
[Fujimaki et al. 1985]	Musculoskeletal pain	Piroxicam 0.5% gel, indomethacin 1% gel, placebo gel	n = 271 multicentre parallel group 7 days	1. 4-pt verbal rating scale pain on rest & movement. 2. Patient global.	1 g 3 times a day	1. Both actives better than placebo in producing marked improvement. 2. Overall improvement better & much better 44/92 piroxicam, 44/90 indomethacin, 40/89 placebo.	1/92 piroxicam, 6/90 indomethacin 2/89 placebo.	Withdrawals: 0/92 piroxicam, 1/90 indomethacin, 0/89 placebo AE: 0/92 piroxicam, 2/90 indomethacin, 0/89 placebo.	3
[Haig 1986]	Acute soft tissue injuries	Benzydamine 3% cream, placebo cream	n = 43 parallel group 2, 4, 6 days	4-pt verbal rating scale: spontaneous pain & pain on movement.	6 times a day	1. Improved day 6 pain on movement, NSD 18/21 benzydamine, 13/22 placebo. 2. Improved day 6 spontaneous pain, sig diff 20/21 benzydamine, 14/22 placebo.	0/21 benzydamine, 0/22 placebo.	Withdrawals & AE: 0/21 benzydamine, 0/22 placebo.	4
[Julien 1989]	Tendinitis	Ketoprofen 0.5% gel, placebo gel	n = 60 parallel group 7 days	1. Patient VAS-PI on rest & movement. 2. Overall patient assessment.	5 cm twice daily	Overall patient assessment (recovery, improvement) on day 7: 25/30 ketoprofen, 13/30 placebo.	1/30 ketoprofen, 0/30 placebo.	Withdrawals & AE: 0/30 ketoprofen, 0/30 placebo.	4
[Kockelbergh et al. 1985]	Acute-soft tissue injuries <1 wk	Ketoprofen 2.5% gel, placebo gel	n = 74 parallel group baseline & one wk	1. 4-pt verbal rating visual analogue pain intensity. 2. Global.	7.5 g gel twice daily	1. Ketoprofen > placebo in producing improved symptoms. 2. Patient global good: 30/38 ketoprofen, 22/36 placebo.	1/38 ketoprofen, 1/36 placebo.	Withdrawals & AE: 0/38 ketoprofen, 0/36 placebo.	2
[Kockelbergh et al. 1985]	Acute low back pain <10 days	Ketoprofen 2.5% gel, placebo gel	n = 40 parallel group 2 wk	1. VAS pain & 5-pt verbal rating. 2. Patient global rating.	15 g gel with physiotherapy & ultrasound 10 sessions.	1. Sig more patients with moderate/ severe pain at end in placebo group. 2. Global rating good, 13/20 ketoprofen, 9/20 placebo.	4/20 ketoprofen, 1/20 placebo.	Withdrawals & AE: 1/20 ketoprofen, 0/20 placebo.	3
[Lester 1983]	Sprained ankle	Salicylic acid 2% cream, placebo cream	n = 42 parallel group 7 days	1. Ankle movement. 2. Swelling. 3. Pain. 4. Return to normal activity.	NS	Pain relieved by 7 days: 18/20 salicylic acid, 13/22 placebo.	0/20 salicylic acid, 2/22 placebo.	Not rep	3
[Linde et al. 1985]	Sprained ankle	Benzydamine 5% cream, placebo cream	n = 100 parallel group 8 days	1. Swelling. 2. Pain on walking. 3. Fit for work.	3 times a day	Sig reduction in swelling with benzydamine NSD for pain. Free of walking pain day 8: 35/50 benzydamine, 40/50 placebo.	Not rep	Not rep	2
[McLatchie et al. 1989]	Acute soft tissue injury	Felbinac 3% gel, placebo gel	n = 231 parallel group baseline & 7 days	1. VAS-PI rest, movement, night pain. 2. Investigator global.	3 cm gel 3 times a day	Good/very good treatment response (physician assessment): 85/118 felbinac, 46/113 placebo.	3/118 felbinac, 2/113 placebo.	Withdrawals & AE: 0/118 felbinac, 0/113 placebo.	4
[Morris et al. 1991]	Acute soft tissue sports injuries	Felbinac 3% gel, placebo gel	n = 100 multicentre parallel group baseline & 7 days	1. Multiple global rating. 2. VAS pain.	1 cm gel 3 times a day	1. Felbinac > placebo. 2. No. of patients with good/ very good results (pt global: 23/50 felbinac, 13/50 placebo.	0/50 felbinac, 0/50 placebo.	Withdrawals & AE: 0/50 felbinac, 0/50 placebo.	4

Ref.	Condition	Drug	No., study design & follow-up	Outcome measures	Dose regimen	Analgesic outcome results	Skin irritation	Withdrawals & adverse effects	Quality score
[Noret et al. 1987]	Minor sports injuries	Ketoprofen 2.5% gel, placebo gel	n = 98 multicentre parallel group 1, 3, 8 days	1. VAS-PI. 2. 4-pt pain on pressure. 3. Global.	7.5 gel twice daily	1. Ketoprofen > placebo on many many indices. 2. Patient global good or better, 39/51 ketoprofen, 9/47 placebo.	1/51 ketoprofen, 0/47 placebo.	Withdrawals & AE: 1/51 ketoprofen, 0/47 placebo.	3
[Parrini et al. 1992]	Soft tissue injuries	Ketoprofen 15% foam placebo foam	n = 169 parallel group 7 days	1. Cat for spontaneous pain, on movement. 2. Cat global physician.	2 g 3 times a day	1. Ketoprofen > placebo for pain on pressure, movement & at rest. 2. Physician global excellent/good: 67/83 ketoprofen, 38/86 placebo.	0/83 ketoprofen, 0/86 placebo.	Withdrawals & AE: 0/83 ketoprofen, 0/86 placebo.	4
[Ramesh et al. 1983]	Soft tissue trauma	Ibuprofen 5% cream, placebo cream	n = 80 parallel group 0, 3, 7, 10 days	1. Pain on rest, pressure & movement, 4-pt scale. 2. Investigator global 3-pt.	5–10 cm 3–4 times a day	Pain on movement day 7 none/slight: 28/40, 16/40.	1/40 ibuprofen, 1/40 placebo.	Withdrawals & AE: 0/40 ibuprofen, 0/40 placebo.	4
[Russell 1991]	Soft tissue injuries	Piroxicam 0.5% gel, placebo gel	n = 214 parallel group 7 days up to 21 days	1. VAS pain on rest & movement. 2. Global 4-pt. 3. Daily pain charts.	1 g 4 times a day	1. Piroxicam > placebo at reducing pain by day 8. 2. Better joint mobility with piroxicam. 3. Global assessment of good/excellent: 79/100 piroxicam, 45/100 placebo.	4/102 piroxicam, 10/12 placebo.	Withdrawals: 1/102 piroxicam, 8/102 placebo AE: 4/102 piroxicam, 7/102 placebo.	5
[Sanguinetti 1989]	Soft tissue traumas	Biphenyl acetic acid 3% gel, placebo gel	n = 82 parallel group 7 days	Various scales.	3 times a day	Patient global: good or very good: 34/42 BPAA, 11/40 placebo.	0/42 BPAA, 0/40 placebo.	AE: 0/42 BPAA, 0/40 placebo.	4
[Sinneger & Blanchard 1981]	Sport microtrauma	Fentiazac 5% cream, placebo cream	n = 20 parallel group 10 days	Pain at rest, pressure, movement by physician	2 or 3 times a day	Total pain relief achieved within 10 days: 7/10 fentiazac, 1/10 placebo	0/10 fentiazac, 0/10 placebo.	Withdrawals & AE: 0/10 fentiazac, 0/10 placebo.	2
[Taboada 1992]	Acute musculoskeletal pain	Piroxicam gel, placebo gel	n = 40 parallel group 5–10 applications	Patient global	Dose of drug or duration not stated gels used with ultrasound with infrared	Excellent or good: 16/20 piroxicam, 6/20 placebo.	Not rep	Not rep	2
[Thorling et al. 1990]	Sport injuries	Naproxen 10% gel, placebo gel	n = 120 parallel group 7 days	1. Physician scoring of pain at rest, movement, swelling. 2. Patient & physician global.	2–6 times a day	Patient global, good or very good on day 7: 38/60 naproxen, 27/60 placebo.	1/60 naproxen, 0/60 placebo	Withdrawal & AE: 0/60 naproxen, 0/60 placebo.	3
[Vecchiet & Colozzi, 1989]	Soft tissue injuries	Meclofenamic acid 5% gel, placebo gel	n = 60 parallel group 5, 10 days	1. Cat for spontaneous pain on movement. 2. Patient & doctor global.	4 g twice daily	1. Meclofenamic acid > placebo. 2. Patient global: 30/30 meclofenamic acid, 19/30 placebo.	0/30 meclofenamic acid, 0/30 placebo.	Withdrawals & AE: 0/30 meclofenamic acid, 0/30 placebo.	3
[Wanet et al. 1979]	Traumatic rheumatological injuries	Diethylamine salicylate placebo gel	n = 56 parallel group 15 days	Pain on rest & movement.	3 times a day	Global assessment at end of treatment, good/very good: 20/32 salicylate, 9/24 placebo.	Not rep	Not rep	3
[Zerbi et al. 1992]	Painful traumatic injuries	Ketoprofen foam, ketoprofen gel, placebo foam	n = 154 parallel group 7 days	1. Pain at rest, under pressure, movement. 2. Global evaluation.	Twice daily application equivalent to 200 mg each time	1. Both active formulations sig better than placebo. 2. Patient global (positive result) 33/46 foam 35/49 gel 13/42 placebo.	2/46 ketoprofen foam, 0/49 ketoprofen gel, 0/42 placebo.	0/46 ketoprofen foam, 0/49 ketoprofen gel, 1/42 placebo, no AE withdrawals.	2

AE, adverse effects; cat, categorical; NS, not stated; NSD, no significant difference; VAS, visual analogue scale; VAS-PI, visual analogue scale of pain intensity; Not rep, not reported.

Appendix 1B
Details of trial design, outcome measures, and results in active controlled trials in acute painful conditions

Ref.	Condition	Drug	No., study design & follow-up	Outcome measures	Dose regimen	Analgesic outcome results	Skin irritation	Withdrawals & adverse effects	Quality score
[Arioli et al. 1990]	Acute musculoskeletal disorders	Piroxicam 1% cream, diclofenac 1% gel	n = 75 parallel group open design 3, 7, 14 days	1. Cat & VAS scales for pain on movement, at rest etc. 2. Patient global.	1 g piroxicam cream, 4 g diclofenac gel 4 times a day	1. Piroxicam > diclofenac on some measures. 2. Patient global 7 days (better/much better): 34/38 piroxicam, 27/37 diclofenac.	0/38 piroxicam, 0/37 diclofenac.	0/38 piroxicam, 0/37 diclofenac	2
[Baixauli et al. 1990]	Acute soft tissue trauma <24 h	Naproxen 10% gel, ketoprofen 10% gel	n = 30 parallel group 3, 7 days	1. Patient & investigator global rating 5-pt. 2. Improved 3-pt.	5 cm naproxen 3–5 cm ketoprofen twice a day	1. Cured or improved day 3 10/15. naproxen, 12/14 ketoprofen. 2. Cured or improved day 7 15/15 naproxen, 13/15 ketoprofen. 3. Patient global (good or very good) 13/15 naproxen 9/15 ketoprofen	0/15 naproxen, 0/15 ketoprofen.	Withdrawals & AE: 0/15 naproxen, 0/15 ketoprofen.	3
[Bouchier-Hayes et al. 1990]	Acute soft tissue injuries	Diclofenac 1% gel, felbinac 3% gel	n = 386 multicentre parallel group 3, 7 days	VAS pain on rest pressure, & movement.	4 g gel 3 times a day	1. Diclofenac > felbinac on some measures 2. ≥50% improvement in pain on movement on day 7: 110/191 diclofenac 100/195 felbinac	Not rep	0/191 diclofenac, 2/195 felbinac.	1 Probably not double-blind
[Butron et al. 1994]	Sprains & contusions	Naproxen 10% gel, diclofenac 1% gel	n = 64 parallel group 4 days	1. VAS pain on rest, movement. 2. Patient & physician global.	As required	Patient global good or excellent 30/34 naproxen, 28/30 diclofenac.	3/34 naproxen, 4/30 diclofenac.	0/34 naproxen, 0/30 diclofenac.	2
[Commandre et al. 1993]	Acute sprains or tendinitis	Niflumic acid 2.5% gel, piroxicam 0.5% gel	n = 100 parallel group 7, 14 days	1. Patient VAS. 2. Investigator categorical. 3. Patient global.	15 g of each per day	1. Niflumic acid sig better than piroxicam days 8 & 15 2. Patient global day 8: 41/51 niflumic acid 23/49 piroxicam	3/51 niflumic acid, 4/49 piroxicam.	0/51 niflumic acid, 0/49 piroxicam. AE withdrawals: 1/51 niflumic acid, 1/49 piroxicam	2
[Curioni et al. 1985]	Soft tissue injuries	Ibuproxam, ketoprofen, etofenamate	n = 60 parallel group 10 days	1. Pain: spontaneous, on palpation, movement. 2. Patient global.	twice daily application	Some diff between groups	2/20 ibuproxam, 3/20 ketoprofen, 1/20 etofenamate.	No info	4
[Diebschlag et al. 1992]	Acute ankle sprain	Indomethacin 1% gel (A) Indomethacin 1% gel (B) (diff vehicles)	n = 42 parallel group 2 wk	Swelling pain	3 times a day	No diff in swelling or pain between the two preparations. Patient global, excellent or good: 19/19 (A) 21/22 (B)	0/19 (A) 1/22 (B).	No diff	3
[Gallachi et al. 1990]	Painful inflammatory symptoms	Diclofenac 1% gel, diclofenac 1.16% gel	n = 50 parallel group 7, 14 days	1. Spontaneous pain. 2. Pain on pressure. 3. Patient global.	2 g 4 times a day	1. NSD. 2. NSD. 3. 19/25 both groups good/excellent.	0/25 both groups.	No data	2
[Governali & Casalini 1995]	Soft tissue injuries	Ketoprofen 5% gel, ketoprofen 1% cream	n = 30 parallel group 7, 14 days	1. Pain: spontaneous, movement, pressure. 2. Patient global.	2–3 g of gel or cream 3 times a day	1. Gel sig better than cream 2. On day 7, excellent or good: 14/15 ketoprofen gel 9/15 ketoprofen cream	0/15 ketoprofen gel, 0/15 ketoprofen cream.	Withdrawals & AE: 0/15 ketoprofen gel, 0/15 ketoprofen cream.	2
[Gualdi et al. 1987]	Soft tissue injuries	Flunoxaprophene gel, ketoprofen gel	n = 60 parallel group 1, 4, 7, 10 days	1. Pain intensity. 2. Function. 3. Patient global.	3–5 cm of gel, twice daily	NSD between groups	1/30 flunoxaprophene, 3/30 ketoprofen.	No info	2
[Hallmeier & Michelbach 1986]	Sports injuries	Etofenamate 10% gel plus dressing heparin/dexpanthenol/ dimethylsulphoxide	n = 60 parallel group 4 days	1. Oedema. 2. Erythema. 3. Movement. 4. Patient global 'success'.	Not given	4. Patient global: 26/30 etofenamate 10/30 heparin	0/30 etofenamate, 2/30 heparin.	Withdrawals: 0/30 etofenamate, 0/30 heparim.	2
[Hallmeier 1988]	Sprains & contusions	Etofenamate 10% gel, diclofenac 1% gel	n = 60 parallel group single-blind 7 days	Patient global.	2–4 times a day	Patient global very good or good: 27/30 etofenamate, 13/30 diclofenac.	0/30 etofenamate, 0/30 diclofenac.	Withdrawals & AE: 0/30 etofenamate, 0/30 diclofenac.	1
[Hosie 1993]	Acute lower back injury	Felbinac 3% foam, ibuprofen 400 mg tablets	n = 287 multicentre parallel group double dummy 7, 14 days	1. Pain 5-pt scale. 2. Investigator global.	2 g gel 3 times a day 1 tablet 3 times a day	1. No diff between the two groups in symptom severity. 2. Both showed sig improvement. 3. No or mild pain on movement at 14 days: 99/140 felbinac foam, 109/147 ibuprofen oral.	1/140 felbinac foam, 3/147 ibuprofen oral.	25/140 felbinac foam, 19/147 ibuprofen oral.	4

Ref.	Condition	Drug	No., study design & follow-up	Outcome measures	Dose regimen	Analgesic outcome results	Skin irritation	Withdrawals & adverse effects	Quality score
[Kroll et al. 1989]	Sprains & tendinitis	Piroxicam 0.5% gel, diclofenac 1.16% gel	n = 173 parallel group open to 14 days	1. Patient score of pain on movement (21 point VAS). 2. Patient global.	1 g piroxicam 2–4 g diclofenac 4 times daily	Patient global excellent or good: 63/84 piroxicam, 62/89 diclofenac.	4/84 piroxicam, 3/89 diclofenac.	Withdrawal: 2/84 piroxicam, 1/89 diclofenac, AE: 2/84 proxicam, 0/89 diclofenac.	2
[Montagna et al. 1990]	Painful musculoskeletal disorders	Meclofenamic acid 5% gel naproxen 10% gel	n = 40 parallel group 4, 8, 15 days	1. Pain—spontaneous & on movement 2. Patient global	Prescribed amounts twice daily	1. No statistical diff between groups 2. Exellent/good on day 8: 13/20. meclofenamic acid, 10/20 naproxen.	no data	no data.	1
[Oakland 1993]	Acute injuries of lateral ankle ligaments	Felbinac plus placebo, ultrasound placebo, gel plus ultrasound, felbinac plus ultrasound	n = 220 parallel group days 3, 5, 7	1. Pain at rest. 2. Investigator global.	1–2 g gel 2–3 times a day	NSD.	3/147 felbinac, 3/73 placebo.	0/147 felbinac, 2/73 placebo.	3
[Picchio et al. 1981]	Acute sports injuries	Ibuprofen 10% gel, ketoprofen 1% gel	n = 40 parallel group 4, 8, 12, 16 days	5-pt pain for pain at rest, on movement, spontaneous.	3 times a day	1. Ibuprofen sig better & faster than ketoprofen. 2. No. with no pain on movement at 12 days: 16/20 ibuprofen, 10/20 ketoprofen.	not rep	0/20 ibuprofen, 0/20 ketoprofen.	3
[Pineda et al. 1983]	Acute soft tissue injuries	Felbinac 3% gel, piroxicam gel (?0.5%)	n = 172 multicentre parallel group 3 & 7 days	1. Multiple 10-pt pain on rest movement & night pain. 2. Global 5-pt.	3 times a day felbinac 180 mg/day piroxicam 18 mg/day	1. Felbinac > piroxicam for complete recovery at 7 days (P = 0.008). 2. Good/very good global: 68/86 felbinac, 65/86 piroxicam.	5/86 felbinac, 1/86 piroxicam.	1/86 felbinac, 0/86 piroxicam.	1
[Rosemeyer 1991]	Distortion of ankle joint	Diclofenac 1% gel, piroxicam 0.5% gel	n = 91 parallel group 3, 7, 10, 14 days	1. Pain at rest. 2. Pain on pressure. 3. Patient global.	10 cm diclofenac 3 cm piroxicam 4 times a day	1/2 NSD at any time. 3. Patient global excellent/good: 35/44 diclofenac, 40/47 piroxicam.	4/44 diclofenac, 5/47 piroxicam.	AE withdrawal: 0/44 diclofenac, 1/47 piroxicam.	4
[Dreiser 1989]	Acute soft tissue injury	Ketoprofen gel, piroxicam gel,	n = 1575 parallel group 5 days	Patients global assessment of injury	Ketoprofen 4–5 g piroxicam 1 g diclofenac 2–4 g three times daily for 5 days	Greatly improved: 396/1048 ketoprofen, 69/263 piroxicam, 80/264 diclofenac.	Not rep	Not rep	2
[Selligra & Inglis 1990]	Soft tissue injuries	Naproxen 10% gel, flufenamic acid 3% gel	n = 100 parallel group single blind 7 days	Patients global	2–6 times a day	Good or very good: 31/49 naproxen, 28/51 flufenamic acid.	1/49 naproxen, 0/51 flufenamic acid.	Withdrawals: 1/49 naproxen, 0/51 flufenamic acid AE: 0/49 naproxen, 0/51 flufenamic acid.	2
[Sugioka et al. 1984]	Non traumatic disease of muscle or tendon	Piroxicam 0.5% gel, indomethacin 1% gel	n = 366 multicentre parallel group 1 & 2 wk	Multiple pain 4-pt. 7-pt symptom improvement	1 g 3 or 4 times a day	Piroxicam > indomethacin 1. patient self-assessment better & much better: 85/183 piroxicam, 55/183 indomethacin.	1/183 piroxicam, 12/183 indomethacin	Withdrawals: 1/183 piroxicam, 12/183 indomethacin AE: 6/183 piroxicam, 26/183 indomethacin.	4
[Tonutti 1994]	Soft tissue trauma	Ketoprofen 5% gel, etofenamate 5% gel	n = 30 parallel group 7 days	1. Pain—spontaneous, on movement, pressure.	2–3 g gel 3 times a day for up to 3 wk	1. Comparable efficacy. good/excellent: 10/15 ketoprofen, 11/15 etofenamate.	0/15 ketoprofen, 0/15 etofenamate.	0/15 ketoprofen, 0/15 etofenamate.	4
[Vanderstraeten & Scheumans 1990]	Strains & sprains of lower limbs within 3 days	Etofenamate 10% gel naproxen 275 mg tablets	n = 60 parallel group 7, 17 days	1. Cat scales for spontaneous pain & pain on palpation.	5 cm gel 3 times a day, 1 tablet 3 times a day	1. Day 7 no or slight pain: 13/30 etofenamate gel, 15/30 naproxen oral. 2. Clinical global good or excellent improvement: 12/30 etofenamate gel, 13/30 naproxen oral.	1/30 etofenamate gel, 0/30 naproxen oral.	0/30 etofenamate gel, 6/30 naproxen oral, Withdrawals: 1/30 etofenamate gel, 2/30 naproxen oral.	2

See Appendix 1A for key to abbreviations.

Appendices 1A and 1B references

Airaksinen O, Venäläinen J, Pietil/ainen T. Ketoprofen 2.5% gel versus placebo gel in the treatment of acute soft tissue injuries. *International Journal of Clinical Pharmacology, Therapy and Toxicology* 1993; **31**:561–3.

Åkermark C, Forsskåhl B. Topical indomethacin in overuse injuries in atheletes. A randomized double blind study comparing Elmetacin® with oral indomethacin and placebo. *International Journal of Sports Medicine* 1990; **11**:393–6.

Aoki T *et al*. Comparative study of piroxicam gel with indomethacin gel and piroxicam placebo gel in the treatment of pain from orthopedic trauma. *Japanese Pharmacology and Therapeutics* 1984; **12**:101–17.

Arioli G, Scaramelli M, Pillosu W. [Topical therapy of acute skeletal muscle diseases. Results of a comparative study on piroxicam cream 1% versus diclofenac emulgel 1%] La terapia topica delle affezioni acte musculoscheletriche. Risultati di uno studio comparativo sul piroxicam crema 1% versus diclofenac emulgel 1%. *Clinica Terapeutica* 1990; **134**:363–9.

Auclair J, Georges M, Grapton X, Gryp L, D'Hooghe M, Meisser RG *et al*. A double-blind controlled multicenter study of percutaneous niflumic acid gel and placebo in the treatment of achilles heel tendinitis. *Current Therapeutics Research* 1989; **46**:782–8.

Baixauli F, Inglés F, Alcántara P, Navarrete R, Puchol E, Vidal F. Percutaneous treatment of acute soft tissue lesions with naproxen gel and ketoprofen gel. *Journal of International Medical Research* 1990; **18**:372–8.

Baracchi G, Messina Denaro S, Piscini S. [Experience of the topical use of isobutylfenylproprionic acid (Ibuprofen) in traumatic inflammation. A double-blind comparison with placebo] Esperienza sull'impiego topico dell'acido isobutil-fenil-proprioico (Ibuprofen) nell flogosi traumatica. Confronto a doppia cecità con placebo. *Gazzetta Medica Italiana* 1982; **141**:691–4.

Bouchier-Hayes TA, Rotman H, Darekar BS. Comparison of the efficacy and tolerability of diclofenac gel (Voltarol Emulgel) and felbinac gel (Traxam) in the treatment of soft tissue injuries. *British Journal of Clinical Practice* 1990; **44**:319–20.

Boutrón F, Galicia A, Zamora G, Martinez-Zurita F. Single-blind study to evaluate the efficacy and safety of naproxen gel compared with diclophenac emulgel in the treatment of soft tissue injuries. *Proceedings of the West Pharmacology Society* 1994; **37**:153–6.

Campbell J, Dunn T. Evaluation of topical ibuprofen cream in the treatment of acute ankle sprains. *Journal of Accident and Emergency Medicine* 1994; **11**:178–82.

Candela V, Bagarone A. Studio in cieco semplice sull'attivita terapeutica del 'Fastum Gel' nelle lesioni traumatiche da sport. *Medicina dello Sport* 1986; **39**:57–63.

Chatterjee DS. A double-blind clinical study with benzydamine 3% cream on soft tissue injuries in an occupational health centre. *Journal of International Medical Research* 1977; **5**:450–8.

Commandre F, Zakarian H, Corriol-rohou S. Comparison of the analgesic and anti-inflammatory effects of topical niflumic acid gel versus piroxicam gel in the treatment of musculoskeletal disorders. *Current Therapeutic Research* 1993; **53**:113–21.

Curioni GB, Di Domenica F, Daolio P, Spignoli G. Valutazione dell'efficacia terapeutica di ibudros gel in traumatologia. *Clinica Europa* 1985; **24**:456–60.

Diebschlag W. [Diclofenac in blunt traumatic ankle joint swelling. Volumetric monitoring in a placebo controlled double blind trial] Diclofenac bei stumpf-traumatischen Sprunggelenkschwellungen. Volumetrische Verlaufsbestimmung im plazebokontrollierten Doppelblindversuch. *Fortschritte der Medizin* 1986; **104**:437–40.

Diebschlag W, Nocker W, Bullingham R. A double-blind study of the efficacy of topical ketorolac tromethamine gel in the treatment of ankle sprain, in comparison to placebo and etofenamate. *Journal of Clinical Pharmacology* 1990; **30**:82–9.

Diebschlag W, Nocker W. [The effect of topical treatment in the treatment of disease in ankle sprains] Einfluß einer topischen Behandlung auf den Krankheitsverlauf bei Sprunggelenks-Distorsionen. *Arzneimittel Forschung [Drug Research]* 1987; **37**:1076–81.

Diebschlag W, Nocker W, Lehmacher W. Treatment of acute sprains of the ankle joint. A comparison of the effectiveness and tolerance of two gel preparations containing indomethacin. *Fortschritte der Medizin* 1992; **110**:64–72.

Dreiser RL. Clinical trial of efficacy and tolerability of topical ibuprofen in the treatment of tendinitis. *Journal International de Médecine* 1988; **119**:15–31.

Dreiser RL. Clinical trial—Fastum gel FG-6. (unpublished) 1989.

Dreiser RE, Charlot J, Lopez A, Ditisheim A. Clinical evaluation of niflumic acid gel in the treatment of uncomplicated ankle sprains. *Current Medical Research* 1990; **12**:93–9.

Dreiser RL, Roche R, De Sahbe R, Thomas F, Leuteneger E. Flurbiprofen local action transcutaneous: clinical evaluation in the treatment of acute ankle sprains. *European Journal of Rheumatology and Inflammation* 1994; **14**:9–13.

Fantato S, De Gregorio M. Clinical evaluation of topical benzydamine in traumatology. *Arzneimittel Forschung [Drug Research]* 1971; **21**:1530–5.

Frahm E, Elsasser U, Kämmereit A. Topical treatment of acute sprains. *British Journal of Clinical Practice* 1993; **47**:321–2.

Fujimaki E *et al*. Clinical evaluation of piroxicam gel versus indomethacin gel and placebo in the treatment of muscle pain: a double-blind, multicenter study. *Japanese Pharmacology and Therapeutics* 1985; **12**:119–37.

Gallacchi G, Mautone G, Lualdi P. Painful inflammatory conditions. Topical treatment with diclofenac hydroxyethylpyrrolidine. *Clinical Trials Journal* 1990; **27**:58–64.

Governali E, Casalini D. Ricerda clinica controllata tra ketoprofene gel 5% e ketoprofene crema 1% in pazienti con postumi di lesioni traumatiche. *La Riabilitazione* 1995; **28**:61–69.

Gualdi A, Bonollo L, Martini A, Forgione A. Antinflammatori no steroidi per uso topico in traumatologia: studio clinico con flunoxaprofene e chetoprofene. *Riforma Medica* 1987; **102**:401–404.

Haig G. Portable thermogram technique for topically applied benzydamine cream in acute soft-tissue injuries. *International Journal of Tissue Reactions* 1986; **8**:145–7.

Hallmeier B. Efficacy and tolerance of etofenamate and diclofenac in acute sports injuries. *Rheumatism* 1988; **8**:183–6.

Hallmeier B, Michelbach B. Etofenamat unter tapeverbänden. *Die Medizinische Welt* 1986; **37**:1344–8.

Hosie GAC. The topical NSAID, felbinac, versus oral ibuprofen: a comparison of efficacy in the treatment of acute lower back injury. *British Journal of Clinical Research* 1993; **4**:5–17.

Julien D. Clinical trial—Fastum gel FG-8. (unpublished) 1989.

Kockelbergh M, Verspeelt P, Caloine R, Dermaux F. [Local anti inflammatory treatment with a ketoprofen gel: current clinical findings] Traitement anti-inflammatoire local par un gel de kétoprofène: données cliniques récentes. *Acta Belgica Medica Physica* 1985; **8**:205–13.

Kroll MP, Wiseman RL, Guttadauria M. A clinical eveluation of piroxicam gel: an open comparative trial with diclofenac gel in the treatment of acute musculoskeletal disorders. *Clinical Therapeutics* 1989; **11**:382–91.

Lester AA. Management of sprained ankles. *Practitioner* 1983; **225**:935–6.

Linde F, Hvass I, Jürgensen U, Madsen F. Ankelforstuvninger behandlet med benzydamin 5% creme. *Ugeskrift for Laeger* 1985; **148**:12–3.

McLatchie GR, McDonald M, Lawrence GF, Rogmans D, Lisai P, Hibberd M. Soft tissue trauma: a randomised controlled trial of the topical application of felbinac, a new NSAID. *British Journal of Clinical Practice* 1989; **43**:277–80.

Montagna CG, Turroni L, Martinelli D, Orlandini MC. Single-blind comparative study of meclofenamic acid gel versus naproxen gel in acute musculoskeletal disorders. *Current Therapeutic Research* 1990; **47**:933–9.

Morris WD, Scott HV, Peters WA, Ketelbey JW. Felbinac topical gel for acute soft tissue sports injuries. *New Zealand Journal of Sports Medicine* 1991; **19**:45–7.

Noret A, Roty V, Allington N, Hauters P, Zuinen C, Poels R. Ketoprofen gel as topical treatment for sport injuries. *Acta Therapeutica* 1987; **13**:367–78.

Oakland C. A comparison of the efficacy of the topical NSAID felbinac and ultrasound in the treatment of acute ankle injuries. *British Journal of Clinical Research* 1993; **4**:89–96.

Parrini M, Cabitza P, Arrigo A, Vanasia M. [Efficacy and tolerability of ketoprofen lysine salt foam for topical use in the treatment of traumatic pathologies of the locomotor apparatus] Efficacia e tollerabilità del ketoprofene sale di lisina schiuma per uso topico nel trattamento di alcune patologie traumatiche dell'apparato locomotore. *Clinica Terapeutica* 1992; **141**:199–204.

Picchio AA, Volta S, Longoni A. Studio clinico controllato sull'impiego dell'ibuprofen per uso topico in traumatologica sportiva. *Medicina dello Sport* 1981; **34**:403–6.

Pineda MD, Capulong OM, De Guzman DL, Te CV. The topical NSAIDs, felbinac and piroxicam: a comparison of efficacy and safety in the treatment of acute soft tissue trauma. *British Journal of Clinical Research* 1993; **4**:63–72.

Ramesh N, Steuber U. Dolgit® cream in accident- and sports-related injuries in medical practice. Results of a double blind study. *Therapiewoche* 1983; **33**:4563–70.

Rosemeyer B. Behandlung von distorsionen des sprunggelenkes. *Die Medizinische Welt* 1991; **42**:166–70.

Russell AL. Piroxicam 0.5% topical gel compared to placebo in the treatment of acute soft tissue injuries: a double-blind study comparing efficacy and safety. *Clinical and Investigative Medicine* 1991; **14**:35–43.

Sanguinetti C. Trattemento con BPAA gel dei traumi dei tessuti moli. *Clinical Terapeutica* 1989; **130**:255–8.

Seligra A, Inglés F. A comparative study of naproxen gel and flufenamic acid gel in the treatment of soft tissue injuries. *Current Medical Research* 1990; **12**:249–54.

Sinniger M, Blanchard P. Controlled clinical trial with fentiazec cream in sport microtraumatology. *Journal of International Research* 1981; **9**:300–2.

Sugioka Y *et al*. Multicenter clinical evaluation of piroxicam gel vs. indomethacin gel in the treatment of non-traumatic diseases of tendon or muscle. *Japanese Pharmacology and Therapeutics* 1984; **12**:139–53.

Taboada A. Experencia controlada con gel de piroxicam asociado a ultrasonidos en afecciones agudas del aparato locomotor. *Prensa Medica Argentina* 1992; **79**:630–2.

Thorling J, Linden B, Berg R, Sandahl A. A double-blind comparison of naproxen gel and placebo in the treatment of soft tissue injuries. *Current Medical Research* 1990; **12**:242–8.

Tonutti A. Utilizzazione del ketoprefene gel 5% (Oridis gel) nella pratica traumatologica: studio in doppio cieco controllato verso etofenamato. *Ortopedica Traumatologica* 1994; **XIV**:119–25.

Unknown. Comparative clinical efficacy of Oruvail, piroxicam and diclofenac gels in soft tissue injury. Unpublished 1993.

Vanderstraeten G, Schuermans P. Study on the effect of etofenamate 10% cream in comparison with an oral NSAID in strains and sprains due to sports injuries. *Acta Belgica Medica Physica* 1990; **13**:139–41.

Vecchiet L, Colozzi A. Effects of meclofenamic acid in the treatment of lesions deriving from minor traumatology. *Clinical Journal of Pain* 1991; **7**:S54–9.

Wanet G. [Controlled clinical study of a topic associating nopoxamine with diethylamine salicylate (Algésal suractivé) in physical medicine and rehabilitation (author's transl)] Etude clinique contrôlée. d'un topique associant la nopoxamine au salicylate de diéthylamine (Algésal suractivé) en médecine physique et réhabilitation. *Journal Belge de Médecine Physique et de Réhabilitation* 1979; **2**:119–26.

Zerbi E, Pace A, Demarchi F, Bassi F, Arrigo A, Garagiola U. Ketoprofen lysine salt in a new foam formulation for the topical treatment of traumatic injuries: a controlled, between-patient, clinical trial. *Current Therapeutic Research* 1992; **51**:823–9.

Appendix 2A

Details of trial design, outcome measures, and results in placebo controlled trials in chronic painful conditions

Ref.	Condition	Drug	No., study design & follow-up	Outcome measures	Dose regimen	Analgesic outcome results	Skin irritation	Withdrawals & adverse effects	Quality score
[Algozzini et al. 1982]	Osteoarthritis of the knee	Trolamine salicylate 10% cream, placebo cream	n = 26 cross-over 1 wk	1. 4-pt pain intensity. 2. Numerical rating 0–10.	3.5 g cream 4 times a day	1. NSD. 2. Patient preference 8/26 salicylate, 6/26 placebo, 11/26 no preference. 3. No. with pain relief from diaries 9/26 salicylate, 6/26 placebo.	0/26 salicylate, 0/26 placebo.	Withdrawals & AE: 0/26 salicylate, 0/26 placebo.	4
[Bolten 1991]	Acute extra-articular rheumatic disorders	Felbinac 3% gel, placebo gel	n = 281 parallel group 0, 7, 14 days	1. Cat & VAS on rest & movement. 2. VAS. 3. Investigator global rating	1 g 3 times a day	1. Felbinac sig better than placebo. 2. Global estimation of good/very good responses (P <0.001); 67/142 felbinac, 39/139 placebo.	2/142 felbinac, 4/139 placebo	Withdrawals & AE: 0/142 felbinac, 0/139 placebo.	3
[Camus 1975]	Rheumatic disorders	Diethylamine salicylate cream, placebo cream	n = 20 parallel group 10 days	4-pt verbal rating.	3 times a day	1. Salicylate > placebo in giving relief over 10 days. 2. Pain reduced: 8/10 salicylate, 3/10 placebo.	0/10 salicylate, 0/10 placebo.	Withdrawals & AE: 0/10 salicylate, 0/10 placebo.	2
[Dreiser & Tisne-Camus 1993]	Osteoarthritis of the knee	Diclofenac plasters, placebo plasters	n = 155 parallel group 4, 7, 15 days	1. VAS. 2. Global rating 5-pt.	Applied twice daily (each plaster contained 180 mg diclofenac derivative)	1. Diclofenac > placebo from day 4. 2. Global rating excellent or good 55/78 diclofenac, 21/77 placebo.	1/78 diclofenac, 3/77 placebo.	Withdrawals: 0/78 diclofenac, 0/77 placebo. AE: 0/78 diclofenac, 1/77 placebo.	4
[El-Hadidi & El-Garf 1991]	Painful rheumatic conditions	Diclofenac gel, ultrasound coupling gel	n = 120 parallel group 4 wk	Physician judgement + VAS-PI by patient at rest & on movement patient global.	3 times a wk	Diclofenac sig better than regular coupling gel on all measures. Complete relief of pain on passive movement at 2 wk: 26/60 diclofenac, 18/60 regular.	2/60 diclofenac, 1/60 regular.	Withdrawals: 1/60 diclofenac, 0/60 regular. AE: 0/60 diclofenac, 0/60 regular.	3
[Fotiades & Bach 1976]	Cervical, lumbar & shoulder pain & gonarthroses	Flufenamate 3% + salicylate 2% gel, placebo gel	n = 100 parallel group up to 20 days	Point scoring system including pain at rest, on pressure, pain relief, muscle spasm & movement.	3 or 4 times a day for 6–20 days	Scoring very good & good 43/48 active, 26/52 placebo.	0/48 active, 0/52 placebo.	Withdrawals & AE: 0/48 active, 0/52 placebo.	3
[Galiazzi & Marcolongo 1993]	Rheumatological disorders	Diclofenac plaster (slow release), placebo plaster	n = 60 parallel group 3, 5, 7, 14 days	1. Multiple 4-pt verbal rating & VAS. 2. Investigator global scale.	Applied twice daily (each plaster contained 180 mg diclofenac derivative)	1. Diclofenac > placebo in reducing pain. 2. Assessment of good/excellent response: 26/30 diclofenac, 2/30	0/30 diclofenac, 0/30 placebo.	0/30 diclofenac, 0/30 placebo.	3
[Ginsberg & Famaey 1991]	Tendinitis	Indomethacin 4% spray, placebo spray	n = 30 cross-over 2 × 2 wk	1. VAS. 2. 4-pt verbal rating.	2–4 sprays 3–5 times a day lightly massaged into skin	1. Indomethacin > placebo on various pain indices. 2. Subjective improvement 26/30 indomethacin, 18/30 placebo.	2/30 indomethacin, 0/30 placebo.	0/30 indomethacin, 0/30 placebo.	2
[Gui et al. 1982]	Osteoarthritis	Ibuprofen cream, placebo cream	n = 40 parallel group 21 days	Spontaneous pain & pain on pressure & movement	Application twice daily	1. No. improved spontaneous pain: 17/19 ibuprofen, 9/20 placebo. 2. No. improved pain on movement: 14/19 ibuprofen, 7/20 placebo.	0/19 ibuprofen, 0/20 placebo.	0/19 ibuprofen, 0/20 placebo.	3
[Hohmeister 1983]	Cervical & lumber back pain	Flufenamate 3% + salicylate 2% gel, placebo gel.	n = 100 parallel group 7, 14, 21 days	Symptom improvement, complete pain relief	3 times a day	Complete pain relief at 21 days: 38/49 active gel, 3/51 placebo.	8/49 active, 0/51 placebo.	Withdrawals: 0/49 active, 0/51 placebo.	4
[Mattara et al. 1994]	Scapulohumoral periarthritis	Flurbiprofen 40 mg patch, placebo patch.	n = 80 parallel group 14 days	VAS pain intensity for extention, flexion & abduction	Twice daily	Day 14 no pain or slight pain: 14/40 flurbiprofen, 13/40 placebo.	4/40 flurbiprofen, 1/40 placebo.	Withdrawals: 0/40 flurbiprofen, 0/40 placebo. AE: 5/40 flurbiprofen, 2/40 placebo.	4
[Rose et al. 1991]	Gonarthrosis	Piroxicam 0.5% gel, placebo gel.	n = 30 parallel group 14 days	1. Pain on movement. 2. Pain at rest. 3. Patient global.	1 g gel 4 times a day	1. No pain 7/15 piroxicam, 2/15 placebo. 3. Excellent or good 8/15 piroxicam, 5/15 placebo.	1/15 piroxicam, 1/15 placebo.	0/15 piroxicam, 0/15 placebo.	2
[Roth 1995]	Osteoarthritis breakthrough pain	Diclofenac gel, placebo gel.	n = 119 parallel group 14 days	1. Overall pain.	4 times a day 2 wk	NSD	12/59 diclofenac, 26/60 placebo.	AE withdrawals: 3/59 diclofenac, 4/60 placebo.	4

AE, adverse effects; Cat, categorical; NSD, no significant difference; VAS, visual analogue scale; VAS-PI, visual analogue scale of pain intensity.

Appendix 2B
Details of trial design, outcome measures, and results in active controlled trials in chronic painful conditions

Ref.	Condition	Drug	No., study design & follow-up	Outcome measures	Dose regimen	Analgesic outcome results	Skin irritation	Withdrawals & adverse effects	Quality score
[Ammer 1991]	Soft tissue rheumatism with pain of medium intensity	Diclofenac gel, Indomethacin 1% gel	n = 227 parallel group 14 days	1. Pain at rest & on movement. 2. General efficacy.	2–4 days a wk	1. NSD. 2. Good/excellent: 76/89 diclofenac, 62/84 indomethacin.		AE withdrawal: 1/89 diclofenac, 0/84 indomethacin.	2
[Balthazar-Letawe 1987]	Rheumatological disorders	Diclofenac gel, indomethacin gel	n = 50 parallel group 7, 14 day	1. Symptom intensity 3-pt scale. 2. Investigator global.	Twice daily	No. improved at 14 days: 15/25 diclofenac, 17/25 indomethacin.	0/25 diclofenac, 0/25 indomethacin.	Withdrawals & AE: 0/25 diclofenac, 0/25 indomethacin.	4
[Browning & Johson 1994]	Mild to moderate osteoarthritis	Normal oral NSAID half normal oral plus piroxicam	n = 91 parallel group open study 14–28 days	1. Patients assessment of pain & stiffness. 2. Patients overall assessment of efficacy day.	3–4 times a day piroxicam	1. Sig reduction in mean score for tenderness & restriction of active movement for topical. 2. Patients' overall assessment of efficacy day, excellent or good: 54/85 oral alone, 71/106 oral plus topical.	1/106 piroxicam.	Withdrawal: 1/106 piroxicam. AE: 1/106 piroxicam, 1/85 oral alone.	2
[Dickson 1991]	Chronic osteoarthritis of the knee	Piroxicam 0.5% gel ibuprofen	n = 235 multicentre parallel group double-dummy 4 wk	1. Pain 9-pt scale. 2. Analgesic consumption. 3. Global 4-pt scale.	1 g gel 3 times a day 400 mg ibuprofen 3 times a day	NSDs between the treatments patient global rating good or better: 68/117 piroxicam, 65/118 ibuprofen.	3/117 piroxicam, 4/118 ibuprofen.	AE: 30/117 piroxicam, 27/118 ibuprofen. Withdrawals: 9/117 piroxicam, 7/118 ibuprofen.	4
[Geller 1980]	Chronic disorders	Diethylamine salicylate 10% gel etofenamate 5% gel	n = 50 cross-over 7 days 4-day washout	1. Pain in rest & movement 4-pt scale. 2. Global 5-pt scale patient.	Not rec	1. Diethylamine salicylate > etofenamate on all scores. 2. After first phase, good or very good results patient global: 24/25 salicylate, 8/25 etofenamate.	2 local effects, but drug responsible not given.	Not rep	2
[Giacovazzo 1992]	Osteoarthritis	Diclofenac gel, felbinac gel (BPAA)	n = 40 parallel group 1 wk	VAS-PI	Diclofenac 160 mg/day, felbinac 90 mg/day 3 times a day	No diff between the two treatments. Improvement in pain scores: 14/20 diclofenac, 14/20 felbinac.	0/20 diclofenac, 0/20 felbinac	0/20 diclofenac, 0/20 felbinac.	1
[Golden 1978]	Rheumatic pain	Triethylamine salicylate 10% cream, oral aspirin 325 mg tablet	n = 40 parallel group double dummy 7 days	Daily diaries, cat scales.	Application of cream 4 times a day 2 tablets 4 times a day	Good/excellent results: 13/20 salicylate cream, 10/20 oral aspirin.	1/20 salicylate cream, 1/20 oral aspirin.	2/20 salicylate cream, 6/20 oral aspirin	3
[Matucci-Cerinic & Casini 1988]	Soft tissue rheumatic disorders	Ketoprofen 2.5% gel, etofenamate 5% gel	n = 36 parallel group 3, 7 days	VAS-PI & tenderness.	Twice daily	1. Ketoprofen > etofenamate for pain on active & passive movement.	0/18 ketoprofen, 0/18 etofenamate,	0/18 ketoprofen, 0/18 etofenamate	2
[Reginster et al. 1990]	Rheumatoid arthritis	Indomethacin 1% gel, indomethacin 4% spray	n = 20 cross-over 14 days	% improvement: on swelling & pain at rest on flexion	3 times a day, 100 mg a day total	Both improved sig from baseline.	2/20 2/20	Withdrawals & AE: 0/20 0/20	2
[Ritchie 1996]	Soft tissue rheumatism of shoulder or elbow	Flurbiprofen patch, piroxicam 0.5% gel	n = 131 cross-over at 4 days 4, 8, 14 days	Pain, tenderness.	Flurbiprofen patch 40 mg twice daily 3 cm piroxicam gel 4 times a day	Statistically more pain relief with flurbiprofen		AE withdrawals: 1/133 flurbiprofen, 3/133 piroxicam.	2
[Rosenthal & Bahous 1993]	Periarticular, tendinous inflammations	DHEP 1% plaster, diclofenac 1% gel	n = 190 parallel group 14 days	Spontaneous pain, pain on pressure, patient global.	Plaster twice daily gel 4 times a day	Patient global, good or excellent: 79/96 plaster, 39/94 gel.	2/96 plaster, 3/94 gel.	Withdrawals & AE: 0/96 plaster, 0/94 gel.	3
[Vitali 1980]	Orthopaedic	Ketoprofen 1, 2.5 & 5% gel	n = 62 parallel group 14 days	Spontaneous pain, palpation, movement.	5–15 cm twice daily 6–13 days	1. The 2.5% gel was the most useful. 2. Spontaneous pain better/much better: 13/20 1% gel, 18/20 2.5% gel, 16/20 5% gel.	Not rep	Not rep	3

See Appendix 2A for key to abbreviations.

Appendices 2A and 2B references

Algozzine GJ, Stein GH, Doering PL, Araujo OE, Akin KC. Trolamine salicylate cream in osteoarthritis of the knee. *Journal of the American Medical Association* 1982; **247**:1311–13.

Bolten W. [Felbinac gel for treatment of localized extra-articular rheumatic diseases–a multicenter, placebo controlled, randomized study] Felbinac-Gel zur Behandlung lokalisierter extra-artikulärer rheumatischer Beschwerden—eine multizentrische, placebokontrollierte, randomisierte Studie. *Zeitschrift für Rheumatologie* 1991; **50**:109–13.

Camus J. Action de la Myrtécaïne associée au Salicylate de Diéthylamine, en traitement local, dans diverses affections rheumatismales. *Rheumatologie* 1975; **27**:61–6.

Dreiser RL, Tisne-Camus M. DHEP plasters as a topical treatment of knee osteoarthritis—a double-blind placebo-controlled study. *Drugs Under Experimental and Clinical Research* 1993; **19**:117–23.

El-Hadidi T, El-Garf A. Double-blind study comparing the use of Voltaren Emulgel versus regular gel during ultrasonic sessions in the treatment of locaized traumatic and rheumatic painful conditions. *Journal of International Medical Research* 1991; **19**:219–27.

Fotiades P, Bach GL. Wirkung einer flufenaminsäurehaltigen salbe bei verschiedenen rheumatischen erkrankungen. *Fortschritte der Medizin* 1976; **94**:1036–8.

Galeazzi M, Marcolongo R. A placebo-controlled study of the efficacy and tolerability of a nonsteroidal anti-inflammatory drug, DHEP plaster, in inflammatory peri- and extra-articular rheumatological diseases. *Drugs Under Experimental and Clinical Research* 1993; **19**:107–15.

Ginsberg F, Famaey JP. Double-blind, randomized crossover study of the percutaneous efficacy and tolerability of a topical indomethacin spray versus placebo in the treatment of tendinits. *Journal of International Medical Research* 1991; **19**:131–6.

Gui L, Pellacci F, Ghirardini G. Impiego dell'ibuprofen crema in pazienti ambulatoriali di interesse ortopedico. Confronto in doppia cecità con placebo. *Clinica Terapeutica* 1982; **101**:363–9.

Hohmeister R. Die behandlung von weichteilrheumatischen erkrankungen mit mobilisin gel. *Fortschritte der Medizin* 1983; **101**:1586–8.

Mattara L, Trotta F, Biasi D, Cervetti R. Evaluation of the efficacy and tolerability of a new locally acting preparation of flurbiprofen in scapulohumeral periarthritis. *European Journal of Rheumatology and Inflammation* 1994; **14**:15–20.

Rose W, Manz G, Lemmel E-. Behandlung der akitivierten gonarthrose mit topisch appliziertum piroxicam-gel. *München Medizinische Wochenschift* 1991; **133**:562–6.

Ammer K. Perkutane antirheumatische therapie beim weichteil-rheumatismus. *Rheumatologie* 1991; **6**.

Balthazar-Letawe D. [Voltaren Emulgel in rheumatological practice. A comparative trial with Indocid gel] Voltaren Emulgel en pratique rheumatologique. Essai comparatif avec Indocid gel. *Acta Belgical Medica Physica* 1987; **10**:109–10.

Browning RC, Johson K. Reducing the dose of oral NSAIDs by use of feldene gel: an open study in elderly patients with osteoarthritis. *Advances in Therapeutics* 1994; **11**:198–206.

Dickson DJ. A double-blind evaluation of topical piroxicam gel with oral ibuprofen in osteoarthritis of the knee. *Current Therapeutic Research* 1991; **49**:199–207.

Geller O. [Comparison of a salicylate heparin gel with a monosubstance preparation. Results of a double blind cross over study] Vergleich eines Salizylat/Heparin-Gels mit einem Mono-Substanzpräparat. Ergebnisse einer Doppelblind-cross-over-Studie. *MMW. Munchener Medizinesche Wochenschrift* 1980; **122**:1231–2.

Giacovazzo M. Clinical evaluation of a new NSAID applied topically (BPAA Gel) vs. diclofenac emulgel in elderly osteoarthritic patients. *Drugs Under Experimental and Clinical Research* 1992; **18**:201–3.

Golden EL. A double-blind comparison of orally ingested aspirin and a topically applied salicylate cream in the relief of rheumatic pain. *Current Therapeutic Research* 1978; **24**:524–9.

Matucci-Cerinic M, Casini A. Ketoprofen vs etofenamate in a controlled double-blind study: evidence of topical effectiveness in soft tissue rheumatic pain. *International Journal of Clinical Pharmacology Research* 1988; **8**:157–60.

Reginster JY, Crommen J, Renson M, Franchimont P. Percutaneous administration of indomethacin in rheumatoid arthritis. *Current Therapeutic Research* 1990; **47**:548–53.

Ritchie LD. A clinical evaluation of flurbiprofen LAT and piroxicam gel: a multicentre study in general practice. *Clinical Rheumatology* 1996; **15**:243–7.

Rosenthal M, Bahous I. A controlled clinical study on the new topical dosage form of DHEP plasters in patients suffering from localized inflammatory diseases. *Drugs Under Experimental and Clinical Research* 1993; **19**:99–105.

Vitali G. [Controlled clinical experiment with the topical use of 2-(3-benzoyl-phenyl) proprionic acid at 3 different concentrations] Sperimentazione clinica controllata sull'impiego topico dell'acido 2-(3-benzoil-fenil) proprionico a tre diverse concentrazioni. *Clinica Terapeutica* 1980; **94**:257–73.

13

Injected morphine in postoperative pain

Summary

This systematic review examined pain relief after injected morphine compared with placebo in patients with moderate or severe pain after surgery, and related the efficacy of injected morphine to that of oral analgesics. MEDLINE, EMBASE ('morphine', 'diamorphine', 'heroin', a combination of free text words and MeSH terms, no language restriction), Cochrane Library, reference lists, review articles, and specialist textbooks were searched for randomized single dose placebo controlled trials.

Pain relief or pain intensity difference over 4 to 6 hours, and adverse effects were extracted. The number of patients with at least 50% pain relief was derived, and then used to calculate the relative benefit and the number-needed-to-treat (NNT) for one patient to achieve at least 50% pain relief for 4 to 6 hours.

Fifteen trials compared intramuscular morphine 10 mg (486 patients) with placebo (460 patients) and the NNT was 2.9 (95% confidence interval 2.6–3.6). One in three patients with moderate or severe postoperative pain achieved at least 50% pain relief who would not have done had they been given placebo. Minor adverse effects were commoner with morphine (34%) than with placebo (23%) (relative risk 1.49, 1.09–2.04), but drug-related study withdrawal was rare and not different from placebo. Ten mg of intramuscular morphine gives analgesia equivalent to oral non-steroidal anti-inflammatory drugs (NSAIDs) in keeping with historic results from single trials. For patients who can swallow, oral NSAIDs may be the best choice.

Introduction

Perhaps, understandably, we all tend to believe that injecting drugs provides better pain relief than taking the same drug by mouth. Indeed, it took generations to persuade doctors that oral morphine was effective in cancer pain—they all wanted to inject. This chapter focuses on the postoperative pain relief produced by injection of morphine, using the same methods as for the oral drugs. What we wanted to achieve was an estimate of the analgesic efficacy of injected morphine which we could compare with the estimates for the oral drugs. Did injected morphine perform better?

Methods

Single dose randomized placebo controlled trials of injectable (intramuscular, subcutaneous, and intravenous) morphine in acute postoperative pain were sought. A number of different search strategies were used to identify eligible reports in MEDLINE (1966–97), EMBASE (1980–97), the Cochrane Library (1997 issue 2) and the Oxford Pain Relief Database (1950–94) [2]. The last electronic search was conducted in March 1997. The words 'morphine', 'diamorphine', 'heroin' were used to identify relevant reports, using a combination of free text words and MeSH (Medical Standardized Heading) terms, and without restriction to language. Additional reports were identified from reference lists of retrieved reports, review articles, and specialist textbooks.

Excluded and included reports

We screened reports to eliminate those without pain outcomes, those which were definitely not randomized, or were abstracts or reviews. Each report which could possibly be described as a randomized controlled trial was read independently by each of the authors and scored using a three-item, 1–5 score, quality scale [3]. Consensus was then achieved. The maximum score of an included study was 5 and the minimum score was 1.

Inclusion criteria were full journal publication of randomized controlled trials which included single dose treatment groups of injected (intravenous, intramuscular, or subcutaneous) morphine and placebo, acute postoperative pain, blinded design, baseline pain of moderate to severe intensity, adult patients, and assessments of pain intensity or pain relief over 4 to 6 hours with results for total pain relief (TOTPAR), summed pain intensity difference (SPID), visual analogue total pain relief (VAS-TOTPAR), or visual analogue summed pain intensity difference (VAS-SPID), or with data from which these could be calculated. Review articles, letters, or abstracts were not included.

Data extraction and analysis

Data extracted from the reports were the pain setting, study treatment groups, numbers of patients treated, study duration, the route and dose of morphine, and mean or derived

The topic discussed in this chapter is also published in full in McQuay *et al.* [1].

TOTPAR, SPID, VAS-TOTPAR, VAS-SPID, or any dichoto-mous global pain relief outcome. Information on minor and major adverse events as defined by the authors of the original reports was also extracted.

For each report with mean TOTPAR, SPID, VAS-TOTPAR, or VAS-SPID values for morphine and placebo, the data was converted to percentage of maximum by division into the calculated maximum value [4]. The proportion of patients in each treatment group who achieved at least 50%maxTOTPAR was calculated using verified equations [5–7]. These proportions were then converted into the number of patients achieving at least 50%maxTOTPAR by multiplying by the total number of patients in the treatment group [5].

Information on the number of patients with >50%maxTOTPAR for morphine and placebo was used to calculate relative risk (or benefit) and NNT by pooling data when available from at least three comparisons between morphine and placebo with a particular dose and route of administration. Relative risk or benefit estimates were calculated with their 95% confidence intervals (CI) using a random effects model [8] for analgesic data which were not homogeneous ($P < 0.1$) and a fixed-effects model [9] for adverse effect data which were homogeneous ($P > 0.1$). Homogeneity of the analgesic results was also explored graphically [10]. NNT [11] was calculated with 95% confidence interval [12]. A statistically significant difference from control was assumed when the 95% confidence intervals of the relative risk/benefit did not include 1. Statistical difference between NNTs was assumed when confidence intervals did not overlap.

Results

Eighteen reports of 20 trials fulfilled the inclusion criteria; 696 patients were given morphine and 563 placebo. No trials of subcutaneous morphine or of diamorphine by any route of administration met the inclusion criteria. Morphine was given by intramuscular injection in all reports except one [13] in which it was given intravenously. Morphine doses were 5 mg [14, 15], 8 mg [13, 16], 10 mg [14, 15, 17, 18–29], 12.5 mg [30] and 20 mg [28]. Details of these studies are given in Table 1.

Two studies [18, 30] included a mixed population of patients with postoperative and other acute pain. Trials otherwise investigated pain relief predominantly after orthopaedic and gynaecological surgery. Pain outcomes were over 6 hours except for two studies in which they were over 4 hours [22, 30]. Quality scores were 2 for two reports, 3 for six, 4 for nine, and 5 for one.

Nine reports that appeared to fulfill inclusion criteria were omitted. Three studies [31–33] had pain relief or intensity information for one hour or less. Two reports [34, 35] appeared to duplicate previously published information. Four reports [36–39] used non-standard assessments which could not be used.

Only for 10 mg of intramuscular morphine was data available from at least three trials to be pooled for meta-analysis. In 15 comparisons 486 patients were given 10 mg intramuscular morphine and 460 placebo (Table 2). The size of the active treatment group in these trials varied between 9 and 51 patients (mean 33 patients, median 30).

The placebo response rate (i.e. the proportion of patients given placebo experiencing at least 50% pain relief) varied from 0% to 47% (mean 15%), and the response rate with 10 mg intramuscular morphine was 7% to 93% (mean 46%; Fig. 1). Of the 15 comparisons between 10 mg intramuscular morphine and placebo, eight were statistically superior to placebo and had a lower confidence interval of the relative benefit above 1 (Table 2). The pooled relative benefit was 2.8 (95% CI 2.0–3.8).

The pooled NNT for 10 mg intramuscular morphine compared with placebo was 2.9 (2.6–3.6). Omitting the trial which included acute non-surgical pain [18] did not affect the result. The pooled NNTs without this study were 3.1 (2.7–3.8). Trials which had fewer than the median number of patients given morphine (fewer than 32 patients treated) gave an NNT of 2.9 (2.3–4.1), the same as larger trials (32 patients or more) with an NNT of 3.0 (2.5–3.8).

Minor adverse effects occurred in 34% of patients given intramuscular morphine compared with 23% of patients given placebo. This was a significantly increased rate with a relative risk of 1.49 (1.09–2.04). Major adverse effects (drug-related study withdrawal) were rare (overall 1.2%) and did not differ between morphine and placebo (Table 2).

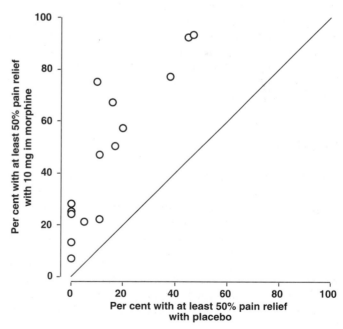

Fig. 1 Relation between the proportion of patients achieving at least 50% pain relief with 10 mg intramuscular (IM) morphine in 15 trials.

Table 1 Details of patients, methods, outcomes, treatments, and results for included studies

Ref.	Condition & no. of patients	Design, study duration, & follow-up	Outcome measures	Treatment groups	Analgesic outcome results (morphine vs. placebo)	Withdrawals & exclusions	Adverse effects	Comment	Quality score
[16]	General & gynae surgery $n = 96$ Age: not given	RCT, double-blind, single dose, parallel group. Assessments by single nurse observer, hourly assessments up to 6 h. Moderate to severe baseline pain.	Standard 4-pt PI; standard 5-pt PR; 9 item tension/ anxiety questionnaire.	1. IM morphine 8 mg $n = 24$. 2. placebo $n = 24$. 3. IM hydroxyzine 100 mg $n = 24$. 4. IM hydroxyzine + morphine $n = 24$.	Morphine superior to placebo PID (Fig. 1).	Withdrawals not reported.	Sedative AE M 19/24 vs. P 3/24.	Morphine better than placebo.	3
[20]	Various surgical procedures $n = 90$ Age: Adults 18–68	RCT, double-blind, single dose, parallel group, double-dummy. Assessed by single nurse observer at 0, 0.5, 1 h then hourly intervals for 6 h. Med taken when baseline pain was at least moderate.	PI (5-pt) none, slight, moderate, severe, very severe. PR (5-pt) none, poor, fair, good, very good. 50% pain relief at 6 h Time to next analgesic.	1. IM morphine 10 mg $n = 30$. 2. placebo $n = 30$. 3. po naproxen 550 mg $n = 30$.	SD between morphine & placebo for most outcomes. 1. % patients with > 50% pain relief P 37% vs. M 77% $P = 0.002$. 2. Mean h in study (SD) P 3.2 (1.5) vs. M 4.7 (1.4). 3. 6 h mean SPID P 2.1 vs. M 5.5. 4. 6 h mean TOTPAR values not given. (NB 5-pt SPID).	No. of patients remaining in study at 6 h P 5 (17%) vs. M13 (43%) $P = 0.01$ early termination due to inadequate relief M 16 (20%) vs. P 25 (83%) $P = 0.01$.	No study withdrawals reported due to AE. NSD between treatments. No. of patients reporting one or more AE P 14 (47%) vs. M 22 (73%) vs. N 13 (43%)	NSAID better than morphine.	4
[27]	Various surgical procedures $n = 150$ Age: 18–66	Study 3 only. RCT, double-blind, single dose, double-dummy, parallel group. Assessed by single nurse observer at 0, 0.5, 1 h then hourly intervals for 6 h. Med taken when baseline pain was at least moderate.	PI (5-pt) 1 = none, 2 = slight, 3 = moderate, 4 = severe, 5 = very severe. PR (5-pt) 5 = none, 4 = poor, 3 = fair, 2 = good, 1 = very good. Pain half gone at end of study, or at time of withdrawal.	1. IM morphine 10 mg $n = 30$. 2. placebo $n = 30$. 3. po anirolac 600 mg $n = 30$. 4. po anirolac 125 mg $n = 30$. 5. po anirolac 5 mg $n = 30$.	1. 6 h SPID mean (SE) M 5.2 (0.6) vs. P 0.9 (1.0) $P < 0.003$. 2. 6 h TOTPAR mean (SE) M 17.7 (1.0) vs. P 24.1 (1.1) $P < 0.003$. NB wrong calculation 50% not reported for TOTPAR.	% completing 6 hr study M 43% P 30%.	No study withdrawals reported due to AE. NSD % patients reporting AE M 41% vs. P 23%.	NSAID better than morphine. Wrong calculations used for Fig. 2 TOTPAR	4
[18]	Various acute and medical patients (2 part studies) $n = 120$ (each study) Age: Adults	RCT, single dose, parallel group, double-blind. Assessments by single nurse observer at 0, 30 min, 1, 2, 3, 4, 5 & 6 h. Baseline pain at least moderate.	Standard 4-pt PI; Pain relief 50%.	1. IM morphine 10 mg $n = 30$. 2. placebo $n = 30$. 3. IM nefopam 20 mg $n = 30$. 4. IM diphenhydramine 20 mg $n = 30$.	1. SPID M 12.32 vs. P 6.48. 2. 50% pain relief M 76% vs. P 49.6%.	Patients completing M 28/30 vs. P 23/40. No. reporting no relief at 2 h. M 1/30 vs. P 6/30. No. dropped out for other reasons M1 vs. P1.	No. reporting AE M 66 vs. P 20	Morphine better than placebo.	3
[13]	Various day surgery procedures $n = 90$ Age: 23–69 yr	RCT, single dose, parallel group, double-blind. Assessments by single observer at 0, 30 min, 1, 2, 3, 4, 5 & 6 h. Baseline pain at least moderate.	VAS-PI 10 cm.	1. IV Morphine 8 mg $n = 30$. 2. placebo $n = 30$. 3. po fenoprofen 200 mg $n = 30$.	Morphine gave significantly less pain than placebo at all assessment times. No VAS-SPID, but data can be calculated from Table.	Withdrawals at 2 h M 3/30 vs. P 20/30 vs. F 8/30.	No. reporting AE M 4 vs. P 3 vs. F 2.	Morphine better than placebo	4

Table 1 *continued*

Ref.	Condition & no. of patients	Design, study duration, & follow-up	Outcome measures	Treatment groups	Analgesic outcome results (morphine vs. placebo)	Withdrawals & exclusions	Adverse effects	Comment	Quality score
[14]	Orthopaedic surgery (hip & knee replacement) n = 176 Age: Adults	RCT, double-blind, single dose, parallel group, double-dummy? Assessed by patients at 0, 0.5, 1 h then hourly intervals for 6 h. Med taken when baseline pain was at least moderate.	PI (5-pt) 0 = none, 1 = mild, 2 = moderate, 3 = severe, 4 = very severe. VAS-PI 100 mm 0–99. PR (5-pt) 0 = none, 1 = a little, 2 = some, 3 = a lot, 4 = complete patient & investigator global evaluation end of study.	1. IM morphine 10 mg n = 51. 2. IM morphine 5 mg n = 50. 3. placebo n = 25. 4. po ketorolac 10 mg n = 50.	1. 6 h mean SPID (SD) M 10 7.2 (3.9) vs. M 5 6.7 (4.6) vs. P 2.4 (3.8) P < 0.01. 2. 6 h mean TOTPAR (SD) M 10 14.0 (6.0) vs. M 5 12.4 (6.7) vs. P 5.0 (7.3) P < 0.01.	105 remaining in study at 6 h M 10 33 vs. M 5 32 vs. P 7 P < 0.01.	5 patients withdrew due to AE: M 2 vs. P 1 M 10 sig > AE than P P 0.01 (Table 4) No. of patients reporting AE M 10 26/51 vs. M 5 17/50 vs. P 5/25	NSAID comparable to morphine. Diff in sample size active vs. placebo controls.	4
[24]	Gynae surgery n = 92 Age: Not stated	RCT, double-blind, single dose, parallel group, double-dummy. Assessed by patients at 0, 1 h then hourly intervals for 6 h. Med taken when baseline pain was at least moderate.	Standard 4-pt PI; investigator rating end of treatment poor/fair = no effect, good/excellent = effective. Pain relief derived score half gone. Need for additional analgesia.	1. IM morphine 10 mg n = 30. 2. placebo n = 30. 3. po flurbiprofen 50 mg n = 30.	1. 6 h mean SPID M 5.17 vs. P 1.80 P < 0.01. 2. Pain more than half gone at 6 h M 6 (20%) vs. P 0 (0%). 3. 6 h mean TOTPAR M 16.98 vs. P 10.80 P < 0.01.	Cumulative drop out rate shown in Table II. No. of patients dropped out at 6 h M 21 (70%) vs. P 66 (74%).	Study withdrawals due to AE not stated. No. of patients reporting AE M 4 vs. P 4	NSAID comparable to morphine.	4
[19]	Orthopaedic & major gynae surgery n = 139 Age: 18–65	RCT, double-blind, single dose, parallel group, double-dummy. Assessed by single observer at 0, 15, 30 min, 1 h then hourly intervals for 6 h. Med taken when baseline pain was at least moderate. Injections into deltoid muscle.	Standard 4-pt PI; PR (5-pt) -1 = worse, 0 = none, 1 = a little, 2 = moderate, 3 = a lot, 4 = complete. VAS-PI 10 cm. Patient rating end of treatment (4-pt) 1 = poor, 2 = fair, 3 = good, 4 = excellent 50% relief (derived).	1. IM morphine 10 mg n = 36. 2. placebo n = 35. 3. IM tramadol 30 mg n = 34. 4. IM tramadol 60 mg n = 34.	1. 6 h mean SPID M 5.0 vs. P 1.6. 2. 6 h mean TOTPAR M 10.1 vs. P 3.6. Fig. 1 shows % patients with > 50% pr at each time point	Cumulative drop-out rate shown in Fig. 2.	Study withdrawals due to AE not reported No. of patients reporting AE not given. Nausea M 5 vs. P 1. Vomit M 4 vs. P 1.	Morphine better than synthetic mixed agonist antagonist control.	3
[21]	Postop wound pain n = 160 Age: 19–70	RCT, double-blind, single dose, parallel group. Assessed by more than 1 observer at 0, 15, 30 min, 1 h then hourly intervals for 6 h. Med taken when baseline pain was at least moderate.	Standard 4-pt PI; PR (6-pt) -1 = worse, 0 = slight, 2 = moderate, 3 = substantial, 4 = complete. VAS-PI 100 mm. Patient rating of treatment (4-pt) poor, fair, good, excellent. Investigator rating of treatment (satisfactory/unsatisfactory).	1. IM morphine 10 mg n = 40. 2. placebo n = 40. 4. IM dezocine 10 mg n = 40. 5. IM dezocine 15 mg n = 40.	1. Pain intensity scores mean shown in Table 3. 2. Pain Relief mean scores shown in Fig. 2. 3. No. of patients with moderate to complete relief by time shown in table. 4. No. of patients rating treatment as good or excellent M 15/36 vs. P 6/24	Not given.	No study. withdrawals reported due to AE. NSD reported between groups	High dose of dezocine better than morphine.	3
[17]	Acute postop pain n = 9/17 (completed cross-over each treatment) Age: 22–65	RCT, double-blind, single dose, cross-over design. Assessed by nurse observer at 0, 30 min, 1 h then hourly intervals for 6 h. Med taken when baseline pain was at least moderate.	Standard 4-pt PI; PR (5-pt) VAS-PI. VAS-PR. VAS-mood.	1. IM morphine 10 mg n = 9. 2. placebo n = 9. 3. oral cocaine 10 mg n = 9. 3. oral cocaine 10 mg + morphine n = 9.	1. VAS-TOTPAR: P 90 vs. M 135 vs. C 70 vs. C + M 161. 2. VAS-SPID: P 58 vs. M 99 vs. C 35 vs. C + M 108.	9 of 17 postop patients completed cross-over.	No. of patients reporting AE's: P 2/12 vs. M 6/13 vs. C 4/16 vs. M + C 7/13.	Morphine better than placebo.	3

Table 1 *continued*

Ref.	Condition & no. of patients	Design, study duration, & follow-up	Outcome measures	Treatment groups	Analgesic outcome results (morphine vs. placebo)	Withdrawals & exclusions	Adverse effects	Comment	Quality score
[30]	Postop & acute traumatic pain n = 250 Age: 21–75	RCT, double-blind, 4 doses of same drug given over 2 days. Nurse observers. assessments at 0, 30 min, 1 h then hourly intervals for 4 h. Med taken when baseline pain was at least moderate.	Standard 4-pt PI; No. of patients with > 50% pain relief.	1. IM morphine 12.5 mg n = 50. 2. placebo n = 49. 3. po codeine 90 mg n = 50. 4. po pentazocine 75 mg n = 50. 5. po oxycodone compound (oxycodone hydrochloride 4.5 mg, oxycodone terephthalate 0.30 mg, aspirin 224 mg, phenacetin 160 mg, caffeine 32 mg) n = 49	1. Derive SPID data for dose 1 day 1 from Fig. 1. 2. SPID for day 1 M 4.90 vs. P 1.20 vs. pentazocine 3.43 vs. cod 3.63 vs. oxycodone 4.35	Not reported.	Total side effects per dose M n = 14/50 34 p n = 4/49.9 pentazocine n = 12/50 cod n = 11/50 25 oxycodone n = 2/49 3.	Morphine better than placebo.	4
[26]	Major abdominal & orthopaedic surgery n = 151 Age: 18–65	RCT, double-blind, parallel group. Assessments at 0, 30 min, 1 h then hourly intervals for 6 h. Med taken when baseline pain was at least moderate.	PI (4-pt) 0 = none, 1 = slight, 2 = moderate, 3 = severe. PR (scale not described). Additional analgesia treatment effective/partially effective/ineffective (derived score).	1. IM morphine 10 mg n = 30. 2. IM placebo n = 30. 3. IM tonazocine 2 mg n = 29. 4. IM tonazocine 4 mg n = 30. 5. IM tonazocine 2 mg n = 31.	Morphine superior to placebo for most outcomes, as were other active treatments. 1. SPID see Fig. 4. 2. TOTPAR see Fig. 3.	See Fig. 6 for % remed by time.	Patients with no AE M 10/30 vs. P 25/30.	High dose of mixed agonist antagonist better than morphine, only extractable.	2
[25]	Major obstetric & gynae surgery n = 181 Age: 19–65	RCT, double-blind, single dose, parallel group. Assessments at 0, 30 min, 1 h then hourly intervals for 6 h. Med taken when baseline pain was at least moderate.	Standard 4-pt PI; PR 1 = unchanged/worse, 2 =< half gone, 3 = half gone, 4 = > half gone, 5 = completely gone. Investigator global 1 = no effect, 2 = poor, 3 = fair, 4 = good, 5 = excellent. Need for supplementary analgesia.	1. IM morphine 10 mg n = 51. 2. placebo n = 55. 3. po flurbiprofen 50 mg n = 53. 4. po zomepirac 100 mg n = 22.	1. SPID mean 6 h M 10.7 vs. 5.07 (see Fig. 2). 2. TOTPAR mean 6 h M 23.91 vs. P 14.54 (see Fig. 2). 3. No. requesting additional analgesia M 12/47 vs. 34/50.	No. of dropped out at 6 h M 15 vs. P 34.	1 patient reported AE with M, no other AE.	No diff between NSAID and morphine. Zomepirac treatments incomplete.	3
[28]	3rd molar extraction n = 252 Age: 18–40	RCT, double-blind, double dummy, parallel group. Assessments at 0, 15, 30, 45 min, 1 h then hourly intervals for 8 h. Med taken when baseline pain was at least moderate.	PI (5-pt) 0 = gone, 1 = slight, 2 = moderate, 3 = severe, 4 = unbearable. PR (11-pt) 0–10. PR (5-pt) 0 = none to 4 = complete. Patient rating of treatment 4 & 8 h 1–5. Onset of relief. Duration of relief. Remed time.	1. IM morphine 10 mg n = 37. 2. IM morphine 20 mg n = 37. 3. IM placebo n = 37. 4. IM lornoxicam 4 mg n = 33. 5. IM lornoxicam 8 mg n = 38. 6. IM lornoxicam 16 mg n = 38. 7. IM lornoxicam 20 mg n = 37.	1. 4 h mean SPID (SD) M 10 mg 1.9 (2.7) vs. M 20 mg 3.9 (3.0) vs. P–5 (2.5). 2. 4 h mean TOTPAR (SD) M 10 mg 5.1 (3.8) vs. M 20 mg 8.8 (3.6) vs. P 1.2 (2.3). 8 h values available.	Time to remed (median + range) M 10 mg 185 65–540, M 20 mg 540 100–540, P 80 30–540 min.	No. of patients reporting AE M 10 mg 32/37 M 20 mg 37/37 P 22/37.	No diff between NSAID and morphine. Extractable data—global rating?	5
[29]	Obstetric & gynae surgery n = 53 Age: 26–61	RCT, double-blind, single dose, parallel group. Assessments at 0, 15, 30 min, 1 h then hourly intervals for 6 h. Med taken when baseline pain was at least moderate.	PI 0–3 4 h & 8 h SPID. PR 0–4. Pain reduced by half. Patient rating of treatment at end of study.	1. IM morphine 10 mg n = 14. 2. IM placebo n = 12. 3. IM enadoline 15 mg n = 14 (kappa agonist). 4. IM enadoline 25 mg n = 13.	1. 6 h mean SPID values not given only levels of sig. 2. 6 h mean TOTPAR (SE?) M 2.7 (1.1) vs. P 0.9 (1.2).	Study stopped early due to neuro-psychiatric effects from enadoline. No. of patients completing study M 1 vs. P 0.	No AE reported with M or P.	No diff between enadoline and morphine. Problems with methods study 2.	4

Table 1 *continued*

Ref.	Condition & no. of patients	Design, study duration, & follow-up	Outcome measures	Treatment groups	Analgesic outcome results (morphine vs. placebo)	Withdrawals & exclusions	Adverse effects	Comment	Quality score
[22]	Orthopaedic, gynae & general surgery $n = 190$ Age: 26–61	RCT, double-blind, single dose, parallel group. Single observer, assessments at 0, 15, 30 min, 1 h then hourly intervals for 4 h. Med taken when baseline pain was at least moderate.	PI (3-pt) mild, moderate, severe. % PR 0 = none, 1 = < 50%, 2 = 50%, 3 = > 50%, 4 = 100% Pain reduced by half.	1. IM morphine 10 mg $n = 39$. 2. IM placebo $n = 38$. 3. IM dezocine 5 mg $n = 38$. 4. IM dezocine 10 mg $n = 37$. 5. IM dezocine 15 mg $n = 38$.	Morphine superior to placebo for some, but not all outcomes. 1. 4 h mean TOTPAR M 5.8 vs. P 3.1. 2. 50% relief at 4 h M 36.8% vs. P 11.4%. 3. Diff in proportion of patients with adequate relief at 2 & 4 h only M vs. P.	Not stated.	% patients reporting AE M 10% P 8%	Dezocine (mixed agonist antagonist) better than morphine on some outcomes. Check Table III—whose judgement?	4
[23]	Orthopaedic, gynae & general surgery $n = 160$ Age: 18–65	RCT, double-blind, multiple dose, parallel group, more than one observer, assessments at 0, 15, 30 min, 1 h then hourly intervals for 6 h. Med taken when baseline pain was at least moderate.	Standard 4-pt PI; PR −1 = worse, 0 = none, 1 = a little, 2 = moderate, 3 = a lot, 4 = complete. Patient rating end of treatment 1 = poor, 2 = fair, 3 = good, 4 = excellent.	1. IM morphine 10 mg $n = 40$. 2. IM placebo $n = 40$. 3. IM ciramadol 30 mg $n = 40$. 4. IM ciramadol 60 mg $n = 40$.	Morphine superior to placebo for all outcomes, as were other active treatments 1. TOTPAR see Figs 2. SPID see Figs 3. VAS-SPID see Figs 4. Patient rating of good or excellent M 48.7% vs. P 26%. Global on p 1106 = M 85% vs. P 26%.	% remed at 6 h M 48.7 vs. P 90%.	% patients reporting AE M 6 (15%) P 7 (18%).	Little diff between ciramadol and morphine. Extractable data—TOTPAR from figs	4
[15]	Orthopaedic, gynae & general surgery $n = 100$ Age: 18–65	RCT, double-blind, single, parallel group, medical observer, assessments at 0, 15, 30 min, 1 h then hourly intervals for 6 h. Med taken when baseline pain was at least moderate.	Standard 4-pt PI; PR −1 = worse, 2 = moderate, 1 = a little, 2 = moderate, 3 = a lot, 4 = complete. VAS-PI 10 cm. Sedation 0–3. Patient & investigator rating of treatment poor, fair, good, excellent.	1. IM morphine 5 mg $n = 20$. 2. IM morphine 10 mg $n = 20$. 3. IM placebo $n = 20$. 4. IM ciramadol 30 mg $n = 40$. 5. IM ciramadol 60 mg $n = 40$.	Morphine superior to placebo for most outcomes. 1. 6 h TOTPAR M 10 13.6 vs. M 5 9.5 vs. P 1.1. 2. 6 h SPID M 10 9.3 vs. M 5 6.3 vs. P 1.3. 3. 6 h VAS-SPID M 10 262.4 vs. M 5 132.0 vs. P 37.9. Other data available.	Mean drop-out rate p 106.	Incidence of AE M 10 0/2 M 5 4/20 P 4/20.	Ciramadol better than morphine on some outcomes.	2

AE, adverse effect; F, fenoprofen; IM, intramuscular; M, morphine; NSD, no significant difference; P, placebo; PI, pain intensity; PID, pain intensity difference; po, oral; PR, pain relief; SD, single dose; SPID, summed pain intensity differences; TOTPAR, total pain relief; VAS-PI, visual analogue scale of pain intensity; VAS-PR, visual analogue scale of pain relief; VAS-TOTPAR, visual analogue scale of total pain relief; VAS-SPID, visual analogue scale of summed pain intensity differences. Standard 4-pt PI; 0, none; 1, slight; 2, moderate; 3, severe. Standard 5-pt PR; 0, none; 1, slight; 2, moderate; 3, good; 4, complete. References to Tables and Figures refer to the original reports.

Table 2   Analgesia and adverse effects of 10 mg intramuscular morphine

Trial (date order)	Ref.	At least 50% pain relief with morphine	At least 50% pain relief with placebo	Relative benefit or relative risk (95% CI)			NNT or NNH (95% CI)		
Campos *et al.* 1980	[18]	28/30	14/30	2.0	1.4	3.0	2.1	1.5	3.7
van den Abeele & Camu 1983	[15]	15/20	2/20	7.5	2.0	28.6	1.5	1.1	2.4
Fragen *et al.* 1983	[19]	17/36	4/35	4.1	1.5	11.1	2.8	1.8	6.1
Brown *et al.* 1984	[20]	23/30	11/29	2.0	1.2	3.4	2.6	1.6	6.5
Gravenstein 1984	[21]	10/40	0/40	101	0.2	>250	4.0	2.6	8.8
Pandit *et al.* 1985	[22]	8/39	2/38	3.9	0.9	17.2	6.7	3.4	138
Powell 1985	[23]	11/39	0/40	114	0.2	>250	3.6	2.4	7.1
DeLia *et al.* 1986	[24]	15/30	5/30	3.0	1.3	7.2	3.0	1.8	9.1
Morrison *et al.* 1986	[25]	47/51	25/55	2.0	1.5	2.7	2.1	1.6	3.2
Kaiko *et al.* 1987	[17]	2/9	1/9	2.0	0.2	18.8	9.1	2.2	∞
Lippmann *et al.* 1989	[26]	4/30	0/30	41	0.1	>250	7.7	3.9	85
Brown *et al.* 1991	[27]	17/30	6/30	2.8	1.3	6.2	2.7	1.7	7.2
DeAndrade *et al.* 1994	[14]	34/51	4/25	4.2	1.7	10.5	2.0	1.4	3.2
Nørholt *et al.* 1996	[28]	9/37	0/37	91	0.2	>250	4.2	2.6	9.5
Pande *et al.* 1996	[29]	1/14	0/12	9.4	0.0	>250	14.3	4.8	∞
Combined analgesic data		241/486	74/460	2.8	2.0	3.8	2.9	2.6	3.6
Trials with <32 treated patients		101/293	40/198	2.2	1.8	2.8	2.9	2.3	4.1
Trials with >32 treated patients		136/293	35/270	4.0	1.6	9.8	3.0	2.5	3.8
Minor adverse effects		108/320	68/295	1.49	1.09	2.04	9.1	5.6	27.7
Major adverse effects		2/334	6/304	0.31	0.07	1.38			

Comment

Morphine is the archetypal analgesic for use in moderate or severe pain. It is also the 'gold standard' against which other injected analgesics are tested. It was surprising, therefore, that rigorous searching revealed so few placebo controlled trials in which morphine had been given by intravenous, intramuscular, or subcutaneous injection, and with testing of single-dose analgesic efficacy using standard, validated methods. We found no subcutaneous studies, one intravenous study, and only for 10 mg intramuscular morphine was there sufficient information (494 treated patients) for information to be pooled for analysis. We found no diamorphine studies that met the criteria.

A single intramuscular dose of morphine 10 mg had an NNT of 2.9 for at least 50% pain relief compared with placebo. This means that one out of every three patients with pain of moderate to severe intensity will experience at least 50% pain relief with morphine which they would not have had with placebo. Sensitivity analysis found that size of trial did not make a difference (Table 2). Sensitivity analysis was not performed for quality of trials, since all but two reports had quality scores of 3 or more. Overestimation of the effect of treatment has been shown in trials with quality scores of 2 or less using the same validated quality scale as here [40].

The NNT for morphine can be compared with those of other analgesics from similar meta-analyses which compared the efficacy of analgesics with placebo in patients with moderate or severe postoperative pain. While there is as yet no comparable information available for other injected anal-

gesics, the NNT of 2.9 (2.6–3.8) for 10 mg intramuscular morphine can be compared with those obtained for oral tramadol 100 mg of 4.8 (3.4–8.2) [41], for oral paracetamol 1000 mg of 4.6 (3.9–5.4), and paracetamol 600/650 mg plus codeine 60 mg of 3.1 (2.6–3.8) [42], and 400 mg ibuprofen 400 mg of 2.7 (2.5–3.0). The equivalence of the NNTs for oral NSAIDs and 10 mg of intramuscular morphine is supported by the repeated failure to separate them in analgesic trials [43, 44]. A crucial issue here is dose. Clearly, with opioids there should be dose titration against effect. The NNT of 2.9 is for 10 mg of intramuscular morphine, and giving 20 mg improved the NNT [28].

Rank ordering the analgesics in this way is potentially less accurate than having the relative efficacy of the individual drugs from within one very large trial with a single randomization. In the absence of such 'head-to-head' comparisons, we would argue that this indirect ranking, the relative efficacy of the drugs against placebo, is helpful for our clinical decisions.

At first sight, the fact that the analgesia from 10 mg of intramuscular morphine is no better than the analgesia from a therapeutic dose of oral NSAID is surprising. We all think of injected drugs as more 'powerful' than oral drugs. In reality, there is a considerable body of direct evidence that confirms the indirect ranking. For many years investigators have been unable to distinguish the analgesia from 10 mg intramuscular morphine and oral NSAID (where comparisons were within the same trial and hence randomization).

This is a clinically helpful observation for patients who can swallow and who have no contra-indication to NSAID. Oral

NSAID appears to be the best analgesic choice. There is no advantage to giving that dose of NSAID by a suppository or injection [45]. If the patient can swallow, but speedy analgesia is required, then intravenous rather than intramuscular analgesia seems more logical. If the patient cannot swallow, then we know that 10 mg of intramuscular morphine gives analgesia equivalent to oral NSAID, and that doubling the dose does indeed increase the analgesia [28]. We do not yet have the ranking of injected NSAID compared with injected opioid.

References

1. McQuay HJ, Carroll D, Moore RA. Injected morphine in postoperative pain; a quantitative systematic review. submitted.

2. Jadad AR, Carroll D, Moore A, McQuay H. Developing a database of published reports of randomised clinical trials in pain research. *Pain* 1996; **66**:239–46.

3. Jadad AR, Moore RA, Carroll D, Jenkinson C, Reynolds DJM, Gavaghan DJ et al. Assessing the quality of reports of randomized clinical trials: is blinding necessary? *Controlled Clinical Trials* 1996; **17**:1–12.

4. Cooper SA. Single-dose analgesic studies: the upside and downside of assay sensitivity. In: Max MB, Portenoy RK, Laska EM, ed. *The design of analgesic clinical trials (Advances in pain research and therapy*, Vol. 18). New York: Raven Press, 1991:117–24.

5. Moore A, McQuay H, Gavaghan D. Deriving dichotomous outcome measures from continuous data in randomised controlled trials of analgesics. *Pain* 1996; **66**:229–37.

6. Moore A, Moore O, McQuay H, Gavaghan D. Deriving dichotomous outcome measures from continuous data in randomised controlled trials of analgesics: Use of pain intensity and visual analogue scales. *Pain* 1997; **69**:311–15.

7. Moore A, McQuay H, Gavaghan D. Deriving dichotomous outcome measures from continuous data in randomised controlled trials of analgesics: Verification from independent data. *Pain* 1997; **69**:127–30.

8. DerSimonian R, Laird N. Meta-analysis of clinical trials. *Controlled Clinical Trials* 1986; **7**:177–88.

9. Gardner MJ, Altman DG. Confidence intervals rather than p values: estimation rather than hypothesis testing. *British Medical Journal* 1986; **292**:746–50.

10. L'Abbé KA, Detsky AS, O'Rourke K. Meta-analysis in clinical research. *Annals of Internal Medicine* 1987; **107**:224–33.

11. Laupacis A, Sackett DL, Roberts RS. An assessment of clinically useful measures of the consequences of treatment. *New England Journal of Medicine* 1988; **318**:1728–33.

12. Cook RJ, Sackett DL. The number needed to treat: a clinically useful measure of treatment effect. *British Medical Journal* 1995; **310**:452–4.

13. Davie IT, Slawson KB, Burt RA. A double blind comparison of parenteral morphine, placebo, and oral fenoprofen in management of postoperative pain. *Anesthesia and Analgesia* 1982; **61**:1002–5.

14. de Andrade JR, Maslanka MA, Maneatis T, Bynum L, Burchmore M. The use of ketorolac in the management of postoperative pain. *Orthopedics* 1994; **17**:157–66.

15. Van Den Abeele G, Camu F. Comparative evaluation of ciramadol (WY 15.705), morphine and placebo for treatment of postoperative pain. *Acta Anaesthesiologica Belgica* 1985; **36**:97–110.

16. Beaver WT, Feise G. Comparison of the analgesic effects of morphine, hydroxyzine, and their combination in patients with postoperative pain. *Advances in Pain Research and Therapy* 1976; **1**:553–7.

17. Kaiko R, Kanner R, Foley K, Wallenstein S, Canel A, Rogers A et al. Cocaine and morphine interaction in acute and chronic cancer pain. *Pain* 1987; **31**:35–45.

18. Campos VM, Solis EL. The analgesic and hypothermic effects of nefopam, morphine, aspirin, diphenhydramine, and placebo. *Journal of Clinical Pharmacology* 1980; **20**:42–9.

19. Fragen RJ, Kouzmanoff C, Caldwell NJ. Intramuscularly administered ciramadol for management of postoperative pain: a comparative study. *Journal of Clinical Pharmacology* 1983; **23**:219–26.

20. Brown CR, Sevelius H, Wild V. A comparison of single doses of naproxen sodium, morphine sulfate, and placebo in patients with postoperative pain. *Current Therapeutic Research* 1984; **35**:511–518.

21. Gravenstein JS. Dezocine for postoperative wound pain. *International Journal of Clinical Pharmacology, Therapy and Toxicology* 1984; **22**:502–5.

22. Pandit SK, Kothary SP, Pandit UA, Kunz NR. Double blind placebo controlled comparison of dezocine and morphine for post operative pain relief. *Canadian Anaesthesia Society Journal* 1985; **32**:583–91.

23. Powell W. A double blind comparison of multiple intramuscular doses of ciramadol, morphine, and placebo for the treatment of postoperative pain. *Anaesthesia and Analgesia* 1985; **64**:1101–17.

24. de Lia JE, Rodman KC, Jolles CJ. Comparative efficacy of oral flurbiprofen, intramuscular morphine sulfate, and placebo in the treatment of gynecologic postoperative pain. *American Journal of Medicine* 1986; **80**:60–4.

25. Morrison J, Harris J, Sherrill J, Heilman C, Bucovaz E, Wiser W. Comparative study of flurbiprofen and morphine for post-surgical gynecologic pain. *American Journal of Medicine* 1986; **80**:55–9.

26. Lippmann M, Mok M, Farinacci J, Lee J. Tonazocine mesylate in postoperative pain patients: a double blind placebo controlled analgesic study. *Journal of Clinical Pharmacology* 1989; **29**:373–8.

27. Brown CR, Schwartz KE, Wild VM, Koshiver JE. Comparison of anirolac with morphine and placebo for postoperative pain. *Current Therapeutic Research* 1991; **50**:379–85.

28. Norholt S, SindetPedersen S, Larsen U, Bang U, Ingerslev J, Nielsen O et al. Pain control after dental surgery: A double-blind, randomised trial of lornoxicam versus morphine. *Pain* 1996; **67**:335–43.

29. Pande AC, Pyke RE, Greiner M, Wideman GL, Benjamin R, Pierce MW. Analgesic efficacy of enadoline versus placebo or morphine in postsurgical pain. *Clinical Neuropharmacology* 1996; **19**:451–6.

30. Kantor TG, Hopper M, Laska E. Adverse effects of commonly ordered oral narcotics. *Journal of Clinical Pharmacology* 1981; **21**:1–8.

31. Rice A, Lloyd J, Miller C, Bullingham RE, O'Sullivan G. A double-blind study of the speed of onset of analgesia following intramuscular administration of ketorolac tromethamine in comparison to intramuscular morphine and placebo. *Anaesthesia* 1991; **46**:541–4.

32. Whitehead EM, O'Sullivan GM, Lloyd J, Bullingham RES. A new method for rate of analgesic onset: two doses of intravenous morphine compared with placebo. *Clinical Pharmacology and Therapeutics* 1992; **52**:197–204.

33. Verborgh C, Camu F. Post surgical pain relief with zero order intravenous infusions of meptazinol and morphine: a double blind placebo controlled evaluation of their effects on ventilation. *European Journal of Clinical Pharmacology* 1990; **38**:437–42.

34. Maslanka MA, de Andrade JR, Maneatis T, Bynum L, DiGiorgio E. Comparison of oral ketorolac, intramuscular morphine, and placebo for treatment of pain after orthopedic surgery. *Southern Medical Journal* 1994; **87**:506–13.

35. Brown CR, Moodie JE, Dickie G, Wild VM, Smith BA, Clarke PJ *et al*. Analgesic efficacy and safety of single dose oral and intramuscular ketorolac tromethamine for postoperative pain. *Pharmacotherapy* 1990; **10**:59S–70.

36. Cohen RI, Edwards WT, Kezer EA, Ferrari DA, Liland AE, Smith ER. Serial intravenous doses of dezocine, morphine, and nalbuphine in the management of postoperative pain for outpatients. *Anesthesia and Analgesia* 1993; **77**:533–9.

37. Lasagna L, Mosteller F, von Felsinger JM, Beecher HK. A study of the placebo response. *American Journal of Medicine* 1954; 770–779.

38. Levine J, Gordon N, Smith R, Fields H. Analgesic responses to morphine and placebo in individuals with post-operative pain. *Pain* 1981; **14**:379–88.

39. Foley WL, Edwards RC, Jacobs L3. Patient-controlled analgesia: a comparison of dosing regimens for acute postsurgical pain. *Journal of Oral Maxillofacial Surgery* 1994; **52**:155–9; discussion 159–60.

40. Khan KS, Daya S, Jadad AR. The importance of quality of primary studies in producing unbiased systematic reviews. *Archives of Internal Medicine* 1996; **156**:661–6.

41. Moore RA, McQuay HJ. Single-patient data meta-analysis of 3453 postoperative patients: Oral tramadol versus placebo, codeine and combination analgesics. *Pain* 1997; **69**:287–94.

42. Moore A, Collins S, Carroll D, McQuay H. Paracetamol with and without codeine in acute pain: a quantitative systematic review. *Pain* 1997; **70**:193–201.

43. Mansfield M, Firth F, Glynn C, Kinsella J. A comparison of ibuprofen arginine with morphine sulphate for pain relief after orthopaedic surgery. *European Journal of Anaesthesiology* 1996; **13**:492–7.

44. Schachtel BP, Thoden WR, Baybutt RI. Ibuprofen and acetaminophen in the relief of postpartum episiotomy pain. *Journal of Clinical Pharmacology* 1989; **29**:550–3.

45. McQuay HJ, Justins D, Moore RA. Treating acute pain in hospital. *British Medical Journal* 1997; **314**:1531–5.

14

Dihydrocodeine in postoperative pain

Summary

This systematic review aimed to determine the analgesic efficacy and adverse effects of oral and injectable dihydrocodeine from single dose studies in moderate to severe postoperative pain. Published studies were identified by searching electronic databases (e.g. MEDLINE) and checking reference lists of retrieved reports. Summed pain relief and pain intensity data were extracted and converted to dichotomous information yielding the number of patients with at least 50% pain relief. This was used to calculate the relative benefit (RB) and number-needed-to-treat (NNT) for one patient to achieve at least 50% pain relief.

Three reports (194 patients) compared oral dihydrocodeine with placebo and one (120 patients) compared oral dihydrocodeine (30 mg or 60 mg) with ibuprofen 400 mg. For a single dose of dihydrocodeine 30 mg in moderate to severe postoperative pain the NNT for at least 50% pain relief was 9.7 (95% confidence interval 4.5–∞) when compared with placebo over a period of 4 to 6 hours. Pooled data showed no significant difference in adverse effect incidence for dihydrocodeine 30 mg compared with placebo.

The confidence intervals (CIs) of the NNTs included no benefit of dihydrocodeine 30 mg over placebo. A statistical superiority of ibuprofen 400 mg over dihydrocodeine (30 mg or 60 mg) was shown.

Introduction

Opioids are used extensively in the management of pain and are believed capable of relieving severe pain more effectively than non-steroidal anti-inflammatory drugs (NSAIDs) [2]. The aim of this quantitative systematic review was to assess the efficacy and safety of a single dose of oral dihydrocodeine in the management of postoperative pain of moderate to severe intensity.

Dihydrocodeine is a synthetic opioid analgesic which was developed in the early 1900s. Its structure and pharmacokinetics are similar to that of codeine [3] and it is used for the treatment of postoperative pain or as an antitussive. In 1995, nearly a tenth of all analgesic prescriptions (opioid, non-opioid, and NSAID) issued in England were for dihydrocodeine [4]. The proportion of dihydrocodeine used for the treatment of postoperative pain is not known.

Methods

MEDLINE (1966–February 1997), EMBASE (1980–97), the Cochrane Library (January 1997), Biological Abstracts (1985–97), and the Oxford Pain Relief Database (1950–94) [5] were searched for randomized controlled trials of dihydrocodeine in postoperative pain. The words: 'dihydrocodeine', 'random*', 'clinical trial', 'trial', 'analgesi*', 'pain' and 36 brand names and preparations [6] were used in a broad free text search without restriction to language. Additional reports were identified from reference lists of retrieved articles. Unpublished data were not sought.

Included reports

The inclusion criteria used were: full journal publication, postoperative pain, postoperative administration, adult patients, baseline pain of moderate to severe intensity, double-blind design, and random allocation to treatment groups which included dihydrocodeine and placebo. Pain outcomes used were TOTPAR or SPID over 4 to 6 hours or sufficient data provided to allow their calculation. Pain measures allowed for the calculation of TOTPAR were a standard five-point pain relief scale (none, slight, moderate, good, complete) and for SPID a standard four-point pain intensity scale (none, mild, moderate, severe).

Data extraction and analysis

From each study we extracted: the number of patients treated, the mean TOTPAR or SPID, study duration, the dose of dihydrocodeine, and information on adverse effects. Mean TOTPAR or SPID values were converted to %maxTOTPAR or %maxSPID by division into the calculated maximum value [7]. The referenced equations were used to estimate the proportion of patients achieving at least 50%maxTOTPAR [8, 9]. This was then converted to the number of patients achieving at least 50%maxTOTPAR by multiplying by the total number of patients in the treatment group. The number of patients with at least 50%maxTOTPAR was then used to calculate estimates of relative benefit and NNT.

Estimates of relative benefit (RB) and risk (RR), with 95% confidence intervals (CIs) were calculated using a random effects model [10]. Homogeneity was assumed when $P > 0.1$. A statistically significant benefit of active treatment over

The topic discussed in this chapter is also published in full in Edwards *et al.* [1].

control was assumed when the confidence interval did not include 1. A statistically significant benefit of control over active treatment was assumed when the upper limit of the 95% CI of the relative benefit was < 1. Number-needed-to-treat (NNT) and number-needed-to-harm (NNH) with 95% confidence intervals were calculated [11]. The confidence interval of the NNT indicates no benefit of one treatment over the other when the upper limit includes infinity.

Results

Forty-eight published reports of dihydrocodeine in postoperative pain were identified; two could not be obtained from the British Library. Of the retrieved reports, 18 studies were not randomized and were excluded. Twenty-eight studies were randomized. Of the randomized controlled studies two included other pain conditions, five had no extractable pain outcome data, seven were not double-blind, four used dihydrocodeine as a rescue analgesic only, and six did not specify baseline pain of moderate to severe intensity. These reports were excluded. Details of the included studies are given in Table 1.

Four studies met our inclusion criteria: three were placebo controlled and one used ibuprofen 400 mg as an active control. All four studies examined the effects of oral dihydrocodeine. Three trials [12, 13, 14] compared dihydrocodeine 30 mg with placebo, and one [15] compared dihydrocodeine (30 mg or 60 mg) with ibuprofen 400 mg.

Oral dihydrocodeine vs. placebo

No reports comparing dihydrocodeine 60 mg with placebo met our inclusion criteria. Three reports compared dihydrocodeine tartrate 30 mg (91 patients) with placebo (85 patients). One trial investigated dental pain [12], one orthopaedic pain [13], and one pain following minor day-case surgery [14].

The proportion of patients experiencing at least 50% pain relief with dihydrocodeine varied between 14% and 50%, with a mean value of 35%. The proportion of patients experiencing at least 50% pain relief with placebo varied between 5% and 50%, with a mean of 23% (Fig. 1). The data sets were homogeneous, $P = 0.12$. Dihydrocodeine 30 mg was not significantly different from placebo, relative benefit 1.7 (0.7–4.0) (Table 2). For a single dose of dihydrocodeine 30 mg compared with placebo the NNT was 9.7 (4.5–∞) for at least 50% pain relief over a period of 4 to 6 hours in postoperative pain of moderate to severe intensity.

Adverse effects

Details of adverse effects are given in Table 3. The incidence of adverse effects with dihydrocodeine was not significantly different than with placebo. All adverse effects were mild and transient in nature and no patients withdrew as a result.

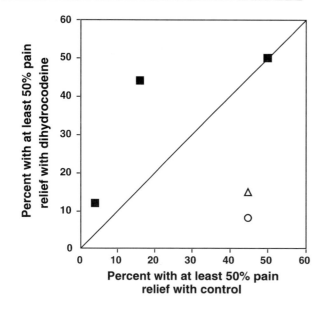

Dihydrocodeine 30 mg
vs. placebo:
RB = 1.7 (0.7 – 4.0)
NNT = 9.7 (4.5 – ∞)

Dihydrocodeine 30 mg
vs. ibuprofen 400 mg:
RB = 0.2 (0.1 – 0.5)
NNT = –2.7 (–1.8 – –5)

Dihydrocodeine 60 mg
vs. ibuprofen 400 mg:
RB = 0.3 (0.2 – 0.8)
NNT = –3.3 (–2.1 – –9)

Fig. 1   Trials of oral dihydrocodeine. (RB, relative benefit; NNT, number-needed-to-treat.)

Table 1 Details of included reports

Ref.	Condition & no. of patients	Design, study duration, & follow-up	Outcome measures	Dose regimen	Analgesic outcome results	Remedication	Withdrawals & exclusions	Adverse effects
[12]	Impacted 3rd molar removal *n* = 148 Age: Adults	RCT, DB, single oral dose, parallel groups. Assessed at t = 30 min, 1 h, and then hourly for 5 h. Med taken when pain of moderate to severe intensity.	PI (9-pt scale) non-standard PR (5-pt scale) standard	Dihydrocodeine 30 mg, *n* = 49 Placebo, *n* = 50	Dihydrocodeine 30 mg was not significantly different to placebo. 4-h TOTPAR: Dihydrocodeine 30 mg 0.5 Placebo 0.3.	Remed allowed at t > 2 h. If remed patients were withdrawn and their PR set to zero for all further time points.	18 withdrew: 9 insufficient pain, 7 did not return assessment forms, 1 did not complete assessment forms, 1 postop complication.	No serious AE were reported and no patients withdrew as a result. Dihydrocodeine 30 mg: 1/49 with 1 AE. Placebo: 1/50 with 3 AE.
[13]	Orthopaedic surgery *n* = 89 Age: 18–80	RCT, DB, multiple oral dose, parallel groups. Assessed at t = 30 min, 1 h and then hourly for 6 h. Med taken when pain of moderate to severe intensity.	PI (5-pt scale) nonstandard PR (5-pt scale) standard VAS 100 mm ('no pain'—'worst pain I have ever felt')	Dihydrocodeine 30 mg, *n* = 30 Placebo, *n* = 28	Dihydrocodeine was NSD to placebo. Mean TOTPAR at 6 h: Dihydrocodeine 11.3. Placebo 11.1.	Multiple dose study 2nd dose given as required. If remed patients were excluded from the analysis.	9 withdrew because of inadequate analgesia after the first dose. Dihydrocodeine 30 mg, *n* = 3 Placebo, *n* = 6.	No patients experienced AE in the single dose analysis.
[14]	Minor day-case surgery (general) *n* = 54 Age: Adults	RCT, DB, multiple oral dose, parallel groups. Assessed at t = 30 min, 1 h, and then hourly for 4 h. Med taken when pain of moderate to severe intensity.	PI (4-pt scale) standard PR (5-pt scale) standard VAS 100 mm	Dihydrocodeine 30 mg, *n* = 18 Placebo, *n* = 19	4 h SPID and TOTPAR presented. TOTPAR: Dihydrocodeine was significantly better than placebo (*P* < 0.05). Dihydrocodeine 30 mg 6.5. Placebo 3.2.	Allowed after 1 h. If remed patients initial PI & PR scores were used for all further timepoints.	Single dose analysis: All AE were mild & no patients withdrew as a result. NSD was found between dihydrocodeine & placebo. Dihydrocodeine 30 mg: 6/18 with 6 AE. Placebo: 3/19 with 3 AE.	
[15]	Lower 3rd molar removal *n* = 68 Age: Adults	RCT, DB, multiple oral dose, cross-over design. Self-assessed at t = 30 min, 1 h, & then hourly for 6 h Med allowed when pain of moderate to severe intensity.	PI (4-pt scale) standard PR (5-pt scale) standard Global rating (5-pt scale) standard	Dihydrocodeine 30 mg, *n* = 40 Dihydrocodeine 60 mg, *n* = 40 Placebo, *n* = 40	TOTPAR at 6 h: Dihydrocodeine 30 mg 3.3. Dihydrocodeine 60 mg 4.7. Ibuprofen 400 mg 10.0. Ibuprofen was significantly better than dihydrocodeine 30 mg or 60 mg (*P* <0.01).	If remed at t < 6 h the initial PI score & PR score of zero were used for all further timepoints.	3 patients withdrew.	Single dose AE data was not presented.

AE, adverse effects; DB, double-blind; NSD, no significant difference; PI, pain intensity; PR, pain relief; SPID, summed pain intensity differences; TOTPAR, total pain relief; VAS, visual analogue scale.

Table 2 Summary of relative benefit and number-needed-to-treat (NNT) for trials of oral dihydrocodeine vs. placebo and ibuprofen 400 mg

No. of trials	Dihydrocodeine dose (mg)	No. of patients with > 50% pain relief: dihydrocodeine	No. of patients with > 50% pain relief: placebo	Relative benefit (95% CI)	NNT (95% CI)
vs. placebo					
3	30	29/97	19/97	1.7 (0.7–4.0)	9.7 (4.5–∞)
vs. ibuprofen			No. of patients with > 50% pain relief: ibuprofen 400 mg		
1	30	3/40	18/40	0.2 (0.1–0.5)	−2.7 (−1.8 to −5)
1	60	6/40	18/40	0.3 (0.2–0.8)	−3.3 (−2.1 to −9)

Negative NNTs in the comparison with ibuprofen mean that ibuprofen is better than dihydrocodeine.

Table 3 Summary of adverse effects of oral dihydrocodeine and placebo

No. of trials	Adverse effect	No. of patients with adverse effects: dihydrocodeine	No. of patients with adverse effects: placebo	Relative risk (95% CI)	NNH (95% CI)
3	Nausea or vomiting	7/97	0/97	25 (0.7–907)	NC
3	Headache	3/97	0/97	1.05 (0.3–4.4)	NC
3	Dizziness, drowsiness, or confusion	5/97	1/97	4.2 (0.6–28)	NC

NC, not calculated, because no significant difference from placebo was shown for relative risk.

Oral dihydrocodeine vs. ibuprofen

One study [15] compared the efficacy and safety of either dihydrocodeine tartrate 30 mg (40 patients) or 60 mg (40 patients) with ibuprofen 400 mg (40 patients) in dental pain.

The proportion of patients experiencing at least 50% pain relief with dihydrocodeine 30 mg was 8%, with dihydrocodeine 60 mg it was 15%, and with ibuprofen 400 mg (active control) it was 45% (Fig. 1). A statistical superiority of ibuprofen 400 mg over dihydrocodeine 30 mg and dihydrocodeine 60 mg was shown, relative benefit 0.2 (0.1–0.5) and 0.3 (0.2–0.8), respectively.

Ibuprofen 400 mg was significantly better than dihydrocodeine 30 mg or dihydrocodeine 60 mg (Fig. 1). When compared with ibuprofen 400 mg, for a single dose of dihydrocodeine 30 mg the NNT was −2.7 (−1.8 to − 5) for at least 50% pain relief over a period of 4 to 6 hours in postoperative pain of moderate to severe intensity (Table 2). Similarly, for a single dose of dihydrocodeine 60 mg the NNT was − 3.3 (− 2.1 to −9) for at least 50% pain relief over a period of 4 to 6 hours.

Adverse effects

No single dose adverse effects data was presented [15].

Comment

Dihydrocodeine is the second most commonly prescribed opioid in England, with 1.5 million prescriptions issued for dihydrocodeine tartrate tablets alone in 1995. This increased to 1.6 million in 1996. We found no papers which investigated injected dihydrocodeine in the evaluation of postoperative pain with standard analgesic measurement methods.

For a single dose of oral dihydrocodeine tartrate 30 mg compared with placebo the NNTs were 9.7 (4.5–∞) for at least 50% pain relief over a period of 4 to 6 hours in postoperative pain of moderate to severe intensity. This means that one in every ten patients with moderate to severe postoperative pain would experience at least 50% pain relief with dihydrocodeine 30 mg who would not have done so with placebo. However, the estimate of relative benefit showed no significant difference between dihydrocodeine 30 mg and placebo.

A number of analgesics have demonstrated greater efficacy than dihydrocodeine 30 mg, although the confidence intervals of the NNTs for many of these overlap. The confidence intervals for ibuprofen 200 mg (2.8–4.0) and 400 mg (2.5–3.0), and diclofenac 50 mg (2.0–2.7) did not overlap with those of dihydrocodeine 30 mg indicating greater analgesic efficacy.

This rank order of relative efficacy against placebo is supported by a head-to-head comparison with ibuprofen. The analgesic efficacy of a single dose of oral dihydrocodeine (30 mg or 60 mg) was significantly inferior to ibuprofen 400 mg. For a single dose of dihydrocodeine 30 mg compared with ibuprofen 400 mg the NNT was –2.7 (–1.8 to –5) for at least 50% pain relief over a period of 4 to 6 hours in postoperative pain of moderate to severe intensity. This means that for every three patients with moderate to severe postoperative pain treated with ibuprofen 400 mg, one will experience at least 50% pain relief who would not have done if given dihydrocodeine 30 mg.

Similarly, for a single dose of dihydrocodeine 60 mg compared with ibuprofen 400 mg the NNT was –3.3 (–2.1 to –9) over a period of 4 to 6 hours. So, one in every three patients with moderate to severe postoperative pain treated with ibuprofen 400 mg would experience at least 50% pain relief who would not have done if given dihydrocodeine 60 mg.

Nausea, vomiting, headache, dizziness, drowsiness, and confusion were the most commonly reported adverse effects for a single dose of oral dihydrocodeine 30 mg when compared with placebo. The incidence of adverse effects was not significantly different for dihydrocodeine 30 mg than for placebo (Table 3).

Our results suggest dihydrocodeine to be less effective than other analgesics when administered as a single oral dose. Few of the retrieved reports investigating oral dihydrocodeine met the criteria for inclusion in this quantitative systematic review. This resulted in very little patient data being available for analysis, particularly for dihydrocodeine 60 mg which is often the preferred dose. Administering dihydrocodeine in multiple doses may improve its analgesic efficacy, but may also increase the incidence of adverse effects.

References

1. Edwards JE, McQuay HJ, Moore RA. Systematic review: dihydrocodeine in postoperative pain. submitted.
2. Alexander JI, Hill RG. *Postoperative pain*. London: Blackwell Scientific Publications, 1987.
3. Rowell FJ, Seymour RA, Rawlins MD. Pharmacokinetics of intravenous and oral dihydrocodeine and its metabolites. *European Journal of Clinical Pharmacology* 1983; 25:419–24.
4. Government Statistical Service. *Prescription cost analysis for England 1995*. London: Department of Health, 1996.
5. Jadad AR, Carroll D, Moore A, McQuay H. Developing a database of published reports of randomised clinical trials in pain research. *Pain* 1996; 66:239–46.
6. Reynolds JEF. *Martindale: the extra pharmacopoeia*, (30th edn). London: Pharmaceutical Press, 1993:292–314.
7. Cooper SA. Single-dose analgesic studies: the upside and downside of assay sensitivity. In: Max MB, Portenoy RK, Laska EM, ed. *The design of analgesic clinical trials (Advances in pain research and therapy*, Vol. 18). New York: Raven Press, 1991:117–24.
8. Moore A, McQuay H, Gavaghan D. Deriving dichotomous outcome measures from continuous data in randomised controlled trials of analgesics: Verification from independent data. *Pain* 1997; 69:127–30.
9. Moore A, Moore O, McQuay H, Gavaghan D. Deriving dichotomous outcome measures from continuous data in randomised controlled trials of analgesics: Use of pain intensity and visual analogue scales. *Pain* 1997; 69:311–15.
10. DerSimonian R, Laird N. Meta-analysis of clinical trials. *Controlled Clinical Trials* 1986; 7:177–88.
11. Cook RJ, Sackett DL. The number needed to treat: a clinically useful measure of treatment effect. *British Medical Journal* 1995; 310:452–4.
12. Frame J, Evans C, Flaum G, Langford R, Rout P. A comparison of ibuprofen and dihydrocodeine in relieving pain following wisdom teeth removal. *British Dental Journal* 1989; 166:121–4.
13. Galasko C, Russel S, Lloyd J. Double-blind investigation of the efficacy of multiple oral doses of ketorolac tromethamine compared with dihydrocodeine and placebo. *Current Therapeutic Research* 1989; 45:844–52.
14. McQuay HJ, Bullingham RE, Moore RA, Carroll D, Evans PJ, O'Sullivan G *et al.* Zomepirac, dihydrocodeine and placebo compared in postoperative pain after day-case surgery. The relationship between the effects of single and multiple doses. *British Journal of Anaesthesia* 1985; 57:412–19.
15. McQuay HJ, Carroll D, Guest PG, Robson S, Wiffen PJ, Juniper RP. A multiple dose comparison of ibuprofen and dihydrocodeine after third molar surgery. *British Journal of Oral and Maxillofacial Surgery* 1993; 31:95–100.
16. Moore A, Collins S, Carroll D, McQuay H. Paracetamol with and without codeine in acute pain: a quantitative systematic review. *Pain* 1997; 70:193–201.
17. Collins SL, Moore A, McQuay HJ, Wiffen PJ. Oral ibuprofen and diclofenac in postoperative pain: a quantitative systematic review. submitted.
18. Collins SL, Edwards J, Moore A, McQuay HJ. Oral dextropropoxyphene in postoperative pain: a quantitative systematic review. *European Journal of Clinical Pharmacology*. in press.

15

Dextropropoxyphene in postoperative pain

Summary

This systematic review aimed to determine the analgesic efficacy and adverse effects of oral dextropropoxyphene alone and in combination with paracetamol for moderate to severe postoperative pain. Published reports were identified from a variety of electronic databases including MEDLINE, Biological Abstracts, EMBASE, the Cochrane Library, and the Oxford Pain Relief Database. Additional studies were identified from the reference lists of retrieved reports.

Summed pain intensity and pain relief data were extracted and converted into dichotomous information to yield the number of patients with at least 50% pain relief. This was used to calculate the relative benefit (RB) and number-needed-to-treat (NNT) for one patient to achieve at least 50% pain relief. Six reports (440 patients) compared dextropropoxyphene with placebo and five (963 patients) compared dextropropoxyphene plus paracetamol 650 mg with placebo.

For a single dose of dextropropoxyphene 65 mg in postoperative pain the NNT for at least 50% pain relief was 7.7 (95% confidence interval 4.6–∞) in when compared with placebo over 4 to 6 hours. For the equivalent dose of dextropropoxyphene in combination with paracetamol 650 mg the NNT was 4.4 (3.5–5.6) when compared with placebo. Pooled data showed increased incidence of central nervous system adverse effects for dextropropoxyphene plus paracetamol compared with placebo.

Dextropropoxyphene 65 mg plus paracetamol 650 mg has a similar analgesic efficacy to tramadol 100 mg but with a lower incidence of adverse effects. Ibuprofen 400 mg has a lower (better) NNT than both dextropropoxyphene 65 mg plus paracetamol 650 mg and tramadol 100 mg.

Introduction

Dextropropoxyphene is an opioid analgesic which has been widely available since the 1950s. It is commonly used both alone, and in combination with paracetamol under such brand names as co-proxamol and distalgesic. In 1996, there were 10 million prescriptions in England for co-proxamol alone representing one-fifth of all analgesics prescribed (opioid, non-opioid, and non-steroidal anti-inflammatory drugs—NSAIDs) although it is not clear how much was used for postoperative pain [2].

The topic discussed in this chapter is also published in full in Collins *et al.* [1].

Patient surveys have shown that postoperative pain is often not managed well [3] and there is a growing need to assess the efficacy and safety of commonly used analgesics as newer treatments become available. Judging relative analgesic efficacy is difficult as clinical trials use a variety of comparators. It can, however, be determined indirectly by comparing analgesics with placebo in similar clinical circumstances to produce a common analgesic descriptor such as number-needed-to-treat (NNT) for at least 50% pain relief. Using this method we have produced a quantitative systematic review of the analgesic efficacy of dextropropoxyphene, both with and without paracetamol, allowing comparison with other analgesics.

Methods

MEDLINE (1966–November 1996), EMBASE (1980–96), the Cochrane Library (November 1996), Biological Abstracts (1985–96), and the Oxford Pain Relief Database (1950–94) [4] were searched for randomized controlled trials (RCTs) of dextropropoxyphene, and its combinations in postoperative pain. The words: 'dextropropoxyphene', 'd-propoxyphene', 'propoxyphene', 'random*', 'clinical trial', 'trial', 'study', 'analgesi*', 'pain', and 41 brand names (including distalgesic and co-proxamol) [5] were used in a broad free text search without restriction to language. Additional reports were identified from reference lists of retrieved articles and reviews. Unpublished data were not sought.

Included reports

The inclusion criteria used were: full journal publication, postoperative pain, postoperative oral administration, adult patients, baseline pain of moderate to severe intensity, double-blind design, and random allocation to treatment groups, which included dextropropoxyphene and placebo or a combination of dextropropoxyphene plus paracetamol and placebo. Pain outcomes used were TOTPAR or SPID over 4 to 6 hours or sufficient data provided to allow their calculation. Pain measures allowed for the calculation of TOTPAR or SPID were a standard five-point pain relief scale (none, slight, moderate, good, complete) or a standard four-point pain intensity scale (none, mild, moderate, severe).

Data extraction and analysis

From each study we extracted: the number of patients treated, the mean TOTPAR or mean SPID, study duration, the dose of dextropropoxyphene and paracetamol where appropriate, and information on adverse effects. Mean TOTPAR and mean SPID values were converted to %maxTOTPAR or %maxSPID by division into the calculated maximum value [6]. The referenced equations were used to estimate the proportion of patients achieving at least 50%maxTOTPAR [7, 8]. The proportions were converted to the number of patients achieving at least 50%maxTOTPAR by multiplying by the total number of patients in the treatment group. The number of patients with at least 50%maxTOTPAR was then used to calculate relative benefit and NNT.

Relative benefit (RB) and relative risk (RR) estimates with 95% confidence intervals (CIs) were calculated using the random effects model which provides a more conservative estimate of relative benefit than the fixed-effects model [9]. Homogeneity was assumed when $P > 0.1$. A statistically significant benefit of active treatment over placebo was assumed when the lower limit of the 95% confidence interval of the relative benefit was > 1. A statistically significant benefit of placebo over active treatment was assumed when the upper limit of the 95% CI of the relative benefit was < 1. Number-needed-to-treat (NNT) and number-needed-to-harm (NNH) with 95% confidence intervals were calculated [10]. The confidence interval includes no benefit of one treatment over the other when the upper limit is represented as infinity.

Dextropropoxyphene is available as either the hydrochloride or napsylate salt. Equivalent molar doses are 65 mg of dextropropoxyphene hydrochloride and 100 mg of dextropropoxyphene napsylate.

Results

A total of 130 published articles were identified. Two could not be obtained and attempts to contact the authors were unsuccessful. Five citations obtained from reference lists of retrieved reports could not be traced by the British Library. Of the 123 retrieved reports, 33 were not randomized controlled trials, 24 were not postoperative pain models or included other pain conditions, 21 were not placebo controlled, and in five, dextropropoxyphene was used as a rescue analgesic only.

Of the 40 RCTs that were placebo controlled, patients did not have baseline pain of at least moderate severity in 10 studies, in 16 there were no pain outcomes that were compatible with our inclusion criteria, and two trials were not double-blind. The data from one study was duplicated and therefore one of the duplicates [11] was excluded. Eleven reports met our inclusion criteria and were included in the analysis. Details of the individual studies are in Table 1.

Dextropropoxyphene vs. placebo

Six reports compared dextropropoxyphene hydrochloride 65 mg (214 patients) with placebo (226 patients), and one trial also compared a dose of 130 mg (25 patients) with placebo (25 patients).

Two trials [12, 13] investigated postpartum pain (episiotomy), one pain following peridontal surgery [14], one post-urogenital surgery [15], one post-gynaecological surgery [16], and one pain after various surgical interventions [17].

The placebo response rate (the proportion of patients experiencing at least 50% pain relief with placebo) varied between 4% and 76%. The dextropropoxyphene response rate (the proportion of patients experiencing at least 50% pain relief with dextropropoxyphene) varied between 19% and 84% (Fig. 1). Data were homogeneous, $P = 0.13$. Dextropropoxyphene 65 mg was not significantly different from placebo, relative benefit 1.4 (0.97–2.0) (Table 2).

For a single dose of 65 mg dextropropoxyphene the NNT was 7.7 (4.6–∞) for at least 50% pain relief over a period of 4 to 6 hours compared with placebo for pain of moderate to severe intensity.

One trial [17] used a dose of 130 mg of dextropropoxyphene (25 patients). The relative benefit estimate for dextropropoxyphene 130 mg compared with placebo was 10 (1.4–73). The NNT was 2.8 (1.8–6.5) for at least 50% pain relief over a period of 5 hours compared with placebo for pain of moderate to severe intensity.

Adverse effects

Details of adverse effects are given in Table 3. No patients withdrew as a result of adverse effects and all were reported as transient and of mild to moderate severity. One study reported no adverse effects with either placebo or active treatment [12].

In one study, the authors reported both dextropropoxyphene 65 mg and 130 mg to have a significantly higher incidence of grogginess, sleepiness, and lightheadedness than placebo ($P = 0.05$) [17]. However, pooled data from the four trials reporting either drowsiness, sleepiness, or somnolence [13–15, 17] showed no significant difference in incidence between dextropropoxyphene 65 mg (18/115) and placebo (15/121), with a relative risk of 1.3 (0.7–24). No other trial reported lightheadedness or grogginess in the dextropropoxyphene group.

Dextropropoxyphene plus paracetamol vs. placebo

Four reports compared dextropropoxyphene napsylate 100 mg plus paracetamol 650 mg with placebo, and one used dextropropoxyphene hydrochloride 65 mg plus paracetamol 650 mg. A total of 478 patients received dextropropoxyphene plus paracetamol, and 485 patients received placebo.

Table 1 Details of included reports

Ref.	Condition & no. of patients	Design, study duration, & follow-up	Outcome measures	Dose regimen	Analgesic outcome results	Remedication	Withdrawals & exclusions	Adverse effects
[19]	Dental surgery n = 248 Age: Adult	RCT, DB, single oral dose, parallel groups, GA or LA. Self-assessed at home at 0, 1 h then hourly for 4 h. Med given when pain of moderate to severe intensity.	PI (4-pt scale) standard. PR (5-pt scale) standard. Global evaluation by patient (5-pt scale) at 4 h.	Dextropropoxyphene napsylate 100 mg + paracetamol 650 mg n = 42. Placebo n = 37.	Combination of dextropropoxyphene with paracetamol was significantly better than placebo for SPID & TOTPAR ($P < 0.001$). 4 h TOTPAR: Dextropropoxyphene + paracetamol: 8.31. Placebo: 3.38.	Allowed at t > 1 h; if remed before patient withdrawn from study. If remed PR recorded as 0, & last PI score prior to remed taken for all further timepoints.	200 analysed. 48 excluded: 31 violated protocol, 17 did not take med.	None serious & no patients withdrew as a result. Dextropropoxyphene + paracetamol: 5/42 with 5 AE. Placebo: 4/37 with 5 AE.
[18]	Dental surgery n = 179 Age: Adult	RCT, DB, single oral dose, parallel groups, mostly LA. Self-assessed at 0, 1 h then hourly for 4 h. Med given when pain of moderate to severe intensity.	PI (4-pt scale) standard. PR (5-pt scale) standard. Global evaluation by patient (5-pt scale) at 4 h.	Dextropropoxyphene napsylate 100 mg + paracetamol 650 mg n = 40 Placebo n = 48.	Combination of dextropropoxyphene with paracetamol was significantly better than placebo for SPID & TOTPAR ($P = < 0.05$). 4 h TOTPAR: Dextropropoxyphene + paracetamol: 5.65. Placebo: 4.17.	Did not state when remed allowed. If remed last PR & PI score before remed were used for all further timepoints.	179 analysed. No withdrawals rep.	None serious & no patients withdrew as a result. Dextropropoxyphene + paracetamol: 10/40 with 13 AE. Placebo: 13/48 with 17 AE.
[20]	Minor orthopaedic surgery n = 120 Age: Adult	RCT, DB single oral dose, parallel groups, GA. Assessed by same nurse observer at 0, 1/2, 1 h then hourly for 4 h. Med given when pain of moderate to severe intensity.	PI (4-pt scale) standard. PR (5-pt scale) standard.	Dextropropoxyphene HCl 65 mg + paracetamol 650 mg n = 30. Placebo n = 30.	Dextropropoxyphene + paracetamol was significantly better than placebo ($P <0.05$) for TOTPAR. 4 h TOTPAR: Dextropropoxyphene + paracetamol: 7.37. Placebo: 4.70.	If remed before 4 h, last PI & PR score prior to remed were used for all further timepoints.	120 analysed. No withdrawals were rep.	None serious & no patients withdrew as a result. Dextropropoxyphene + paracetamol: 16/30 with 16 AE. Placebo: 13/30 with 13 AE.
[21]	Postop, primarily orthopaedic n = 196 Age: 19–74	RCT, DB, single oral dose, parallel groups. Assessed by nurse observer at 0, 1/2, 1 h then hourly for 6 h. Med given when pain of moderate to severe intensity.	PI (4-pt scale) standard. PR (5-pt scale) nonstandard. Global evaluation by patient at 5 h (5-pt).	Dextropropoxyphene napsylate 100 mg + paracetamol 650 mg n = 50. Placebo n = 48.	Combination of dextropropoxyphene with paracetamol was significantly better than placebo ($P < 0.05$) for SPID & TOTPAR. 6-h TOTPAR: Dextropropoxyphene + paracetamol: 8.04. Placebo: 5.49.	If remed within 6 h patient's overall rating of the drug was taken at time of remed.	196 analysed. No withdrawals rep.	Authors did not give details of AE but rep that there was NSD between active & placebo groups.
[22]	Dental & postop pain n = 638 Age: Adult	Individual patient data from 18 DB, RCTs. Study duration 8 h. Single oral dose, parallel groups. Med was given when pain of moderate to severe intensity.	No. of patients with at least 50% of max TOTPAR.	Dextropropoxyphene napsylate 100 mg + paracetamol 650 mg n = 316. Placebo n = 322.	No. of patients with at least 50% of max TOTPAR: Dextropropoxyphene napsylate 100 mg + paracetamol 650 mg n = 112/316. Placebo n = 41/322.	None rep.	None rep.	None serious & no withdrawals. Dextropropoxyphene + paracetamol: 88/316 AE. Placebo: 66/322 AE. Significantly higher incidence of AE with active treatment than placebo for: Dizziness: RR 2.0 (1.1–4). Drowsiness/somnolence: RR 2.16 (1.5–3.2).

AE, adverse effect; DB, double-blind; GA, general anaesthetic; LA, local anaesthetic; NSD, no significant difference; PI, pain intensity; PR, pain relief; SPID, summed pain intensity differences; TOTPAR, total pain relief.

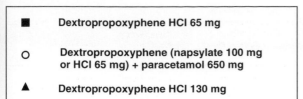

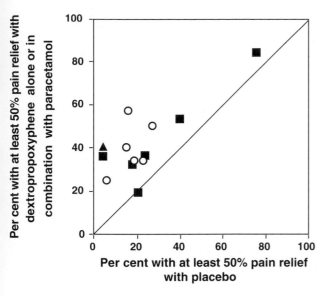

Dextropropoxyphene
65 mg alone:
RB = 1.4 (0.97 – 1.96)
NNT = 7.7 (4.6 – 23)

In combination with
paracetamol 650 mg:
RB = 2.4 (2.0 – 3.2)
NNT = 4.4 (3.5 – 5.6)

Fig. 1 Trials of oral dextropropoxyphene. (RB, relative benefit.)

Table 2 Summary of relative benefit and NNT for trials of dextropropoxyphene and dextropropoxyphene plus paracetamol vs. placebo

No. of trials	Dextropropoxyphene dose (mg)	No. of patients with >50% pain relief: dextropropoxyphene	No. of patients with >50% pain relief: placebo	Relative benefit (95% CI)	NNT (95% CI)
Dextropropoxyphene alone vs. placebo					
6	65	85/214	60/226	1.4 (0.97–2.0)	7.7 (4.6–∞)
1	130	10/25	1/25	10.0 (1.4–73)	2.8 (1.8–6.5)
Dextropropoxyphene + paracetamol vs. placebo					
5	65 mg hydrochloride or 100 mg napsylate	184/478	74/485	2.4 (1.9–3.1)	4.4 (3.5–5.6)

One report [7] was a meta-analysis of individual patient data from 18 studies with dichotomous information (the number of patients achieving at least 50%maxTOTPAR); eight investigated dextropropoxyphene napsylate 100 mg plus paracetamol 650 mg. Only one of the studies had been published and we excluded the duplicate publication [11].

Two reports [18, 19] studied pain following dental surgery (impacted third molar), two [20, 21] post-orthopaedic surgery, and one [7] pain following both dental and general surgery (abdominal, orthopaedic, and gynaecological).

The placebo response rate varied between 6% and 27%. The dextropropoxyphene plus paracetamol response rate varied between 25% and 57% (Fig. 1). The trial results were homogeneous (*P* = 0.35). Dextropropoxyphene (65 mg

hydrochloride or 100 mg napsylate) plus paracetamol 650 mg was significantly superior to placebo, relative benefit 2.4 (1.9–3.1) (Table 2). For a single dose of dextropropoxyphene (65 mg hydrochloride or 100 mg napsylate) plus paracetamol 650 mg the NNT was 4.4 (3.5–5.6) for at least 50% pain relief over 4 to 6 hours compared with placebo for pain of moderate to severe intensity.

Adverse effects

Details of adverse effects are given in Table 3. No patients withdrew as a result of adverse effects and all were reported as transient and of mild to moderate severity. One trial [21]

Table 3 Summary of adverse effects for trials of dextropropoxyphene and dextropropoxyphene plus paracetamol vs. placebo

No. of trials	Adverse effect	No. of patients with adverse effects: drug	No. of patients with adverse effects: placebo	Relative risk (95% CI)	NNT (95% CI)
Dextropropoxyphene					
2	Nausea	3/75	2/81	1.6 (0.3–9.4)	NC
3	Drowsiness/sleepiness/ somnolence	18/115	15/121	1.3 (0.7–2.4)	NC
2	Headache	5/75	3/81	1.6 (0.5–4.9)	NC
Dextropropoxyphene + paracetamol					
3	Nausea	12/405	33/799	0.7 (0.4–1.4)	NC
1	Vomiting	2/323	6/714	1.4 (0.3–6.7)	NC
4	Dizziness	17/435	16/829	2.2 (1.1–4.3)	50 (24–∞)
3	Drowsiness/somnolence	57/405	55/799	2.2 (2.0–2.4)	14 (9.1–30)
4	Headache	14/435	51/829	0.5 (0.4–0.6)	–33 (–170 to –19)

NC, not calculated because no significant difference from placebo was shown for relative risk.
Negative NNTs indicate that fewer headaches occur with dextropropoxyphene plus paracetamol than with placebo.

did not give details of adverse effects but reported that there was no significant difference between active and placebo groups. The individual patient meta-analysis [7] pooled data on adverse effects from all 18 placebo groups; 714 patients received placebo.

Three studies reported the incidence of drowsiness or somnolence [7, 18, 19]. The pooled data indicated a significantly higher incidence in the dextropropoxyphene combination group (57/405) than in the placebo group (55/799), with a relative risk of 2.2 (2.0–2.4) and a NNH of 14 (9.1–30).

Four trials reported dizziness [7, 18–20]. Pooled data indicated a significantly higher incidence of dizziness with dextropropoxyphene plus paracetamol (17/435) than with placebo (16/829), with a relative risk of 2.2 (1.1–4.3) and a NNH of 50 (24–∞).

Four trials reported the incidence of headache [18–21]. The pooled data showed dextropropoxyphene plus paracetamol (14/435) to have a significantly lower incidence of headache than placebo (51/829), with a relative risk of 0.5 (0.4–0.6) and an NNH of –33 (–170 to –19).

Three trials reported the incidence of nausea [7, 18, 19]. Pooled data showed no significant difference with dextropropoxyphene plus paracetamol (12/405) than with placebo (33/799), relative risk 0.7 (0.4–1.4).

Vomiting was reported in one study [7]. The incidence of vomiting with dextropropoxyphene plus paracetamol (2/323) was not significantly different from placebo (6/714), relative risk 1.4 (0.3–6.7).

Comment

For a single dose of dextropropoxyphene 65 mg the NNT was 7.7 (4.6–∞) for at least 50% pain relief compared with placebo. This means that one in every eight patients with

pain of moderate to severe intensity would experience at least 50% pain relief with dextropropoxyphene hydrochloride 65 mg who would not have done so with placebo. The confidence interval included no benefit. The equivalent NNT for a single dose of dextropropoxyphene (65 mg hydrochloride or 100 mg napsylate) plus paracetamol 650 mg was 4.4 (3.5–5.6), indicating higher efficacy. The confidence intervals of dextropropoxyphene alone and the combination with paracetamol overlapped. The dextropropoxyphene/paracetamol combination had an NNT similar to that of paracetamol 1000 mg and ibuprofen 200 mg. Both ibuprofen 400 mg and diclofenac 50 mg had NNTs whose confidence intervals were lower (better) than that of the combination and did not overlap with it.

For a single dose of dextropropoxyphene 130 mg the NNT was 2.8 (1.8–6.5). This appears to show a dose-response for dextropropoxyphene. However, given the overlapping confidence intervals and the very small number of patients in the dextropropoxyphene 130 mg trial (50), this conclusion is not robust.

A single dose of dextropropoxyphene 65 mg plus paracetamol 650 mg showed a significantly higher incidence of central nervous system adverse effects (somnolence, dizziness) than placebo (Table 3). These adverse effects have also been shown for tramadol 100 mg with a lower (worse) NNH for both dizziness and somnolence [7]. Tramadol 100 mg also showed a significantly higher incidence of nausea and vomiting than placebo. These adverse effects were reported with dextropropoxyphene 65 mg plus paracetamol 650 mg but the incidence was not significantly different from placebo.

The combination of dextropropoxyphene 65 mg with paracetamol 650 mg showed similar efficacy to tramadol 100 mg for single dose studies in postoperative pain with a lower incidence of adverse effects.

References

1. Collins SL, Edwards J, Moore A, McQuay HJ. Oral dextropropoxyphene in postoperative pain: a quantitative systematic review. *European Journal of Clinical Pharmacology*. in press.
2. Government Statistical Service. *Prescription cost analysis for England 1995*. London: Department of Health, 1996.
3. Bruster S, Jarman B, Bosanquet N, Weston D, Erens R, Delbanco TL. National survey of hospital patients. *British Medical Journal* 1994; **309**:1542–6.
4. Jadad AR, Carroll D, Moore A, McQuay H. Developing a database of published reports of randomised clinical trials in pain research. *Pain* 1996; **66**:239–46.
5. Reynolds JEF. *Martindale: the extra pharmacopoeia*, (30th edn). London: Pharmaceutical Press, 1993:292–314.
6. Cooper SA. Single-dose analgesic studies: the upside and downside of assay sensitivity. In: Max MB, Portenoy RK, Laska EM, ed. *The design of analgesic clinical trials (Advances in pain research and therapy*, Vol. 18). New York: Raven Press, 1991, 117–24.
7. Moore A, McQuay H, Gavaghan D. Deriving dichotomous outcome measures from continuous data in randomised controlled trials of analgesics: Verification from independent data. *Pain* 1997; **69**:127–30.
8. Moore A, Moore O, McQuay H, Gavaghan D. Deriving dichotomous outcome measures from continuous data in randomised controlled trials of analgesics: Use of pain intensity and visual analogue scales. *Pain* 1997; **69**:311–15.
9. DerSimonian R, Laird N. Meta-analysis of clinical trials. *Controlled Clinical Trials* 1986; **7**:177–88.
10. Cook RJ, Sackett DL. The number needed to treat: a clinically useful measure of treatment effect. *British Medical Journal* 1995; **310**:452–4.
11. Sunshine A, Olson NZ, Zighelboim I, DeCastro A, Minn FL. Analgesic oral efficacy of tramadol hydrochloride in postoperative pain. *Clinical Pharmacology and Therapeutics* 1992; **51**:740–6.
12. Berry FN, Miller JM, Levin HM, Bare WW, Hopkinson JH3, Feldman AJ. Relief of severe pain with acetaminophen in a new dose formulation versus propoxyphene hydrochloride 65 mg. and placebo: a comparative double blind study. *Current Therapeutic Research* 1975; **17**:361–8.
13. Bloomfield SS, Barden TP, Mitchell J. Nefopam and propoxyphene in episiotomy pain. *Pharmacology and Therapeutics* 1980; **27**:502–7.
14. Cooper SA, Wagenberg B, Zissu J, Kruger GO, Reynolds DC, Gallegos L.T. *et al.* The analgesic efficacy of suprofen in peridontal and oral surgical pain. *Pharmacotherapy* 1986; **6**:267–76.
15. Coutinho A, Bonelli J, Nanci de Carvelho P. A double-blind study of the analgesic effects of fenbufen, codeine, aspirin, propoxyphene and placebo. *Current Therapeutic Research* 1976; **19**:58–65.
16. Van Staden MJ. The use of gilfanan in postoperative pain. *South African Medical Journal* 1971; **45**:1235–7.
17. Trop D, Kenny L, Grad BR. Comparison of nefopam hydrochloride and propoxyphene hydrochloride in the treatment of postoperative pain. *Canadian Anaesthesia Society Journal* 1979; **26**:296–304.
18. Cooper SA. Double-blind comparison of zomepirac sodium, propoxyphene/acetaminophen, and placebo in the treatment of oral surgical pain. *Current Therapeutic Research* 1980; **28**:630–8.
19. Cooper SA, Breen JF, Giuliani RL. The relative efficacy of indoprofen compared with opioid-analgesic combinations. *Journal of Oral Surgery* 1981; **39**:21–5.
20. Evans PJ, McQuay HJ, Rolfe M, O'Sullivan G, Bullingham RE, Moore RA. Zomepirac, placebo and paracetamol/dextropropoxyphene combination compared in orthopaedic postoperative pain. *British Journal of Anaesthesia* 1982; **54**:927–33.
21. Honig S, Murray KA. Surgical pain: zomepirac sodium, propoxyphene/acetaminophen combination, and placebo. *Journal of Clinical Pharmacology* 1981; **21**:443–8.
22. Moore RA, McQuay HJ. Single-patient data meta-analysis of 3453 postoperative patients: Oral tramadol versus placebo, codeine and combination analgesics. *Pain* 1997; **69**:287–94.

16

Oral tramadol versus placebo, codeine, and combination analgesics

Summary

The analgesic effectiveness and safety of oral tramadol was compared with standard analgesics using a meta-analysis of individual patient data from randomized controlled trials in patients with moderate or severe pain after surgery or dental extraction. Calculation of %maxTOTPAR from individual patient data, and the use of at least 50%maxTOTPAR defined clinically acceptable pain relief. Number-needed-to-treat (NNT) for one patient to have at least 50%maxTOTPAR compared with placebo was used to examine the effectiveness of different single oral doses of tramadol and comparator drugs.

Eighteen randomized, double-blind, parallel-group single dose trials with 3453 patients using categorical pain relief scales allowed the calculation of %maxTOTPAR. The use of at least 50%maxTOTPAR was a sensitive measure to discriminate between analgesics.

Tramadol and comparator drugs gave significantly more analgesia than placebo. In postsurgical pain tramadol 50, 100, and 150 mg had NNTs for at least 50%maxTOTPAR of 7.3 (95% confidence intervals 4.6–18), 4.8 (3.4–8.2), and 2.4 (2.0–3.1), comparable with aspirin 650 mg plus codeine 60 mg (NNT 3.6; 2.5–6.3) and paracetamol 650 mg plus propoxyphene 100 mg (NNT 4.0; 3.0–5.7). With the same dose of drug postsurgical patients had more pain relief than those having dental surgery. Tramadol showed a dose-response for analgesia in both postsurgical and dental pain patients.

With the same dose of drug postsurgical pain patients had fewer adverse events than those having dental surgery. Adverse events (headache, nausea, vomiting, dizziness, somnolence) with tramadol 50 mg and 100 mg had a similar incidence to comparator drugs. There was a dose-response with tramadol, tending towards higher incidences at higher doses.

Single patient meta-analysis using more than half pain relief provides a sensitive description of the analgesic properties of a drug, and NNT calculations allow comparisons to be made with standard analgesics.

Introduction

Study of analgesics still poses problems, some 40 years after Beecher first described methods of measuring pain and pain relief [2, 3]. Problems can be of different types, starting with the obvious but important, for instance, the many possible comparisons of drugs, doses, routes of administration, and pain condition which makes meaningful comparison difficult. Many controlled trials have been performed, and many published; some 10 000 randomized controlled trials (over 4000 in pharmacological interventions in acute pain) have been identified [4].

Quantitative systematic reviews pool data from a number of trials; while individual trials may have relatively small numbers of patients receiving a particular treatment, meta-analysis allows the result to be confirmed using data from many patients in many trials, thereby increasing the power to determine the 'true' result. It can therefore provide a higher quality of evidence on which to base decisions by prescribers, policy-makers, and patients.

Choice of randomized, controlled trials for systematic reviews is essential. Randomization (and concealment) of treatment allocation limits selection bias, and blinding of treatments controls observer bias. Inadequacies of randomization or blinding exaggerate estimates of treatment effect [5]. In randomized controlled trials in pain relief, standard methods of measuring pain relief and trial conduct appear to be effectively blinded [6].

Results of systematic reviews have to be easily understood to be useful and used. The elegant numbers-needed-to-treat (NNT) approach [7] involves defining a clinical endpoint, and comparing the rate of that event in a treatment group with the rate in a comparator group; NNT calculations require dichotomous data. NNTs derived for particular benefits or harm can provide a useful starting point for simple verbal and numerical results accessible to any doctor or patient [8].

Meta-analysis using individual patient data sometimes produces lower estimates of effect of treatment than does meta-analysis using group descriptions [9], though the generality of this has been challenged [10]. Using individual patient information may not always be possible, but where possible it is preferred [11] because it is claimed to have the least bias of any meta-analytical method.

Studies of pain relief may present an additional complication. The classic design of single dose oral medication with both placebo and active controls to demonstrate analgesic sensitivity [3] is explanatory [12]. Such trials provide evidence that a drug is an analgesic, rather than about the best

The topic discussed in this chapter is also published in full in Moore *et al.* 1997 [1].

way to use the compound in practice. In this context, NNT methods are useful as indicators of relative efficacy [13].

Tramadol has been used in many European countries since the late 1970s, in many different pain conditions. Since most studies with tramadol in Europe had not been conducted according to US regulatory requirements, a completely new programme of clinical studies for registration in the United States of an oral tramadol formulation took place in the late 1980s and early 1990s. Eighteen single dose studies were conducted, nine in dental pain models and nine in postsurgical pain, and the results of the studies have been summarized [14].

We performed a single patient data meta-analysis of these 18 studies, and any others (published or unpublished) which could be found and which had categorical pain relief scales, allowing the calculation of the percentage of maximum pain relief obtained by individual patients. Combining data from many studies will help shed additional light on the debate [15, 16] about the conflicting results of tramadol in postoperative pain [17, 18].

Methods

Primary trials

Individual patient data from 18 primary trials was made available by Grünenthal GmbH, Aachen, Germany and Robert Wood Johnson Pharmaceutical Research Institute, Spring House, Pennsylvania. One of these had been published [17]. Other studies which used single doses of oral tramadol with categorical pain relief scoring in acute painful conditions were sought by reference to the in-house data from Grünenthal GmbH, from Searle (UK) Ltd, and by searching MEDLINE (1960–5) and the Oxford Pain Relief Database (1950–5) [4] using tramadol as a free text term.

There was a prior hypothesis that analgesic drugs may produce different analgesic responses in painful dental procedures (such as third molar extractions) than postsurgical procedures (such as abdominal, orthopaedic, or gynaecological operations). The prior intention, therefore, was to analyse these conditions separately. Included reports were scored for inclusion and methodological quality using a three-item scale [19].

Protocols for the Robert Wood Johnson studies of postsurgical pain and of pain due to the extraction of impacted third molars were essentially identical. Trials were of double-blind, single dose, parallel-group design; randomization was by computerized random-number generation, stratified on pre-treatment pain intensity. Criteria for patient selection were moderate or severe pain and that the patient's condition was appropriate for management with a centrally acting analgesic and paracetamol. The age range was 18 to 70 years. Patients had to be co-operative, reliable, and motivated, and be able to take oral medication. Exclusion criteria included patients with mild or no pain, those who had taken analgesic drugs within three hours of study drug administration, those needing sedatives during the observation period and those with known contraindications or medical conditions which might interfere with observations.

Drugs were given as single oral doses, of placebo (695 evaluable patients), codeine 60 mg (649), tramadol 50 mg (409), tramadol 75 mg (281), tramadol 100 mg (468), tramadol 150 mg (279), tramadol 200 mg (50), aspirin 650 mg plus codeine 60 mg (305), and paracetamol 650 mg plus propoxyphene 100 mg (316).

Patients were given the study drug if they had moderate or severe pain on a four-point categorical scale (0 = no pain, 1 = slight, 2 = moderate, 3 = severe). Thereafter, observations were made at 30 minutes, and 1, 2, 3, 4, 5, and 6 hours after administration. Pain intensity was measured using the same categorical scale, together with a five-point categorical scale of pain relief (0 = no relief, 1 = a little, 2 = some, 3 = a lot, 4 = complete). Time of remedication was also recorded, as well as a global assessment of therapy (excellent, very good, good, fair, or poor) at the final evaluation.

Adverse experiences volunteered by the patient after non-directive questioning were recorded regardless of any rescue medication used.

Calculations

For each patient the area under the curve of pain relief (categorical scale) against time was calculated (TOTPAR) for six hours after the study drug was given. If patients remedicated, pain relief scores reverted to zero and pain intensity scores to the initial value; adverse event recording, but not pain evaluations, continued after remedication. The percentage of the maximum possible for this summary measure was then calculated (%maxTOTPAR) [20]. The number of patients on each treatment who achieved more than 50% of %maxTOTPAR was determined.

Relative benefit (which indicates how much more likely is an individual given a particular treatment to have a specific outcome than someone not given the treatment) and its 95% confidence intervals were calculated for individual trials using a fixed-effects model [21], and number-needed-to-treat (NNT) using the method of Cook and Sackett [7]. The same method was used to calculate the number-needed-to-harm (NNH) for adverse effects. Relative risk and NNT are given with 95% confidence intervals in text and tables. Significance testing for dose-response of tramadol was done using the Kruskal–Wallis test unstratified for type of surgery.

Results

Search results

Individual patient data for 3453 patients from 18 studies was supplied. It consisted of pain intensity and pain relief scores from start of study to 8 hours post dose and aggregate adverse effect information. Studies with their codes, drug treatments and numbers of patients, are detailed in Table 1. Data on pain measurements and adverse effects for these single dose, parallel-group double-blind studies was provided. Of the nine post-surgical pain studies, two (TR and TV) followed Caesarean section, and one (TX) was conducted with outpatients. Of the nine dental pain studies, three (TI, TI2 and TO) were conducted with outpatients. Tramadol 200 mg was given in only one study in dental pain, and these data were excluded. Study reports were of high methodological quality, scoring the maximum of 5 points on a validated scale [19].

Literature searches through MEDLINE found two relevant studies of oral tramadol in postoperative pain [17, 18]. The former formed part of the data set supplied. The latter, which did not show a significant difference between tramadol 50 and 100 mg and placebo, used a pain intensity scoring system rather than pain relief, and therefore had to be excluded from this analysis. Another study [22] of several dose levels of oral tramadol after dental surgery was multiple dose and used only pain intensity scoring. It showed significant differences between all tramadol doses and placebo, but again could not be used. No other relevant studies were identified.

Analgesic efficacy

The relative benefits and NNT for each drug tested are shown in Table 2, for dental and postsurgical pain separately and combined. The proportions achieving at least 50%maxTOTPAR are shown in Fig. 1. There was a clear dose-response for tramadol ($P < 0.0001$, Kruskal–Wallis test).

Dental pain

Among the dental studies all treatments showed significantly greater pain relief (greater proportion of patients with at least 50% of %maxTOTPAR) than with placebo (relative risk lower confidence interval > 1), except codeine 60 mg. There was a clear dose-response for tramadol, with greater relative benefit and lower NNT values with the higher doses. Tramadol doses of 100 and 150 mg produced NNT values of 4.6 (3.6–6.4) and 4.1 (2.9–7.3), respectively, lower than aspirin/ codeine with an NNT of 6.3 (4.5–9.8) and paracetamol/ propoxyphene with an NNT of 5.3 (3.4–11.4).

Postsurgical pain

All treatments showed statistically significantly superior analgesia to placebo. There was a clear dose-response for tramadol; tramadol 100 mg had a NNT of 4.8 (3.4–8.2) and tramadol 150 mg had a NNT of 2.4 (2.0–3.1). This was lower than aspirin/codeine and paracetamol/propoxyphene combinations with NNT values of 3.5 (2.5–6.3) and 4.0 (3.0–5.7), respectively.

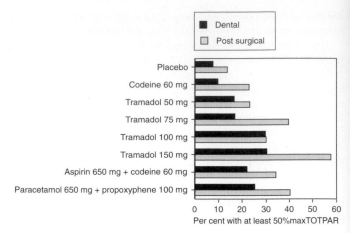

Fig. 1   Proportion of patients with at least 50%maxTOTPAR.

Dental and postsurgical pain models compared

With the exception of tramadol 100 mg, NNT was lower in postsurgical pain than in dental pain. When the numbers of patients with more than 50% pain relief were compared for each treatment between postsurgical and dental pain (Fig. 1), some treatments produced significantly more pain relief in postsurgical pain. This was the case for codeine 60 mg (relative benefit 2.4; 1.6–3.5), tramadol 75 mg (2.4; 1.5–3.8) and 150 mg (1.9; 1.4–2.6), aspirin plus codeine (1.6; 1.04–2.3), and paracetamol plus propoxyphene (1.6; 1.1–2.4).

This difference was not due to a greater proportion of postsurgical patients with more moderate than severe initial pain intensity. The ratio of moderate to severe initial (base-line) pain intensity was 931:663 (1.40:1) in postsurgical pain, compared with 1294:505 (2.56:1) in dental pain (significantly less severe initial pain in the dental group, relative risk 0.81; 0.77–0.85). Initial pain intensity stratification produced no consistent or significant differences in the proportion of patients with at least 50%maxTOTPAR, or in NNT (data not shown). For postsurgical pain, 44 of 323 patients (13.6%) given placebo had at least 50%maxTOTPAR, compared with 28 of 373 patients (7.5%) for dental pain patients given placebo (relative benefit 1.8; 1.2–2.8).

Combined data

NNT with dental and postsurgical patients combined is also shown in Table 2. Few data sets have sufficient information to allow calculation of analgesic efficacy for dental and postsurgical pain models separately. These numbers are those used for comparisons with other analgesic drugs from published reports without individual meta-analysis.

Choice of half pain relief

In order to test the effect of choices other than half pain relief, NNT was calculated using dichotomous data for 20% to 80%maxTOTPAR (combined data). The results are shown in Fig. 2.

Table 1 Trials, drug treatments, and patient numbers

	Post-surgical			Dental	
Trial	Drug	No. of patients	Trial	Drug	No. of patients
TA	Tramadol 50 mg	52	TE	Tramadol 50 mg	28
	Tramadol 100 mg	58		Tramadol 100 mg	30
	Codeine 60 mg	26		ASA650 & C60	28
	Placebo	28		Codeine 60 mg	28
				Placebo	29
TC	Tramadol 50 mg	40			
	Tramadol 100 mg	39	TE2	Tramadol 50 mg	23
	ASA650 & C60	40		Tramadol 100 mg	21
	Codeine 60 mg	39		ASA650 & C60	22
	Placebo	40		Codeine 60 mg	24
				Placebo	21
TR	Tramadol 75 mg	40			
	Tramadol 150 mg	40	TF	Tramadol 50 mg	47
	APAP650 & P100	41		Tramadol 100 mg	49
	Placebo	40		ASA650 & C60	45
				Codeine 60 mg	47
TV	Tramadol 50 mg	31		Placebo	49
	Tramadol 100 mg	31			
	ASA650 & C60	30	TG	Tramadol 50 mg	50
	Codeine 60 mg	29		Tramadol 100 mg	49
	Placebo	28		ASA650 & C60	41
				Codeine 60 mg	33
TW	Tramadol 50 mg	40		Placebo	27
	Tramadol 100 mg	40			
	APAP650 & P100	39	TH	Tramadol 50 mg	47
	Codeine 60 mg	39		Tramadol 100 mg	51
	Placebo	40		ASA650 & C60	51
				Codeine 60 mg	48
TW2	Tramadol 75 mg	41		Placebo	50
	Tramadol 150 mg	40			
	APAP650 & P100	39	TI	Tramadol 50 mg	51
	Codeine 60 mg	41		Tramadol 100 mg	50
	Placebo	40		ASA650 & C60	48
				Codeine 60 mg	50
TX	Tramadol 75 mg	35		Placebo	49
	Tramadol 150 mg	36			
	APAP650 & P100	37	TI2	Tramadol 75 mg	45
	Codeine 60 mg	33		Tramadol 150 mg	45
	Placebo	36		APAP650 & P100	42
				Codeine 60 mg	47
TY	Tramadol 75 mg	31		Placebo	44
	Tramadol 150 mg	28			
	APAP650 & P100	31	TO	Tramadol 100 mg	50
	Codeine 60 mg	30		Tramadol 200 mg	50
	Placebo	30		Codeine 60 mg	47
				Placebo	53
TZA	Tramadol 75 mg	39			
	Tramadol 150 mg	40	TQ	Tramadol 75 mg	50
	APAP650 & P100	38		Tramadol 150 mg	50
	Codeine 60 mg	38		APAP650 & P100	49
	Placebo	41		Codeine 60 mg	50
				Placebo	51

ASA650 & C60, aspirin 650 mg plus codeine 60 mg; APAP650 & P100, paracetamol 650 mg plus proproxyphene 100 mg.

Table 2 Analgesic effectiveness

Drug treatment	Improved on active drug	Improved on control	Relative benefit (95% CI)	NNT (95% CI)
Dental				
Codeine 60 mg	36/374	28/373	1.3 (0.8–2.1)	47.2 (16.3–∞)
Tramadol 50 mg	41/246	13/225	2.9 (1.6–5.2)	9.2 (6.1–18.8)
Tramadol 75 mg	16/95	6/95	2.7 (1.1–6.5)	9.5 (5.1–64.5)
Tramadol 100 mg	89/300	22/278	3.8 (2.4–5.8)	4.6 (3.6–6.4)
Tramadol 150 mg	29/95	6/95	4.8 (2.1–11.1)	4.1 (2.9–7.3)
Paracetamol 650 mg + propoxyphene 100 mg	23/91	6/95	4.0 (1.7–9.4)	5.3 (3.4–11.4)
Aspirin 650 mg + codeine 60 mg	52/235	13/225	3.8 (2.2–6.8)	6.3 (4.5–9.8)
Post-surgical				
Codeine 60 mg	*63/275*	*35/283*	*1.9 (1.3–2.7)*	*9.5 (6–23.4)*
Tramadol 50 mg	38/163	13/136	2.4 (1.4–4.4)	7.3 (4.6–17.9)
Tramadol 75 mg	74/186	31/187	2.4 (1.7–3.5)	4.3 (3.1–7)
Tramadol 100 mg	51/168	13/136	3.2 (1.8–5.6)	4.8 (3.4–8.2)
Tramadol 150 mg	106/184	31/187	3.5 (2.5–4.9)	2.4 (2–3.1)
Paracetamol 650 mg + propoxyphene 100 mg	91/225	34/227	2.7 (1.9–3.8)	3.9 (3–5.7)
Aspirin 650 mg + codeine 60 mg	24/70	4/68	5.8 (2.1–15.9)	3.5 (2.5–6.3)
Combined				
Codeine 60 mg	99/649	63/656	1.6 (1.2–2.1)	16.7 (11–48)
Tramadol 50 mg	79/409	26/361	2.7 (1.8–4.1)	8.3 (6.0–13)
Tramadol 75 mg	90/281	37/282	2.4 (1.7–3.5)	5.3 (3.9–8.2)
Tramadol 100 mg	140/468	35/414	3.5 (2.5–5.0)	4.8 (3.8–6.1)
Tramadol 150 mg	135/279	37/282	3.7 (2.7–5.1)	2.9 (2.4–3.6)
Paracetamol 650 mg + propoxyphene 100 mg	114/316	40/322	2.9 (2.1–4.0)	4.2 (3.3–5.8)
Aspirin 650 mg + codeine 60 mg	76/305	17/293	4.3 (2.6–7.1)	5.3 (4.1–7.4)

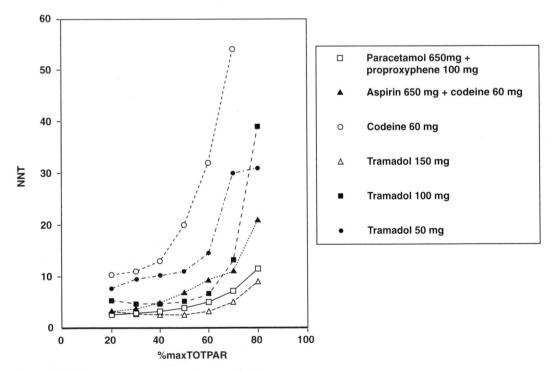

Fig. 2 Effect of %maxTOTPAR on number-needed-to-treat (NNT)

NNT for an effective drug, tramadol 150 mg, was essentially the same at about 2–3 over a wide range of decision points. Those for a slightly less effective analgesic (aspirin 650 mg plus codeine 60 mg) rose slightly with pain relief cut-off values above 50%maxTOTPAR, but for codeine 60 mg NNT values which started at about 10 for > 20%maxTOTPAR rose rapidly and were not significantly different from placebo by >60%maxTOTPAR.

Adverse effects

The incidence of the more common adverse events reported is shown in Fig. 3 for dental and postsurgical pain. Headache, vomiting, nausea, dizziness, and somnolence were the most commonly reported adverse effects, although predominantly of mild intensity.

For dental, but not postsurgical pain, the adverse effect incidence was generally sufficiently high to achieve a statistical difference from placebo for vomiting, nausea, dizziness, and somnolence, but not headache. For tramadol there was a distinct dose-response in dental pain, with higher doses producing greater incidence of adverse effects; this trend was not present in postsurgical pain. Numbers-need-to-harm (NNH) can be calculated for adverse effects in dental patients because their incidence was sufficiently high. The clear dose-response is shown in Fig. 4.

Comment

Tramadol is an effective analgesic in postoperative pain. All doses of tramadol were statistically superior to placebo in both postsurgical and dental pain, and there was a significant dose-response. Single oral doses of tramadol 75 mg to 150 mg had analgesic efficacy equivalent to combinations of paracetamol plus propoxyphene and aspirin plus codeine. Internal sensitivity was demonstrated by two comparator analgesics being statistically superior to placebo, and by the dose-response for tramadol. The study methodology—randomized, double-blind trials—avoided known sources of major bias.

Search strategies identified a total of 20 randomized trials of oral tramadol in postoperative acute pain with standardized measurements of pain intensity and pain relief. Only two of these had been published in full [17, 18] with one other in press [22]. Results of the other trials had been published in summary form only [14]. Meta-analytic tools so far developed have concentrated on patients achieving at least 50% pain relief as a single dichotomous measure of clinical effectiveness [13], so the two studies which used pain intensity and not pain relief scales could not be included. Of the two studies excluded, one, [18], could not distinguish oral tramadol from placebo after orthopaedic surgery; the other [22] found oral tramadol effective in dento-alveolar surgical pain.

Because the only two studies published in full [17, 18] came to contrary conclusions about the efficacy of oral tramadol in postoperative pain, a controversy has arisen about its analgesic properties [15, 16]. Examining all the available information (published and unpublished) has demonstrated clear analgesic efficacy; three standard analgesics were distinguished from placebo, as were tramadol 50 mg, 100 mg and 150 mg. Larger doses of tramadol produced more analgesia. This was done in a single patient meta-analysis, a method which is claimed to be more conservative than aggregating mean data [9].

Sunshine [14], Cooper [20], and others have pointed out the variability that can occur in clinical trials of analgesics even in standard settings. This variability may have a number of causes. One is almost certain to be due to the random play of chance in clinical trials where group sizes are of the order of 30 patients, although there may also be systematic causes. These causes may be apparent only in the systematic examination of large numbers of clinical trials with common endpoints.

The other consideration is that analgesic trial designs are explanatory [12]. They are designed to demonstrate that a particular compound is an analgesic in single doses in acute pain. They cannot in themselves determine the value of the intervention in clinical practice, although meta-analysis of such trials may be helpful in determining relative efficacy [13].

This unique opportunity to use the individual patient data from 18 trials conducted to a common protocol allowed several questions to be addressed. The first, the original purpose of the studies, was to compare the efficacy and adverse effects of the novel analgesic with placebo and standard oral analgesics. The data also allowed the confirmation of the usefulness of at least 50% pain relief as an indicator of efficacy, comparison of the various analgesics in patients with either moderate or severe baseline pain and comparison of dental with postsurgical pain.

As a clinical outcome, 50% relief of pain has historical provenance over 40 years [2], and is more readily clinically interpretable than the summary TOTPAR measure. For comparisons of analgesics the question arises whether the 50% relief is a better cut-off than 20% or 80% relief. The best performing analgesic, tramadol 150 mg, had NNT values of 2–3 across a range of cut-offs, from 30% to 60%maxTOTPAR (Fig. 2). The least analgesic drug, codeine 60 mg, showed a rapid rise in NNT beyond 50%maxTOTPAR, and the aspirin–plus codeine combination showed a gradual rise in NNT with higher cut-offs. This provides some empirical support for the use of 50% as the cut-off. Not only does it have a clinically useful resonance, but it also provides sensible discrimination between the best and worst analgesics.

That NNT (the reciprocal of the absolute risk reduction, or risk difference) should be relatively unaffected by choice of cut-off is not unexpected. With placebo, the proportion of patients achieving a particular level of pain relief falls quickly as %maxTOTPAR increases. For effective analgesics, this proportion falls slowly until high %maxTOTPAR levels are reached. The difference will remain largely unaltered over a wide range of %maxTOTPAR—generating stable NNTs.

The imposition of an arbitrary dichotomous outcome, at least 50%maxTOTPAR, on continuous data—a spectrum of response between no pain relief and complete pain relief—is

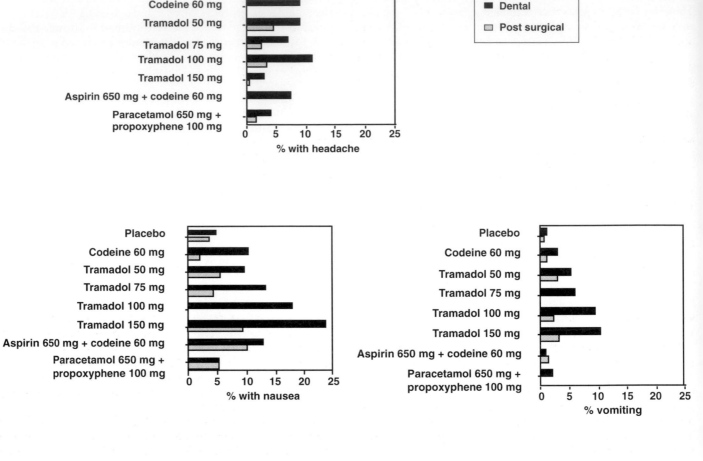

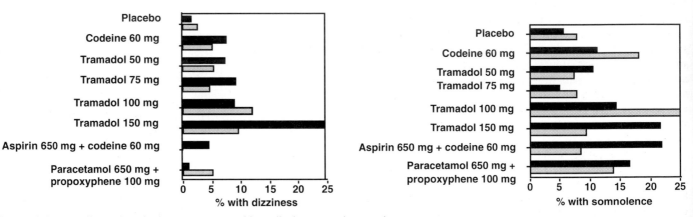

Fig. 3   Adverse effects: headache, nausea, vomiting, dizziness, and somnolence.

justified because it allows analgesics to be compared across many different trials. However, it should not be over-interpreted; patients with less than 50%maxTOTPAR can also obtain useful pain relief; conversely, those with at least 50%maxTOTPAR may have near maximal pain relief. The reality, however, is that multiple dosing is the norm in pain management, where adverse effects may drive practice as much as analgesia.

It has been suggested that differences might be seen between analgesics when tested on pain of initial moderate as opposed to severe intensity. This was not supported by these data. Stratification by initial pain intensity revealed no con-

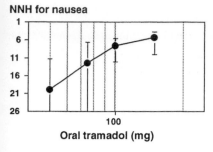

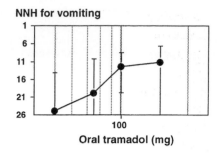

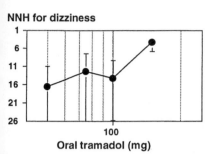

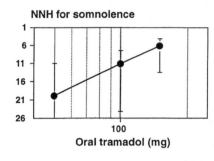

Fig. 4   Number-needed-to-harm (NNH) for adverse effects in dental patients.

sistent or significant differences in the proportion of patients with at least 50%maxTOTPAR.

In these trials the analgesics were more effective in postsurgical pain than in dental pain (Table 2), producing lower NNT despite significantly more patients with severe pain intensity at baseline in postsurgical pain. In postsurgical trials, significantly more patients given placebo (14%) had at least 50% pain relief that was the case with dental models (8%). These average figures for nine trials in each group are lower than those found by Cooper [20].

Cooper's figures were derived from study mean TOTPAR. McQuay *et al.* [6] have pointed out that means are inadequate descriptors of asymmetrically distributed pain measurements, making comparison between estimates derived by single patient meta-analysis difficult. What Cooper's data did show was the great between-trial variability of placebo and active responses. This variability is not limited to acute pain studies, and is seen also in chronic pain studies [23], as well as in studies with more objective outcomes like postoperative vomiting [24], and in the response of infants to pulmonary surfactant [25].

Despite analysing results on nearly 3500 patients, there were only 18 trials, 9 each in dental and postsurgical pain. In order to make definitive statements about differences between pain models information from many more trials would need to be available. Cooper's 1991 analysis had information from as many as 63 studies. The differences in analgesic efficacy and adverse events seen in this study support the view that dental and postoperative pain should be considered separately in meta-analytical comparisons of analgesic efficacy, at least when opioid analgesics or combinations with opioids are used.

Analyses of other analgesics in postsurgical and dental pain models are needed to allow comparisons to be made of relative effectiveness. This will not be easy, partly because few studies report data in ways which allow meta-analysis from the published reports, and partly because many patients are needed to obtain estimates with narrow confidence intervals. Single patient meta-analysis is the most useful way of generating comparative information, though that will involve much co-operation between investigators and sponsoring pharmaceutical companies.

Authors of reports of trials of analgesics can aid future meta-analysis by including dichotomous outcomes as part of their analysis and report. This can easily be done as an addition to, not to the exclusion of, classical pain measures and analysis [6].

References

1. Moore RA, McQuay HJ. Single-patient data meta-analysis of 3453 postoperative patients: Oral tramadol versus placebo, codeine and combination analgesics. *Pain* 1997; **69**:287–94.
2. Denton J, Beecher H. New analgesics. *Journal of the American Medical Association* 1949; **141**:1051–7.
3. Houde R, Wallenstein S, Beaver W. Clinical measurement of pain. In: G. De Stevens, ed. *Analgesics*. New York/London: Academic Press, 1965:75–122.
4. Jadad AR, Carroll D, Moore A, McQuay H. Developing a database of published reports of randomised clinical trials in pain research. *Pain* 1996; **66**:239–46.
5. Schulz KF, Chalmers I, Hayes RJ, Altman DG. Empirical evidence of bias: dimensions of methodological quality associated with estimates of treatment effects in controlled trials. *Journal of the American Medical Association* 1995; **273**:408–12.
6. McQuay H, Carroll D, Moore A. Variation in the placebo effect in randomised controlled trials of analgesics: All is as blind as it seems. *Pain* 1996; **64**:331–5.
7. Cook RJ, Sackett DL. The number needed to treat: a clinically useful measure of treatment effect. *British Medical Journal* 1995; **310**:452–4.

8. Chalmers I. 'Applying overviews and meta-analyses at the bedside'. *Journal of Clinical Epidemiology* 1995; **48**:67–70.

9. Stewart LA, Parmar MKB. Meta-analysis of the literature or of individual patient data: is there a difference? *Lancet* 1993; **341**:418–22.

10. Harvey I, Peters TJ, Toth B. Meta-analysis [letter]. *Lancet* 1993; **341**:964.

11. Oxman AD, Clarke MJ, Stewart LA. From science to practice. Meta-analyses using individual patient data are needed. *Journal of the American Medical Association* 1995; **274**:845–6.

12. Schwartz D, Lellouch J. Explanatory and pragmatic attitudes in therapeutic trials. *Journal of Chronic Disease* 1967; **20**:637–48.

13. Moore A, McQuay H, Gavaghan D. Deriving dichotomous outcome measures from continuous data in randomised controlled trials of analgesics. *Pain* 1996; **66**:229–37.

14. Sunshine A. New clinical experience with tramadol. *Drugs* 1994; **47**(Suppl 1):8–18.

15. Vielvoye-Kerkmeer APE. Comments on Stubhaug, Grimstad and Breivik: *Pain*, **62** (1995) 111–118 (letter). *Pain* 1996; **64**:401–2.

16. Stubhaug A, Grimstad J, Breivik H. Reply to Vielvoye-Kerkmeer (letter). *Pain* 1964; 1996:402.

17. Sunshine A, Olson NZ, Zighelboim I, DeCastro A, Minn FL. Analgesic oral efficacy of tramadol hydrochloride in postoperative pain. *Clinical Pharmacology and Therapeutics* 1992; **51**:740–6.

18. Stubhaug A, Grimstad J, Breivik H. Lack of analgesic effect of 50 and 100 mg oral tramadol after orthopaedic surgery: a randomized, double-blind, placebo and standard active drug comparison. *Pain* 1995; **62**:111–18.

19. Jadad AR, Moore RA, Carroll D, Jenkinson C, Reynolds DJM, Gavaghan DJ *et al*. Assessing the quality of reports of randomized clinical trials: is blinding necessary? *Controlled Clinical Trials* 1996; **17**:1–12.

20. Cooper SA. Single-dose analgesic studies: the upside and downside of assay sensitivity. In: Max MB, Portenoy RK, Laska EM, ed. *The design of analgesic clinical trials (Advances in pain research and therapy*, Vol. 18). New York: Raven Press, 1991:117–24.

21. Gardner MJ, Altman DG. *Statistics with confidence.* London: British Medical Journal, 1989.

22. Collins M, Young I, Sweeney P, Fenn GC, Stratford ME, Wilson A *et al*. The effect of tramadol on dento-alveolar surgical pain. *British Journal of Oral and Maxillofacial Surgery* 1997; **35**:54–8.

23. McQuay HJ, Tramer M, Nye BA, Carroll D, Wiffen PJ, Moore RA. A systematic review of antidepressants in neuropathic pain. *Pain* 1996; **68**:217–227.

24. Tramer M, Moore A, McQuay H. Prevention of vomiting after paediatric strabismus surgery: a systematic review using the numbers-needed-to-treat method. *British Journal of Anaesthesia* 1995; **75**:556–61.

25. Soll JC, McQueen MC. Respiratory distress syndrome. In: Sinclair JC, Bracken ME, ed. *Effective care of the newborn infant.* Oxford University Press, 1992: Ch. 15, 333.

17

Pain relief with intra-articular morphine after knee surgery

Summary

Reduction of postoperative pain by injecting opioid into the knee joint is believed to support the hypothesis of peripheral opioid receptor activation in inflammation. This systematic review of randomized controlled trials (RCTs) was designed to examine the evidence for this. Main outcomes were pain intensity and the use of supplementary analgesics. Efficacy of intra-articular bupivacaine versus placebo was used as an index of internal sensitivity. Evidence of efficacy was sought in both early (0–6 hours after intra-articular injection) and late (6–24 hour) periods.

Thirty-six RCTs in knee surgery were found. Six had both a local anaesthetic control and placebo; four showed internal sensitivity. All four sensitive studies had at least one outcome showing efficacy of intra-articular morphine versus placebo. Six studies compared intra-articular morphine with intravenous or intramuscular morphine or with intra-articular saline without a bupivacaine control. Four of the six studies showed greater efficacy for intra-articular morphine. There was no dose-response evident. No quantitative analysis of pooled data was done.

Intra-articular morphine may have some effect in reducing postoperative pain intensity and consumption of analgesics. These studies had significant problems in design, data collection, statistical analysis, and reporting. Trials of better methodological quality are needed for a conclusive answer that intra-articular morphine is analgesic, and that any analgesia produced is clinically useful.

Introduction

Intra-articular morphine has been used as a clinical test of the hypothesis that peripheral opioid receptors are activated in inflammation [2]. The judgement that exogenous opioids can provide effective postoperative analgesia has been taken as confirmation of the hypothesis [2]. Even though many studies and reviews have been published on this subject, consensus on whether intra-articular opioids offer clinically relevant pain relief is still lacking.

Particularly important is the issue of the sensitivity of analgesic measurement. Over 40 years ago, Beecher [3] and Houde [4] described methods for measuring analgesic drugs which were sensitive and reproducible. Sensitive analgesic assays depended on patients experiencing pain of moderate or severe intensity before test drug administration.

This systematic review, using the evidence from all relevant randomized controlled trials (RCTs), was undertaken to investigate the evidence for an analgesic effect of intra-articular morphine and to examine those features of trial methodology which influence judgement of experimental or clinical effectiveness.

Methods

Randomized controlled trials (RCTs) of intra-articular opioids were sought systematically. A number of different search strategies in both MEDLINE (1966–May 1996), EMBASE, and the Oxford Pain Relief Data-base (1950–94) were used, without language restriction. Search terms used included: 'intra-articular', 'opioids', 'opioids', 'morphine', and 'random*' [5]. Additional reports were identified from the reference lists of retrieved reports and from review articles. Unpublished reports, abstracts, and reviews were not considered. Authors were not contacted for original data.

Reports considered

Reports were considered if they were randomized comparisons of intra-articular morphine with placebo (saline), or different doses of intra-articular morphine, or comparisons of intra-articular morphine with systemic (intravenous or intramuscular) morphine. Reports of direct comparisons of intra-articular morphine and local anaesthetic agents [6, 7] were not considered. Reports of pethidine [8] were not considered because of potential confounding due to its local anaesthetic properties.

Each report which could possibly be described as an RCT was read independently by each of the authors and scored using a three item quality scale [9]. The scale takes into account proper randomization, double-blinding, and reporting of drop-outs and withdrawals. Consensus was then achieved. Information about the treatments and controls, types of surgery and anaesthesia, number of patients enrolled and analysed, study design, observation periods, outcome

The topic discussed in this chapter is also published in full in Kalso *et al.* 1997 [1].

measures used for pain intensity, and consumption of supplementary analgesics and adverse effects was taken from each report.

Validity and inclusion criteria

Pre-hoc validity criteria were number of patients per treatment group ≥ 10 [10], standardized methods of measuring pain intensity, and general anaesthesia. Spinal or epidural anaesthetics were not accepted, nor infiltrations of local anaesthetic into the joints, because we judged that low pain scores in the immediate postoperative period could render studies insensitive.

Two periods: early (up to 6 hours from the intra-articular injection) and late (from 6 to 24 hours) were defined for the evaluation of effectiveness.

Effectiveness was defined as a significant difference (as reported in the original trials) between the active and the control in pain intensity (early and late) or total consumption of rescue analgesics.

There was a *pre-hoc* agreement that an adequate description of internal sensitivity was a requirement for the demonstration of an analgesic action of intra-articular morphine. Such sensitivity would be derived (not necessarily exclusively) from a statistically significant difference between a known analgesic (intra-articular local anaesthetic) and placebo, from intra-articular morphine being different from placebo, or from a dose-response for intra-articular morphine.

Quantitative analysis of morphine against placebo was planned.

Results

Thirty-three RCTs were found in 31 reports, studying nearly 1500 patients (about 900 of whom received morphine). All were in knee surgery. Two reports were in Danish, one in German, and the rest in English.

The following papers were excluded: duplicate publications [11, 12]; the influence of tourniquet time on the efficacy of intra-articular morphine as the only outcome [13]; number of patients per group less than ten [14, 15]; double-dummy technique not used for intramuscular administration [16] study 2; control group not blinded [17]; controls were intra-articular bupivacaine and unblinded lumbar plexus block only [18]; spinal anaesthesia [19, 20] study 1, epidural anaesthesia [21], operative intra-articular local anaesthetic [11, 20, 22, 23] study 2 [24], non-standardized anaesthesia (general anaesthesia, spinal, or epidural anaesthesia) [25], and inadequate standardization of the timing of pain measurements [26].

Details of the included studies are shown in Table 1. In all these trials morphine (0.5–5 mg) was used as the intra-articular opioid. Controls used were bupivacaine (0.25–0.5%) as the only intra-articular local anaesthetic, intra-articular saline or intravenous or intramuscular morphine 1–2 mg. No quantitative analysis of pooled data was done because results were presented as means, which are inadequate descriptors of assymmetrically distributed data [27].

Morphine vs. saline in studies where bupivacaine was an index of internal sensitivity

Six studies compared intra-articular morphine with both bupivacaine and saline (Table 1). One [28] was only analysed for an early effect (fewer than 10 evaluable patients in the late period).

In two studies [16, 39], intra-articular bupivacaine could not be differentiated from intra-articular saline and the sensitivity of the analgesic assay was not proven. There was no difference between intra-articular morphine and saline in either.

Four of the trials [28–31] showed significantly lower visual analogue scale pain intensity (VASPI) scores with intra-articular bupivacaine compared with intra-articular saline during the early period (0–6 hours) and so had internal sensitivity.

All four sensitive studies reported early outcomes. Three of the four studies showed significantly lower early pain intensity scores after intra-articular morphine compared with intra-articular saline [28, 29, 31] (Fig. 1A).

In the late period from 6 hours onwards intra-articular morphine produced significantly lower pain intensity scores compared with placebo in all three evaluable sensitive studies [29, 30, 31] (Fig. 1B). Total consumption of supplementary analgesics over 24 hours was significantly lower after intra-articular morphine compared with saline in the two sensitive studies which analysed it [30, 31].

Morphine vs. saline, no active (bupivacaine) control

Three studies compared only intra-articular morphine with intra-articular saline [32, 40, 41].

In the early period morphine visual analogue scale pain intensity (VAS-PI) scores were significantly lower in two of the three studies which reported early outcomes [32, 41] (Fig. 1C).

In the late period, the same two studies [32, 41] indicated that intra-articular morphine produced significantly lower pain intensity scores compared with saline. Two of the three studies [32, 40] had significantly lower total consumption of analgesics over 24 hours after morphine.

Morphine vs. systemic morphine control

Three studies compared intra-articular with intravenous or intramuscular morphine [33–35].

In the early period one showed greater efficacy of intra-articular morphine compared with 1 mg intravenous morphine [35] (Fig. 1C).

Table 1 Study details

Ref.	Included or reason for exclusion	Drugs, routes & (no. of patients)	Results: compared with placebo (saline)					Quality score
			VAS-PI: early bupivacaine	VAS-PI: late bupivacaine	VAS-PI: early morphine	VAS-PI: late morphine	Analgesic consumption (total in 24 h)	
Included studies: active control (bupivacaine) and placebo								
[16]	Included.	ia 1 mg M in 20 ml S (21) ia 20 ml S (19) ia 0.25% bup 20 ml (19) ia 0.25% bup 20 ml + 1 mg M (19)	No diff between bup & S at 0.5, 1, 1.5, or 2 h.	No diff at 8, 24, or 48 h.	No diff between M & S: at 0.5, 1, 1.5, or 2 h.	No diff at 8, 24, or 48 h.	No diff.	2
[28]	Included in early (0–6 hrs) excluded from late analysis (inadequate no. of patients per group).	ia 40 ml S (10) ia 1 mg M in 39 ml S (10) ia 0.25% bup 40 ml + 1 in 200 k adr (10) ia 0.25% bup 40 ml + 1 in 200 k adr + 1 mg M (10)	bup better than S: at 2 h. $P = 0.01$; at 4 h $P < 0.05$; at 6 h $P < 0.05$.	$n < 10$.	M better than S: at 2 h. $P = 0.01$; at 4 h $P < 0.05$; at 6 h $P < 0.05$.	$n < 10$.	$n < 10$.	3
[29]	Included.	ia 5 mg M in 25 ml (10) ia 0.25% bup 25 ml (10) ia 5 mg M in 0.25% bup 25 ml (10) ia 25 ml S (10).	bup better than S at 1, 2, 4 h. No P-values given.	NSD (8 or 24 h).	M better than S at 1, 2, 4 h & statistics as for bup.	M better than NS at 8, 24 h & statistics as for bup.	Sig. is not mentioned.	2
[30]	Included.	ia 1 mg M in 20 ml (10) ia 0.375% bup 20 ml (10) ia 1 mg M in 0.375% bup 20 ml (10) ia 20 ml S (10).	bup better than S at 2, 4, 6 h. No actual P-values given.	NSD (24 or 48 h).	NSD (2, 4, 6 h).	M better than S at 24, 48 h & statistics as for bup.	M sig, better than S (0–24 h & 24–48 h). No P-value given.	4
[31]	Included.	ia 5 mg M in 0.25% bup 12.5 ml + 12.5 ml S (10) ia 0.25% bup 25 ml (10) ia 5 mg M in 25 ml S (10) ia 25 ml S (10).	bup better than S at 0.5, 1, 1.5, 2, 4 h. No sem/sd-bars; no P-values.	bup better than S at 8, 12 h; no sem/sd-bars; no P-values.	M better than S at 0.5, 1, 1.5, 2, 4 h; no sem/sd-bars; no P-values.	M better than S at 8, 12, 24 h; no sem/ sd-bars; no P-values.	M & bup sig ($P < 0.05$) better than NS.	2
Included studies: placebo but no local anaesthetic as active control								
[11]	Included.	ia 1 mg M in 5 ml (26) ia 5 ml S (26)			NSD (2 or 4 h).	ia M better than ia S at 8 & 24 h, $P < 0.05$.	ia M better than ia S; $P < 0.05$.	2
[32]	Included.	ia M better than ia 5 mg M in 25 ml (10) ia 25 ml S (10)			ia M better than ia S at 0, 0.5, 1, 1.5, 2, & 4 h; $P < 0.05$	ia M better than ia S at 8 & 12 h; $P < 0.05$.	ia M better than ia S; $P < 0.05$.	2
[15]	Included.	ia 5 mg M in 25 ml (11) ia 25 ml S (9)			NSD (1, 2, or 4 h).	NSD (8 or 24 h).	ia M better than ia S; $P < 0.01$.	2

Table 1 *continued*

Ref.	Included or reason for exclusion	Drugs, routes & (no. of patients)	Results: compared with placebo (saline)					Quality score
			VAS-PI: early bupivacaine	VAS-PI: late bupivacaine	VAS-PI: early morphine	VAS-PI: late morphine	Analgesic consumption (total in 24 h)	
Included studies: cross-route morphine comparison								
[33]	Included.	ia 2 mg M in 40 ml S + IM 1 ml S (18) 40 ml S + IM 2 mg M (15)			NSD (1, 2, 4, 6 h)	Not evaluated.	Not evaluated.	4
[34]	Included.	ia 1 mg M in 10 ml + 10 ml S IV (29) iv 1 mg M in 10 ml + 10 ml S ia (30)			NSD (1, 2, 3, 4, 6 h)	NSD (8 or 24 h)	No diff.	3
[35]	Included (low dose morphine excluded), inadequate no. of patients.	ia 1 mg M in 40 ml S + 1 ml IV S (18) 40 ml S + 1 mg IV M (15) ia 0.5 mg M in 40 ml S + 1 ml IV S (10) ia 1 mg M + 0.1 mg naloxone in 40 ml S + 1 ml IV			ia M better than IV M at 3, 4, & 6 h $P < 0.05$.	NSD (24 h)	ia M sig (P?) better than IV M.	2
Included studies: morphine dose-response								
[36]	Included.	ia 0.25% bup 30 ml (30) ia 1 mg M in 30 ml S (30) ia 2 mg M in 30 ml S (30) ia 1 mg M in 0.25% bup 30 ml (30) ia 20 ml 0.5% bup (11)						5
[37]	Included.	ia M 1 mg in 0.5% bup 20 ml (10) ia M 3 mg in 0.5% bup 20 ml (10)						2
[23]	Included.	ia 2 mg M in 5 ml (25) ia 4 mg M in 5 ml (25)						3
[38]	Included.	ia 5 mg M in 0.25% bup 40 ml (20) ia 2 mg M in 0.25% bup 40 ml (20) ia 0.25% bup 40 ml (18)						4
Included studies: not analysed								
[6]	Included (early), excluded (late) inadequate no. of patients per group	ia 1 mg M in 20 ml (11) ia 0.25% bup 20 ml (11) ia 1 mg M + 0.25% bup 20 ml (11)						3
[7]	Included.	ia 0.25% bup 30 ml + 1 in 200 k adr (41) ia 2 mg M (2 ml) + 28 ml S (40)						1

bup, bupivacaine; ia, intra-articular; NSD, no significant difference; S, saline; sem/sd, standard error/deviation of mean; M, morphine.

1. Studies with active (local anaesthetic) control

A. Early (4 h) pain intensity

B. Late (24 h) pain intensity

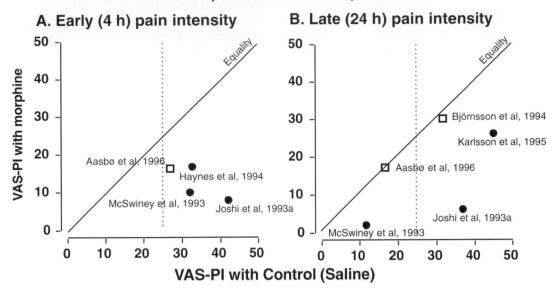

2. Studies without active (local anaesthetic) control

C. Early (4 h) pain intensity

D. Late (24 h) pain intensity

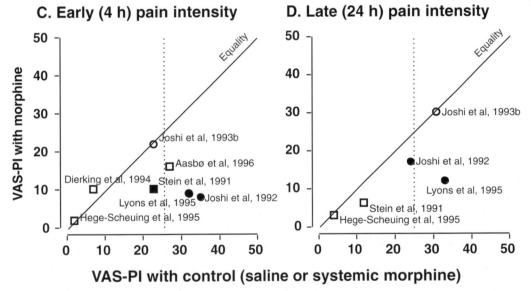

Fig. 1   L'Abbé plots for intra-articular morphine trials. Mean visual analogue scale pain intensity (VAS-PI, mm) for intra-articular morphine vs. control. Each point represents an individual trial. Internal sensitivity was assumed when intra-articular bupivacaine was significantly better than saline. The dotted vertical line is at control VAS-PI 25% of maximum. (1A and B): ○, sensitive studies; □, insensitive study; ●, morphine significantly better than saline. (1C and D): ○, placebo control; □, systemic morphine control; ● and ■, morphine significantly better than control.

In the late period, no study indicated that intra-articular morphine had statistically lower pain intensity scores, though one had no evaluations beyond 6 hours [33] (Fig. 1D). Lower total consumption of analgesics over 24 hours was found in only one study [35].

Combination of morphine plus bupivacaine vs. saline

All four sensitive studies which compared intra-articular morphine with both saline and bupivacaine also included a group with a combination of intra-articular morphine plus bupivacaine. All the studies which were sensitive to bupivacaine alone and showed a positive effect for morphine also showed a significant effect for the combination compared with placebo, both early and late [28–31]. The two studies which were insensitive for bupivacaine and morphine showed no efficacy for the combination [16, 39].

Dose-response

Two studies addressed the question of a dose response with intra-articular morphine alone [35, 36]. One study [35] could differentiate 1 mg intra-articular morphine, but not 0.5 mg, from control; it could not differentiate 0.5 mg from 1 mg of morphine. The other [36] showed a reversed dose-response between 1 mg and 2 mg. Neither had evidence of internal sensitivity.

Two studies compared different doses of morphine in combination with a standard dose of bupivacaine [37, 38]. No dose-response was detected between either 1 mg and 3 mg or 2 mg and 5 mg morphine.

Adverse effects

No adverse effects that could have been attributed to the intra-articular treatment were reported.

Comment

These reports of intra-articular morphine emphasize the importance of considering potential bias and issues of validity in clinical studies before interpreting results.

Bias

It is now well recognized that studies that are either not randomized or randomized without concealment of treatment allocation, or which are not adequately blinded result in an overestimation of the effect of treatment [42]. Method and concealment of randomization, double-blinding, and description of withdrawals, and drop-outs were inadequately described in all these studies. The method of randomization was explicit in three studies [30, 36, 38]. In many, it was unclear who was blinded.

Design and validity

Classic analgesic trial design includes both active and placebo controls. The reason is to ensure that if no difference is found between test analgesic and placebo, the correct interpretation of a negative result can be made if the standard (active control) analgesic gives a significant difference from placebo. This is particularly important when pain is of only mild to moderate intensity. The mean pain intensities

after placebo were with one exception less than 50% of the maximum possible [30], both early and late, and frequently below 25% of maximum (Fig. 1). If there is no pain, reduction in pain intensity cannot be measured. The reduced sensitivity of analgesic studies with low pain intensity has been evaluated [43].

For this reason we chose a hierarchy of evidence. The highest rank was when active (bupivacaine) control was used as well as placebo, and analgesic efficacy of intra-articular morphine was interpreted only when intra-articular bupivacaine was better than placebo (i.e. established internal sensitivity). Intra-articular bupivacaine is known to provide reliable analgesia of predictable duration following knee surgery [44, 45] and it was therefore a valid active control.

Outcome measures

The special feature of these studies was that necessarily the intervention was made before the patient had pain, analogous to pre-emptive studies [46]. The VAS-PI levels were low for several reasons. Diagnostic arthroscopies were included in the primary studies, and opioids and non-steroidal anti-inflammatory drugs (NSAIDs) were given both pre- and perioperatively. Diagnostic arthroscopies may not cause enough postoperative pain to be sufficiently sensitive for an analgesic assay. Figure 1 indicates that studies that were sensitive generally had VAS-PI levels above 30% of the maximum possible VAS-PI in the control group in the early period (and most had high VAS-PI values in the late period also). We excluded studies that used spinal or epidural anaesthesia or infiltration of the knee joint with high doses of local anaesthetic, because these measures further reduce postoperative pain and hence sensitivity.

VAS-PI was usually measured at rest; sensitivity might have been increased by assessing VAS-PI on movement. Arthroscopic surgery is usually performed as day-case surgery. Sensitivity might have been increased by following the patients in hospital for a longer period. Patients were instructed in the use of VAS-PI before anaesthesia in only a minority of studies. Most patients were sent home with a questionnaire within 2 to 6 hours from the end of surgery. Few studies mentioned that VAS-PI assessment was done by a trained, or even the same, observer. All these issues should be addressed in study design. Sensitivity of the analgesic assay is crucial.

Consumption of supplementary analgesics within the first 24 hours after surgery was the second commonest outcome measure, but usually not standardized. Other indicators of pain and pain relief, such as time to first analgesic, time to weight bearing or time to discharge, were also used, but only in a minority of studies. VAS-PI and the total consumption of supplementary analgesics were therefore used as primary outcome measures in the analysis.

Early and late periods

Analysis by early and late periods was used for several reasons. During the first 2 to 6 hours patients were still in hospital where VAS-PI measurements were made by researchers or (trained) nurses at predetermined intervals. Secondly, the effect of intra-articular bupivacaine, the index of internal trial sensitivity, should have been most pronounced during this time. Thirdly, any systemic effect of morphine should have been obvious during this period rather than later. The late period was considered to be important as several studies suggested a prolonged effect of intra-articular morphine. Most studies provided information on VAS-PI values at 24 hours and consumption of supplementary analgesics was reported as a total amount taken in 24 hours.

No biological reason for suspecting a late rather than an early effect was apparent in the original study on intra-articular morphine [35]. That indicated that 1 mg of intra-articular morphine provided significantly better analgesia after knee surgery than the same dose given intravenously at 3, 4, or 6 hours. No difference was found between the VASPI values at 24 hours, although the total consumption of supplementary analgesics during the 24-hour period was significantly less after intra-articular morphine.

Studies with both active and placebo controls

Only six studies included groups receiving saline, bupivacaine, and morphine. Four of them were sensitive as defined by significant analgesic effect of bupivacaine compared with saline. All four demonstrated significant analgesic effect of intra-articular morphine compared with placebo at both early and late times (Fig. 1). This provides some evidence for a prolonged biological effect of morphine in the knee joint. The two negative studies [16, 39] failed the sensitivity test.

Studies with no active control

Three studies of morphine versus saline showed an analgesic effect, two in the early period and all three in the late period. Comparisons of intra-articular with intravenous or intramuscular morphine were less compelling; only one [35] of the three showed a significant effect, both early and late. These results again provide some evidence for an analgesic effect of morphine in the knee joint, while raising the issue of whether this is a systemic as opposed to a local effect.

Dose-response studies

No dose response was detectable in any study, over a dose range of 0.5–5 mg. The minimum dose tested (0.5 mg) did not show analgesic efficacy [35]. A dose of 1 mg did [28, 30, 35]. No greater effect was found using morphine doses of 2 mg compared with 1 mg [36]. In combination with local anaesthetic, morphine doses of 3 mg compared with 1 mg [37], and 5 mg compared with 2 mg [38] showed no increased efficacy. None of these studies had proven internal sensitivity. Failure to demonstrate dose-response may therefore have been due to lack of sensitivity in the methods.

However, the lowest effective dose used, of 1 mg morphine, would, in a 20 ml injection, be equivalent to a concentration of about 200 μmol/l (50 μg/ml). Typical blood or tissue levels after systemic injections of analgesic doses of morphine are found at concentrations of nmol/l, at least 1000 times lower [47]. The very high concentrations of morphine in the knee joint would be expected to saturate any opioid receptors present. If morphine is acting on local opioid receptors, then the minimal effective dose may well be much less than 1 mg. Failure to demonstrate a dose-response might then be because the doses tested were at the top end of the dose-response curve. Late efficacy might be a consequence of residual high morphine concentrations.

Is intra-articular morphine effective?

Taken together, these results render some support for the hypothesis that intra-articular morphine provides pain relief after knee surgery [2]. Using a simple 'vote-counting' approach on Fig. 1, the points from the majority of the trials fall in the lower right quadrant, indicating greater efficacy with morphine than control. Convincing evidence for an early effect is lacking. There was more consistent evidence for a prolonged analgesic effect, mostly a single estimate of pain intensity at 24 hours or consumption of analgesic. These are weak measures.

The problem is that this evidence rests on four trials that fulfilled the sensitivity requirements but which had only 10 patients per treatment group, and two other trials that were methodologically weak but did distinguish morphine from saline. Against these studies stands the failure to demonstrate a dose-response for intra-articular morphine.

Overall, the evidence is not compelling. The lessons for future studies are obvious, but the current agenda is one of research rather than clinical utility.

References

1. Kalso E, Tramèr M, Carroll D, McQuay H, Moore RA. Pain relief from intra-articular morphine after knee surgery: A qualitative systematic review. *Pain* 1997; **71**:642–51.
2. Stein C. The control of pain in peripheral tissue by opioids. *New England Journal of Medicine* 1995; **332**:1685–90.
3. Beecher HK. The powerful placebo. *Journal of American Medical Association* 1955; **159**:1602–6.
4. Houde R. On appraising pain and analgesic drugs. In: Keele C, Smith R, ed. *The assessment of pain in man and animals.* Edinburgh: Churchill Livingstone, 1962:202–12.
5. Jadad AR, McQuay HJ. A high-yield strategy to identify randomized controlled trials for systematic reviews. *Online Journal of Current Clinical Trials* [serial online] 1993; Doc No 33:3973 words; 39 paragraphs. 5 tables.
6. Khoury GF, Chen ACN, Garland DE, Stein C. Intaarticular morphine, bupivacaine, and morphine/bupivacaine for pain control after knee videoarthroscopy. *Anesthesiology* 1992; **77**:263–6.
7. VanNess SA, Gittins ME. Comparison of intra-articular morphine and bupivacaine following knee arthroscopy. *Orthoptics Review* 1994; **23**:743–7.

8. Ekblom A, Westman L, Söderlund A, Valentin A, Eriksson E. Is intra-articular pethidine an alternative to local anaesthetics in arthroscopy? A double-blind study comparing prilocaine with pethidine. *Knee Surgery, Sports Traumatology Arthroscopy* 1993; 1:189–94.

9. Jadad AR, Moore RA, Carroll D, Jenkinson C, Reynolds DJM, Gavaghan DJ *et al.* Assessing the quality of reports of randomized clinical trials: is blinding necessary? *Controlled Clinical Trials* 1996; 17:1–12.

10. L'Abbé KA, Detsky AS, O'Rourke K. Meta-analysis in clinical research. *Annals of Internal Medicine* 1987; 107:224–33.

11. Dalsgaard J, Felsby S, Juelsgaard P, Frokjaer J. [Analgesic effect of low-dose intra-articular morphine after ambulatory knee arthroscopy] Analgesi af lavdosis intraartikulaer morfin efter ambulant knaeartroskopi. *Ugeskrift for Laeger* 1993; 155:4166–9.

12. Lehrberger K, Stein C, Hassan A, Yassouridis A. Opioids as novel intra-articular agents for analgesia following arthroscopic knee surgery. *Knee Surgery Sports Traumatology Arthroscopy* 1994; 2:174–5.

13. Klinken C. Effects of tourniquet time in knee arthroscopy patients receiving intraarticular morphine combined with bupivacaine. *CRNA* 1995; 6:37–42.

14. Boden BP, Fassler S, Cooper S, Marchetto PA, Moyer RA. Analgesic effect of intraarticular morphine, bupivacaine, and morphine/bupivacaine after arthroscopic knee surgery. *Arthroscopy* 1994; 10:104–7.

15. Joshi GP, McCarroll SM, Brady OH, Hurson BJ, Walsh G. Intra-articular morphine for pain relief after anterior cruciate ligament repair. *British Journal of Anaesthesia* 1993; 70:97–8.

16. Björnsson A, Gupta A, Vegfors M, Lennmarken C, Sjöberg F. Intraarticular morphine for postoperative analgesia following knee arthroscopy. *Regional Anesthesia* 1994; 19:104–8.17. Chan ST. Intra-articular morphine and bupivacaine for pain relief after therapeutic arthroscopic knee surgery. *Singapore Medical Journal* 1995; 36:35–7.

18. De Andrés J, Bellver J, Barrera L, Febre E, Bolinches R. A comparative study of analgesia after knee surgery with intraarticular bupivacaine, intraarticular morphine, and lumbar plexus block. *Anesthesia and Analgesia* 1993; 77:727–30.

19. Ho ST, Wang JJ, Liaw WJ, Wong CS, Cherng CH. Analgesic effect of intra-articular morphine after arthroscopic knee surgery in Chinese patients. *Acta Anaesthesiologica Sinica* 1995; 33:79–84.

20. Niemi L, Pitkänen M, Tuominen M, Björkenheim JM, Rosenberg PH. Intraarticular morphine for pain relief after knee arthroscopy performed under regional anaesthesia. *Acta Anaesthesiologica Scandinavica* 1994; 38:402–5.

21. Raja SN, Dickstein RE, Johnson CA. Comparison of postoperative analgesic effects of intraarticular bupivacaine and morphine following arthroscopic knee surgery. *Anesthesiology* 1992; 77:1143–7.

22. Jaureguito JW, Wilcox JF, Cohn SJ, Thisted RA, Reider B. A comparison of intraarticular morphine and bupivacaine for pain control after outpatient knee arthroscopy. A prospective, randomized, double-blinded study. *American Journal of Sports Medicine* 1995; 23:350–3.

23. Juelsgaard P, Dalsgaard J, Felsby S, Frokjaer J. Analgetisk effekt af to doser intraartikulaer morfin efter ambulant knaeartroskopi. Et randomiseret, prospektivt, dobbeltblindt studie. *Ugeskrift for Laeger* 1993; 155:4169–72.

24. Reuben SS, Connelly NR. Postarthroscopic meniscus repair analgesia with intraarticular ketorolac or morphine. *Anesthesia and Analgesia* 1996; 82:1036–9.

25. Heard SO, Edwards WT, Ferrari D, Hanna D, Wong PD, Liland A *et al.* Analgesic effect of intraarticular bupivacaine or morphine after arthroscopic knee surgery: a randomized, prospective, double-blind study. *Anesthesia and Analgesia* 1992; 74:822–6.

26. Ruwe PA, Klein I, Shields CL. The effect of intraarticular injection of morphine and bupivacaine on postarthroscopic pain control. *American Journal of Sports Medicine* 1995; 23:59–64.

27. McQuay H, Carroll D, Moore A. Variation in the placebo effect in randomised controlled trials of analgesics: All is as blind as it seems. *Pain* 1996; 64:331–335.

28. Haynes TK, Appadurai IR, Power I, Rosen M, Grant A. Intra-articular morphine and bupivacaine analgesia after arthroscopic knee surgery. *Anaesthesia* 1994; 49:54–6.

29. Joshi GP, McCarroll SM, O'Brien TM, Lenane P. Intraarticular analgesia following knee arthroscopy. *Anesthesia and Analgesia* 1993; 76:333–6.

30. Karlsson J, Rydgren B, Eriksson B, Jarvholm U, Lundin O, Sward L *et al.* Postoperative analgesic effects of intra-articular bupivacaine and morphine after arthroscopic cruciate ligament surgery. *Knee Surgery, Sports Traumatology Arthroscopy* 1995; 3:55–9.

31. McSwiney MM, Joshi GP, Kenny P, McCarroll SM. Analgesia following arthroscopic knee surgery. A controlled study of intra-articular morphine, bupivacaine or both combined. *Anaesthesia and Intensive Care* 1993; 21:201–3.

32. Joshi GP, McCarroll SM, Cooney CM, Blunnie WP, O'Brien TM, Lawrence AJ. Intra-articular morphine for pain relief after knee arthroscopy. *Journal of Bone and Joint Surgery [Br.]* 1992; 74:749–51.

33. Dierking GW, Østergaard MD, Dissing CK, Kristensen JE, Dahl JB. Analgesic effect of intra-articular morphine after arthroscopic meniscectomy. *Anaesthesia* 1994; 49:627–9.

34. Hege-Scheuing G, Michaelsen K, Bühler A, Kustermann J, Seeling W. Analgesie durch intraartikuläres Morphin nach Kniegelenks-arthroskopien? *Anaesthesist* 1995; 44:351–8.

35. Stein C, Comisel K, Haimerl E, Yassouridis A, Lehrberger K, Herz A *et al.* Analgesic effect of intraarticular morphine after arthroscopic surgery. *New England Journal of Medicine* 1991; 325:1123–6.

36. Allen GC, St. Amand MA, Lui ACP, Johnson DH, Lindsay MP. Postarthroscopy analgesia with intraarticular bupivacaine/morphine. *Anesthesiology* 1993; 79:475–480.

37. Heine MF, Tillet ED, Tsueda K, Loyd GE, Schroeder JA, Vogel RL *et al.* Intra-articular morphine after arthroscopic knee operation. *British Journal of Anaesthesia* 1994; 73:413–15.

38. Laurent SC, Nolan JP, Pozo JL, Jones CJ. Addition of morphine to intra-articular bupivacaine does not improve analgesia after day-case arthroscopy. *British Journal of Anaesthesia* 1994; 72:170–3.

39. Aasbø V, Raeder JC, Grøgaard B, Røise O. No additional analgesic effect of intra-articular morphine or bupivacaine compared with placebo after elective knee arthroscopy. *Acta Anaesthesiologica Scandinavica* 1996; 40:585–8.

40. Joshi GP, McCarroll SM, McSwiney M, O'Rourke P, Hurson BJ. Effects of intraarticular morphine on analgesic requirements after anterior cruciate ligament repair. *Regional Anesthesia* 1993b; 18:254–7.

41. Lyons B, Lohan D, Flynn CG, Joshi GP, O'Brien TM, McCarroll M. Intra-articular analgesia for arthroscopic meniscectomy. *British Journal of Anaesthesia* 1995; 75:552–5.

42. Schulz KF, Chalmers I, Hayes RJ, Altman DG. Empirical evidence of bias: dimensions of methodological quality associated

with estimates of treatment effects in controlled trials. *Journal of the American Medical Association* 1995; **273**:408–12.

43. Stubhaug A, Grimstad J, Breivik H. Lack of analgesic effect of 50 and 100 mg oral tramadol after orthopaedic surgery: a randomized, double-blind, placebo and 1 standard active drug comparison. *Pain* 1995; **62**:111–18.

44. Chirwa SS, MacLeod BA, Day B. Intraarticular bupivacaine (Marcaine) after arthroscopic meniscectomy: a randomized double blind controlled study. *Arthroscopy* 1989; **5**:33–5.

45. Kaeding CC, Hill JA, Katz J, Benson L. Bupivacaine use after knee arthroscopy: pharmacokinetics and pain control study. *Arthroscopy* 1990; **6**:33–9.

46. McQuay HJ. Pre-emptive analgesia: a systematic review of clinical studies. *Annals of Medicine* 1995; **27**:249–56.

47. Moore RA, Hand CW, McQuay HJ. Opioid metabolism and excretion. In: Budd K, ed. *Update in opioids. Clinical anaesthesiology.* London: Baillière Tindall, 1987:829–58.

18

Analgesic efficacy of peripheral opioids

Summary

Anaesthetists, using basic scientific concepts of peripheral opioid activity, try to improve regional anaesthesia and post-operative analgesia by injecting opioids, with or without local anaesthetic, close to nerve trunks or nerve endings. This systematic review set out to test the evidence that peripherally applied opioids (all except intra-articular) have an analgesic effect outside the knee joint.

A systematic search was carried out for published reports of randomized controlled trials 1966–96 (MEDLINE, EMBASE, Oxford Data Base, reference lists) which compared efficacy of peripheral opioids with placebo, local anaesthetic, or systemic opioids in acute pain. Reports of pethidine or intraarticular opioids were not included. Data on intraoperative efficacy (onset, quality, duration of sensory block), and postoperative efficacy (pain intensity, analgesic consumption) were extracted. Statistical significance as indicated in the original reports and clinical relevance of differences between opioids and controls were taken into account to estimate qualitatively overall efficacy.

Twenty-six trials with data from 952 patients were analysed. Opioids used were morphine (16 trials), fentanyl (8), alfentanil (1), buprenorphine (1), and butorphanol (1). Of four experimental pain trials, two reported a statistically significant difference in favour of the opioid. In 22 clinical trials efficacy of opioid injections into the brachial plexus (10), Bier's block (4), perineural (3), or other sites (5) was tested.

Five of 10 clinical trials measuring intraoperative efficacy reported statistically significant efficacy with opioids compared with control; none of them were judged to be clinically relevant. Five of 17 clinical trials measuring postoperative efficacy reported a significant difference in favour of the opioid; none was judged to be clinical relevant. Trials of lower quality were more likely to report increased efficacy with opioids. Adverse events related to the route of administration were not reported.

These trials provide no evidence for clinically relevant peripheral analgesic efficacy of opioids in acute pain.

Introduction

For over 10 years anaesthetists have been trying to improve efficacy of regional anaesthesia and postoperative analgesia by injecting opioids close to the nerve trunks or the nerve endings. The biological basis for this approach is the presence of opioid receptors and their endogenous ligands in the peripheral nervous system, and their effect on modulation of inflammatory pain [2].

There are several distinct clinical approaches to this topic. First, do opioids when injected in combination with local anaesthetics improve the quality and duration of a sensory block? This could lead to improved surgical conditions. Second, does this method allow the dose of the local anaesthetic to be reduced? This would minimize the risk of systemic toxicity of local anaesthetics. Third, do opioids, when applied alone in peripheral sites, decrease postoperative pain intensity and analgesic requirements? This is a purer test of the biological question of whether opioids have analgesic effects peripherally.

The aim of this systematic review was to test the evidence that peripheral opioids (all except intra-articular) improve the quality of either intraoperative regional anaesthesia or postoperative analgesia.

Methods

Full published reports of randomised controlled trials (RCTs) of peripheral opioids were sought systematically. A number of different search strategies in MEDLINE (1966 to September 1996), EMBASE (1981–96), and the Oxford Pain Relief Database (1950–94) were used, without language restriction. Additional reports were identified from the reference lists of retrieved reports and from review articles. Unpublished reports and abstracts were not considered. Authors were not contacted for original data. Reports were included if they were randomized comparisons of peripheral opioids with either local anaesthetics, placebo (saline), no treatment, or an opioid given by a different route, or comparisons of different doses of peripheral opioids. Reports of analgesic efficacy of intra-articular opioids were not considered because these have already been the subject of a recent systematic review [3].

Inclusion criteria

Each report which could possibly be described as a randomized controlled trial (RCT) was read independently by each of the authors and scored using a three-item, 1–5 score, quality scale [4]. Consensus was then achieved. Reports which were described as randomized were given one point,

The topic discussed in this chapter is also published in full in Picard *et al.* [1].

and a further point if the method of randomization was described and was adequate (such as a table of random numbers). There was a prior agreement that reports without randomization would be excluded. Reports which were described as double-blind were given one point. If blinding was considered to be adequate (double-dummy design, for instance), one additional point was given. Reports which described the numbers of, and reasons for, withdrawals were given a further point. Thus, the maximum score of an included RCT was 5 and the minimum score was 1.

Information about doses and routes of administration of opioids and controls, types of surgery and anaesthesia, number of patients enrolled and analysed, study design, observation periods, outcome measures, and adverse effects was taken from each report.

Validity criteria

Validity criteria for included studies were number of patients per treatment group ≥ 10, any opioid except pethidine, which has shown local anaesthetic properties [5], any peripheral site of injection except intra-articular [3], and standardized methods of measuring sensory block and pain intensity.

Intraoperative efficacy was estimated by comparing onset and quality (loss of pinprick and touch sensation), and duration of a sensory block with opioid compared with control. Post-operative efficacy was estimated by comparing pain intensity, delay until first analgesic, and total analgesic consumption with opioid compared with control. Pain intensity measurement was analysed when reported as visual analogue scale (VAS) or verbal rating scale (VRS).

Data showing any statistically significant difference ($P < 0.05$) between opioid and control, as indicated in the original report, were extracted. Authors then met to achieve consensus (vote-counting procedure) whether such a statistically significant difference was of clinical relevance. Finally, our decision (i.e. our vote counting) on clinical relevance was compared with the original authors' conclusion of efficacy.

Results

Forty-five trials were considered for analysis. Seventeen were subsequently excluded (Table 1). Two further reports were not considered because no copies were available in the United Kingdom [6, 7].

Data from 26 RCTs, published in 25 reports, were analysed. A total of 952 patients, 485 of whom received an opioid, was studied (Table 2).

The average size was 15 patients per group (range 10–32). The median quality score was 2 (range 1–4). Four trials (8%) included a treatment arm with an analgesic method of proven efficacy and, therefore, had an index of internal sensitivity [31, 32 (study I and II), 34]. Eight trials (16%) used a double-dummy design [15, 32, 34, 36, 40, 42, 44].

Efficacy of peripheral opioids was tested in experimental pain trials in healthy volunteers, and in a large variety of surgical settings with intravenous regional anaesthesia (Bier's block), intrapleural, intraperitoneal, incisional, and dental injections, perineural blocks (femoral, ankle block, intercostal), and brachial plexus sheath injections (axillary, supraclavicular, and interscalene approaches). Opioids used were morphine (16 trials), fentanyl (8), alfentanil (1), buprenorphine (1), and butorphanol (1). Intraoperative efficacy assessments were done in 10 clinical trials. Postoperative efficacy was evaluated in 17 clinical trials.

Experimental pain trials ($n = 4$)

In one trial, morphine was applied perineurally [21]; sensory and pain thresholds were significantly increased compared

Table 1 Trials excluded from analysis

Trial	Ref.	Reason for exclusion
Acalovschi & Cristea 1995	[8]	Pethidine
Armstrong *et al.* 1993	[5]	Pethidine
Davidas *et al.* 1992	[9]	Pethidine
El Bakry *et al.* 1989	[10]	Pethidine
Oldroyd *et al.* 1994	[11]	Pethidine
Gobeaux & Landais, 1988	[12]	Pethidine, not random
Arendt-Nielsen *et al.* 1990	[13]	Not random
Kepplinger *et al* 1995	[14]	Not random
Moore *et al.* 1994, study II	[15]	No. of patients/group < 10
Pere 1993	[16]	No. of patients/group < 10
Wajima *et al.* 1995b	[17]	No. of patients/group < 10
Welte *et al.* 1992	[18]	No. of patients/group < 10
Tenant *et al.* 1993	[19]	No. of patients/group < 10
Ben-Ameur *et al.* 1993	[20]	No pain outcomes
Arendt-Nielsen *et al.* 1991, study II	[21]	No opioid evaluated
Bullingham *et al.* 1984	[22]	Not analysable
Mays *et al.* 1987	[23]	Chronic pain

Table 2   Analgesic efficacy of peripheral opioids: analysed randomized controlled trials (RCTs)

Ref.	Treatment & no. of patients	Setting	Efficacy intraoperatively ('anaesthesia')	Efficacy postoperatively ('analgesia')	Adverse effects
Experimental					
[21] study I	1. mo 4 mg (10 ml) (10) 2. saline (10 ml) (10)	Left and right ulnar nerve block. Laser stimulation.	**Pain and sensory thresholds and brain potentials:** mo > saline at 1 15 min only.	NA	None.
[5]	1. prilo 0.5% (40 ml) + fenta 100 μg (2 ml) (15) 2. prilo 0.5% (40 ml) + saline (2 ml) (15)	Bier's block. Needle and temperature stimulation.	**Onset, speed of recovery & quality of sensory block:** Fenta = saline.	NA	**Nausea:** fenta 7, saline 1.
[24]	1. ligno 0.5% 100 mg (40 ml) + 2 ml saline (10) 2. ligno 0.5% 100 mg (40 ml) + fenta 100 μg (2 ml) (10) 3. fenta 100 μg (2 ml) + saline (40 ml) (10)	Bier's block. Needle, temperature. Grip strength.	**Sensory and motor block (quality and onset):** fenta < ligno = ligno + fenta.	NA	**Nausea:** ligno + fenta 2, fenta 1.
[25]	1. mo 2 mg (5 ml) (12) 2. saline (5 ml) (12)	Drugs injected SC in the injury. Burn injury (49°C) on calf bilaterally.	NA	**Heat pain threshold:** mo > saline (T30'–330'). **Pressure pain threshold:** mo > saline at T30'.	**Erythema at the site of injection:** mo 5.
Bier's block					
[26]	1. ligno 100 mg (40 ml) (15) 2. ligno 100 mg + fenta 50 μg (15) 3. ligno 100 mg + pancuronium 0.5 μg (15) 4. ligno 100 mg + fenta 50 μg + pancuronium 0.5 mg (15)	Upper limb surgery.	**VRS:** (4) > (1); (4) > (3) No sig result for (2). **Neuromuscular block:** (3) and (4) > (1) or (2).	NA	None.
[27]	1. prilo 1% (30 ml) + saline (10 ml) (10) 2. prilo 1% (30 ml) + mo 6 mg (10 ml) (10)	Upper limb surgery.	**Onset and recovery of sensory block:** mo > saline.	NA	None.
[28]	1. prilo 0.5% (3 mg/kg) + saline (5 ml) (20) 2. prilo 0.5% (3 mg/kg) + mo 1 mg/5 ml (17)	Upper limb surgery.	NA	**VAS-PI, total analgesic consumption:** mo = saline.	**Mild localized urticaria:** mo 1.
[29]	1. prilo 0.5% (40 ml) + saline (4 ml) (12) 2. prilo 0.5% (40 ml) + fenta 100 μg (4 ml) (13) 3. prilo 0.5% (40 ml) + fenta 200 μg (4 ml) (12)	Minor surgery of upper extremity.	**At T15' loss of pinprick:** fenta 200 > fenta 100 = saline. **Time to develop analgesia:** fenta 200 = fenta 100 = saline.	NA	**Nausea and dizziness:** Saline 1, fenta (100) 7, fenta (200) 6.
Other peripheral sites of injection: all drugs were injected postoperatively					
[30]	1. mo 20 mg intrapleural (20 ml) (14) 2. mo 20 mg IV (ml NA) (14)	Thoracotomy (lobectomy for lung cancer). Mo injected after pleural closure.	NA	**VRS:** intrapleural > IV. **Blood levels:** IV > intrapleural.	**Confusion:** intrapleural 4, IV 4. **Urinary retention:** intrapleural 3, IV 6. **Respiratory depression:** IV 1.
[15] Study I	1. mo 30 ng local (0.3 ml) + oral placebo (10) 2. placebo local (0.3 ml) + mo 50 ng per os (10)	Bilateral 3rd molar surgery. Locally applied morphine.	NA	**VAS-PI, analgesic consumption:** mo = saline.	None.
[31]	1. mo 5 mg (6 ml) incisionally (10) 2. mo 5 mg (1 ml) IV (10) 3. mo 5 mg (6 ml) SC (10) 4. saline (6 ml) incisionally (10)	Inguinal herniotomy. Incisional morphine postop.	NA	**VAS-PI (rest, movement), analgesic consumption:** mo incision = IV = SC = saline.	Not rep.
[32] Study I	1. mo 1 mg intraperitoneal + saline IV (18) 2. saline intraperitoneal + mo 1 mg IV (17) 3. bupi 0.25% intraperitoneal + saline IV (15) (all drugs diluted in 20 ml)	Laparoscopic cholecystectomy. Intraperitoneal injection at the end of surgery. intraperitoneal.	NA	**VAS-PI, VRS, McGill, analgesic consumption:** mo intraperitoneal = mo IV = bupi.	Not rep.
[32] Study II	1. mo 1.5 mg intrapleural + saline IV (20) 2. saline intrapleural + mo 1.5 mg IV (20) 3. bupi 0.25% intrapleural + saline IV (20) (all drugs diluted in 30 ml)	Laparoscopic cholecystectomy. Intrapleural injection at the end surgery.	NA	**VAS-PI, VRS, McGill, analgesic consumption:** mo intrapleural = mo IV < bupi. intrapleural.	Not rep.

Table 2 *continued*

Ref.	Treatment & no. of patients	Setting	Efficacy intraoperatively ('anaesthesia')	Efficacy postoperatively ('analgesia')	Adverse effects
Perineural (drugs were injected pre- or postoperatively)					
[33]	1. mo 0.02% one side + saline other side [10]; 2. mo 0.04% one side + mo 0.02% other side [10] (volume: 15–20 ml per injection)	Ankle nerve block (4 nerves). Bilateral foot minor surgery.	NA	**VAS-PI and pain relief:** mo 0.02% = mo 0.01% = saline.	Not rep.
[34]	1. mo 4 mg epidural (10 ml) + saline femoral (10 ml) [10]; 2. saline epidural (10 ml) + mo 4 mg femoral (10 ml) [10]	Femoral block and epidural catheter after knee surgery. Treatment reversed for the next 24 h	NA	**VAS-PI:** epidural > femoral; **mo consumption:** epidural = femoral.	**Nausea, vomiting:** epidural > femoral.
[35]	1. bupi 0.5% (20 ml) [24]; 2. bupi 0.5% (20 ml) + mo 4 mg (26) (ml NA)	Intercostal block (4 ml per 5 ribs). Biliary surgery.	NA	**VAS-PI, delay for analgesic, analgesic consumption:** bupi + mo = bupi.	None.
Brachial plexus					
[36]	1. ligno 1.5% (0.55 ml/kg) + mo 0.1 mg/kg (ml NA) + saline IV (0.1 ml/kg) [20]; 2. ligno 1.5% (0.55 ml/kg) + mo 0.1 mg/kg IV (ml NA) + saline (0.1 ml/kg) [20]	Hand and forearm surgery. Axillary block.	NA	**VAS, recovery of sensory and motor block:** IV = ax; **Analgesic consumption:** ax > IV	**Mild nausea:** ax 1, IV 2.
[37]	1. ligno 1.5% (38 ml) + fenta 100 μg (2 ml) [26]; 2. ligno 1.5% (38 ml) + saline (2 ml) [25]	Orthopaedic surgery. Axillary block.	**Onset and duration of block:** fenta = saline; **Success rate of each nerve block:** fenta = saline	NA	None.
[38]	1. bupi 0.5% (40 ml) + mo 5 mg (5 ml) [20]; 2. bupi 0.5% (40 ml) + saline (5 ml) [20]	Shoulder surgery. Interscalene block.	NA	**VAS-PI, delay until first and total dose of analgesic:** mo = saline	**Nausea, vomiting:** saline 5, mo 10. **Pruritus:** saline 3, mo 0. **Urine retention:** saline 1, mo 1.
[12]	1. ligno 1.5% (30 ml) [12]; 2. ligno 1.5% (30 ml) + fenta 100 μg (12) (ml NA)	Upper limb surgery. Axillary block.	**Onset and intensity of block:** fenta > no treatment between T5' and T10'.	NA	None.
[39]	1. ligno 1.5% (7 mg/kg) + alfentanil 10 μg/kg (10 ml) [28]; 2. ligno 1.5% (7 mg/kg) + saline (10 ml) [32]	Upper limb surgery. Axillary block.	**Duration of sensory and motor block:** Alfentanil > saline (T0' to T40').	**VAS:** alfentanil > saline (h 3); **Delay for first analgesic, block recovery:** alfentanil = saline	None.
[40]	1. mepi 1.5% (30 ml) + fenta 75 μg + saline IM (1.5 ml) [10]; 2. mepi 1.5% (30 ml) + fenta 75 μg IM (1.5 ml) + saline (1.5 ml) [10]	Upper limb surgery. Supraclavicular block.	**Onset, duration of sensory, & motor block:** ax > IM	**VAS-PI:** ax > IM (0–1 h)	None.
[41]	1. mepi 1% (40 ml); 2. mepi 1% (40 ml) + fenta 100 μg (ml NA); 3. as (1) + fenta 100 μg SC	Upper limb surgery. Axillary block.	**Onset and quality of block:** (1) = (2) = (3)	**Delay until first analgesia:** (1) = (2) = (3)	None.
[42]	1. bupi 0.5% + ligno 1% (40 ml) + mo 5 mg (1 ml) [19]; 2. bupi 0.5% + ligno 1% (40 ml) + mo 5 mg IM (1 ml) [21]	Arm and forearm minor surgery. Axillary block.	**Onset and quality of sensory and motor block:** ax = IM	**VAS-PI, delay until first analgesic:** ax = IM	None.
[43]	1. bupi 0.5% (40 ml) + mo 50 μg/kg [20]; 2. bupi 0.5% (40 ml) + buprenorphine 3 μg/kg [20]	Upper limb surgery. Supraclavicular block.	**Sensory and motor block:** buprenorphine > mo	**Quality, duration of analgesia:** Buprenorphine > mo	**Pruritus:** mo 1. **Nausea, vomiting:** buprenorphine 1.
[17]	1. butorphanol 83 μg/h + saline IV [12]; 2. butorphanol 83 μg/h IV + saline [10] (all perfusion 50 ml/72 h)	Upper extremity surgery. Axillary block (postoperatively continuous infusion).	NA	**VAS-PI at h 9, 12, 18, 20:** ax > IV; **Supplemental analgesia:** IV = ax	**Nausea:** IV 6, ax 4. **Vomiting:** IV 2, ax 2. **Drowsiness:** IV 1, ax 2.

<, less effective ($P < 0.05$); >, more effective ($P < 0.05$); =, no difference; bupi, bupivacaine; fenta, fentanyl; ligno, lignocaine; mepi, mepivacaine; mo, morphine; prilo, prilocaine; SC, subcutaneous; IM, intramuscular; IV, intravenous; NA, not applicable; Tx, x minutes; VAS-PI, visual analogue scale of pain intensity; VRS, verbal rating scale; ax, axillary.

with saline but for no longer than 15 minutes. One trial used morphine subcutaneously at the site of injury and reported higher heat and pain thresholds compared with saline [25]. Two other trials failed to demonstrate any benefit from adding fentanyl to a local anaesthetic in a Bier's block [24, 45].

The experimental nature of these reports makes it difficult to judge clinical relevance. Therefore we did not take them into account in estimating overall efficacy of peripheral opioids.

Bier's block (*n* = 4)

Fentanyl was used in two trials [26, 29]. Abdulla and Fadhil could not demonstrate any significant difference between the combination of fentanyl plus local anaesthetic and local anaesthetic alone [26], but nevertheless concluded that the method was of clinical relevance. We disagreed with the authors because they did not comment on the comparison of interest to us (i.e. opioid vs. no treatment) but rather based their conclusion on the comparison between opioid plus curare vs. no treatment or curare alone.

Pitkanen *et al.* reported a significantly improved quality of the sensory block after 15 minutes with fentanyl 200 μg compared with either saline or fentanyl 100 μg [29]. No measurements were taken after 15 minutes. Nausea and dizziness were more frequent with fentanyl. These authors concluded that their finding was not clinically relevant.

Morphine was used in two trials [27, 28]. In one of them there was no significant difference between morphine and saline, and the authors concluded that morphine was of no value in Bier's block [28]. In the other trial, both onset of and recovery from anaesthesia and analgesia were significantly better with morphine compared with local anaesthetic alone [27]. These authors concluded that the differences of one and two minutes, respectively, were clinically relevant. We disagreed, because the difference between the two groups was of very short duration only, and therefore of no practical importance.

Other peripheral sites (*n* = 5)

All five trials used morphine. Four of them could not demonstrate any difference in the postoperative period between morphine and control when applied into a tooth socket [15], into a surgical wound [31], or by intraperitoneal or intrapleural block [32] (study I and II). The fifth trial reported a statistically significant improvement with morphine 20 mg given intrapleurally compared with the same drug and dose given intravenously [30]; verbal pain rating scores were lower for 20 hours in the intrapleural group. Morphine plasma levels were lower in the intrapleural group. This was considered to be of clinical relevance by these authors. Analgesic consumption was not reported. We considered the outcome to be of little clinical relevance because of the unconventional (high) dose of morphine used.

Perineural (*n* = 3)

None of these trials reported any significant difference between the opioid and control [33–35].

Brachial plexus (*n* = 10)

Opioids were given by interscalene (1 trial), supraclavicular (2) or axillary (7) approaches to the brachial plexus sheath.

In three trials, morphine was combined with a local anaesthetic and applied either by axillary [36, 42] or interscalene route [38]. Comparators were systemic morphine or axillary saline. No intraoperative or postoperative improvement could be demonstrated with peripheral morphine in two of the three trials [38, 42]. The third trial (axillary route) reported similar pain scores in the groups, but a significantly lower postoperative analgesic consumption (number of tablets of oxycodone 5 mg plus acetaminophen 500 mg) with the opioid; the authors concluded that this difference was of clinical importance [36]. The median number of tablets was two with axillary morphine and was four with systemic morphine. We did not consider this difference to be of clinical importance in this acute setting.

Four trials combined fentanyl with a local anaesthetic and compared it with a local anaesthetic alone or with another route of injection [37, 40, 41, 46]. Two of them reported a significant improvement with fentanyl [40, 46]. Gobeaux *et al.* concluded that a faster speed of onset of the sensory block with the opioid was clinically relevant [46]. However, this difference was only five minutes. Kardash *et al.* reported a lower VAS for pain intensity for the first postoperative hour with fentanyl but did not consider this as being clinically important [40].

Alfentanil added to a local anaesthetic led to a significant improvement compared with the local anaesthetic plus placebo [39]; duration of sensory and motor block after surgery was 40 minutes longer with the opioid. This was considered to be clinically relevant by these authors, although there was no difference between the two groups in the delay until the first analgesic rescue medication.

Butorphanol perfusion into the plexus sheath led to significantly lower VAS scores for pain intensity up to the 24th postoperative hour compared with the same butorphanol perfusion given intravenously [44]. There was no difference in postoperative analgesic requirements. The authors concluded that this difference was clinically relevant. However, average VAS scores were very low irrespective of the route of administration (i.e. axillary route 6–7% of the maximum on a VAS pain intensity scale; intravenous route 17–33%).

Buprenorphine 3 μg/kg was compared with morphine 50 μg/kg in one trial; both opioids were added to the same local anaesthetic before supraclavicular injection [43]. A placebo group was lacking in this trial. Duration and quality of postoperative analgesia were significantly better with buprenorphine; 'good' pain relief, as judged by the patients, was 35 hours with buprenorphine and 18 hours with morphine. Authors concluded that buprenorphine is efficacious and long acting as an analgesic when injected into the brachial plexus sheath. However, they did not take into account equianalgesic dosing.

There was a relationship between quality scores of the reports and original authors' conclusions on efficacy of peripheral opioids (Fig. 1). Authors of 10 trials (2 experimental and 8 clinical) reported positive estimates of efficacy. Quality scores of these 10 trials were 2 or below [21, 25–27, 30, 36, 39, 43, 44, 46]. In the 16 remaining trials (2 experimental and 14 clinical) conclusions were negative. Seven of them had a score of 3 or 4 [28, 37, 38, 42, 45] and [32] (study I and II).

Adverse effects

No adverse effects attributable to the route of administration were reported.

Comment

The aim of this systematic review was to test the evidence for an analgesic action of peripheral opioids and the clinical relevance of such action. Twenty-six randomized control trials (RCTs) with data from more than 950 patients were analysed. These trials described a variety of surgical procedures and experimental designs. Five different opioids with several different doses were administered with 10 different regional anaesthetic techniques. Trials were not consistent in either analysing or reporting quality of surgical blocks, postoperative analgesia, or observation periods. Estimation of efficacy based on data of such methodological and clinical heterogeneity was, therefore, difficult. Quantitative analysis was impossible. Unfortunately the different procedures or blocks operate, or may operate, in different ways, so that a negative result from one procedure does not preclude a positive result with another.

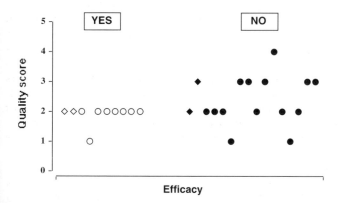

Fig. 1 Efficacy of peripheral opioids. (Relationship between quality of trials and overall estimation of efficacy as stated in the original reports). ○ and ●, clinical trials; ◇ and ◆, experimental pain trials.

We chose to judge the studies in two ways—those that had any result which was statistically in favour of a peripheral action of opioid, and those where the result was of a sufficient magnitude or importance to be clinically relevant. Because most of the studies had a number of different measurements at different times, the possibility that some statistical differences could occur by chance was high. Use of the conventional level of statistical significance in clinical and scientific studies of the 95th centile implies that if 20 different measurements are made, one will show significance just by chance. Thus, in 26 different studies with a large number of outcome measurements, some statistically significant differences with opioid would be expected. Judging clinical relevance may be easier or more difficult. Most practising clinicians would claim they could tell when a result was going to benefit their patients. Codifying what that entails is not easy. In coming to consensus on clinical efficacy of peripheral opioids we were influenced by whether all the measures in a study showed statistically significant differences, or whether the magnitude of any difference shown in a trial was sufficiently large to make change in practice a reasonable consideration. We are conscious that others might come to different conclusions.

Of 26 trials, 14 were unequivocally negative. The other 12 [21, 25, 26, 27, 29, 30, 36, 39, 40, 43, 44, 46] reported at least one statistically significant result in favour of the peripheral opioid. Of these 12 positive trials, 2 were in experimental pain [21, 25]; their results may not be directly applicable to clinical practice. Of the remaining 10 positive trials, authors of 2 [29, 40] did not regard their findings as being clinically relevant. This means that results from only 8 out of the 26 reports (31%) were judged by their original authors to be clinically relevant.

We could not, for different reasons, support the conclusions of any of these positive reports. An isolated significant outcome in favour of the opioid, such as a longer duration of a sensory block which was not correlated with a delay until the patient needed a first analgesic, was not judged clinically relevant by us [39]. Differences of doubtful clinical importance were reported, such as the shortening of the onset of a surgical block by a few minutes [27, 46] or a minimal difference in the average analgesic consumption [36]. A significant difference between two opioids was shown but without a placebo control [43], so that clinical relevance of this greater efficacy of buprenorphine relative to morphine remains questionable. Furthermore, in this trial the two opioids were compared in non-equianalgesic doses, and a systemic analgesic effect of buprenorphine with its long duration of action cannot be ruled out. Other drawbacks in studies with positive findings were the very low pain intensity scores irrespective of the treatment [44], the unconventional dose of opioids used [30], or the comparison of treatment arms which were of no interest to this review [26]. Such trials cannot be regarded as valid assays for evaluation of analgesic efficacy.

Do these trials represent evidence of a lack of efficacy of peripheral opioids, or rather a lack of evidence of their efficacy? In the systematic review of the relevant published literature on the analgesic efficacy of intra-articular morphine, only a minority of the analysed data could be regarded as valid [3]. However, this limited amount of data provided some evidence for the analgesic efficacy of intra-articular morphine [3]. Validity in those trials was assumed when baseline pain was sufficiently high to allow measurement of pain relief, when an index of internal sensitivity was given, and when blinding was adequate [3]. Most of the trials in the present review did not meet these criteria.

As well as the issue of validity, there is the issue of methodological quality. There are other examples where trials with low scores (two or below on a scale of 1–5) on the validated quality scale [4] used in this review, have overestimated the effectiveness of treatment [47]. In the present review none of the 10 trials that claimed efficacy of peripheral opioids had a score above two (Fig. 1). Seven of the 14 unequivocally negative reports had a score of three or four. This means that the trials of highest methodological quality in this data set could not show any difference between peripheral opioid and control.

This subgroup analysis by trial quality emphasizes that in these clinical models peripheral opioids have no efficacy. The question is then why good quality trials showed some efficacy of morphine in the knee joint but no efficacy of different opioids in peripheral sites outside the knee joint. This may be because the knee joint model better reflects the inflammatory process which is thought to be of importance in sensitizing peripheral opioid receptors [48]. It may also be related to inadequately low doses of opioids used in these trials. Doses of morphine between 0.5 mg and 5 mg tested in the confined space of the knee joint produced very high local concentrations [3]. Similar doses of morphine injected into the peritoneal or pleural cavity, or into an isolated limb would produce much lower local concentrations than in the knee joint.

This qualitative analysis of pain trials highlights the importance of critical appraisal of the written literature, and some of the difficulty encountered in doing it. Authors of original reports tended to over-interpret their findings and to confuse statistical significance with clinical relevance. Inattentive or uncritical readers may be misled into a false perception of treatment efficacy. Thirty years ago Schwartz and Lellouch distinguished between explanatory studies, designed to prove a hypothesis, and pragmatic studies, designed to tell us whether instigating a change was of benefit [49]. The distinction is still important, and the clinical use of peripheral opioids requires much more evidence than we have at present.

References

1. Picard PR, Tramèr MR, McQuay HJ, Moore RA. Analgesic efficacy of peripheral opioids (all except intraarticular): A qualitative systematic review of randomised controlled trials. *Pain* 1997; **72**:309–18.
2. Stein C. The control of pain in peripheral tissue by opioids. *New England Journal of Medicine* 1995; **332**:1685–90.
3. Kalso E, Tramer M, Carroll D, McQuay H, Moore RA. Pain relief from intra-articular morphine after knee surgery: A qualitative systematic review. *Pain* 1997; **71**:642–51.
4. Jadad AR, Moore RA, Carroll D, Jenkinson C, Reynolds DJM, Gavaghan DJ et al. Assessing the quality of reports of randomized clinical trials: is blinding necessary? *Controlled Clinical Trials* 1996; **17**:1–12.
5. Armstrong PJ, Morton CPJ, Nimmo AF. Pethidine has a local anaesthetic action on peripheral nerves in vivo. *Anaesthesia* 1993; **48**:382–6.
6. Mocavero G. Analgesia selettiva con morfina perinervosa. *Incontri Di Anestesia Rianimazione e Scienze Affini* 1981; **16**:1–3.
7. Vinoles CM, Cuenca P, Monsegur JC, Valloba FC. Adicion de fentanilo a la mepivacaina en el bloqueo axilar del plexo braquial. *Revista Espanola de Anestesiologica y Reanimacion* 1991; **38**:87–89.
8. Acalovschi I, Cristea T. Intravenous regional anesthesia with meperidine. *Anesthesia and Analgesia* 1995; **81**:539–43.
9. Davidas JL, Blond JL, Rochette A, Manchon M, Degoute CS, Bansillon V. Action analgésique locale par effet directe sur les troncs nerveux de la péthidine. *Thérapie* 1992; **47**:485–7.
10. El Bakry MS, El-Shafei SB, Seyam EM, El-Kobbia NM, Ebrahim UH. Use of pethidine as an intravenous regional anesthetic. *Middle East Journal of Anesthesia* 1989; **10**:189–94.
11. Oldroyd GJ, Tham EJ, Power I. An investigation of the local anaesthetic effects of pethidine in volunteers. *Anaesthesia* 1994; **49**:503–6.
12. Gobeaux D, Landais A. Utilisation de deux morphiniques dans les blocs du plexus brachial. *Cahiers d'Anesthesiologie* 1988; **36**:437–40.
13. Arendt-Nielsen L, Oberg B, Bjerring P. Laser-induced pain for quantitative comparison of intravenous regional anesthesia using saline, morphine, lidocaine, or prilocaine. *Regional Anesthesia* 1990; **15**:186–93.
14. Kepplinger B, Schmid H, Rettensteiner G, Derfler C, Papst H, Erhart H et al. Wirkungsvergleich zwischen intramuskulär und periradikulär verabreichtem Tramadol. *Neuropsychiatrie* 1995; **9**:196–200.
15. Moore UJ, Seymour A, Gilroy J, Rawlins MD. The efficacy of locally applied morphine in post-operative pain after bilateral third molar surgery. *British Journal of Clinical Pharmacology* 1994; **37**:227–30.
16. Pere P. The effect of continuous interscalene brachial plexus block with 0.125% bupivacaine plus fentanyl on diaphragmatic motility and ventilatory function. *Regional Anesthesia* 1993; **18**:93–7.
17. Wajima Z, Shitara T, Nakajima Y, Kim C, Kobayashi N, Kadotani H et al. Comparison of continuous brachial plexus infusion of butorphanol, mepivacaine and mepivacaine-butorphanol mixtures for postoperative analgesia. *British Journal of Anaesthesia* 1995; **75**:548–51.
18. Welte M, Haimerl E, Groh J, Briegel J, Sunder-Plassmann L, Herz A et al. Effect of intrapleural morphine on postoperative pain and pulmonary function after thoracotomy. *British Journal of Anaesthesia* 1992; **69**:637–9.
19. Tenant F, Moll D, De Paulo V. Topical morphine for peripheral pain. *Lancet* 1993; **342**:1047–48.
20. Ben-Ameur M, Ecoffey C, Kuhlman G, Mazoit X, Gobeaux D. Réponse ventilatoire au dioxyde de carbone après bloc axillaire avec fentanyl et lidocaïne. *Annales Françaises d' Anesthesie et de Reanimation* 1993; **12**:22–6.
21. Arendt-Nielsen L, Bjerring P, Berg Dahl J. A quantitative double-blind evaluation of the antinociceptive effects of peri-

neurally administered morphine compared with lidocaine. *Acta Anaesthesiologica Scandinavica* 1991; 35:24–29.

22. Bullingham RE, McQuay HJ, Moore RA. Studies on the peripheral action of opioids in postoperative pain in man. *Acta Anaesthesiologica Belgica* 1984; 35:(suppl.)285–90.

23. Mays KT, Lipman JJ, Schnapp M. Local analgesia without anesthesia using peripheral, perineural morphine injections. *Anesthesia and Analgesia* 1987; 66:417–20.

24. Arthur JM, Heavner JE, Tanmian MB, Rosenberg PH. Fentanyl and lidocaine versus lidocaine for Bier block. *Regional Anesthesia* 1992; 17:223–7.

25. Moniche S, Dahl JB, Kehlet H. Peripheral antinociceptive effects of morphine after burn injury. *Acta Anaesthesiologica Scandinavica* 1993; 37:710–12.

26. Abdulla WY, Fadhil NM. A new approach to intravenous regional anesthesia. *Anesthesia and Analgesia* 1992; 75:597–601.

27. Erciyes N, Akturk G, Solak M, Dohman D. Morphine/prilocaine combination for intravenous regional anesthesia. *Acta Anaesthesiologica Scandinavica* 1995; 39:845–6.

28. Gupta A, Bjornsson A, Sjoberg F, Bengtsson M. Lack of peripheral analgesic effect of low dose morphine during intravenous regional anesthesia. *Regional Anesthesia* 1993; 18:250–3.

29. Pitkanen MT, Rosenberg PH, Pere PJ, Tuominen MK, Seppala TA. Fentanyl-prilocaine mixture for intravenous regional anaesthesia in patients undergoing surgery. *Anaesthesia* 1992; 47:395–8.

30. Aykac B, Erolcay H, Dikmen Y, Oz H, Yillar O. Comparison of intrapleural versus intravenous morphine for post thoracotomy pain management. *Cardiothoracic and Vascular Anesthesia* 1995; 9:538–40.

31. Rosenstock C, Andersen G, Antonsen K, Rasmussen H, Lund C. Analgesic effect of incisional morphine following inguinal herniotomy under spinal anesthesia. *Regional Anesthesia* 1996; 21:93–8.

32. Schulte-Steinberg H, Weninger E, Jokisch D, Hofstetter B, Misera A, Lange V *et al*. Intraperitoneal versus interpleural morphine or bupivacaine for pain after laparoscopic cholecystectomy. *Anesthesiology* 1995; 82:634–40.

33. Bullingham R, O'Sullivan G, McQuay H, Poppleton P, Rolfe M, Evans P *et al*. Perineural injection of morphine fails to relieve postoperative pain in humans. *Anesthesia and Analgesia* 1983; 62:164–7.

34. Dahl JB, Daugaard JJ, Kristoffersen E, Johannsen HV, Dahl JA. Perineuronal morphine: a comparison with epidural morphine. *Anaesthesia* 1988; 43:463–5.

35. Sternlo IE, Hagerdal M. Perineuronal morphine in intercostal block. *Anaesthesia* 1992; 47:613–15.

36. Bourke DL, Furman WR. Improved postoperative analgesia with morphine added to axillary block solution. *Journal of Clinical Anesthesia* 1993; 5:114–17.

37. Fletcher D, Kuhlman G, Samii K. Addition of fentanyl to 1.5% lidocaine does not increase the success of axillary plexus block. *Regional Anesthesia* 1994; 19:183–8.

38. Flory N, Van Gessel E, Donald F, Hoffmeyer P, Gamulin Z. Does the addition of morphine to brachial plexus block improve analgesia after shoulder surgery? *British Journal of Anaesthesia* 1995; 75:23–6.

39. Gormley WP, Murray JM, Fee JPH, Bower S. Effect of the addition of alfentanil to lignocaine during axillary brachial plexus anaesthesia. *British Journal of Anaesthesia* 1996; 76:802–5.

40. Kardash K, Schools A, Concepcion M. Effects of brachial plexus fentanyl on supraclavicular block: a randomized, double-blind study. *Regional Anesthesia* 1995; 20:311–15.

41. Morros Vinoles C, Perez Cuenca MD, Castillo Monsegur J, Cedo Valloba F. Adicion de fentanilo a la mepivacaina en el bloqueo axilar del plexo braquial. *Revista Espanola de Anestesiologica y Reanimacion* 1991; 38:87–9.

42. Racz H, Gunning K, Della Santa D, Forster A. Evaluation of the effect of perineuronal morphine on the quality of postoperative analgesia after axillary plexus block: a randomised double-blind study. *Anesthesia and Analgesia* 1991; 72:769–72.

43. Viel EJ, Eledjam JJ, De La Coussaye JE, D'Athis F. Brachial plexus block with opioids for postoperative pain relief: comparison between buprenorphine and morphine. *Regional Anesthesia* 1989; 14:274–8.

44. Wajima Z, Nakajima Y, Kim C, Kobayashi N, Kadotami H, Adachi H *et al*. I.v. compared with brachial plexus infusion of butorphanol for postoperative analgesia. *British Journal of Anaesthesia* 1995; 74:392–395.

45. Armstrong PJ, Power I, Wildsmith JAW. Addition of fentanyl to prilocaine for intravenous regional anesthesia. *Anaesthesia* 1991; 46:278–80.

46. Gobeaux D, Landais A, Bexon G, Cazaban J, Levron JC. Adjonction de fentanyl à la lidocaïne adrénalinée pour le blocage du plexus brachial. *Cahiers d' Anesthesiologie* 1987; 35:195–9.

47. Khan KS, Daya S, Jadad AR. The importance of quality of primary studies in producing unbiased systematic reviews. *Archives of Internal Medicine* 1996; 156:661–6.

48. Nagasaka H, Awad H, Yaksh T. Peripheral and spinal actions of opioids in the blockade of the autonomic response evoked by compression of the inflamed knee joint. *Anesthesiology* 1996; 85:808–16.

49. Schwartz D, Lellouch J. Explanatory and pragmatic attitudes in therapeutic trials. *Journal of Chronic Disease* 1967; 20:637–48.

19

Pre-emptive analgesia: a systematic review of clinical studies: 1950–94

Summary

Basic science evidence suggests that an analgesic intervention made before surgery will produce a better outcome than the same intervention made after surgery. The evidence from randomized controlled trials (RCTs) which tested this hypothesis in patients is reviewed.

Four studies with paracetamol or non-steroidal anti-inflammatory drugs (NSAIDs) did not show any pre-emptive effect. Of seven studies with local anaesthetic six did not show a pre-emptive effect. In the four studies with opioids there was weak evidence of a pre-emptive effect in three.

There are few perfect RCTs, and unfortunately this rule applies in the pre-emptive analgesia field. Many of the studies which did not show a pre-emptive effect lacked power. The opioid studies which did show a pre-emptive effect had other technical weaknesses.

One way to combat lack of power would be to combine data (meta-analysis). This is very difficult in this field because of the outcome measures which investigators are using.

Introduction

Pre-emptive analgesia is analgesia given before the painful stimulus begins. The reason for giving analgesia before the painful stimulus is to prevent or reduce subsequent pain. The concept that pre-emptive analgesia might provide better pain control came from basic science studies. The initial observations were that noxious stimuli induced changes in neural function [1], such as hyperexcitability, in the spinal cord. Later studies suggested that analgesia given *before* the nociceptive stimulus began was more effective than the same dose given *after* the stimulus.

Professor Wall's editorial focused clinicians' attention on pre-emptive analgesia, and linked fundamental work to clinical studies [2]. He related the findings in fundamental studies, the ways in which the central nervous system changed following nociceptive stimuli and the methods which could preempt these changes, to clinical management of postoperative pain. Since that editorial the issues have become much more focused.

The central question is whether an intervention made before the pain starts has greater analgesic effect than the same intervention (same dose, same route) made after the pain. The aim of this chapter is to define the questions we need to ask, and, by reviewing the clinical evidence systematically, to see whether or not we have definitive answers. This is a very active area of clinical research, so that any conclusions may be overtaken by new evidence.

The concept is a simple one. The effect of the pre-emptive analgesia is to prevent or reduce the development of any 'memory' of the pain stimulus in the nervous system. Preventing or reducing the pain memory should lower any subsequent analgesic needs [3]. The scientific interest in this phenomenon is in the underlying mechanism. The clinical interest is in the potential for improving postoperative pain management.

The concept, and the explanation, are very attractive. Management of postoperative pain has rightly been criticized many times over the last thirty years. Despite the advent of increasingly high-tech approaches it is doubtful that most patients are any better served. If pre-emptive analgesia worked then these patients' pain might be reduced. Unfortunately, there are difficulties with the details, and difficulties in interpreting conflicting evidence from clinical studies.

We have been slow to distinguish that pre-emptive treatment with one kind of analgesic intervention, for instance opioids, may not give the same answer as pre-emptive treatment with another, such as non-steroidal anti-inflammatory drugs (NSAIDs). We have also been slow to distinguish between two very different outcomes, the outcome of a pre-emptive treatment on nociceptive pain and the outcome of a pre-emptive treatment on neuropathic pain.

Problems with the fundamental evidence

Timing is one critical problem. If pre-emptive treatment reduces the memory of the subsequent noxious stimulus how long does this effect last? Evidence of any pre-emptive effect is of great academic interest, but a very short-lived effect, such as less than two hours, might be of little clinical relevance, particularly if the pre-emptive treatment carried any risk of increased morbidity. Conversely, pre-emptive treatments which lasted for 10 hours with minimal increase in morbidity would be of immense clinical importance. Extrapolating from brief effects demonstrated in various animal models to clinical pain is not easy.

A second problem is whether any pre-emptive effect is an effect on acute postoperative pain (nociceptive pain), or on the development of long-term sequelae such as phantom limb pain (neuropathic pain) or on both. Different pre-emptive interventions might be required to tackle these two different problems. Positive or negative evidence of an effect of a particular intervention on nociceptive pain might not apply to neuropathic pain, and vice versa.

One animal model (rat) in which pre-emptive analgesic effects have been shown is the formalin test. Subcutaneous injection of formalin into the paw gives rise to two 'peaks' of nociceptive input. Interventions may be made at various times relative to the injection of formalin, and the relative efficacy of the same intervention made before the formalin injection may be compared with the same injection made after the formalin injection. With **opioids** intrathecal injection of DAMGO *before* the formalin produced 70% greater inhibition of the C-fibre response than the same dose injected intrathecally *after* the formalin [4, 5]. With peripheral infiltrations of **local anaesthetic**, one *before* and one *after* the formalin injection, the behavioural response to the formalin was abolished [6]. Infiltration with local anaesthetic 25 min *after* the formalin made the hindpaw anaesthetic but did not abolish the behavioural response. Intrathecal injection of local anaesthetic *before* the formalin abolished the behavioural response; the same intrathecal dose 5 min *after* the formalin had no effect [6]. **NSAIDs** injected systemically or intrathecally *before* the formalin injection produce a reduction in the behavioural response [6, 7]; it is not clear whether the same dose of NSAIDs given *after* the formalin is less effective.

The 'end' of the second peak of the formalin model occurs within an hour. This is very brief when compared with clinical pain. In another animal model, however, the development of autotomy after peripheral nerve section, longer term 'preemptive' effects have been reported with the use of **local anaesthetic**. The speed with which autotomy developed in response to nerve section, and the severity of the autotomy, was altered by applying local anaesthetic to the nerve fibre before the operation [8]. Pre-emptive use of local anaesthetic delayed the onset of autotomy (42 days vs. 23 days) and reduced its severity (15% vs. 41%). Similarly, 50 μg of intrathecal morphine reduced autotomy following unilateral sciatic nerve section [9]. These studies are perhaps more analogous to chronic rather than acute pain. The effect of such nerve injury is believed to be analogous to neuropathic as opposed to nociceptive pain.

From basic science then comes the idea that the same dose of an analgesic given by the same route may be more effective if given *before* surgery compared with *after*. Neither of these models operates on a time scale which is a totally convincing analogy of the clinical operative and postoperative states. The formalin model is perhaps too brief and the autotomy model too long. The formalin model involves inflammatory change, the autotomy model nerve damage. Clinical procedures may involve both inflammatory response and nerve damage. Could pre-emptive analgesia alter outcome in all pain contexts, or is it limited, operating for example in somatic but not visceral pain, and are the underlying mechanisms the same? Clinical demonstration of pre-emptive analgesia might fail if the wrong setting was chosen. The secondary issue is which is the pertinent outcome? For clinical postoperative pain the outcome is measured over hours to days. The prevention of chronic pain development requires outcome measurement over weeks, months, and perhaps years.

Clinical evidence

The aim is to provide a systematic review of the evidence that an intervention given before the pain starts has greater effect than the same intervention (same dose, same route) given after the pain. This review is done separately for each of three classes of intervention, NSAIDs, local anaesthetics, and opioids.

The inclusion criterion for the review was randomized controlled trials (RCTs) which addressed the question of pre-emptive versus the same treatment given after the pain had begun (Fig. 1). Randomized studies reduce the chance of selection bias; studies which are not randomized have no such protection. Ideally, the studies should be double-blind, and double-dummy if different routes are to be compared in the treatment and control groups. Studies were excluded from the review if they were not RCTs and if they were RCTs which did not compare pre-emptive with post-treatment (Fig. 1).

Studies were identified by a MEDLINE search and by a manual search. The MEDLINE search (Silver Platter MEDLINE version 3.0 and 3.1) was done for 1966 to May 1993. The strategy was designed to identify the maximum number of randomized and/or double-blind reports by using a combination of text words, 'wild cards', and MeSH terms as described previously [10]. Medical journals were manually searched. They were selected from a list of the 50 journals with the highest number of reports in MEDLINE, and 9 specialist journals which were not included in that list or which were not indexed. The search process included volumes published between 1950 and 1994. The studies included (and excluded) are shown in Table 1.

Excluded studies

Comparisons of pre-emptive treatment with no treatment (± not RCT)

Several of the excluded papers (Table 1) are often quoted as showing evidence of a pre-emptive effect. They were, however, designed to show that an analgesic intervention

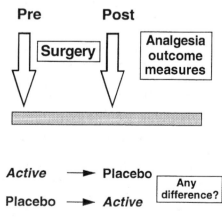

Fig. 1   Design required to show pre-emptive effect.

Table 1 References for studies excluded or included from review

NSAID	Local anaesthetic	Opioid

Excluded studies

Pre-emptive treatment with no postop comparison ± not RCT

[27]	[28]	[29]
[30]	[31]	[32]
[33]	[34]	
[35]	[36]	
	[37]	

RCT but pre-emptive treatment + postop treatment compared with postop only

[38]
[39]
[40]

Included studies

[11]	[12]	[13]
[14]	[15]	[16]
[17]	[18]	[19]
[20]	[21]	[22]
	[23]	
	[24]	
	[25]	

NSAID + local anaesthetic + opioid [26]

made before surgery was more effective than no intervention at all, and did not ask whether an analgesic intervention made *before* surgery is more, less or as effective than the same intervention made *after* surgery. Nonetheless, reviewers have reached the conclusion that these studies produce evidence of a pre-emptive effect. Although a positive result in such studies suggests a worthwhile clinical benefit it is not evidence for or against a pre-emptive effect. Such evidence requires the control of the same intervention made after surgery (Fig. 1).

Comparisons of pre-emptive treatment with pre-emptive plus post-treatment

These studies (all were NSAID studies) were designed to compare NSAIDs given before surgery with the same NSAID given both before and after surgery. It is not possible from these studies to answer the question of whether an analgesic intervention made *before* surgery is more, less, or as effective than the same intervention made *after* surgery.

Included studies

NSAIDs and paracetamol

Three RCTs with NSAIDs and one with paracetamol met the inclusion criterion. All were in oral surgery patients. Flath *et al.* [11] studied four groups of 30 patients each having endodontic surgery (Table 2). One of these four groups had preoperative flurbiprofen and postoperative placebo. A second group had preoperative placebo and postoperative flurbiprofen. The preoperative dose was given 30 minutes before surgery and the postoperative dose 3 hours after surgery. On the outcome measures of categorical pain intensity (cat PI) and visual analogue pain intensity (VAS-PI) there was no evidence of a pre-emptive effect. The study had adequate sensitivity to detect a difference because one of the groups had preoperative and postoperative placebo, and the pain scores in that group were significantly higher than those in the groups who had flurbiprofen.

Sisk *et al.* [14] compared diflunisal 1 g with placebo in 20 patients having third molar extraction (Table 2). The design was cross-over, as shown in Fig. 1. Over eight hours there was no significant difference between preoperative and postoperative dosing, using catPI and VAS-PI scales. Sisk and Grover [17] used a similar design to investigate naproxen 550 mg in third molar extraction (Table 2). Again, there was no significant difference between preoperative and postoperative dosing, using catPI and VAS-PI scales.

Table 2 NSAID and paracetamol studies reviewed

Study	Design	No. of patients	Procedure	Treatment	Outcome measures	Timing (pre)	Timing (post)	Outcome (pre vs. post)
[11]	Parallel	120	Endodontic	Flurbiprofen 100 mg vs. placebo	catPI & VAS-PI	15 min preop	3 h postop	NSD
[14]	Cross-over	20	Third molar	Diflunisal 1 g vs. placebo	catPI & VAS-PI	30 min preop	30 min postop	NSD
[17]	Cross-over	36	Third molar	Naproxen 550 mg vs. placebo	catPI & VAS-PI	30 min preop	30 min postop	NSD
[20]	Cross-over	50	Third molar	Paracetamol 1 g vs. placebo	VAS-PI & TFA	45 min preop	35 min postop	NSD

NSD, no significant difference; catPI, categorical pain intensity scale; TFA, time to first analgesic; VAS-PI, visual analogue pain intensity scale.

Gustafsson *et al.* [20] also used a two occasion cross-over design in third molar extraction, comparing paracetamol 1 g with placebo (Table 2). Using a VAS-PI scale and time to first analgesic as outcome measures there was no significant difference between preoperative and postoperative dosing.

These four studies provide a consistent answer to the question. No measurable difference was found between the same dose given preoperatively and postoperatively. All four studies necessarily used local anaesthetic; none used opioids. The balance of the evidence is therefore that at normal therapeutic oral doses of NSAID no pre-emptive effect was demonstrable.

Local anaesthetic

Studies of pre-emptive effect with local anaesthetics may be divided into trials of epidural (spinal), nerve block, and infiltration (Table 3).

Epidural

Dahl *et al.* [12] used a parallel group design on 32 colonic surgery patients (Table 3). Epidural bolus and infusion of a local anaesthetic and opioid combination was given 40

minutes before surgery for the preoperative group, and after surgery for the postoperative group (some 2 hours after the preoperative). There was no dummy injection. On cat PI and VA-SPI scales there was no evidence of a pre-emptive effect.

Pryle *et al.* [15] used a similar design in 36 abdominal hysterectomy patients (Table 3). Local anaesthetic with adrenaline was given as a lumbar epidural bolus either 40 minutes before incision or after surgery (75 minutes after the preoperative group). On the outcome measures of cat PI and VAS-PI scales, time to first use of intravenous morphine via patient-controlled analgesia (PCA) and amount of intravenous morphine via PCA, there was no demonstrable pre-emptive effect.

Rice *et al.* [21] compared caudal blocks pre-and post-surgery (Table 3) in 40 children having outpatient surgery (mean operation time 30 minutes). An objective pain score did not show any pre-emptive effect. Gunter *et al.* [23] used a similar design in 24 boys having hypospadias repair (Table 3). The caudal block before surgery did reduce operating time and blood loss significantly compared with the same block after surgery, but there was no significant difference on the pain outcomes of time to first analgesic (TFA) or on overall analgesic consumption.

Table 3 Local anaesthetic studies reviewed

Study	Design	No. of patients	Procedure	Treatment	Outcome measures	Timing (pre)	Timing (post)	Outcome (pre vs. post)
Epidural								
[12]	Parallel	32	Major colonic surgery	Epidural (T9–T12) Bupivacaine & morphine	VAS-PI & catPI at rest, cough & sitting up	Bolus + infusion 40 min preop	Bolus + infusion after surgery (still asleep)	NSD
[15]	Parallel	36	Abdominal hysterectomy	Epidural (lumbar) bupivacaine + adrenaline	VAS-PI, catPI, PCA IV morphine	40 min pre incision	After surgery (still asleep)	NSD
[21]	Parallel	40	Hernia, orchidopexy	Caudal bupivacaine	Paediatric objective score, TFA	After induction	After surgery	NSD
[23]	Parallel	24	Distal hypospadias	Caudal bupivacaine	TFA analgesic needs	After induction	After surgery	NSD
Nerve block								
[18]	Parallel	32	Herniorrhaphy	Inguinal field block lignocaine	VAS-PI & catPI at rest, cough & moving	15 min preop	After closure	NSD
Infiltration								
[24]	Parallel	37	Herniorrhaphy	Infiltration lignocaine	TFA, analgesic needs	5 min pre incision (19)	Before closure (18)	Significantly delayed remed time in pre gp
[25]	Parallel	90	Appendicectomy (29 controls with no infiltration)	Infiltration lignocaine	VAS-PI lying & sitting, PCA	3 min pre incision (29)	At closure (32)	NSD on VAS-PI or on PCA

NSD, no significant difference; catPI, categorical pain intensity scale; IV, intravenous; PCA, patient-controlled analgesia; TFA, time to first analgesic; VAS-PI, visual analogue pain intensity scale; gp, group.

Nerve block

Dierking *et al.* [18] compared inguinal field block preoperatively and postoperatively in 32 patients having herniorrhaphy (Table 3). Using categorical and VAS-PI scales there was no evidence of a pre-emptive effect.

Infiltration

Ejlersen *et al.* [24] investigated preoperative and postoperative wound infiltration in 37 herniorrhaphy patients (Table 3). Using time to remedication as the outcome measure the patients who had the infiltration 5 minutes before incision had significantly longer time until remedication, clear evidence of a pre-emptive effect.

Turner and Chalkiadis [25] compared infiltration after induction (29 patients) with infiltration after surgery (32 patients) and with no infiltration (29 patients) in appendicectomy (Table 3). The outcome measures were VAS-PI scores and PCA consumption. They found no significant difference between the groups.

The study which did show a pre-emptive effect is the least subject to criticism [24], but it is still balanced by six negative studies, one of which is an infiltration study of similar design. The two paediatric studies [21, 23] both had the problem of pain scoring in children, but both showed no pre-emptive effect. Importantly, neither study involved the use of opioid, and both studies therefore sought, and did not find, a pre-emptive effect of local anaesthetic alone. It is difficult to understand why one infiltration study should have produced a positive result [24] when the other did not [25].

In all the negative studies the local anaesthetic intervention worked well, whether given before or after surgery. The power of these studies (is the lack of difference a true result?), becomes a major issue. We also do not know whether these studies were sufficiently sensitive to measure an effect if there was one. The one study which did use a no treatment control [25] did not measure any significant difference between infiltration (pre or post) and no infiltration. We now have a set of negative studies, without internal sensitivity checks, none of which is of adequate size to be totally convincing.

Opioids

Four opioid studies (Table 4) conform to the design required to answer the pre-emptive question. Katz *et al.* [13] looked at spinal opioid, while Richmond *et al.* [16], Amanor-Boadu *et al.* [19] and Wilson *et al.* [22] investigated the intravenous route.

Katz *et al.* [13] randomized 30 thoracic patients to lumbar epidural fentanyl infusion, either preoperatively or intraoperatively (Table 4). The infusion in the post-incision group was started 15 minutes after incision. Using a VAS-PI scale and PCA intravenous morphine as outcome measures they found significantly lower VAS-PI scores at 6 hours in the preoperative group (with no significant difference in the PCA

Table 4 Opioid studies reviewed

Study	Design	No. of patients	Procedure	Treatment	Outcome measures	Timing (pre)	Timing (post)	Outcome (pre vs. post)
Epidural								
[13]	Parallel	30	Thoracotomy	Lumber epidural fentanyl	VAS-PI & PCA IV morphine	30 min infusion started 55 min pre incision	30 min infusion started 15 min after incision	SD (VAS-PI lower at 6 h and PCA morphine lower 12–24 h in pre gp
Intravenous								
[16]	Parallel	76	Total abdominal hysterectomy	10 mg IV or IM morphine	VAS-PI & PCA IV morphine	IM premed (16) or IV at induction (23)	IV at closure (21)	SD (PCA morphine lower to 24 h in IV pre gp at equivalent VAS-PI)
[19]	Parallel	41	Body surface	5 mg IV morphine	VAS-PI & catPI at TFA	At induction (21)	At closure (20)	SD (catPI lower at TFA in pre gp)
[22]	Parallel	40	Total abdominal hysterectomy	40 μg/kg IV alfentanil	VAS-PI & PCA IV morphine	IV at induction (20)	IV 1 min after incision (20)	SD (VAS-PI rest) higher in pre-emptive gp at same PCA

SD, significant difference; catPI, categorical pain intensity scale; IM, intramuscular; IV, intravenous; PCA, patient-controlled analgesia; TFA, time to first analgesic; VAS-PI, visual analogue pain intensity scale; gp, group. Numbers in parenthesis are the number of patients.

morphine consumption). From 12 to 24 hours they found significantly lower PCA morphine consumption in the preoperative group with no significant difference in the VAS-PI score.

Richmond *et al.* [16] randomized 76 total abdominal hysterectomy patients to 10 mg intramuscular morphine as pre-medication, 10 mg intravenous morphine at induction, or 10 mg intravenous morphine at closure (Table 4). Analgesic outcome measures were VAS-PI scores and PCA intravenous morphine consumption. They found significantly lower PCA intravenous morphine consumption in the group who had received intravenous morphine at induction compared with the group who received the same dose by the same route at closure.

Amanor-Boadu *et al.* [19] in a similar design looked at the effect of 5 mg of intravenous morphine given at induction or at closure to 41 body surface surgery patients (Table 4). Outcome measures were the time to first analgesic and the VAS-PI and catPI scores at that time. CatPI scores were significantly lower at the time of remedication in the group given morphine at induction compared with the group given morphine at closure.

Wilson *et al.* [22] randomized 40 total abdominal hysterectomy patients to 40 μg/kg intravenous alfentanil at induction or after skin incision (Table 4). Analgesic outcome measures were VAS-PI scores and PCA intravenous morphine consumption. They found no significant difference in PCA morphine consumption but significantly higher pain scores at rest in the pre-emptive group.

Three studies suggest that opioids may have a pre-emptive effect. Unfortunately, none of the studies is perfect. In the epidural study there was a significant pre-emptive effect at only one of the six VAS-PI scale measurement points. In the 10 mg intravenous study the PCA morphine consumption was reversed in the subsequent 24 hours [16]. In the 5 mg intravenous study only one of the two outcomes showed a significant effect. These three studies showing a weak positive pre-emptive effect with opioid are balanced by a negative [22]. The negative study is difficult to interpret because difference in pain score at the same PCA consumption may mean a failure of study sensitivity.

Using pre-emptive NSAIDs, local anaesthetic, and opioids together

Kavanagh *et al.* [26] compared a premedication of intramuscular morphine (0.15 mg/kg), perphenazine (0.03 mg/kg), and rectal indomethacin (100 mg) coupled with intercostal local anaesthetic with intramuscular midazolam premedication (0.05 mg/kg) and saline intercostal blocks. Thirty thoracotomy patients were randomized to pre-emptive or control, and were compared using VAS-PI and PCA morphine consumption. There were no significant differences on VAS-PI. PCA consumption was significantly lower at 6 hours in the pre-emptive group, there was no significant difference at 12 hours, and at 24 and 48 hours the pre-emptive group morphine consumption was significantly greater than control. This study did not compare the same intervention made before and after, but is included because it is the clearest example of an RCT using multiple (three drug classes) interventions to demonstrate a pre-emptive effect.

Comment

The evidence for pre-emptive effects should be answered separately for each of the three drug classes reviewed, because the answers may be different. For NSAIDs and paracetamol there are four good studies, all with no evidence of a pre-emptive effect. If there is a pre-emptive effect of NSAID it is unlikely to be seen with conventional dosing. For local anaesthetics one infiltration study showed a pre-emptive effect, another of similar design did not. Five other studies, spinal and nerve block, did not show any effect. These negative local anaesthetic studies have been criticized [41] because they were 'contaminated' by opioid, but in two of the studies [21, 23] patients received no opioid. Perhaps a stronger criticism of these negative studies is that they lacked power.

The evidence with opioids is inconclusive. The evidence from fundamental studies for a pre-emptive effect of opioid [4, 9] is stronger than the equivalents for local anaesthetic and NSAID. Inevitably, we now need studies of adequate design and size to establish whether or not there is indeed a measurable pre-emptive effect of opioid in man. If the intravenous route can be used to answer the question studies are easier to do than if the effect was only found with spinal routes. The caveat must be that the dose used in the (intrathecal) basic studies was large (up to 50 μg), and that the effect was demonstrated via the intrathecal route. This makes the human findings with relatively small intravenous doses all the more remarkable. Evidence of a pre-emptive effect with opioid would offer great potential benefit to patients with postoperative pain. It would also be important to know if such a pre-emptive effect applied to neuropathic pain [9, 36].

One important methodological issue is that increasingly investigators are using two postoperative outcomes, a VAS-PI scale and PCA consumption. The assumption is made that patients will use PCA to achieve similar levels of VAS-PI. If the VAS-PI values for pre-emptive and control are not significantly different, but the PCA consumption does show a significant difference, that is a valid result. The corollary is not valid. There may also be advantage (at least to the systematic reviewer) to using pain relief rather than pain intensity outcomes. Combining data across studies is much more valid for pain relief than pain intensity [42]. Ideally, such combination would increase power and help to answer the clinical pre-emptive question.

One final point which we keep forgetting is that acute tolerance is well known with opioids. Two of the pre-emptive studies [16, 26] showed that pre-emptive treatment led to significant increase in postoperative analgesic consumption. It may be that any pre-emptive effect of opioids would be counteracted by induction of acute tolerance. This, however, does not gel with the basic science demonstration of a pre-emptive opioid effect.

References

1. Woolf CJ. Evidence for a central component of post-injury pain hypersensitivity. *Nature* 1983; 306:686–8.

2. Wall PD. The prevention of postoperative pain. *Pain* 1988; 33:289–90.

3. McQuay HJ, Dickenson AH. Implications of nervous system plasticity for pain management. *Anaesthesia* 1990; 45:101–12.

4. Dickenson AH, Sullivan AF. Subcutaneous formalin-induced activity of dorsal horn neurones in the rat: differential response to an intrathecal opioid administered pre or post formalin. *Pain* 1987; 30:349–60.

5. Dickenson AH. Recent advances in the physiology and pharmacology of pain: plasticity and its implications for clinical analgesia. *Journal of Psychopharmacology* 1991; 5:342–51.

6. Coderre TJ, Vaccarino AL, Melzack R. Central nervous system plasticity in the tonic pain response to subcutaneous formalin injection. *Brain Research* 1990; 535:155–8.

7. Malmberg AB, Yaksh TL. Hyperalgesia mediated by spinal glutamate of substance P receptor blocked by spinal cyclooxygenase inhibition. *Science* 1992; 257:1276–9.

8. Selzer Z, Beilin BZ, Ginzburg R, Paran Y, Shimko T. The role of injury discharge in the induction of neuropathic pain behavior in rats. *Pain* 1991; 46:327–36.

9. Puke MJC, Wiesenfeld-Hallin Z. The differential effects of morphine and the alpha2-adrenoreceptor agonists clonidine and dexmedetomidine on the prevention and treatment of experimental neuropathic pain. *Anesthesia and Analgesia* 1993; 77:104–9.

10. Jadad AR, McQuay HJ. A high-yield strategy to identify randomized controlled trials for systematic reviews. *Online Journal of Current Clinical Trials* [serial online] 1993; Doc No 33:3973 words; 39 paragraphs. 5 tables.

11. Flath RK, Hicks ML, Dionne RA, Pelleu GB. Pain suppression after pulpectomy with preoperative flurbiprofen. *Journal of Endodontics* 1987; 13:339–47.

12. Dahl JB, Hansen BL, Hjortsø NC, Erichsen CJ, Møiniche S, Kehlet H. Influence of timing on the effect of continuous extradural analgesia with bupivacaine and morphine after major abdominal surgery. *British Journal of Anaesthesia* 1992; 69:4–12.

13. Katz J, Kavanagh BP, Sandler AN, Nierenberg H, Boylan JF, Friedlander M *et al.* Preemptive Analgesia-Clinical Evidence of Neuroplasticity Contributing to Postoperative Pain. *Anesthesiology* 1992; 77:439–46.

14. Sisk AL, Mosley RO, Martin RP. Comparison of preoperative and postoperative diflunisal for suppression of postoperative pain. *Journal of Oral and Maxillofacial Surgery* 1989; 47:464–8.

15. Pryle BJ, Vanner RG, Enriquez N, Reynolds F. Can preemptive lumbar epidural blockade reduce postoperative pain following lower abdominal surgery? *Anaesthesia* 1993; 48:120–3.

16. Richmond CE, Bromley LM, Woolf CJ. Preoperative morphine pre-empts postoperative pain. *Lancet* 1993; 342:73–5.

17. Sisk AL, Grover BJ. A comparison of preoperative and postoperative naproxen sodium for suppression of postoperative pain. *Journal of Oral and Maxillofacial Surgery* 1990; 48:674–8.

18. Dierking GW, Dahl JB, Kanstrup J, Dahl A, Kehlet H. Effect of pre vs postoperative inguinal field block on postoperative pain after herniorrhaphy. *British Journal of Anaesthesia* 1992; 68:344–8.

19. Amanor-Boadu SD, Jadad AR, Glynn CJ, Jack TM, McQuay HJ. Influence of pre and postoperative morphine administration on pain after body surface surgery: a double-blind randomised controlled study. *Proceedings of 7th World Congress on Pain.* 1993; 538–9.

20. Gustafsson I, Nystrom E, Quiding H. Effect of preoperative paracetamol on pain after oral surgery. *European Journal of Clinical Pharmacology* 1983; 24:63–5.

21. Rice LJ, Pudimat MA, Hannalah RS. Timing of caudal block placement in relation to surgery does not affect duration of postoperative analgesia in paediatric ambulatory patients. *Canadian Journal of Anaesthesia* 1990; 37:429–31.

22. Wilson RJT, Leith S, Jackson IJB, Hunter D. Pre-emptive analgesia from intravenous administration of opioids. *Anaesthesia* 1994; 49:591–3.

23. Gunter JB, Forestner JE, Manley CB. Caudal epidural anesthesia reduces blood loss during hypospadias repair. *Journal of Urology* 1990; 144:517–19.

24. Ejlersen E, Andersen HB, Eliasen K, Mogensen T. A comparison between preincisional and postincisional lidocaine infiltration and postoperative pain. *Anesthesia and Analgesia* 1992; 74:495–8.

25. Turner GA, Chalkiadis G. Comparison of preoperative with postoperative lignocaine infiltration on postoperative analgesia requirements. *British Journal of Anaesthesia* 1994; 72:541–3.

26. Kavanagh BP, Katz J, Sandler AN, Nierenberg H, Roger S, Boylan JF *et al.* Multimodal analgesia before thoracic surgery does not reduce postoperative pain. *British Journal of Anaesthesia* 1994; 73:184–9.

27. Hutchison GL, Crofts SL, Gray IG. Preoperative piroxicam for postoperative analgesia in dental surgery. *British Journal of Anaesthesia* 1990; 65:500–3.

28. Tverskoy M, Cozacov C, Ayache M, Bradley EL, Kissin I. Postoperative pain after inguinal herniorrhaphy with different types of anesthesia. *Anesthesia and Analgesia* 1990; 70:29–35.

29. McQuay HJ, Carroll D, Moore RA. Postoperative orthopaedic pain—the effect of opioid premedication and local anaesthetic blocks. *Pain* 1988; 33:291–5.

30. McGlew IC, Angliss DB, Gee GJ, Rutherford A, Wood AT. A comparison of rectal indomethacin with placebo for pain relief following spinal surgery. *Anaesthesia and Intensive Care* 1991; 19:40–5.

31. Jebeles JA, Reilly JS, Gutierrez JF, Bradley EL, Kissin I. The effect of pre-incisional infiltration of tonsils with bupivacaine on the pain following tonsillectomy under general anesthesia. *Pain* 1991; 47:305–8.

32. Koskinen R, Tigerstedt I, Tammisto T. The effect of peroperative alfentanil on the need for immediate postoperative pain relief. *Acta Anaesthesiologica Scandinavica* 1991; 35 (suppl. 96):021.

33. Smith AC, Brook IM. Inhibition of tissue prostaglandin synthesis during third molar surgery: use of preoperative fenbufen. *British Journal of Oral and Maxillofacial Surgery* 1990; 44:251–3.

34. Bugedo GJ, Cárcamo CR, Mertens RA, Dagnino JA, Muñoz HR. Preoperative percutaneous ilioinguinal and iliohypogastric nerve block with 0.5% bupivacaine for post-herniorrhaphy pain management in adults. *Regional Anesthesia* 1990; 15:130–3.

35. Campbell WI, Kendrick R, Patterson C. Intravenous diclofenac sodium. Does its administration before operation suppress postoperative pain? *Anaesthesia* 1990; 45:763–6.

36. Bach S, Noreng MF, Tjellden NU. Phantom limb pain in amputees during the first 12 months following limb amputation, after preoperative lumbar epidural blockade. *Pain* 1988; 33:297–301.

37. Narchi P, Benhamou D, Fernandez H. Intraperitoneal local anaesthetics for shoulder pain after day-case laparoscopy. *Lancet* 1991; **338:**291–5.

38. Hill CM, Carroll MJ, Giles AD, Pickvance N. Ibuprofen given pre and post operatively for the relief of pain. *International Journal of Oral Maxillofacial Surgery* 1987; **16:**420–4.

39. Dupuis R, Lemay H, Bushnelle MC, Duncan GH. Preoperative flurbiprofen in oral surgery: a method of choice in controlling postoperative pain. *Pharmacotherapy* 1988; **8:**193–200.

40. Murphy DF, Medley C. Preoperative indomethacin for pain relief after thoracotomy: comparison with postoperative indomethacin. *British Journal of Anaesthesia* 1993; **70:**298–300.

41. Katz J. Preop analgesia for acute pain. *Lancet* 1993; **342:**65–6.

42. Jadad-Bechara AR. *Meta-analysis of randomized clinical trials in pain relief.* D. Phil thesis Oxford University, 1994.

20
Transcutaneous electrical nerve stimulation (TENS) in acute postoperative pain

Summary

We set out to examine the evidence for the importance of randomization of transcutaneous electrical nerve stimulation (TENS) in acute postoperative pain. Controlled trials were sought; randomization and analgesic and adverse effect outcomes summarized. Forty-six reports were identified by searching strategies. Seventeen reports with 786 patients could be regarded unequivocally as randomized controlled trials (RCTs) in acute postoperative pain. No meta-analysis was possible. In 15 of 17 RCTs we judged there to be no benefit of TENS over placebo. Of the 29 excluded trials 19 had pain outcomes but were not RCTs; in 17 of these 19 TENS their authors concluded that TENS had a positive analgesic effect. No adverse effects were reported. Non-randomized trials overestimate treatment effects.

Introduction

Transcutaneous electrical nerve stimulation (TENS) was originally developed as a way of controlling pain through the 'gate' theory [2]. There is conflicting professional opinion about the use of TENS in acute postoperative pain. The recommendations of the Agency for Health Care Policy and Research [3] for acute pain management state that TENS is 'effective in reducing pain and improving physical function' while the earlier report of the UK College of Anaesthetists' working party on pain after surgery [4] says that 'TENS is not effective as the sole treatment of moderate or severe pain after surgery'. For postoperative pain some textbooks recommend or strongly recommend TENS [5–9], although one at least is uncertain [10]. TENS is of doubtful benefit in labour pain [11], but we could find no systematic review of its use in chronic pain.

Quality of methods used in clinical trials has been shown to be a key determinant of the eventual results. Schulz and colleagues [12] have demonstrated that trials that are not randomised or which are inadequately randomized exaggerate the estimate of treatment effect by up to 40%. Studies which are not fully blinded can exaggerate the estimate of treatment effect by up to 17%. We sought evidence of the effect of randomization in trials with pain as an outcome in studies of TENS in acute postoperative pain.

Methods

A number of different search strategies were used to identify controlled trials for TENS in acute postoperative pain in both MEDLINE (1966–95: Knowledge Server version 3.25: January 1996) and the Oxford Pain Relief Database (1950–92) [13]. The words 'TENS' and 'transcutaneous electrical nerve stimulation' were used in searching, including combinations of these words. Additional reports were identified from the reference lists of retrieved reports, review articles, and text-books.

Inclusion criteria were full journal publication, TENS, and postoperative pain with pain outcomes. Reports of TENS for the relief of other acute pain conditions, such as labour pain, acute infections, and procedures, or those where the number of patients per treatment group was fewer than 10 were excluded. Abstracts and review articles were not considered. Unpublished reports were not sought. Neither authors of reports nor manufacturers of TENS equipment were contacted.

Two types of control predominated—open studies compared TENS with conventional postoperative analgesia (intramuscular opioid), or with disabled TENS instruments (sham TENS). Some studies used blinded observers. While there was no prior hypothesis that TENS could not be blinded adequately, it was determined that, despite the considerable efforts documented in some reports, adequate blinding was impossible in practice.

Each report which could possibly meet the inclusion criteria was read by each author independently and scored for inclusion and quality using a three-item scale [14]. Included reports had one point for randomization, a further point if this had been done correctly, and a third point if the number and reasons for withdrawals were given. Authors met to agree that studies were randomized, or whether the description of the method of randomization was adequate [12].

Information about the surgery, number of patients, study design, and duration of treatment was extracted from randomized reports. The type of TENS equipment, its settings, and the method and frequency of its use and placement of electrodes was also extracted. Control group design and the use of TENS in these controls was similarly noted. Pain outcomes, overall findings, and conclusions were noted for each report, together with any adverse effect information.

The topic discussed in this chapter is also published in full in Carroll *et al.* [1].

A judgement was then made by us as to whether the overall conclusion of randomized reports was positive or negative for the analgesic effectiveness of TENS. *Post-hoc* subgroup analysis in the original reports was not considered in our judgement of overall effectiveness. Reports that had pain measures but which were not randomized or were inadequately randomized were examined for positive or negative analgesic effectiveness of TENS using the judgement of their authors.

	Analgesic result	
	Positive	**Negative**
Randomized	2	15
Inadequate or not randomized	17	2

Fig. 1   TENS in postoperative pain.

Results

Forty-six reports were considered. Three did not have pain outcomes, three had numbers per group of fewer than 10 patients, three had methodological problems and one reported on pain during rather than after a procedure. These were not considered further.

Nineteen were either not RCTs or the method of randomization was inappropriate (Table 1). Seventeen of the 19 reports with pain measures excluded because they were either not randomized or inadequately randomized were judged by their authors to have positive analgesic results for TENS in acute postoperative pain.

Seventeen randomized studies with pain outcomes were found. Of these, 15 were judged by us to show no analgesic benefit of TENS in acute postoperative pain (Fig. 1).

Randomized studies

The randomized studies had information from 786 patients (Table 2). TENS was used after various operative procedures including cardiothoracic, major orthopaedic, and gastro-intestinal surgery. Ten different TENS machines were used with different control settings and durations of treatment; individual titration of settings took place in six reports. Fourteen reports compared TENS with sham TENS without batteries, with batteries reversed or with sub-threshold stimulation; the other three compared TENS plus intramuscular opioid with intramuscular opioid alone. Quality scores were generally 1 or 2 out of a maximum of 3. The most common outcome measures reported were analgesic consumption and a variety of pain score measurements. Information was not presented in formats that allowed extraction for meta-analysis (Table 2).

TENS vs. sham TENS

Fourteen of the 17 included RCTs compared TENS with sham TENS. Not one found any difference. One of the 14 [49] reported no significant difference between TENS and sham TENS for analgesic consumption, but did report a statistically significant difference for pain intensity in favour of the active TENS; the published results, however, used a one-tailed statistical test which we judged inappropriate.

Table 1   Non-randomized reports

Ref.	Pain condition or type of surgery	Description	Judgement of analgesic effectiveness
[15]	Upper abdominal	Not RCT	Positive
[16]	Cholecystectomy, hernia repair	Retrospective study not RCT	Positive
[17]	Upper abdominal	Inadequate randomization	Positive
[18]	Foot	Not RCT: matched case control	Positive
[19]	Caesarean section	Not RCT	Positive
[20]	General	Not RCT	Positive
[21]	Spinal fusion	Not RCT	Positive
[22]	Foot	Retrospective, not RCT	Positive
[23]	Urological	Not RCT	Positive
[24]	Urological	Not RCT	Positive
[25]	Urological	Not RCT	Positive
[26]	Abdominal, thoracic	Not RCT	Positive
[27]	Cholecystectomy	Not RCT	Negative
[28]	Thoracotomy	Inadequate randomization method	Positive
[29]	Laparotomy	Retrospective, not RCT	Positive
[30]	Low back	Not RCT	Positive
[31]	Lumbar, hip, gynaecological	Retrospective, not RCT	Positive
[32]	Knee and hip joint	Not RCT	Positive
[33]	Gastric bypass	Not RCT	Negative

Table 2 Randomized reports

Ref.	Type of surgery	Study design & duration of treatment	No. of patients	TENS details	TENS control setting	TENS control	Pain outcomes	Results for pain outcomes	Judgement	Quality score
[34]	Appendicectomy	Parallel group: TENS (15); sham TENS (13); standard postop Analgesia (14); 48 h.	42	Dow–Corning–Wright, single channel, electrodes (either side of wound).	Fixed-rate (tingling sensation preop).	Sham TENS (not turned on).	VAS-PI at 48 h, analgesic consumption (24 & 48 h).	NSD sham & active TENS for pain & drug consumption; sig & diff for pain intensity control vs. TENS & sham TENS ($P < 0.01$).	Negative.	1
[35]	Abdominal	Parallel group: sham TENS (53); TENS (53); 72 h.	106	Codman, dual channel, 2 electrodes (either side of wound).	Fixed-rate (tingling sensation preop) rectangular wave form, pulse width (170 ms), pulse rate 80/s, output 15 milliamp.	Sham TENS (batteries reversed).	VAS-PI: average pain twice daily, morphine consumption.	NSD between TENS & sham TENS.	Negative.	2
[36]	Caesarean section	Parallel group (female); GA + TENS (10); Epidural + TENS (11); GA + sham TENS (8); Epidural + sham TENS (6); 24 h.	35	Stim-tec EPC Mini, Model 6011, dual channel (1 channel only used), 2 electrodes (either end of wound).	Amplitude individually titrated, wave fixed (during surgery).	Sham TENS (no batteries).	VAS-PI: hourly, time to first analgesic, analgesic consumption.	No overall diff in analgesic consumption or pain.	Negative.	2
[37]	Coronary artery bypass	Parallel group (males); TENS (15); sham TENS (15); postop analgesia (15); 72 h.	45	Nuwave, Staodyn. 1 pair electrodes (T1–T5). 1 pair (either side of wound).	Individually titrated (tingling sensation).	Sham TENS (no current).	Pain (0–10) on cough & rest, narcotic consumption.	NSD TENS vs. sham TENS.	Negative.	2
[38]	Cholecystectomy	Parallel group: TENS (14); remote TENS (12); postop analgesia (14); 48 h.	40	3M Tenzcare, dual channel, site of electrodes not described.	Individually titrated.	Sham TENS (remote non-segmental).	VAS-PI, catPI (4-pt) at 24 & 48 h, analgesic consumption.	NSD TENS vs. sham TENS for pain or analgesic consumption. Pain but not analgesic consumption significantly worse in control group ($P < 0.05$) immediately after surgery.	Negative.	1
[39]	Herniorrhaphy	Parallel group (males); TENS (20); sham TENS (20); 72 h.	40	Dow–Corning–Wright–Care dual channel, 2 electrodes (either side of wound).	Individually titrated: pulse duration 180 μs, frequency 70 Hz amplitude 7.5.	Sham TENS (no current).	VAS-PI twice daily, analgesic consumption.	NSD TENS vs. sham TENS.	Negative.	1
[40]	Abdominal	Parallel group: TENS (15); sham TENS (15); 48 h.	34	Neuromed 3722, 2 electrodes (either side of wound).	Individually titrated (tingling sensation).	Sham TENS (batteries reversed).	VAS-PI (2, 4, 6, 24, 48 h), analgesic consumption.	NSD TENS vs. sham TENS.	Negative.	2
[41]	Laminectomy	Parallel group: TENS (10); sham TENS (10); 24 h.	20	Dow–Corning–Wright–Care dual channel, 4 electrodes (at each end & on either side of wound).	Individually titrated, 180 μs pulse width, frequency 70 Hz.	Sham TENS (no current).	PCA morphine consumption 24 h.	NSD TENS vs. sham TENS.	Negative.	2
[42]	Cardiac	Parallel group: TENS (14); sham TENS (17); 72 h.	31	3M Tenzcare Model 6240, dual channel, 2 pairs electrodes (either side of the wound & mid-thoracic region).	Individually titrated: pulse rate 5, width control 3, amplitude.	Sham TENS (no batteries).	5-pt catPI, analgesic consumption.	NSD TENS & sham TENS.	Negative.	2
[43]	Total hip replacement	Parallel group: TENS (20); opiate control (20); 24 h.	40	EPC TimeTech clinical stimulator, dual channel, 2 pairs electrodes (1 pr paravertebrally (L2-S2), between trochanter and coccyx, 1 pr above iliac crest, head of fibula).	Individually titrated, continual stimulation.		Global assessment, analgesic consumption.	Sig less pethidine consumed in TENS group on day 1 ($P < 0.001$).	Positive.	1

Table 2 *continued*

Ref.	Type of surgery	Study design & duration of treatment	No. of patients	TENS details	TENS control setting	TENS control	Pain outcomes	Results for pain outcomes	Judgement	Quality score
[27]	Cholecystectomy	Parallel group: TENS (30); opiate control (34).	64	EPC, electrodes placed within 2 cm of the wound.	Pulse rate 50/s, pulse width 170 ms amplitude 0–50 Å.		Daily dose of pethidine for 3 postop days	NSD	Negative.	1
[44]	Inguinal hernia repair	Parallel group (males); TENS (34); sham TENS (28); 48 h.	62	3M Tenzcare dual channel, 2 pairs of electrodes (over first lumbar vertebrae & on either side of wound).	Individually titrated (tingling sensation), 70 Hz rectangular pulse, amplitude.	Sham TENS (controls turned off).	VAS-PI 6, 12, 24, 36, 48 h, opiate consumption.	NSD TENS vs. sham TENS.	Negative.	2
[45]	Thoracotomy	Parallel group: TENS + IM omnopon (20); IM omnopon (20); 48 h.	40	Dow-Corning-Wright-Care 2 channel, 2 electrodes (either side of incision).	Individually titrated, fixed pulse rate 70/s, rectangular wave form, pulse width 180 μs.		5-pt PI 6, 24, 48 h analgesic consumption, time to oral analgesics, length of hospital stay.	NSD TENS vs. sham TENS.	Negative.	1
[46]	Abdominal	Parallel group: TENS (30); sham TENS (22); IM narcotics (25); 72 h	77	MedGen, electrode placement not described.	Fixed-pulse width 80 ms, frequency 40 Hz, amplitude individually titrated.	Sham TENS (no current)	Daily 10-pt PI.	NSD TENS vs. sham TENS, or control.	Negative.	1
[47]	Abdominal & thoracic	Parallel group: TENS (61); sham TENS (39); 24 h post surgery until discharge, TDS × 20 min.	100	Neuromed Model 3700, Meditronic, electrode site individually chosen.	Frequency 100 – 150/s, output 20–35, pulse duration 250–400 ms.	Sham TENS (no batteries).	Pain, analgesic consumption, duration of relief.	Sig diff reported. 2/39 partial relief or complete relief sham TENS vs. 34/61 with active TENS. Analgesic consumption not rep.	Positive.	1
[48]	Total knee replacement	Phase 2: parallel group: TENS (18); sham TENS (18); postop analgesia (12); 72 h.	48	Strodynamics, continuous. No other information given; electrode placement not described.	Amplitude setting individually titrated, pulse duration 100 μs at 70/s.	Sham TENS (sub-threshold stimulation).	Analgesic consumption, hospital stay.	NSD TENS vs. sham TENS or control.	Negative.	1
[49]	Thoracotomy	Parallel group: TENS (12); sham TENS (12); 48 h.	24	3M Tenzcare 6240, 2 electrodes placed on either side of incision.	Continuous stimulation, amplitude 7, pulse rate 3, pulse width 5.	Sham TENS (no current).	Pain intensity 0–10, analgesic consumption.	NSD TENS vs. sham TENS. Positive result reported was with one-tailed test of statistical sig.	Negative.	2

catPI, categorical pain intensity; IM, intramuscular; NSD, no significant difference; PCA, patient-controlled analgesia; PI, pain intensity; VAS-PI, visual analogue scale of pain intensity.

TENS vs. opioid control

Seven of the 17 included RCTs compared opioid plus TENS with opioid alone, four of which also included sham TENS. Of the seven studies, five failed to detect any differences in analgesic consumption or pain measurements between TENS and non-TENS controls. Two reports were judged by their authors and by us to be positive [43, 47].

Pike [43] studied 40 patients after total hip replacement. The study had as its main outcome measure the number of pethidine (meperidine) injections in the first two postoperative days and a retrospective global rating. Patients with active TENS had significantly fewer pethidine injections on the first postoperative day as well as higher scores on global rating of treatment. VanderArk and McGrath [47] recruited 100 patients having abdominal and thoracic surgery in two months, and although there was more success with active TENS used for 20 minutes three times a day, maximal relief was 'almost invariably associated with the first stimulation'. Generally, there were no obvious differences between the use of TENS in these two positive studies and the 15 which showed no benefit.

Adverse events

No report described systematic recording of adverse events, nor were any reported.

Discussion

The gold standard in clinical trials is adequate randomization [12]. Non-randomized studies have for nearly 20 years been shown to yield larger estimates of treatment effects than studies using random allocation [50]. The degree of the exaggeration of treatment effect when randomization is inappropriate can be as much as 40% [12]. These findings underpin the inclusion criteria chosen in systematic reviews.

For TENS in acute postoperative pain, 17 of 19 reports with pain outcomes that were either not randomized or inappropriately randomized claimed TENS to be effective, compared with two of 17 randomized controlled trials (Fig. 1).

The possibility of bias exists. The method of randomization was described in only two reports [17, 28]. The method described was inadequate in both, one using a nurse to randomize patients [17] and the other using alternate allocation [28]. Reports which said only that they were randomized may have used an inadequate method.

That these data represent the lowest common denominator of information, essentially vote counting rather than a more sophisticated analysis, reflects the nature of the analgesic scoring methods that predominated in the original reports. Pain scoring using analogue or categorical scales was reported as means (an unreliable statistic [51]), or mean analgesic consumption or time to first analgesic was used. None of these allowed data extraction for further statistical analysis or comparison between reports. Although more rigorous pain scoring might have been used, there is no evidence that all of the reports suffered a systematic failure in analgesic measurement.

Inadequacy of blinding in clinical trials of analgesic interventions continues to be of concern [52], although this may be less of an issue with pharmacological interventions [51]. Blinding of procedures is much more difficult than blinding of drug studies. Most of the TENS studies did make attempts at blinding, for instance, by removing batteries from the TENS apparatus (sham TENS) or by using staff with no knowledge of the study or allocation to conduct the patient assessments. Lack of blinding has been estimated to exaggerate the estimate of treatment effect of trials by some 17% [12]. Adequate blinding of TENS for both carers and patients is particularly difficult [53]. None of the reports was judged to have been blinded, and this lowered the quality scores given to the seventeen randomized studies. The fact that only two of the reports showed any positive effect of TENS in acute postoperative pain is all the more striking because of this potential overestimation of treatment effect due to lack of blinding.

The clear message of the reports considered in this systematic review is that adequate randomization is an important quality standard in studies with pain outcomes. Including non-randomized studies in reviews may give the wrong answer. The AHCPR guideline on acute pain management included non-randomized reports, and this may explain their more positive attitude towards TENS [3].

References

1. Carroll D, Tramer M, McQuay H, Nye B, Moore A. Randomization is important in studies with pain outcomes: Systematic review of transcutaneous electrical nerve stimulation in acute postoperative pain. *British Journal of Anaesthesia* 1996; **77**:798–803.
2. Melzack R, Wall PD. Pain mechanisms: a new theory. *Science* 1965; **150**:971–8.
3. Acute Pain Management Guideline Panel. *Acute pain management: operative or medical procedures and trauma.* Clinical Practice Guideline No. 1. Agency for Health Care Policy and Research, U.S. Department of Health and Human Services. AHCPR Publication No. 92–0032. Rockville, MD: Public Health Service, 1992:24–5.
4. Royal College of Surgeons of England, the College of Anaesthetists. *Report of the working party on pain after surgery.* London: Royal College of Surgeons, 1990.
5. Charman RA. Physiotherapy for the relief of pain. In: Carroll D, Bowsher D, ed. *Pain management and nursing care.* Oxford: Butterworth-Heinemann, 1993:146–65.
6. Woolf CJ, Thomson JW. Stimulation-induced analgesia: transcutaneous electrical nerve stimulation (TENS) and vibration. In: Wall PD, Melzack R, ed. *Textbook of pain*, (3rd edn). Edinburgh: Churchill Livingstone, 1994:1191–1217.
7. McCaffery M, Beebe A. *Pain: a clinical manual for nursing practice.* St. Louis, MO: C.V. Mosby, 1989.
8. Chaney ES. The management of postoperative pain. In: Wells P, Frampton V, Bowsher D, ed. *Pain: management and control in physiotherapy.* Oxford: Heinemann, 1988:253–68.
9. Park G, Fulton B. *The management of acute pain.* Oxford University Press, 1991.
10. Justins DM, Richardson PH. Clinical management of acute pain. *British Medical Bulletin* 1991; **47**:561–83.

11. Carroll D, Tramer M, McQuay H, Nye B, Moore A. Transcutaneous electrical nerve stimulation in labour pain: A systematic review. *British Journal of Obstetrics and Gynaecology* 1997; **104**:169–75.

12. Schulz KF, Chalmers I, Hayes RJ, Altman DG. Empirical evidence of bias: dimensions of methodological quality associated with estimates of treatment effects in controlled trials. *Journal of the American Medical Association* 1995; **273**: 408–12.

13. Jadad AR, McQuay HJ. A high-yield strategy to identify randomized controlled trials for systematic reviews. *Online Journal of Current Clinical Trials* [serial online] 1993; Doc No 33:3973 words; 39 paragraphs. 5 tables.

14. Jadad AR, Moore RA, Carroll D, Jenkinson C, Reynolds DJM, Gavaghan DJ *et al.* Assessing the quality of reports of randomized clinical trials: is blinding necessary? *Controlled Clinical Trials* 1996; **17**:1–12.

15. Ali J, Yaffe CS, Serrette C. The effect of transcutaneous electric nerve stimulation on postoperative pain and pulmonary function. *Surgery* 1981; **89**:507–12.

16. Bussey JG, Jackson A. TENS for postsurgical analgesia. *Contemporary Surgery* 1981; **18**:35–41.

17. Cooperman AM, Hall B, Mikalacki K, Hardy R, Sadar E. Use of transcutaneous electrical stimulation in the control of postoperative pain. *American Journal of Surgery* 1977; **133**:185–7.

18. Cornell PE, Lopez AL, Malofsky H. Pain reduction with transcutaneous electrical nerve stimulation after foot surgery. *Journal of Foot Surgery* 1984; **23**:326–33.

19. Hollinger JL. Transcutaneous electrical nerve stimulation after cesarean birth. *Physical Therapy* 1986; **66**:36–8.

20. Hymes AC, Raab DE, Yonehiro EG, Nelson GD, Printy AL. Electrical surface stimulation for control of acute postoperative pain and prevention of ileus. *Surgical Forum* 1974; **24**:447–9.

21. Issenman J, Nolan MF, Rowley J, Hobby R. Transcutaneous electrical nerve stimulation for pain control after spinal fusion with Harrington rods. *Physical Therapy* 1985; **65**:1517–20.

22. Lanham RH, Powell S, Hendrix BE. Efficacy of hypothermia and transcutaneous electrical nerve stimulation in podiatric surgery. *Journal of Foot Surgery* 1984; **23**:152–8.

23. Merrill DC. Electroanalgesia in urologic surgery. *Urology* 1987; **29**:494–7.

24. Merrill DC. FasTENS—a disposable transcutaneous electrical nerve stimulator designed specifically for use in postoperative patients. *Urology* 1988; **31**:78–9.

25. Merrill DC. Clinical evaluation of FasTENS, an inexpensive, disposable transcutaneous electrical nerve stimulator designed specifically for postoperative electroanalgesia. *Urology* 1989; **33**:27–30.

26. Neary JM. Transcutaneous electrical nerve stimulation for the relief of post-incisional surgical pain. *American Association Nursing Journal* 1981; **49**:151–5.

27. Reuss R, Cronen P, Abplanalp L. Transcutaneous electrical nerve stimulation for pain control after cholecystectomy: lack of expected benefits. *Southern Medical Journal* 1988; **81**: 1361–3.

28. Rooney SM, Jain S, Goldiner PL. Effect of transcutaneous nerve stimulation on postoperative pain after thoracotomy. *Anesthesia and Analgesia* 1983; **62**:1010–12.

29. Schomberg FL, Carter-Baker SA. Transcutaneous electrical nerve stimulation for postlaparotomy pain. *Physical Therapy* 1983; **63**:188–93.

30. Schuster GD, Infante MC. Pain relief after low back surgery: the efficacy of transcutaneous electrical nerve stimulation. *Pain* 1980; **8**:299–302.

31. Solomon R, Viernstein MC, Long D. Reduction in postoperative pain and narcotic use with transcutaneous electrical nerve stimulation. *Surgery* 1980; **87**:142–6.

32. Stabile ML, Mallory TH. The management of postoperative pain in total joint replacement. *Orthopaedic Review* 1978; **7**:121–3.

33. Strayhorn G. Transcutaneous electrical nerve stimulation and postoperative use of narcotic analgesics. *Journal of the National Medical Association* 1983; **75**:811–16.

34. Conn IG, Marshall AH, Yadav SN, Daly JC, Jaffer M. Transcutaneous electrical nerve stimulation following appendicectomy: the placebo effect. *Annual Review of Royal College of Surgeons, England* 1986; **68**:191–2.

35. Cuschieri RJ, Morran CG, McArdle CS. Transcutaneous electrical stimulation for postoperative pain. *Annual Review of Royal College of Surgeons, England* 1985; **67**:127–9.

36. Davies JR. Ineffective transcutaneous nerve stimulation following epidural anaesthesia. *Anaesthesia* 1982; **37**:453–7.

37. Forster EL, Kramer JF, Lucy SD, Scudds RA, Novick RJ. Effect of TENS on pain, medications, and pulmonary function following coronary artery bypass graft surgery. *Chest* 1994; **106**:1343–8.

38. Galloway DJ, Boyle P, Burns HJ, Davidson PM, George WD. A clinical assessment of electroanalgesia following abdominal operations. *Surgery, Gynecology and Obstetrics* 1984; **159**:453–6.

39. Gilbert JM, Gledhill T, Law N, George C. Controlled trial of transcutaneous electrical nerve stimulation (TENS) for postoperative pain relief following inguinal herniorrhaphy. *British Journal of Surgery* 1986; **73**:749–51.

40. Lim AT, Edis G, Kranz H, Mendelson G, Selwood T, Scott DF. Postoperative pain control: contribution of psychological factors and transcutaneous electrical stimulation. *Pain* 1983; **17**:179–88.

41. McCallum MI, Glynn CJ, Moore RA, Lammer P, Phillips AM. Transcutaneous electrical nerve stimulation in the management of acute postoperative pain. *British Journal of Anaesthesia* 1988; **61**:308–12.

42. Navarathnam RG, Wang IY, Thomas D, Klineberg PL. Evaluation of the transcutaneous electrical nerve stimulator for postoperative analgesia following cardiac surgery. *Anaesthesia and Intensive Care* 1984; **12**:345–50.

43. Pike PM. Transcutaneous electrical stimulation. Its use in the management of postoperative pain. *Anaesthesia* 1978; **33**:165–71.

44. Smedley F, Taube M, Wastell C. Transcutaneous electrical nerve stimulation for pain relief following inguinal hernia repair: a controlled trial. *European Surgery Research* 1988; **20**:233–7.

45. Stubbing JF, Jellicoe JA. Transcutaneous electrical nerve stimulation after thoracotomy. Pain relief and peak expiratory flow rate a trial of transcutaneous electrical nerve stimulation. *Anaesthesia* 1988; **43**:296–8.

46. Taylor AG, West BA, Simon B, Skelton J, Rowlingson JC. How effective is TENS for acute pain? *American Journal of Nursing* 1983; **83**:1171–4.

47. VanderArk GD, McGrath KA. Transcutaneous electrical stimulation in treatment of postoperative pain. *American Journal of Surgery* 1975; **130**:130–8.

48. Walker RH, Morris BA, Angulo DL, Schneider J, Colwell CWJ. Postoperative use of continuous passive motion, transcutaneous electrical nerve stimulation, and continuous cooling pad following total knee arthroplasty. *Journal of Arthroplasty* 1991; **6**:151–6.

49. Warfield CA, Stein JM, Frank HA. The effect of transcutaneous electrical nerve stimulation on pain after thoracotomy. *Annals of Thoracic Surgery* 1985; **39**:462–5.

50. Chalmers TC, Matta RJ, Smith JJ, Kunzler AM. Evidence favoring the use of anticoagulants in the hospital phase of acute myocardial infarction. *New England Journal of Medicine* 1977; 297:1091–6.

51. McQuay H, Carroll D, Moore A. Variation in the placebo effect in randomised controlled trials of analgesics: All is as blind as it seems. *Pain* 1996; 64:331–5.

52. Wall PD. The placebo effect: an unpopular topic. *Pain* 1992; 51:1–3.

53. Deyo RA, Walsh NE, Schoenfeld LS, Ramamurthy S. Can trials of physical treatments be blinded? The example of transcutaneous electrical nerve stimulation for chronic pain. *American Journal of Physical Medicine and Rehabilitation* 1990; 69:6–10.

Transcutaneous electrical nerve stimulation (TENS) in labour pain

Summary

Transcutaneous electrical nerve stimulation (TENS) is used widely for relief of pain in labour. Two previous systematic reviews have questioned the effectiveness of TENS in this context. Reports were sought by searching MEDLINE, EMBASE, CINAHL, and the Oxford Pain Relief Database. Outcomes included pain and adverse effect measures.

There were 10 randomized controlled trials, involving 877 women: 436 received active TENS and 441 acted as controls (sham TENS, or no treatment). There were no significant differences reported for prospective primary pain outcomes in any of the 10 studies. Three studies reported significant differences between active and sham TENS for secondary pain outcomes. The use of additional analgesic interventions was not different with active or sham TENS (relative risk 0.88; 0.72 to 1.07).

The findings of this review suggest that TENS has no significant effect on pain in labour. Women should be offered more effective interventions for the relief of pain in labour.

Methods

Randomized controlled trials (RCTs) of TENS in labour pain were sought. A number of different search strategies were used to identify eligible reports in both MEDLINE (1966–97), EMBASE (1980–97), CINAHL (1982–97), the Cochrane Library (issue 2, 1997), and the Oxford Pain Relief Database (1950–5) [2]. The date of last search was April 1997. The words: 'TENS', 'transcutaneous electrical nerve stimulation', 'labour', and 'childbirth' were used in searching, including combinations of these words, and without language restriction. Additional reports were identified from the reference lists of retrieved reports, review articles [3], and text-books. Manufacturers of TENS equipment were not contacted. Abstracts and review articles were not considered. Unpublished reports were not sought.

Inclusion criteria were full journal publication, TENS, labour pain with pain outcomes, and randomized treatment allocation. Reports of TENS for the relief of other pain conditions or those where the number of patients per treatment group were fewer than 10 were excluded [4].

Each report which could possibly meet the inclusion criteria was read by each author independently and scored for inclusion and quality using a three-item scale [5] which examined randomization, blinding, and withdrawal, and drop-outs. An included report could have a maximum score of 5 and a minimum of 1. Where the method of treatment allocation was unconcealed (alternate allocation, for instance) the report was excluded. A *pre-hoc* judgement was made that it would be difficult to blind TENS and, therefore, quality scores were unlikely to exceed 3.

Information about inclusion criteria for women in labour, stage of labour, cervical dilatation, number of women, study design, and timing and duration of treatment was extracted from the reports, together with information on other analgesic interventions and preferences for future childbirth. The type of TENS equipment, its settings, and the method and frequency of its use and positioning of electrodes was also extracted. Control group design and the use of TENS in these controls was similarly noted, including the methods used to disable TENS devices (e.g. sham TENS with no battery).

The effectiveness of TENS was judged by whether or not a statistically significant difference between TENS and the control group (sham TENS or no treatment) was reported in the original report for at least one of the outcome measures used. Outcomes were judged by us as being either primary or secondary. Primary outcomes were defined as any prospective assessment of pain intensity or pain relief made at the time of labour and when TENS was in use. Secondary outcomes were defined as any retrospective assessment of pain or pain relief or any other measure, or judgement made after delivery, or after TENS had been discontinued. Secondary outcomes included the use of any additional pain interventions, the timing of such interventions, and any retrospective global evaluation of the study treatments. A judgement was then made by us as to whether the overall conclusion of the report was positive or negative for the analgesic effectiveness of TENS on primary and secondary outcomes separately. *Post-hoc* subgroup analysis in the original reports was not considered in our judgement of overall effectiveness. Any adverse effect information given was summarized.

Relative risk or benefit was calculated with the 95% confidence interval (CI) using a random-effect model [6] for analgesic data that were not homogeneous ($P < 0.1$). A statistically significant difference from control was assumed when

The topic discussed in this chapter is also published in full in Carroll *et al.* [1].

the 95% confidence interval of the relative risk did not include 1. Number-needed-to-treat (NNT) was calculated with 95% confidence interval [7] on any comparison which showed significance with relative risk.

Results

Two additional reports were found which were not in a previous review [1]. Ten reports involving 877 women were included; 436 women received active TENS and 441 acted as controls. The methodological details of the study designs, instructions to women before and during labour, TENS details and settings, control conditions, and methods of blinding are given in Table 1. One study [8] used cranial TENS; others used TENS with dorsal or suprapubic stimulation. Nine different TENS devices were used in the 10 studies, predominantly with individual titration.

Three studies used conventional analgesic administration (no TENS) as the control group [8–10]. Seven studies used disabled TENS instruments (sham TENS) as a control group [11–17]. One study used both sham TENS and a no TENS control [13]. Only one study [16] had made sufficiently determined attempts at blinding to be awarded any inclusion points for blinding. This study had an inclusion quality score of 4; seven studies scored 2 and two scored 1.

Pain outcome measures and results for the 10 studies are shown in Table 2. There was no consistency in the method of measuring pain intensity or relief. Some studies measured suprapubic and back pain separately, and some measured pain at different stages of labour, or at different degrees of cervical dilatation. No study recorded any difference in pain intensity or relief scores between TENS and control during Additional analgesic interventions were recorded in 8 of the 10 reports [9, 11–17]. In 2 reports the total number of interventions was noted. Bundsen [9] recorded 17 additional analgesic interventions in 11 women receiving usual obstetric analgesic care compared with 21 additional interventions in 16 women receiving TENS. Nesheim [14] recorded that 35 women with TENS needed 49 analgesic interventions compared with 63 interventions in 35 women with sham TENS. One study [13] reported all analgesic interventions given, other than epidurals, which were discouraged in that study.

Five studies [11–13, 15, 16] gave figures for the number of women who received any other analgesic intervention. The results of this secondary outcome for the comparisons of active TENS with sham TENS, together with the number of women in the comparison, are given in Fig. 1. Overall 227 of 292 women (78%) given active TENS had an additional analgesic intervention compared with 239 of 280 women (85%) having sham TENS. There was no difference between active and sham TENS in the three largest studies (Fig. 1). The combined result of all five studies had a relative risk of 0.88 (95% CI 0.72–1.07; Fig. 2). The lack of any statistical difference made the calculation of an NNT irrelevant.

None of the studies were judged by us to have a positive result for the primary outcome measures, which were prospective measures of pain intensity or pain relief. For the secondary

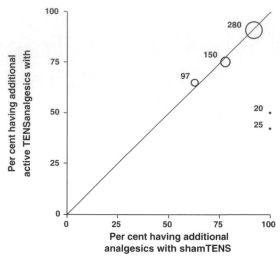

Fig. 1 Additional analgesic requirements. (Number of patients in each trial is given next to the circle, where the diameter is proportional to the number.)

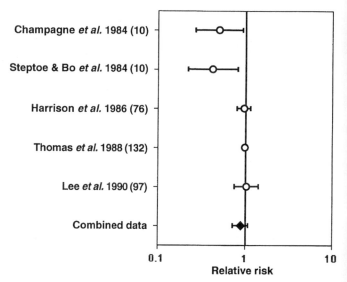

Fig. 2 Relative risk for additional analgesic intervention. Number of patients having active TENS in parenthesis.

outcomes of additional analgesics taken or time to next analgesic three [8, 11, 15] of the 10 studies were judged by us to have a positive result. The three positive studies included a study of cranial TENS in 20 women [16], which only used the single outcome of other analgesics taken, and a comparison of TENS plus epidural compared with epidural alone [17].

There were no reports of adverse events in any of the 10 studies.

Comment

None of the 10 studies included in this review reported any significant difference between the active TENS treatments

Table 1 Details of randomized studies of TENS in labour pain

Ref.	Entry criteria	Study design & duration of treatment	Pre-study instructions	Intra-study instructions	TENS machine	TENS setting	Electrode details	Control group(s)	Binding	Quality score
[9]	Induced labour only (amniotomy ± oxytocin), who did not desire specific alternative pain intervention, all attended antenatal clinic pre-delivery	Parallel group. 1. TENS (16). 2. Control group (11). Dorsal & suprapubic stimulation at 2 diff frequencies; TENS from time of first contraction to parturition.	Standard information about the study & available methods of pain relief. Women requested to try TENS before receiving other pain interventions.	Women in the control group were allowed conventional obstetric analgesia as required.	Custom-built stimulator.	Individually titrated by one author: 2 frequencies (high frequency 50 Hz, pulse train), until paraesthesia to painful areas.	2 electrodes: 1 supra-pubic, 1 low back.	Individually titrated conventional obstetric analgesia (nitrous oxide, epidural, pethidine, diazepam, pudendal block, paracervical block).	Open, no attempt to blind. TENS was given by one of the authors over the painful areas (low back or suprapubic) randomly, if the first method was not effective or caused discomfort then the other site was used after 15–30 min.	2
[11]	Primipara & multipara requiring analgesia during labour & delivery.	Parallel group. 1. Limoge cranio TENS (10): 2 Sham cranio TENS (10). Began when analgesia was requested.	Not described.	Not described.	Anesthelec MPO2 cranial Limoge TENS.	High frequency 166 kHz, 1.2 ms, 20% low frequency 83 Hz, 4 ms, 33%.	3 electrodes: 2 post-mastoid, 1 between eye brows	Sham cranio TENS; (no current).	Described as double-blind, light hidden on both machines, independent person set up machine. Patient and observer blind.	2
[10]	Surgical induction or early labour, primigravida who had not previously experienced other forms of analgesia in labour.	Partial cross-over. 1. TENS (10). 2. Entonox (10). Study began when patients requested analgesia in early stage of labour & was complete once second stage of labour was reached or other form of analgesia was requested.	TENS unit explained and demonstrated before painful contractions midwife taught patients breathing technique for Entonox.	Could use burst mode if needed during painful contractions.	Spembly (Obstetric Pulsar), dual channel.	Individually titrated, fixed pulse rate of 200 ms, amp-48 ma.	2 pairs: 1 either side of midline 5 cm apart. 1 pair at T11, T10, 1 pair upper sacral vertebrae.	Entonox.	Open, no attempt to blind treatments.	2
[12]	Primigravida & third labour, who did not desire specific alternative pain intervention.	Parallel group. 1. Para 0 TENS (49). 2. Para 0 sham TENS (51). 3. Para 3 TENS (27). 4. Para 3 sham TENS (23). From admission to labour ward.	Patients assured that they could use TENS until confident, that other forms of analgesia would be made available, nature of TENS explained.	Titrate controls as contractions increased, they were not made aware of any sensations at site of electrodes.	3M Tenzcare, dual channel.	Individually titrated, pulse width 60–80 μs, repetition rate 80–100/s.	2 pairs, 1 pair T10-L1 dermatome 5 cm away from either side of spine, 1 pair posterior rami S2-L1.	Sham TENS (no current).	Described as double-blind. TENS machine with red light, no current. Neither patient or attending midwife were aware which treatments were allocated, third party changed numbers in attempt to maintain blinding.	1
[13]	Primigravida & second uncomplicated labour, aged 18–35 years.	Parallel group. 1. TENS (38). 2. Sham TENS (33). 3. No treatment control (34).	Patients were given verbal explanation on rationale for TENS. Additional analgesia was given as necessary, but epidurals were not encouraged.	Low frequency TENS was commenced during first stage of labour, high frequency TENS was used during contractions & second stage of labour. Patients were not made aware of sensations at site of stimulation.	Eastleigh Obstetric device.	Biphasic rectangular wave, frequency range 2–200 Hz bursts/s. Amplitude individually titrated by patients.	2 pairs silicone electrodes 4 × 12 cm. T10-L1 & S2-4 spinal level.	Sham TENS (no current); Control (no TENS device).	Neither patients or obstetric staff knew which device were active or inactive.	1

Table 1 *continued*

Ref.	Entry criteria	Study design & duration of treatment	Pre-study instructions	Intra-study instructions	TENS machine	TENS setting	Electrode details	Control group(s)	Binding	Quality score
[14]	Expected birth following normal labour & normal pregnancy, cervical dilation < 4 cm.	Parallel group. 1. TENS (35). 2. Sham TENS (35). Began when dilation < 4 cm.	Aim was to try TENS to determine its effectiveness in labour pain, no risks & alternative methods would be available if pain relief was inadequate.	2 sets of instructions: 1. Explanation of active treatment to patient & partner, encouraged to use when contraction began, to use more intensely as pain increased, free to stop at any time; 2. Sham —to expect no sensation other than warmth.	Travisens, Dan-Sjo Elektronik.	Individually titrated & decreased until comfortable, pulse 0–40 ma frequency 100 Hz, pulse duration 0.25 ms, frequency 50–150 Hz.	2 pairs both, pairs T10-L1.	Sham TENS (no current).	Red light, not blind to observer as patients told different instructions.	2
[15]	Normal vaginal delivery, primigravida, > 3 cm dilation.	Parallel group. 1. TENS (13). 2. Sham TENS (12). Stimulation for 30 min.	Identical short verbal and written information to both groups.	Same to both groups to titrate up to level of comfort or adequate pain relief during first 30 min.	Elpha 500.	Individually titrated over 30 minutes, 0–60 m amp, pulse width 0.2 ms, frequency 1–4 Hz, 100 Hz.	2 pairs carbon rubber: T10-T12, S2-S3.	Sham TENS + standard obstetric analgesia.	Red light, same instruction to both groups.	2
[16]	Early labour in primigravida & multigravida, normal or induced delivery, < 7 cm cervical dilation.	Parallel group. 1. TENS (132). 2. Sham TENS (148). TENS applied when discomfort was reported.	No antepartum instruction given on TENS. Standard protocol given to both groups by instructor who only advised on TENS use.	Both groups advised to increase TENS settings as needed during contractions, patients free to use other analgesia if required. TENS turned off for 2 contractions each hour and assess the diff in pain.	3M, dual channel	Individually titrated.	2 pairs electrodes: 1 pair para-vertebrally on either side of spinous process T10-L1, 1 pair S2-4.	Sham TENS (no current).	Good attempt to blind study, both active and sham machines had flashing light, TENS applied by staff not associated with trial, labour managed by non study staff in normal way. Instructions not given by assessor.	4
[17]	First stage of labour, primiparane multiparae, when analgesia requested.	Parallel group. 1. TENS (46). 2. Sham Tens (48). TENS applied until cervix fully dilated.	Use of TENS explained to expectant parents by attending physician. Patients supervised until competent in the use of TENS.	Low frequency TENS used until contractions when high frequency TENS was used (range 1–6). Titrated by partner (mostly). PCA pethidine and promethazine escape analgesia.	Agar GK (Klinerva Holland).	Individually titrated.	2 pairs electrodes 50 × 100 mm. 1 cm lateral spine L1-L3 & L4-S1.	Sham TENS (identical placebo device).	No description of sham TENS other than identical device.	2
[8]	Primigravid, gestation of at least 38 wks, < 3 cm cervical dilation, expected normal delivery with extradural analgesia.	Parallel group. 1. Epidural (60). 2. Epidural + TENS (60). TENS applied with epidural up to end of labour.	Not described.	Not described.	Anesthelec MPO2.	High frequency 166 kHz, 1 ms, 20%, low frequency 83 Hz, 4 ms, 33%.	3 electrodes: 2 posterior mastoid, 1 between eye brows.	Epidural 0.25% bupivacaine as required, first bolus with fentanyl 100 μg.	None.	2

Ma, milliamps; ms, milliseconds; μs, microseconds.

Table 2 Results of randomized studies of TENS in labour pain

Ref.	Pain outcomes	Results for outcome	Withdrawals & drop-outs	Adverse effects	Significant difference for at least 1 primary/ secondary outcome	Judgement
[9]	1. 5-pt PT (hourly) 2. Use of any other PR interventions. 3. Duration of labour. 4. Questionnaire on day after delivery Abdominal & back pain assessed independently.	Back pain severe: ≤ 5 cm dilated TENS 3/15, control 5/9 > 5 cm dilated TENS 1/7, control 5/6 Suprapubic pain severe: ≤5 cm dilated TENS 10/15, control 7/9 >5 cm dilated TENS 7/8 control 5/6 Stage 2: pudendal block 13/15 TENS, 7/9 control analgesic.	1 in each group excluded due to subsequent Caesarean section 1 in each group received epidural because of special problems which were not described.	No specific effect of TENS on fetal heart rate.	no/no	Negative
[11]	1. Additional PR interventions.	5/10 required additional analgesic intervention active stimulation, 10/10 control group.	None rep.	Not rep	na/yes	Positive secondary.
[10]	1. 3-pt PI pre-escape analgesia. 2. 3-pt PR. 3. Time to next analgesic.	NSD. No relief 11% TENS, 50% Entonox, but contractions significantly higher in Entonox group Additional analgesia not described.	1 woman in Entonox group delivered without further analgesia, and was excluded.	Not rep	no/no	Negative.
[12]	Research midwife assessments. 1. 5-pt PI (hourly). 2. Baseline pain threshold (Mosanto gun). 3. 4-pt PR. 4. Site of pain.	NSD between TENS & sham TENS for pain or for those requiring extra analgesia (12% TENS, 14% sham TENS) Pain score > 50% at 1 h: TENS 63/64, sham TENS 55/59 Additional analgesia needed: 57/76 TENS, 58/74 controls.	Not described.	Not rep	no/no	Negative.
[13]	Every 30 min. 1. VAS-PI 0–10 every 30 minutes. 2. Strength of uterine contractions (weak, moderate, strong). Retrospective questionnaire at 24 h postpartum 1. Did patient find TENS helpful or not? (0–3) 2. future use.	NSD between TENS & Sham TENS use of additional analgesic interventions (excluding epidurals) 40/62 with TENS, 22/35 sham TENS, 28/37 control NSD between the 3 treatments for 30-min pain scores.	Not described.	No AE, rep	no/no	Negative.
[14]	1. Overall 5-pt PR after childbirth. 2. Escape analgesia.	NSD between TENS & sham TENS pain-free: 1/35 TENS, 0/35 sham TENS Good relief: 4/35 TENS 5/35 sham TENS 63 analgesic interventions in TENS, 49 in controls.	Not described	Not rep	na/no	Negative.

Table 2 *continued*

Ref.	Pain outcomes	Results for Ooutcome	Withdrawals & drop-outs	Adverse effects	Significant difference for at least 1 primary/ secondary outcome	Judgement
[15]	1. VAS-PI 0–10 at baseline & 30 min after TENS. 2. Other analgesic interventions. 3. Time of contractions.	No diff in pain measurements. Additional analgesia 5/12 TENS, 13/13 control group.	1/13 excluded in TENS group due to failed battery in device 1/13 in control group had Caesarean section but included in analysis.	0/12 TENS 0/13 sham TENS	no/yes	Positive secondary.
[16]	1. VAS-PI (hourly) for abdominal and back pain. 2. Use of other analgesic interventions. 3. Postpartum overall assessment by patient.	NSD between TENS & sham TENS at <7 cm dilated, 7–10 cm dilated, or during stage 2. No diff in use of other methods of pain relief: Entonox, pethidine or epidural postpartum assessment of excellent/good relief by 29/132 active	52/148 control group requested to withdraw compared with 54/132 in TENS group Only 96 patients could continue with VAS beyond 7 cm & 16 into second stage of labour.	Not rep	no/no	Negative.
[17]	1. VAS-PI (bad = no-good = yes). 2. Other analgesic interventions. 3. Patient's impression on medication during labour. 4. Would patient choose TENS in future deliveries? 5. Patient's impression of effect of TENS on pain.	No sig diff between TENS and sham TENS. Mean no. of requests for other analgesia: 18.2 TENS, 26.2 sham TENS no. of times analgesia administered: 5.9 ± 2.32 TENS, 6.5 ± 1.77 sham TENS amount of pethidine administered (mg): 60.8 ± 21.6 TENS.	2 refused to take part and received standard analgesia. No other details given.	No AE rep	no/no	Negative.
[8]	1. VAS for global pain quality (patient) during labour at 2 h post-delivery. 2. Duration of analgesia after first epidural bolus. 3. Time between epidural boll.	Quality of analgesia during dilatation & at delivery not diff between active and control. Duration of first epidural local anaesthetic bolus was increased in TENS group by a mean of 22 min (P = 0.01) Time between boll significantly prolonged in TENS.	7 withdrawals, 1 Caesarean section, 2 technical problem with epidural, 2 electrodes fell off, 1 had other treatment. (NB not all described)	Not rep	no/yes	Positive

AE, adverse effect; NSD, no significant difference; PI, pain intensity; PR, pain relief; VAS-PI, visual analogue scale of pain intensity; rep, reported.

and controls for any of the primary pain outcome measures used. This strengthens the findings of previous negative reviews on TENS in labour [1,3]. The weak evidence from secondary outcome measures that the need for additional analgesics may be diminished [11] was negated by an additional large trial [13] which found no difference between active TENS and sham TENS. Trial size is likely to be important when assessing even primary outcomes, but for weak secondary pain outcomes such as additional analgesic requirements, the effect of trial size shown in Fig. 1 was dramatic. The two trials that showed TENS to reduce additional analgesic interventions [11, 15] had only 20 and 25 patients in the comparisons compared with 527 patients in the comparisons in the other three trials (Fig. 1). Only one study of moderate size [8] had a secondary outcome judged by us to be positive for cranial TENS. This emphasizes how individual small studies may mislead because of the random play of chance.

The choice of outcome measure is an important determinant of how studies are to be judged. If the objective of TENS is to alleviate pain then it is fair that judgements of its effectiveness are based on prospective subjective measures of pain intensity or pain relief (primary outcomes), and that these assessments are done at appropriate time points. Retrospective measures of pain are notoriously unreliable. Subsequent need for other analgesic interventions is a secondary outcome measure, but one used commonly in these studies. The implications for current practice from these results is that women who are offered TENS are at risk of having their pain inadequately controlled and may experience delays in receiving effective interventions.

We restricted this review to randomized controlled trials, unlike Reeve *et al.* [3]. Randomized controlled trials represent the 'gold standard' in clinical trials of efficacy [18]. Nonrandomized studies have for nearly 20 years been known to yield larger estimates of treatment effects than studies using random allocation [19]. The size of the overestimation of treatment effect when randomization is inappropriate can be as much as 40%. In postoperative pain non-randomized trials of TENS were more likely to show a positive result than randomized trials, with 15 of 17 randomized trials being negative while 17 of 19 non-randomized trials were positive.

The overall methodological quality of the trials reported was low, reflecting the fact that it is difficult, if not impossible, to blind studies of TENS [20]. Inadequate blinding may be an important source of observer bias and may contribute to overestimation of treatment effects. Four studies here made no attempt at blinding, and of the seven that used sham TENS, only one [16] described the method of blinding in sufficient detail to indicate that blinding may have been adequate.

The 1994 Maternity Service Charter [21] tells women: 'you have the right to be given an explanation of any treatment proposed, including the benefits and risks and of any alternatives before you decide whether you will agree with the treatment'. Those involved in the provision of maternity services therefore need to be aware of current research findings concerning effective interventions for the relief of pain, so they can apply these findings in their clinical practice and provide women with accurate information so they can be involved in decisions concerning their care.

On the basis of these findings the continued use of TENS in childbirth needs to be carefully reconsidered. The continued use of TENS in labour pain has considerable implications for maternity services and the women who use TENS in terms of receiving prompt and effective pain relief during child birth. Instead of TENS, women should be given the option of more effective interventions.

References

1. Carroll D, Tramer M, McQuay H, Nye B, Moore A. Transcutaneous electrical nerve stimulation in labour pain: A systematic review. *British Journal of Obstetrics and Gynaecology* 1997; **104**:169–75.
2. Jadad AR, McQuay HJ. A high-yield strategy to identify randomized controlled trials for systematic reviews. *Online Journal of Current Clinical Trials* [serial online] 1993 Feb 27; Doc No 33:3973 words; 39 paragraphs. 5 tables.
3. Reeve J, Menon D, Corabian P. Transcutaneous electrical nerve stimulation (TENS): a technology assessment. *International Journal of Technology Assessment in Health Care* 1996; **12**:299–324.
4. L'Abbé KA, Detsky AS, O'Rourke K. Meta-analysis in clinical research. *Annals of Internal Medicine* 1987; **107**:224–33.
5. Jadad AR, Moore RA, Carroll D, Jenkinson C, Reynolds DJM, Gavaghan DJ, McQuay HJ. Assessing the quality of reports of randomized clinical trials: is blinding necessary? *Controlled Clinical Trials* 1996; **17**:1–12.
6. DerSimonian R, Laird N. Meta-analysis of clinical trials. *Controlled Clinical Trials* 1986; **7**:177–88.
7. Cook RJ, Sackett DL. The number needed to treat: a clinically useful measure of treatment effect. *British Medical Journal* 1995; **310**:452–4.
8. Wattrisse G, Leroy B, Dufossez F, Bui Huu Tai R. Electrostimulation cerebrale transcutanee: etude comparative des effets de son association a l'anesthesie peridurale par bupivacaine-fentanyl au cours de l'analgesie obstetricale. *Cahiers d'Anesthesiologie* 1993; **41**:489–95.
9. Bundsen P, Ericson K, Peterson LE, Thiringer K. Pain relief in labor by transcutaneous electrical nerve stimulation. Testing of a modified stimulation technique and evaluation of the neurological and biochemical condition of the newborn infant. *Acta Obstetrica Gynaecologica Scandinavica* 1982; **61**:129–36.
10. Chia YT, Arulkumaran S, Chua S, Ratnam SS. Effectiveness of transcutaneous electric nerve stimulator for pain relief in labour. *Asia–Oceania Journal of Obstetrics and Gynecology* 1990; **16**:145–51.
11. Champagne C, Papiernik E, Thierry JP, Noviant Y. Electrostimulation cerebrale transcutanee par les courants de Limoge au cours de l'accouchement. *Annales Françaises d'Anesthesie et de Reanimation* 1984; **3**:405–13.
12. Harrison RF, Woods T, Shore M, Mathews G, Unwin A. Pain relief in labour using transcutaneous electrical nerve stimulation (TENS). A TENS/TENS placebo controlled study in two parity groups. *British Journal of Obstetrics and Gynaecology* 1986; **93**:739–46.
13. Lee EWC, Chung IWY, Lee JYL, Lam PWY, Chin RKH. The role of transcutaneous electrical nerve stimulation in management of labour in obstetric patients. *Asia–Oceania Journal of Obstetrics and Gynaecology* 1990; **16**:247–54.

14. Nesheim BI. The use of transcutaneous nerve stimulation for pain relief during labor. A controlled clinical study. *Acta Obstetrica Gynecology Scandinavica* 1981; **60**:13–16.

15. Steptoe P, Bo JO. Transkutan nervestimulations smertelindrende effekt ved fødsler. *Ugeskrift for Laeger* 1984; **146**:3186–9.

16. Thomas IL, Tyle V, Webster J, Neilson A. An evaluation of transcutaneous electrical nerve stimulation for pain relief in labour. *Australian and New Zealand Journal of Obstetrics and Gynaecology* 1988; **28**:182–9.

17. van der Ploeg JM, Vervest HAM, Liem AL, van Leeuwen S. Transcutaneous nerve stimulation (TENS) during the first stage of labour: a randomized clinical trial. *Pain* 1996; **68**:75–8.

18. Schulz KF, Chalmers I, Hayes RJ, Altman DG. Empirical evidence of bias: dimensions of methodological quality associated with estimates of treatment effects in controlled trials. *Journal of the American Medical Association* 1995; **273**:408–12.

19. Chalmers TC, Matta RJ, Smith JJr, Kunzler AM. Evidence favoring the use of anticoagulants in the hospital phase of acute myocardial infarction. *New England Journal of Medicine* 1977; **297**:1091–6.

20. Deyo RA, Walsh NE, Schoenfeld LS, Ramamurthy S. Can trials of physical treatments be blinded? The example of transcutaneous electrical nerve stimulation for chronic pain. *American Journal of Physical Medicine and Rehabilitation* 1990; **69**:6–10.

21. *The patient's charter: maternity services.* London: Department of Health; 1994.

22

Acute pain: conclusion

Interventions

In treating acute pain, as in other areas of medicine, tradition and ill-informed prejudice sometimes hold sway over evidence and common sense. We concentrated on gathering evidence for the treatments that are simple. This chapter draws together that evidence in a wider frame, including interventions for which there are no systematic reviews. Wherever possible we base our recommendations on randomized trials.

Effective pain management is fundamental to quality care, and although we believe that good pain control speeds recovery, there is still no compelling evidence that this is so. Advantage can be shown with proxy measures like mobility or coughing, but evidence that good pain management led to faster recovery would increase the pressure to improve current practice, which is often less than ideal.

Non-opioids: paracetamol, combinations, and non-steroidal anti-inflammatory drugs (NSAIDs)

Effective relief can be achieved with oral non-opioids and non-steroidal anti-inflammatory drugs. These drugs are appropriate for many post-surgical and post-traumatic pains, especially when patients go home on the day of the operation. Figure 1 shows the evolving league table for analgesic efficacy compiled from randomized trials after all kinds of surgery. Analgesic efficacy is expressed as the number-needed-to-treat (NNT), the number of patients who need to receive the active drug for one to achieve at least 50% relief of pain compared with placebo over a six-hour treatment period. The most effective drugs have a low NNT of about 2, meaning that for every two patients who receive the drug one patient will get at least 50% relief because of the treatment (the other patient may obtain relief but it does not reach the 50% level).

For paracetamol 1 g the NNT is nearly 5. Combination of paracetamol 650 mg with dextropropoxyphene 65 mg improves the NNT slightly. Ibuprofen is better at 3 and diclofenac at about 2.5.

These NNT comparisons are versus placebo; the best NNT of 2 means that while 50 of 100 patients will get at least 50% relief because of the treatment, another 20% will have a placebo response which gives them at least 50% relief, so that with diclofenac, 70 of 100 will have effective pain relief.

This alternative way of looking at the effect of the various analgesics is shown in Fig. 2. The range is from about 25%

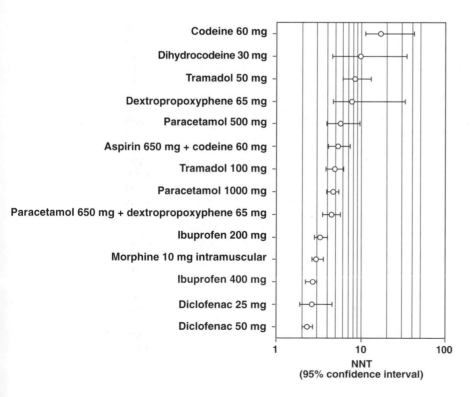

Fig. 1 Oral analgesic number-needed-to-treat (NNT) league table.

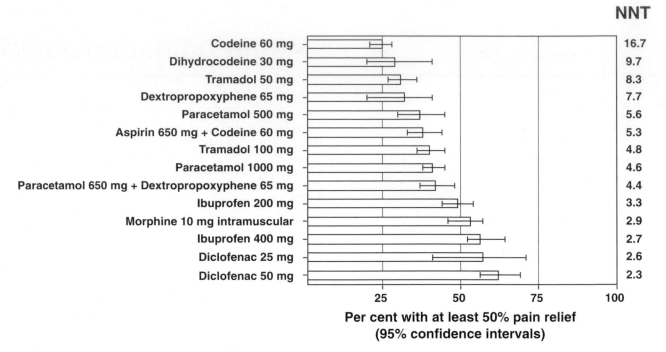

Fig. 2   Oral analgesic league table: percentage of patients with at least 50% pain relief.

of patients getting at least 50% pain relief with codeine 60 mg (largely because of the effect of placebo), to over 70% at the high end of the 95% confidence interval with oral NSAID. For comparison, with 10 mg intramuscular morphine about 53% of patients get more than 50% pain relief. Because the effect of placebo is added in, the comparisons between analgesics are not as stark as with NNT.

The clear message is that of the oral analgesics, non-steroidal anti-inflammatory drugs (NSAIDs) perform best, and that paracetamol alone or in combinations is also effective. Initial prescription of oral NSAIDs can be supplemented with paracetamol. As pain wanes then the prescription should be paracetamol-based, supplemented if necessary by NSAIDs.

There is an old adage that if patients can swallow it is best to take drugs by mouth. There is no evidence that NSAIDs given rectally or by injection perform better (or faster) than the same drug at the same dose given by mouth (Chapter 11). These other routes become appropriate when patients cannot swallow. Topical NSAIDs are effective in acute musculoskeletal injuries—ibuprofen has an NNT of 3 for at least 50% relief at one week compared with placebo (Chapter 12).

Adverse effect data on NSAIDs from long-term dosing, where gastric bleeding is the main worry, rate ibuprofen the safest [1]. In acute pain the main concerns are renal and co-agulation problems. Acute renal failure can be precipitated in patients with pre-existing heart or kidney disease, those on loop diuretics, or those who have lost more than 10% of blood volume. NSAIDs cause significant lengthening (~ 30%) of bleeding time, usually still within the normal range. This can last for days with aspirin, hours with non-aspirin

NSAIDs. Whether or not NSAIDs cause significant increase in blood loss remains contentious.

Other drugs

As yet, we do not have any systematic review evidence for a number of niche analgesic interventions. These include inhaled nitrous oxide, which can provide fast-onset fast-offset analgesia for obstetrics and wound dressings, corticosteroids to reduce pain and swelling after head and neck surgery, and when swelling causes pain in cancer, ketamine in emergency analgesia and anaesthesia and clonidine.

Opioids

For severe acute pain opioids are the first-line treatment, and to date we have only one systematic review, that for injected morphine (Chapter 13). Intermittent opioid injection can provide effective relief of acute pain [2]. Unfortunately, adequate doses are withheld because of traditions, misconceptions, ignorance, and fear. Doctors and nurses fear addiction and respiratory depression. Addiction is not a problem with opioid use in acute pain. Over 11000 patients were followed up a year after opioids were given for acute pain, and just 4 individuals were considered to be addicts [3].

Irrespective of the route, opioids used for people who are not in pain, or in doses larger than necessary to control the pain, can slow or indeed stop breathing. The key principle is to titrate the dose against the desired effect—pain relief—and minimize unwanted effects (Fig. 3). If the patient is still

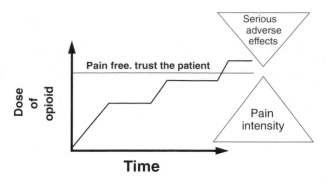

Fig. 3 Titrate opioids to effect.

Principle for safe and effective opioid use: titrate to effect

> If the patient is asking for more opioid then it usually signals inadequate pain control:
> - too little drug
> - too long between doses
> - too little attention paid to the patient
> - too much reliance on rigid (inadequate) prescriptions

complaining of pain and you are sure that the drug has all been delivered and absorbed, then it is safe to give another, usually smaller, dose (5 minutes after intravenous, 1 hour after intramuscular or subcutaneous, 90 minutes after oral). If the second dose is also ineffective, then repeat the process or change the route of administration to achieve faster control. Delayed release formulations, oral or transdermal, should not be used in acute pain, because delayed onset and offset are dangerous in this context.

There is no compelling evidence that one opioid is better than another, but there is good evidence that pethidine has a specific disadvantage [4] and no specific advantage. Given in multiple doses the metabolite norpethidine can accumulate and act as a central nervous system irritant, ultimately causing convulsions, especially in renal dysfunction. Pethidine should not be used when multiple injections are needed. The old idea that pethidine is better than other opioids at dealing with colicky pain is no longer tenable [5].

Morphine (and relatives diamorphine and codeine), have an active rather than a toxic metabolite, morphine-6-glucuronide. In renal dysfunction this metabolite can accumulate and result in greater effect from a given dose, because it is more active than morphine. If you are, as you should be, titrating dose against effect, this will not matter. Less morphine will be needed. Accumulation can be a problem with unconscious intensive care patients on fixed dose schedules when renal function is compromised.

Opioid adverse effects include nausea and vomiting, constipation, sedation, pruritus, urinary retention, and respiratory depression. There is no good evidence that the incidence is different with different opioids at the same level of analgesia. There is good evidence that the risk of adverse events is increased when high-tech approaches are used for drug administration [6].

There are strong arguments, based on minimizing risk, for using one opioid only, so that everyone is familiar with dosage, effects, and problems. Our first choice opioid is morphine. Whichever drug you choose, simple changes to the way opioids are used, good staff education, and implementation of an algorithm for intermittent opioid dosing, can have a powerful impact on pain relief and patient satisfaction [2].

Nurse-administered intermittent opioid injection requires good staffing levels to minimize delay between need and injection. Staffing shortage, ward distractions, and controlled drug regulations all increase the delay. Patient-controlled analgesia overcomes these logistical problems. The patient presses a button and receives a pre-set dose of opioid, from a syringe driver connected to an intravenous or subcutaneous cannula. This delivers opioid to the same opioid receptors as an intermittent injection, but allows the patient to circumvent delays. Not surprisingly, there is little difference in outcome between efficient intermittent injection and patient-controlled analgesia [7]. Good risk management with patient-controlled analgesia should emphasize the same drug, protocols, and equipment throughout the hospital.

Novel routes of opioid administration, intended to improve analgesia and reduce adverse effects, include intra-articular (Chapter 17), nasal, active transdermal, and inhalational. These may prove to have advantage over conventional routes, different kinetic profiles, or greater convenience, but their place in mainstream care is unproved.

Regional analgesia

The perceived advantage of regional analgesia with local anaesthetic is that it can deliver complete pain relief by interrupting pain transmission from a localized area, so avoiding generalized drug adverse effects. This advantage is more obvious when it is possible to give further doses via a catheter, extending the duration of analgesia. Details are given in Table 1.

There is a necessary distinction between blocks done to permit surgery, and blocks done together with a general anaesthetic to provide postoperative pain relief. There is clear evidence that blocks can indeed provide good relief in the initial postoperative period [8], and no evidence to suggest that patients with blocks then experience 'rebound', and need more postoperative pain relief. The risk of neurological damage is the major drawback [9], and ideally, blocks should not be done on anaesthetized patients.

Epidural analgesia

Epidural infusion via a catheter can offer continuous relief after trauma or surgery, for lower limb, spine, abdominal, or chest. The current optimal infusate is an opioid/local anaesthetic mixture. Opioids and local anaesthetics have a synergistic effect, so that lower doses of each are required for equivalent analgesia with fewer adverse effects [10]. Epidurals are widely used for pain relief in labour.

The risks are those of an epidural, (dural puncture, infection, haematoma, nerve damage), those of the local anaesthetic (hypotension, motor block, toxicity) and those of the

Table 1 Regional analgesia summary

	Indications	Advantages	Problems
Low-tech			
Topical	Surface surgery	Simple	Short duration
Wound infiltration	Most wounds	Simple	Short duration
Peripheral nerve blocks	Limb surgery/trauma	Catheter possible	
Plexus blocks	Limb surgery	Catheter possible	Nerve damage, motor block
High-tech			
Epidural (including caudal)	Major surgery (thoracoabdominal, lower limb)	Catheter possible Reduced thromboembolism	Adverse effects, surveillance
Intrathecal	Major surgery (thoracoabdominal, lower limb)	Long duration, relief possible from single injection low dose opioid	Adverse effects, surveillance

opioid, (nausea, sedation, urinary retention, respiratory depression, pruritus) (Table 2). Wrong doses do get given [6], so increased surveillance is mandatory. The risk of persistent neurological sequelae after an epidural is about 1 in 5000 [11]. Debate continues about whether patients with epidural infusions can be nursed on general wards. These techniques are only appropriate for major trauma or surgery when the potential benefits outweigh the risks.

Other techniques

Although experts can obtain good results with specialized procedures, such as paravertebral or interpleural injections, the evidence that in less skilled hands these are better than standard methods (should-do rather than can-do evidence), is often lacking.

Transcutaneous electrical nerve stimulation (TENS) and acupuncture

TENS is not effective for postoperative pain (Chapter 20), and is of limited value for labour pain (Chapter 21). Systematic reviews of acupuncture are confined to chronic pain.

Psychological methods

There is evidence that psychological approaches are beneficial [12]. Cognitive-behavioural methods can reduce pain and distress in burn patients. Preparation before surgery can reduce postoperative analgesic consumption.

Table 2 Adverse effects of regional analgesia

- Needle or catheter damage to nerves, pleura, dura, or viscus
- Intravenous injection of local anaesthetic
- Overdose of local anaesthetic
- Motor block
- Autonomic blockage: hypotension, urinary retention
- Respiratory depression (spinal opioids)

Factors to consider when choosing therapy

- Coexisting illness
- Available staff
- Available equipment
- Risks and unwanted effects of the various options
- Appropriateness of the chosen intervention for that pain
- Evidence of efficacy for the chosen intervention cost

Steps to successful management

- Regular assessment of pain and adverse effects
- Protocols for monitoring and treating pain
- Protocols for monitoring and treating adverse effects titration of doses at short intervals until pain relieved
- Do not be afraid to use more than one approach
- Appropriate back-up by identified personnel
- Continuing in-service training and education

Predictable problems

Patient	**Problems**
Babies and infants	Communication; drug handling
Elderly	Coexisting illness; drug handling
Respiratory disease	Respiratory depression; NSAIDs and asthma
Renal failure	Drug handling; NSAIDs
Head injury or impaired consciousness	Assessment; dose titration
Drug addiction or already taking opioids	Dose titration; weaning; respiratory depression after nerve block which stops pain
Sickle-cell disease	Assessment; varying analgesic needs

Key points for improving acute pain management

1. Opt for safety and simplicity
2. Measure and record pain regularly—be proactive
3. Choose evidence-based interventions
4. Individualize treatment; allow patient control
5. Choose appropriate drug, route, mode of delivery
6. Provide education for staff and patients

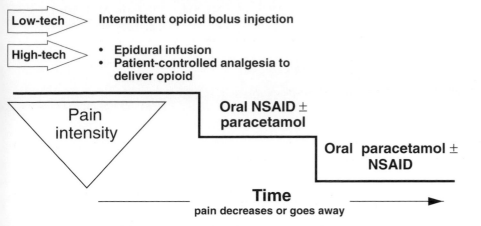

Fig. 4 General strategy for the management of acute pain.

Clinical settings and recommendations

General

The tenets of good management of acute pain are that, with good staff (and patient) education in place, appropriate drug doses are given when needed by the appropriate route and delivery method. Schemes have to be flexible enough to respond to individual patient need and different clinical settings. Figure 4 gives a general strategy.

There is controversy about the optimal timing of initial analgesia. The idea is that analgesia is more effective when given before pain begins than when given after. Most randomized trials comparing the same intervention given before or after pain starts have not shown clinical advantage of so-called pre-emptive analgesia [13]. Whether poorly-controlled acute pain generates chronic pain is also controversial.

Problem pains and patients

Standard interventions and protocols will cope with most acute pain problems, but some patients, particularly in hospital, will require special management. Expertise can be developed in specific units, but if not available seek the advice of your acute pain service. In particular do not let pain in children go untreated.

Comment

The key to successful pain management is education, not new drugs or high-tech delivery systems. Existing tools can do the job if doctors and nurses are educated, both to dispel the myths and misconceptions and to take responsibility for providing good pain control. It is much easier to dispel myths when you have the evidence. For many years, patients were not given adequate analgesia for abdominal pain in case it masked the signs necessary for diagnosis. This was wrong [14].

Pain relief should not be seen as someone else's responsibility, nor just dismissed, because 'in the end the pain and the patient go away'. Freedom from pain is important to patients. In 1846, the first anaesthetic provided pain-free surgery—150 years later patients should not have to endure unrelieved pain anywhere in hospital.

References

1. Henry D, Lim LL, Rodriguez LAG, Gutthann SP, Carson JL, Griffin M *et al.* Variability in risk of gastrointestinal complications with individual non-steroidal anti-inflammatory drugs: results of a collaborative meta-analysis. *British Medical Journal* 1996; **312**:1563–6.
2. Gould TH, Crosby DL, Harmer M, Lloyd SM, Lunn JN, Rees GAD *et al.* Policy for controlling pain after surgery: effect of sequential changes in management. *British Medical Journal* 1992; **305**:1187–93.
3. Porter J, Jick H. Addiction rate in patients treated with narcotics. *New England Journal of Medicine* 1980; **302**:123.
4. Szeto HH, Inturrisi CE, Houde R, Saal S, Cheigh J, Reidenberg M. Accumulation of norperidine, an active metabolite of meperidine, in patients with renal failure or cancer. *Annals of Internal Medicine* 1977; **86**:738–41.
5. Nagle CJ, McQuay HJ. Opioid receptors; their role in effect and side-effect. *Current Anaesthesia and Critical Care* 1990; **1**:247–52.
6. Bates DW, Cullen DJ, Laird N, Petersen LA, Small SD, Servi D *et al.* Incidence of adverse drug events and potential adverse drug events. *Journal of the American Medical Association* 1995; **274**:29–34.
7. Ballantyne JC, Carr DB, Chalmers TC, Dear KB, Angelillo IF, Mosteller F. Postoperative patient-controlled analgesia: meta-analyses of initial randomized control trials. *Journal of Clinical Anesthesia* 1993; **5**:182–93.
8. McQuay HJ, Carroll D, Moore RA. Postoperative orthopaedic pain—the effect of opioid premedication and local anaesthetic blocks. *Pain* 1988; **33**:291–5.
9. Bridenbaugh PO. Complications of local anesthetic neural blockade. In: Cousins MJ, Bridenbaugh PO, ed. *Neural blockade*, (2nd edn). Philadelphia PA: Lippincott, 1988:695–717.
10. McQuay H. Epidural Analgesics. In: Wall P, Melzack R, (ed.) *Textbook of pain*, (3rd edn). London: Churchill Livingstone, 1994:1025–34.
11. Kane RE. Neurologic deficits following epidural or spinal anesthesia. *Anesthesia and Analgesia* 1981; **60**:150–61.

12. Justins DM, Richardson PH. Clinical management of acute pain. *British Medical Bulletin* 1991; 47:561–83.

13. McQuay HJ. Pre-emptive analgesia: a systematic review of clinical studies. *Annals of Medicine* 1995; 27:249–56.

14. Attard AR, Corlett MJ, Kidner NJ, Leslie AP, Fraser IA. Safety of early pain relief for acute abdominal pain. *British Medical Journal* 1992; 305:554–6.

Part III

CHRONIC PAIN

23

Chronic pain: introduction

Summary

In chronic pain relief, just as in other therapeutic areas, there are often many ways to tackle a particular problem. There may be evidence of benefit for each of the alternatives. The task that faces us is to have a way of ranking the relative effectiveness of these interventions, and to couple that with knowledge of any hazards, minor or major. Then we can make informed decisions about which should be selected, purchased and offered to patients.

Perhaps in the ideal world there would be large randomized trials comparing the various interventions. In practice, what we have is a number of small studies. Later chapters will describe the methods used to rank the relative performance of the interventions. The ranking often has to be indirect, how well does each intervention compare with placebo, rather than derived from direct 'head-to-head' comparisons of the treatments (Table 1).

This chapter provides an overview of interventions for chronic pain, and provides references to systematic reviews for some of the interventions which are not covered in detail in the succeeding chapters.

Range of interventions

The range of interventions available for chronic pain management is summarized in Fig. 1.

Table 1   Ranking efficacy

Trial comparator	Data source
• Comparisons with placebo	Individual patient data
• Comparison with other 'active' interventions	Published group data
	• Indirect ranking
	• Direct ranking

The same conventional analgesics, from non-steroidal anti-inflammatory drugs (NSAIDs) through to opioids, are used in chronic as in acute pain. If analgesics relieve the pain to an adequate extent, and with tolerable or controllable adverse effects, then there is little reason to use other interventions. If analgesics are ineffective other methods have to be considered. If analgesics are effective but cause intolerable or uncontrollable adverse effects then again other methods should be considered. The effectiveness and the adverse effects of the analgesics are critical.

We know from audits of cancer pain that using analgesics according to the The World Health Organization (WHO) 'ladder' (Fig. 2) can relieve pain for 80% of patients. For most of the 80% the relief will be good, for a minority it will only be moderate. This presumes that the pain is managed optimally, and we know from audit is often not the case. Optimal management requires that the correct drugs are available, and that they are given in the correct dose by the correct route and at the correct time. This needs staff who are well versed in the problems, and who are available to care for the patient. The second problem is the 20% of patients whose pain is not well managed by intelligent use of analgesic guidelines. The other treatment methods on Fig. 1 are necessary to manage those for whom analgesics fail.

Non-opioid analgesics

Oral NSAIDs, combinations, and others

Choosing the best analgesic for long-term use involves the same decisions as in acute pain. Most comparisons are done using single doses, whereas patients with chronic pain take multiple doses. Historically, the efficacy league table (Chapter 22) for single doses in acute pain has also proved valid in chronic pain. Despite the fact that the drugs in this category are by far the most widely used, there is remarkably little

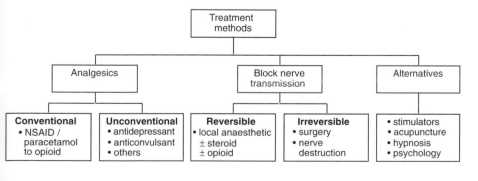

Fig. 1   Chronic pain: interventions.

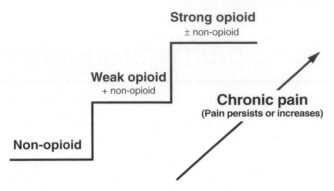

Fig. 2   Schematic WHO 'ladder' for cancer pain management.

good evidence about their relative efficacy and adverse effects after chronic usage.

No single dose trial has shown any efficacy advantage of one NSAID over another [1]. This does not fit well with patients' reports on multiple dosing of increased efficacy from NSAIDs with greater anti-inflammatory action. The adverse effect profile may also be different with chronic dosing. The risk of NSAID-induced gastric bleeding is lowest with ibuprofen, and increases with increasing age [2]. Prophylactic misoprostol should be considered for preventing NSAID-associated gastrointestinal complications when age is greater than 75 years, cardiovascular disease, history of peptic ulcer, or of gastrointestinal bleeding (numbers-needed-to-treat to prevent one serious gastrointestinal complication in one year 105,58,11, and 7 respectively) [3, 4].

The efficacy dose-response curve for NSAIDs is said to be flat compared with the dose-response for adverse effects such as gastrointestinal symptoms, dizziness, and drowsiness [5] (but see Chapter 10). Increasing the dose to improve analgesia is therefore more likely to increase adverse effects than to improve analgesia.

Centrally acting non-opioids include dipyrone and nefopam. Dipyrone is widely used in certain countries, and is an effective analgesic which can produce blood dyscrasias. The lack of comparative evidence makes it hard to rank its risk benefit profile against the other analgesics.

Comparisons

NSAIDs alone produced as good analgesia as single or multiple doses of weak opioids alone or in combination with nonopioid analgesics [5]. Adverse effect incidence and patient drop-out rates were the same for multiple doses of NSAIDs or weak opioids in combination with non-opioid analgesics [5]. Conversely, two studies suggest that there is little advantage in osteoarthritis of either NSAIDs over paracetamol [6] or weak opioids in combination with paracetamol over paracetamol alone [7].

Topical NSAIDs

Many doctors and some pundits are sceptical about the efficacy of topical NSAIDs. Evidence presented in Chapter 12 for both acute and chronic painful conditions suggests that this may not be correct.

Published randomized control trials (RCTs) on chronic pain conditions (mainly knee osteoarthritis) studied over 1000 subjects treated with topical NSAIDs or placebo. For analgesic effects the NNT was 3.1 (2.7–3.8) [8].

Having this evidence shows how we may begin to re-think our treatment options. We might, for instance, want to start with a prescription of paracetamol, moving on to topical nonsteroidals, oral non-steroidal, and oral non-steroidal plus mucosoprotective agent, depending on the severity of the condition and on patient characteristics. Effectiveness of treatment becomes one dimension of treatment to be examined alongside adverse effects and cost. We might even see the evidence to date as setting the research agenda for tomorrow, testing the effectiveness of a package of care.

Opioids

In chronic pain there are two particular problems with opioids [9]. The first is that adequate doses are often not available or are not given, primarily because of fears of addiction. The second is that some (rarer) chronic pain states, particularly when the nervous system is damaged, may not respond fully to opioids.

Opioids used for people who are not in pain can induce physical and psychological dependence. This does not happen to patients who receive them for pain relief, for instance after an operation or for severe pain from osteoporotic vertebral collapse. Some governments restrict medical availability on the grounds that if the drugs are available medically this will worsen the street addiction problem. There is no evidence for this. The casualties are patients who are deprived of adequate pain relief.

In chronic pain, opioids are usually given by mouth. The dose is worked out by titration over a period of days, and then the drug is given regularly, not waiting for the pain to come back. Initial problems with nausea or dizziness commonly settle. If constipation is likely laxatives are given.

Patients who cannot swallow can try sublingual, transdermal, or suppository dosing. Subcutaneous infusion, usually from a small (external) pump is used for terminal patients who cannot manage these other routes. Rarely, the epidural route is used for combination infusion of opioid and local anaesthetic.

If patients' pain starts to increase the dose is increased. If sensible dose increases do not produce pain relief, or if increasing the opioid dose provokes intolerable or unmanageable adverse effects, then other methods have to be considered, either as well as the opioid or instead of it. A working rule is that if the pain is in a numb area, which is a marker for a damaged nervous system, we would be less confident that opioids would necessarily produce pain relief [10], and our threshold for using other strategies would be lower.

Unconventional analgesics

Unconventional analgesics [11] are drugs which have other indications in other medical settings, and are not normally thought of as analgesics. Treating chronic pain in a tertiary hospital setting we use these drugs for about one-third of our patients. The hallmark is pain in a numb area, neuropathic pain.

When the patient has symptoms and signs of nervous system damage in the area of their pain we expect the response to conventional analgesics to be reduced. Conventional analgesics have often failed already, which is why the patient has been referred. If not, we try them, before we embark on empirical testing to see if any of the unconventional analgesics can provide relief.

Antidepressants

Antidepressants work on the nervous system to relieve depression. We use them in much lower dosage (about half) to relieve pain. Classically, they were used to relieve pain that was burning rather than shooting in character, and anticonvulsants were used for shooting pains. Now we tend to use antidepressants as first-line treatment for both types of pain, because we have greater success and we believe (but see Chapter 31) that antidepressants cause fewer adverse effects.

Anticonvulsants

Anticonvulsants have been used for many years to treat the shooting pains of trigeminal neuralgia and of diabetic neuropathy. How they work has never been clear. The catch-all explanation was that they stabilised nerve membranes, preventing them carrying spurious messages. The current fashionable explanation is that these drugs acting as antagonists on the N-methyl-D-aspartate (NMDA) mechanism.

Anticonvulsants can provide good relief in neuropathic pain (Chapter 30). Doses required for analgesic effect are close to the anticonvulsant dosing range, and carry a perceived burden of adverse effects.

Others

Clonidine and other alpha-2 adrenergic agonists have analgesic effects, both in conventional pain and in neuropathic pain [12]. They extend the duration of local anaesthetic effect and have a synergistic effect with opioids. Their clinical utility is limited by the adverse effects of sedation and hypotension. In neuropathic pain single doses of clonidine were effective in postherpetic neuralgia [13], and in cancer pain [14]. Baclofen is used by intrathecal pump to treat the painful spasms of cerebral palsy. Ketamine and dextromethorphan, both drugs with NMDA antagonist action, are being used in severe neuropathic pain.

Block nerve transmission: reversible

Local anaesthetics

Local anaesthetics block nerve conduction reversibly. When the local anaesthetic wears off the pain returns. This is the pharmacologically correct statement, but another old saying, that a series of local anaesthetic blocks can be used to 'break the cycle' of pain and effect a cure, now has some empirical support [15], even if we do not understand the mechanism.

Arner and colleagues showed that the duration of pain relief could far outlast the duration of local anaesthetic action, and that prolonged relief could result from a series of blocks [15]. Local anaesthetic blocks can thus be diagnostic and therapeutic. Diagnosis of pain for instance from a 'trapped' lateral cutaneous nerve of thigh can be confirmed by local anaesthetic block, and a series of blocks may prevent pain recurring.

Pain clinics use such blocks commonly, for shoulder pain (suprascapular nerve block [16] or intra-articular [17]), for intercostal neuralgia, for rectus sheath nerve entrapment, postoperative scar pains and other peripheral neuralgias (Table 2). What is not clear is the extent to which adding steroid to the local anaesthetic makes a difference, either prolonging the duration of effect of a particular procedure or increasing the chance of success of a series of blocks.

Fibromyalgia

Similar injections are done for the trigger points of fibromyalgia, but there do not appear to be any controlled comparisons of injections with other treatments.

Intravenous regional sympathectomy

Intravenous regional sympathetic blocks (IRSBs) are used widely in patients with reflex sympathetic dystrophy (RSD). A systematic review of 7 RCTs of IRSBs found that none of the four guanethidine trials showed significant analgesic effect. Two reports, one using ketanserin and one bretylium with 17 patients in total, showed some advantage of IRSBs over control [18]. Adding guanethidine in IRSBs does not appear to be more effective than local anaesthetic alone (Chapter 26).

Table 2 Common nerve blocks

Block	Common indications
Trigger point	Focal pain (e.g. in muscle)
Peripheral	Pain in dermatomal distribution
• intercostal	
• sacral nerves	
• rectus sheath	
Extradural	Uni- or bilateral pain (lumbosacral, cervical, thoracic, etc.) Midline perineal pain.
Intrathecal	Unilateral pain (neurolytic injection for pain due to malignancy, limbs, chest, etc.). Midline perineal pain.
Autonomic	
Intravenous regional sympathectomy	Reflex sympathetic dystrophy
Stellate ganglion	Reflex sympathetic dystrophy Arm pain Brachial plexus nerve compression
Lumbar sympathetic	Reflex sympathetic dystrophy Lumbosacral plexus nerve compression Vascular insufficiency lower limb Perineal pain
Coeliac plexus	Abdominal pain

Epidural steroids and facet joint blocks

Two other common (for back pain) pain clinic procedures are epidural steroid injection and facet nerve blocks. Epidural steroids in back pain have been studied in two systematic reviews [19, 20], and are covered in Chapter 27.

Classically facet joint injection with local anaesthetic and steroid is indicated when pain is worse when sitting, and pain is provoked by lateral rotation and spine extension. Recent studies suggest that whether or not the injection is actually in the facet joint makes little difference [21], and indeed cast some doubt on long-term utility [22]. Short-lived success (less than six weeks) with local anaesthetic and steroid is said to be improved by use of cryoanalgesia or radiofrequency blocks to the nerves to the joints.

Block nerve transmission: irreversible

The destructive procedures are aimed at cutting, burning, or damaging (Table 1) the nerve fibres carrying the pain signals. The flaw in the logic is that the nervous system can all too often rewire, finding a way around the lesion. If that happens, and the pain returns, then it may be even more difficult to manage—severe neuropathic pain can result. In general, neurolytic blocks in non-malignant pain are not recommended, because they do not last forever, and recurrent pain may be more difficult to manage, and because of the morbidity. In cancer pain, these neurolytic block procedures do have a place, when there is a short (< 3 month) prognosis, or where alternatives, such as pains-taking drug control or long-term epidural infusion, are not possible. Similar distinction between cancer and non-cancer pain holds for coeliac plexus block in pancreatic pain. Pain associated with pancreatic cancer responds well to coeliac plexus block [23], and it may also help those with abdominal or perineal pain from tumour in the pelvis. In chronic pancreatitis results are much less convincing.

The limitation is the potential for motor and sphincter damage. This risk is higher with bilateral and repeat procedures, and higher the lower the cord level of the block. Extradural neurolytics have limited efficacy. Although claims have been made that the paravertebral approach is preferable, patchy results may be attributed to unpredictable injectate spread. Our results of spinal infusion of a combination of local anaesthetic and opioid are superior to neurolytic blocks, providing good analgesia with minimal irreversible morbidity.

Surgery

The relevant neurosurgical interventions for orthopaedic pain include dorsal column stimulation, rhizotomy, cordotomy, and dorsal root entry zone (DREZ) lesions. The indications are usually non-malignant neuropathic pain which has failed to respond to pharmacological measures. The difficulties of trials of uncommon surgical procedures are well known. These procedures are usually documented by glowing case series. Longer-term outcomes may not be so good [24].

Alternative analgesics

TENS, acupuncture

The rationale for transcutaneous nerve stimulation (TENS) is the gate theory [25]. If the spinal cord is bombarded with impulses from the TENS machine then it is distracted from transmitting the pathological pain signal. We know from Chapter 20 that TENS has limited efficacy in acute (and postoperative) pain, and also in labour pain (Chapter 21). Chapter 25 reports an ongoing systematic review of the many trials in chronic pain.

What we do know is that attention to detail makes considerable difference to TENS efficacy in chronic pain [26]. Patients need to be told that it is useless expecting success unless the machine is connected for at least an hour at a time. They need to be told where to put the electrodes, how to put them on, how to manipulate the stimulus to best advantage, and indeed to turn the machine on.

Three systematic reviews discuss acupuncture in chronic non-malignant pain [27–29]. These show an effect, but that effect in clinical practice is often short-lived (3 days), and is therefore expensive in time. It is difficult to know what is the real place of acupuncture, like other complementary interventions, because of the lack of trials comparing complementary with mainstream procedures. In this context, see the systematic review by Puett and Griffin [30].

Physiotherapy and variants

Pain clinics keep a very open mind about other interventions. If patients benefit from alternatives we are only too pleased. The evidence from back pain, however, suggests that on rigorous outcome measures physiotherapy and other forms of manipulation have but limited success. Such analyses often did not include any measure of quality of life. If they make the patient feel better and they are cheap then it is a decision for the third party payer whether or not these physiotherapy manoeuvres should be offered. Systematic reviews include references 31–39.

Behavioural management

Back 'schools' through to behavioural management programmes offer a range of help for patients to cope with their (usually back) pain problems. Making decisions about the benefits of psychologically based treatments of medical problems are not easy, and are especially difficult to compare with other treatments and to measure relative benefit and cost.

Patients whose pain has proved intractable to all reasonable medical and other interventions are chronic consumers of health care—general practitioner or hospital clinic time, analgesic and psychotropic drugs, repeated admissions, and sometimes surgery. If rehabilitation treatment enables these patients to carry on more satisfying lives with minimum medical help, how can it be most effectively and economically offered?

Randomized comparison of the St. Thomas' (London) 4-week inpatient treatment with 8-week half-day outpatient treatment, with fitness training, planned increases in activity,

activity scheduling, drug reduction, relaxation, and cognitive therapy as the pain management methods taught by the same staff team [40] showed that for every three patients treated as inpatients rather than outpatients, one patient fewer was taking analgesic or psychotropic drugs. For every four patients treated as inpatients rather than outpatients, one patient fewer sought additional medical advice in the year after treatment. For every five patients treated as inpatients rather than outpatients, one patient more had a 10-minute walking distance improved by more than 50%. For every six patients treated as inpatients rather than outpatients, one patient fewer was depressed [41, 42].

Systematic reviews in this area include references 43–50.

References

1. Gøtzsche PC. Patients' preference in indomethacin trials: an overview. *Lancet* 1989; **1**:88–91.
2. Henry D, Lim LL, Rodriguez LAG, Gutthann SP, Carson JL, Griffin M *et al.* Variability in risk of gastrointestinal complications with individual nonsteroidal anti-inflammatory drugs: results of a collaborative meta-analysis. *British Medical Journal* 1996; **312**:1563–6.
3. Silverstein FE, Graham D.Y., Senior JR, Davies HW, Struthers BJ, Bittman RM *et al.* Misoprostol reduces serious gastrointestinal complications in patients with rheumatoid arthritis receiving nonsteroidal anti-inflammatory drugs. *Annals of Internal Medicine* 1995; **123**:241–9.
4. Shield MJ, Morant SV. Misoprostol in patients taking nonsteroidal anti-inflammatory drugs. *British Medical Journal* 1996; **312**:846.
5. Eisenberg E, Berkey CS, Carr DB, Mosteller F, Chalmers TC. Efficacy and safety of nonsteroidal antiinflammatory drugs for cancer pain: a meta-analysis. *Journal of Clinical Oncology* 1994; **12**:2756–65.
6. March L, Irwig L, Schwarz J, Simpson J, Chock C, Brooks P.N of 1 trials comparing a non-steroidal antiinflammatatory drug with paracetamol in osteoarthritis. *British Medical Journal* 1994; **309**:1041–6.
7. Kjærsgaard-Andersen P, Nafei A, Skov O, Madsen F, Andersen HM, Krøner K *et al.* Codeine plus paracetamol versus paracetamol in longer-term treatment of chronic pain due to osteoarthritis of the hip. *Pain* 1990; **43**:309–18.
8. Moore RA, Carroll D, Wiffen PJ, Tramèr M, McQuay HJ. A systematic review of topically-applied non-steroidal anti-inflammatory drugs. *British Medical Journal*. in press.
9. McQuay HJ. Opioids in chronic pain. *British Journal of Anaesthesia* 1989; **63**:213–26.
10. Jadad AR, Carroll D, Glynn CJ, Moore RA, McQuay HJ. Morphine responsiveness of chronic pain: double-blind randomised crossover study with patient-controlled analgesia. *Lancet* 1992; **339**:1367–71.
11. McQuay HJ. Pharmacological treatment of neuralgic and neuropathic pain. *Cancer Surveys* 1988; **7**:141–59.
12. McQuay HJ. Is there a place for alpha 2 adrenergic agonists in the control of pain? In: Besson JM, Guilbaud G, ed. *Toward the use of alpha2 adrenergic agonists for the treatment of pain.* Amsterdam: Elsevier, 1992:219–32.
13. Max MB, Schafer SC, Culnane M, Dubner R, Gracely RH. Association of pain relief with drug side effects in postherpetic neuralgia: a single dose study of clonidine, codeine, ibuprofen, and placebo. *Clinical Pharmacology and Therapeutics* 1988; **43**:363–71.
14. Eisenach JC, DuPen S, Dubois M, Miguel R, Allin D. Epidural clonidine analgesia for intractable cancer pain. The Epidural Clonidine Study Group. *Pain* 1995; **61**:391–9.
15. Arner A, Lindblom U, Meyerson BA, Molander C. Prolonged relief of neuralgia after regional anesthetic blocks. A call for further experimental and systematic clinical studies. *Pain* 1990; **43**:287–97.
16. Emery P, Bowman S, Wedderburn L, Grahame R. Suprascapular nerve block for chronic shoulder pain in rheumatoid arthritis. *British Medical Journal* 1989; **299**:1079–80.
17. van der Heijden CJM, van der Windt DAW, Kleijnen J, Koes BW, Bouter LM. Steroid injections for shoulder disorders: a systematic review of randomized clinical trials. *British Journal of General Practice* 1996; **46**:309–16.
18. Jadad AR, Carroll D, Glynn CJ, McQuay HJ. Intravenous regional sympathetic blockade for pain relief in reflex sympathetic dystrophy: a systematic review and a randomized, double-blind crossover study. *Journal of Pain and Symptom Management* 1995; **10**:13–20.
19. Watts RW, Silagy CA. A meta-analysis on the efficacy of epidural corticosteroids in the treatment of sciatica. *Anaesthesia and Intensive Care* 1995; **23**:564–9.
20. Koes BW, Scholten RPM, Mens JMA, Bouter LM. Efficacy of epidural steroid injections for low-back pain and sciatica: a systematic review of randomized clinical trials. *Pain* 1995; **63**:279–88.
21. Lilius G, Laasonen EM, Myllynen P, Harilainen A, Grönlund G. Lumbar facet joint syndrome. *Journal of Bone and Joint Surgery* 1989; **71**:681–4.
22. Carette S, Marcoux S, Truchon R, Grondin C, Gagnon J, Allard Y *et al.* A controlled trial of corticosteroid injections into facet joints for chronic low back pain. *New England Journal of Medicine* 1991; **325**:1002–7.
23. Eisenberg E, Carr DB, Chalmers TC. Neurolytic celiac plexus block for treatment of cancer pain: a meta-analysis. *Anesthesia and Analgesia* 1995; **80**:290–5.
24. Abram SE. 1992 Bonica Lecture. Advances in chronic pain management since gate control. *Regional Anesthesia* 1993; **18**:66–81.
25. Melzack R, Wall PD. Pain mechanisms: a new theory. *Science* 1965; **150**:971–8.
26. Johnson MI, Ashton CH, Thompson JW. Long term use of transcutaneous electrical nerve stimulation at Newcastle Pain Relief Clinic. *Journal of the Royal Society of Medicine* 1992; **85**:267–8.
27. Patel M, Gutzwiller F, Paccaud F, Marazzi A. A meta-analysis of acupuncture for chronic pain. *International Epidemiology* 1989; **18**:900–6.
28. Ter Riet G, Kleijnen J, Knipschild P. Acupuncture and chronic pain: a criteria-based meta-analysis. *Journal of Clinical Epidemiology* 1990; **43**:1191–9.
29. BhattSanders D. Acupuncture for rheumatoid arthritis: an analysis of the literature. *Seminars Arthritis and Rheumatism* 1985; **14**:225–31.
30. Puett DW, Griffin MR. Published trials of nonmedicinal and noninvasive therapies for hip and knee osteoarthritis. *Annals of Internal Medicine* 1994; **121**:133–40.
31. Abenhaim L, Bergeron AM. Twenty years of randomized clinical trials of manipulative therapy for back pain: a review. *Clinical and Investigative Medicine* 1992; **15**:527–35.
32. Anderson R, Meeker WC, Wirick BE, Mootz RD, Kirk DH, Adams A. A meta-analysis of clinical trials of spinal manipulation. *Journal of Manipulative and Physiological Therapeutics* 1992; **15**:181–94.

33. Assendelft WJ, Koes BW, Van der Heijden GJ, Bouter LM. The efficacy of chiropractic manipulation for back pain: blinded review of relevant randomized clinical trials. *Journal of Manipulative and Physiological Therapeutics* 1992; **15**:487–94.

34. Brunarski DJ. Clinical trials of spinal manipulation: a critical appraisal and review of the literature. *Journal of Manipulative and Physiological Therapeutics* 1984; **7**:243–9.

35. Koes BW, Assendelft WJ, van der Heijden GJ, Bouter LM, Knipschild PG. Spinal manipulation and mobilisation for back and neck pain: a blinded review. *British Medical Journal* 1991; **303**:1298–303.

36. Koes BW, Bouter LM, Beckerman H, van der Heijden G, Knipschild PG. Physiotherapy exercises and back pain: a blinded review. *British Medical Journal* 1991; **302**:1572–6.

37. Ottenbacher K, DiFabio RP. Efficacy of spinal manipulation/mobilization therapy. A meta analysis. *Spine* 1985; **10**:833–7.

38. Powell FC, Hanigan WC, Olivero WC. A risk/benefit analysis of spinal manipulation therapy for relief of lumbar or cervical pain. *Neurosurgery* 1993; **33**:73–8; discussion 78–9.

39. Shekelle PG, Adams AH, Chassin MR, Hurwitz EL, Brook RH. Spinal manipulation for low-back pain *Annals of Internal Medicine* 1992; **117**:590–8.

40. Pither CE, Nicholas MK. Psychological approaches in chronic pain management. *British Medical Journal* 1991; **47**:743–61.

41. Bandolier. More wisdom. *Bandolier* Issue 22, December 1995.

42. McQuay HJ, Moore RA, Eccleston C, Morley S, de C Williams AC. Systematic review of outpatient services for chronic pain control. *Health Technology Assessment* 1997; **1**(6).

43. Cohen JE, Goel V, Frank JW, Bombardier C, Peloso P, Guillemin F. Group education interventions for people with low back pain. An overview of the literature. *Spine* 1994; **19**:1214–22.

44. Cutler RB, Fishbain DA, Rosomoff HL, Abdel-Moty E, Khalil TM, Rosomoff RS. Does nonsurgical pain center treatment of chronic pain return patients to work? A review and meta-analysis of the literature. *Spine* 1994; **19**:643–52.

45. Fernandez E, Turk DC. The utility of cognitive coping strategies for altering pain perception: a meta analysis. *Pain* 1989; **38**:123–35.

46. Gebhardt WA. Effectiveness of training to prevent job-related back pain: a meta-analysis. *British Journal of Clinical Psychology* 1994; **33**:571–4.

47. Hyman RB, Feldman HR, Harris RB, Levin RF, Malloy GB. The effects of relaxation training on clinical symptoms: a meta analysis. *Nursing Research* 1989; **38**:216–20.

48. Malone MD, Strube MJ, Scogin FR. Meta analysis of non medical treatments for chronic pain. *Pain* 1988; **34**: 231–44.

49. Mullen PD, Laville EA, Biddle AK, Lorig K. Efficacy of psycho-educational interventions on pain, depression, and disability in people with arthritis: a meta analysis. *Journal of Rheumatology* 1987; **14**(suppl.):33–9.

50. Suls J, Fletcher B. The relative efficacy of avoidant and nonavoidant coping strategies: a meta analysis. *Health and Psychology* 1985; **4**:249–88.

24

Radiotherapy for painful bone metastases

Summary

For this systematic review of randomized controlled trials (RCTs) we assessed pain relief from:

1. Localized bone metastases achieved by radiotherapy, comparing the efficacy of different fractionation schedules.
2. More generalized metastatic disease achieved by radiotherapy or radioisotopes.

Thirteen trials reported on 40 different radiotherapy fractionation schedules and four studies of radioisotopes. Radiotherapy produced complete pain relief at one month in 368/1373 (27%) patients, and at least 50% relief in 628/1486 (42%) patients at some time during the trials. There was no difference between single or multiple fraction schedules in the proportions of patients achieving these outcomes. The number-needed-to-treat (NNT) to achieve complete relief at one month (compared with an assumed natural history of 1 in 100 patients whose pain resolved without treatment) was 3.9 (95% confidence interval 3.5–4.4). No pooled estimates of speed of onset of relief, or of its duration, could be obtained. In the largest trial (759 patients) 52% of those who had complete relief had achieved it within four weeks, and the median duration of complete relief was 12 weeks. For more generalized disease radioisotopes produced similar analgesic results to external irradiation.

Adverse effect reporting was poor. There were no obvious differences between the various fractionation schedules in the incidence of nausea and vomiting, diarrhoea, or pathological fractures.

Radiotherapy is clearly effective at reducing pain from painful bone metastases. There was no evidence of any difference in efficacy between different fractionation schedules, nor indeed of a dose-response with total dose of radiation. For treatment of generalized bone pain both hemibody irradiation and radioisotopes can reduce the number of painful new sites.

Introduction

Radiotherapy is used commonly to provide pain relief for localized painful bone metastases [2]. Received wisdom is that at least 75% of patients achieve pain relief, and that about half of those who achieve relief stay free from pain [3]. The difficulty in providing accurate estimates of the proportion achieving relief, the extent of that relief and its duration stems in part from the variation in the site and extent of the bone metastases, in the primary cancer, and from other contemporaneous interventions. Patients also take analgesics, and the precise contribution from the radiotherapy and the co-interventions may be unclear.

The primary aim of the review was to provide the best estimate of the pain relief which patients with bone metastases can expect from radiotherapy, its extent, onset time, and duration. Secondary aims were to examine differences in effect and in adverse effect incidence between different radiotherapy fractionation schedules.

Methods

Published randomized controlled trials (RCTs) of radiotherapy in the palliative treatment of painful bone metastases were identified; radiotherapy was taken to include both external irradiation and administration of isotopes. A number of different search strategies were used to identify eligible reports in MEDLINE (1966–March 1996), the Oxford Pain Relief Database (1950–94), EMBASE, and the Cochrane Library. The words: 'RANDOM' and 'PAIN' were used with 'RADIOTHERAPY', 'RADIATION', 'ISOTOPE' and 'STRONTIUM' in searching, in a broad free text search including combinations of these words, and without restriction to language. Additional reports were identified from the reference lists of retrieved reports and review articles. Inclusion criteria were full journal articles of the palliative treatment of painful bone metastases with pain outcomes and randomized study.

Abstracts, review articles, and textbooks were not considered. Unpublished reports were not sought. Reports of the relief of pain conditions other than painful bone metastases were excluded. Authors were not contacted.

Each report which could possibly meet the inclusion criteria was read by each author independently and scored for inclusion and methodological quality using a three-item scale [4].

Included reports

Reports compared different fractionation radiotherapy schedules, or radiotherapy versus isotope injection or isotope injection versus placebo. Information about inclusion criteria, number of patients, fractionation schedule, and drugs, route, and doses used was extracted from the reports, together with information on analgesic measurements and

The topic discussed in this chapter is also published in full in McQuay et al. [1].

results. Fractionation schedules are quoted as total dose/ number of fractions/time interval. Adverse effect information was also noted.

Information about pain relief was used in two ways. To estimate the overall efficacy of radiotherapy for palliation of painful bone metastases numbers of patients achieving complete relief (no pain) at one month were compared with an assumed natural history of 1 in 100 patients achieving pain relief without treatment, to obtain the number-needed-to-treat (NNT). The NNT was used to answer the question 'How well does this intervention work compared with nothing?', and was calculated with its 95% confidence intervals [5].

To estimate the relative efficacy of different fractionation schedules, the numbers of patients achieving at least 50% relief at any time during the trial were obtained, by using the top categories of the scales used in the trials, for instance good or excellent on a scale of none, some, good, excellent.

Results

The trials

Thirteen trials were included (Table 1). Ten included reports (40) of different radiotherapy fractionation schedules and four investigated isotopes. Four reports were excluded. Three were excluded because they were not restricted to management of painful bone metastases, MRC 1991 [6] and MRC 1992 [7] investigated lung cancer and Young *et al.* 1980 [8] compared laminectomy with radiotherapy for the treatment of epidural metastases. Poulter *et al.* 1992 [9] studied hemibody plus local field irradiation for bone metastases, but did not have pain outcomes.

The validated quality scale includes points for blinding. Blinding is not possible for radiotherapy interventions. The median quality score of 2 for these studies should be judged against a maximum of 3 rather than 5. In extracting pain data we made no distinction between patient judgement and physician judgement, although in purist terms patient judgement is preferred.

Analgesia one month after radiotherapy: complete pain relief or 50% pain relief

Information about the incidence of complete pain relief at one month was obtained from five trials. Radiotherapy produced complete pain relief at one month in 368/1373 (27%) patients. Compared with an assumed rate of 1 in 100 patients having naturally resolving pain, external irradiation, independent of fractionation schedule, gave an NNT of 3.9 (95% confidence interval 3.5–4.4). One patient in four given radiotherapy will get complete relief at one month who would not have obtained relief without radiotherapy.

An outcome of at least 50% pain relief at one month, rather than complete relief, was achieved by 437/1486 (29%)

patients, with an NNT of 3.6 (3.2–3.9). The slight improvement in NNT, from 3.9 to 3.6, when the less stringent outcome of at least 50% relief at one month rather than complete relief was used, may be due to the fact that there was data from only 113 additional patients for the less stringent outcome.

Analgesic effect of radiotherapy at any time during the study

The number of patients obtaining at least 50% pain relief at any time during the studies was obtained for 23 treatment groups in the various included trials. Overall (independent of fractionation schedule), radiotherapy produced at least 50% relief in 628/1486 (42%) patients (Fig. 1).

Analysing the various fractionation schedules radiotherapy produced at least 50% pain relief in a median of 49% of patients (range 28–81%), with little difference between the schedules (Fig. 1). Taking single fraction schedules only (five treatment groups) the median percentage of patients achieving at least 50% pain relief was 45% (range 36–81%), and for multiple fraction schedules (17 treatment groups) the median was 49% (range 28–68%).

Speed of onset of relief and duration

Taking the trials together did not yield good estimates either of the speed of onset of the analgesia after radiotherapy or of its duration. The estimates from the biggest trial [18], were that half the patients who achieved complete relief took more than 4 weeks to achieve it, and the median duration of relief in that study (759 evaluable patients), was 12 weeks for complete relief.

Radioisotopes and radiotherapy for generalized disease

Radioisotopes alone (192 patients, 3 trials) produced similar extent of relief with similar onset and duration to that provided by radiotherapy. In two trials [22, 23] the striking finding was of significantly fewer new pain sites in the strontium groups compared with controls. Both hemibody irradiation and radioisotopes have the potential to reduce the number of new sites of bone pain [9, 22, 23]. The radioisotopes do have increased haematological toxicity [20]. Quality of life scores were better for radiotherapy plus strontium than for radiotherapy plus placebo [22].

Adverse effects

Adverse effect reporting was poor. There were no obvious differences between the various fractionation schedules in the incidence of nausea and vomiting, diarrhoea, or pathological fractures.

Table 1 Details of reports included

Ref.	Treatments compared total dose/fractions/ time (no.)	Patients & co-interventions	Pain relief & adverse effects	Quality score
Single fraction vs. single fraction				
[10]	4 Gy/1f (137); 8 Gy/1f (133)	Bony metastases; 72% & 81% had moderate or severe baseline pain; median survival 8 months; co-interventions not specified.	Complete response as 3, 2, or 1 to 0 achieved on 4 Gy 25/98 at 4 wks, 31/86 at 8 wks, 27/75 at 12 wks, for 8 Gly 22/96, 21/75 and 26/66. 28 (20%) of 4 Gy were retreated within 12 wks, 12 (9%) of 8 Gly. No clear dose- response, no AE data.	3
Single fraction vs. multiple fractions				
[11]	8 Gy/1f (16); 24 Gy/6f/2–3 wks (13)	Painful bony metastases; no previous RT.	5-pt categorical PI scale. 13/16 single fraction patients improved by more than 2 categories, 8/13 multiple fractions. NSD between sf and mf at 1 or 6 months. Nausea & vomiting in 33% mf 70% sf, diarrhoea and skin problems in 22% mf, 30% sf.	1
[12]	Single f (14) vs. multiple f (13); doses depended on site (31 patients total; 27 followed up for > 8 wks)	Painful bony metastases. Baseline pain intensity score of 2 in 13 patients, and 3 in 10 patients.	Complete response, not defined clearly, was achieved in 12/27. There was NSD between the two schedules. Nausea and vomiting; 2/14 sf 3/13 mf. Diarrhoea 3/14 sf, 2/13 mf.	2
[13]	8 Gy/1f (140); 30 Gy/10f/2wks (148)	Painful bony metastases; hormonal, chemo, or RT in 30/140 sf, 21/148 mf.	Complete response was achieved in 22/49 sf and in 12/43 mf patients at 180 das (NSD). 23 sf and 20 mf had pathological fractures. No diff in 'acute morbidity' between schedules.	2
Multiple fractions vs. multiple fractions				
[14]	25 Gy/5f 1wks; 30 GY/10f/2wks; 128 patients in total	Bony metastases; no co-intervention data.	RTOG pain scores. There was NSD between the pain relief provided by the two schedules. No dichotomous data. Analysed on big field size, lumbar spine and pelvis subgroup only. Significantly more nausea and vomiting on 25 Gy/5f.	2
[15]	20 Gy/2f/1wks (27); 24 Gy/6f/3wks (30);	Painful bony mets; 27/57 had mod/sev pain at baseline (categorized VAS); co-interventions controlled out.	Satisfactory response (at least 1 step down on the category scale for at least 4 wks) in 27/57. Maximal response in 5/27 on 2f, 8/30 on 6f (NSD). Nausea slight 16/57, severe 2. Skin erythema 6, paraparesis 1.	2
[16]	20 Gy/10f/3wks (23); 22.5 Gy/5f/3wks (32); 30 Gy/15f/3wks (25); 80 patients, 92 painful sites	Painful bony metastases.	5-pt catPI, and judging response as excellent (pain disappeared) or good (2 category fall), 47/80 patients achieved excellent or good response. NSD between schedules. ? faster relief with 5 or 10 than with 15f.	2
[17]	15 Gy/3f/2wks (100); 30 Gy/10f/2wks (100);	Painful bony metastases. Breast cancer 217, randomized, 200 evaluable. 80% had moderate or strong PT at baseline.	RTOG criteria; limited (70%) compliance for pain data. Of 127 patients evaluated at 1 mth, 60% had no or light PI, and same for 60% of 27 evaluated at a year. NSD between schedules. 'Very modest' AEs.	2
[18]	Solitary metastases: 266 (146 evaluable) 45 Gy/15f/3wks (74); 20 Gy/5f/1wk (72); Multiple Metastases; 750 (613 evaluable); 15 Gy/5f/1wk (143); 20 Gy/5f/1wk (155); 25 Gy/5f/1wk (148); 30 Gy/10f/2wks (167)	Bony metastases any primary; 99% had pain severity × frequency score of 4; 56% in worst pain category (9); chemotherapy to 28% of the multiple metastases patients and to 12% of the solitary during the 4 wks of the study. Overall, 9% had steroids.	Complete relief (pain score fell to zero) in 325/613 patients ?when, 48% of those with complete relief took >4 wks to achieve it (inc. treatment time). NSD between schedules. Relief for median 12 wks (complete); 54% relapsed.	2

Table 1 *continued*

Ref.	Treatments compared total dose/fractions time (no.)	Patients & co-interventions	Pain relief & adverse effects	Quality score
Strontium (Sr) + Rhenium (Re)				
[20]	Cross-over Sr-89 vs. radioactive placebo.	Cross-over; 32 prostate bony metastases (26 evaluable); additional therapy controlled out.	Using a complicated weighted score at 5 wks 5/19 patients had substantial or dramatic improvement on Sr-89, 1/18 on placebo.	5
[21]	Cross-over Re-186 vs. radioactive placebo (methylene diphosphonate).	Cross-over; 20 painful bony metastases, 13 evaluable.	Using RTOG scoring, the mean decrease on pain scoring with Re was 22% at 3 wks, compared with a mean increase on placebo of 39%.	3
[22]	Radiotherapy + Sr-89 (67) or placebo (58); 3 fractionation schedules: 30 Gy/10f/2wks; 20 Gy/5f/1wk; ≤ 10 Gy/1f (ribs); no data on how many patients on each schedule.	126 painful bony metastases prostate cancer; co-interventions controlled out.	RTOG; Re-186 alone complete relief in 36% at 3 mths, 30% at 6 mths; Re-186 + Sr-89 40% (NSD) New metastases at 3 mths in 41% of Re-186 + Sr-89, 66% R.	5
[23]	Local (20 Gy/5f/1wk; 72) or hemibody (6 Gy/1f upper 1/2; 8 Gy/1f lower 1/2; 80) radiotherapy or Sr-89 (153), 305 recruited, 284 treated.	Metastatic prostate cancer.	Weighted pain score, substantial/dramatic improvement at 12 wks or the time of cross-over in 73/123 Sr-89 patients, 16/48 local Re-186 and 14/46 hemibody R. NSD in efficacy. Sig fewer new pain sites with Sr-89.	2

AE, adverse effect; f, fraction; mf, multiple fractions; sf, single fraction; NSD, no significant difference; PI, pain intensity; RT, radiotherapy; RTOG, radiation therapy oncology group.

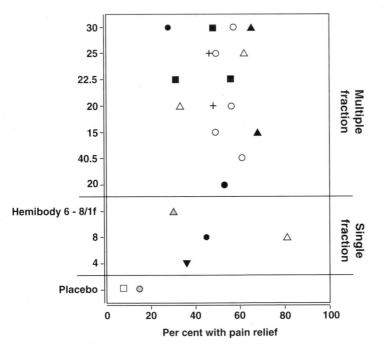 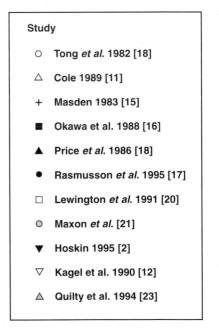

Fig. 1   Percentage of patients achieving at least 50% pain relief (at any time during study) with different radiotherapy schedules (Total dose in Gg).

Comment

Radiotherapy can provide effective analgesia for painful bone metastases. Over 40% of patients can expect at least 50% pain relief, and just under 30% can expect complete pain relief at one month. Given that analgesic drug regimes are often poorly effective for the incident pain associated with bone metastases [24], radiotherapy has a very important role to play.

It is surprising that there is little discernible difference in efficacy between the fractionation schedules and indeed between different doses at the same schedule. It is hoped that an ongoing study [25] will help to untangle this puzzle. We were unable to analyse by histological type. The relationship between radiosensitivity and the probability of successful palliation is unclear.

We wanted to obtain the best possible quantitative estimate, knowing full well that some compromises would have to be made. Radiotherapy for painful bone metastases is not an easy topic. There are many different types of patient with different degrees of illness combined with many different radiotherapy regimens. Placebo treatment is not seen as an ethical option. We believe that a benchmark of current treatment is important as a stimulus to further work, and so that we (and patients) know where we stand.

The rules we adopted were:

1. We used only randomized trials to reduce the largest known source of bias.

2. A quality score is given for each trial using a validated scale. There was no great discrepancy between sizes of trials or their quality so that sensitivity analysis by trial size or quality was irrelevant. Indeed, most studies were of high quality (2 or more on a scale of 1–3, since blinding was not possible).

3. The studies themselves meant that classical pooling was not possible. At the simplest level, there was no common comparator, so it was not possible to pool information between trials. We felt it reasonable to estimate NNT using a sensible estimate of 1% of patients with bone metastases having spontaneously resolving pain. Calculating NNT sums patients from all trials, automatically weighting them.

4. The lack of common comparator meant that we could not use standard approaches such as relative risk or odds ratio, to obtain 'classic' statistical output form meta-analysis.

The compromise is a delicate balance between overcooking inadequate information and overlooking important points.

The clinical choice at present, given equivalent efficacy, must be a balance between adverse effects, the impact of the different schedules on patients' quality of life, prognosis, and cost. Until the pathophysiology of metastatic bone pain and the way in which radiotherapy produces analgesia are understood [2], and until trials of adequate size and quality are reported, these estimates show what clinicians and patients can expect. It is also important to acknowledge the formidable difficulties surrounding clinical trials in this patient group.

References

1. McQuay HJ, Carroll D, Moore RA. Radiotherapy for painful bone metastases: a systematic review. *Clinical Oncology* 1997; 9:150–4

2. Hoskin P. Radiotherapy for bone pain. *Pain* 1995; 63:137–9.

3. Jacox A, Carr DB, Payne R. *Management of cancer pain.* Clinical Practice Guideline No. 9. Agency for Health Care Policy and Research, U.S. Department of Health and Human Services. *AHCPR* Publication No. 94–0592. Rockville, MD: Public Health Service, 1994:41–74.

4. Jadad AR, Moore RA, Carroll D, Jenkinson C, Reynolds DJM, Gavaghan DJ *et al.* Assessing the quality of reports of randomized clinical trials: is blinding necessary? *Controlled Clinical Trials* 1996; 17:1–12.

5. Cook RJ, Sackett DL. The number needed to treat: a clinically useful measure of treatment effect. *British Medical Journal* 1995; 310:452–4.

6. Medical Research Council Lung Cancer Working Party. Inoperable non-small-cell lung cancer (NSCLC): a Medical Research Council randomised trial of palliative radiotherapy with two fractions or ten fractions. Report to the Medical Research Council by its Lung Cancer Working Party. *British Journal of Cancer* 1991; 63:265–70.

7. Medical Research Council Lung Cancer Working Party. A Medical Research Council (MRC) randomised trial of palliative radiotherapy with two fractions or a single fraction in patients with inoperable non-small-cell lung cancer (NSCLC) and poor performance status. *British Journal of Cancer* 1992; 65:934–41.

8. Young RF, Post EM, King GA. Treatment of spinal epidural metastases. Randomized prospective comparison of laminectomy and radiotherapy. *Journal of Neurosurgery* 1980; 53:741–8.

9. Poulter CA, Cosmatos D, Rubin P *et al.* A report of RTOG 8206. *International Journal of Radiation Oncology Biology, Physics* 1992; 23:207–14.

10. Hoskin PJ, Price P, Easton D, Regan J, Austin D, Palmer S *et al.* A prospective randomised trial of 4 Gy or 8 Gy single doses in the treatment of metastatic bone pain. *Radiotherapy and Oncology* 1992; 23:74–8.

11. Cole DJ. A randomized trial of a single treatment versus conventional fractionation in the palliative radiotherapy of painful bone metastases. *Clinical Oncology* 1989; 1:59–62.

12. Kagei K, Suzuki K, Shirato H, Nambu T, Yoshikawa H, Irie G. [A randomized trial of single and multifraction radiation therapy for bone metastasis: a preliminary report]. *Gan No Rinsho* 1990; 36:2553–8.

13. Price P, Hoskin P, Easton D, Austin D, Palmer S, Yarnold J. Prospective randomised trial of single and multifraction radiotherapy schedules in the treatment of painful bony metastases. *Radiotherapy and Oncology* 1986; 6:247–55.

14. Hirokawa Y, Wadasaki K, Kashiwado K, Kagemoto M, Katsuta S, Honke Y *et al.* [A multi institutional prospective randomized study of radiation therapy of bone metastases]. *Nippon Igaku Hoshasen Gakkai Zasshi* 1988; 48:1425–31.

15. Madsen E. Painful bone metastasis: efficacy of radiotherapy assessed by the patients: a randomized trial comparing 4 Gy × 6 versus 10 Gy × 2. *International Journal of Radiation Oncology Biology, Physics* 1983; 9:1775–9.

16. Okawa T, Kita M, Goto M, Nishijima H, Miyaji N. Randomized prospective clinical study of small, large and twice a day fraction radiotherapy for painful bone metastases. *Radiotherapy and Oncology* 1988; 13:99–104.

17. Rasmusson B, Vejborg I, Jensen AB, Andersson M, Banning AM, Hoffmann T *et al.* Irradiation of bone metastases in breast cancer patients: a randomized study with 1 year follow-up. *Radiotherapy and Oncology* 1995; **34**:179–84.

18. Tong D, Gillick L, Hendrickson R. The palliation of symptomatic metastases: Final results of the study by the radiation therapy oncology group. *Cancer* 1982; **50**:893–9.

19. Blitzer PH. Reanalysis of the RTOG study of the palliation of symptomatic osseous metastasis. *Cancer* 1985; **55**:1468–72.

20. Lewington VJ, McEwan AJ, Ackery DM, Bayly RJ, Keeling DH, Macleod PM *et al.* A prospective, randomised double-blind crossover study to examine the efficacy of strontium-89 in pain palliation in patients with advanced prostate cancer metastatic to bone. *European Journal of Cancer* 1991; **27**:954–8.

21. Maxon HR3, Schroder LE, Hertzberg VS, Thomas SR, Englaro EE, Samaratunga R *et al.* Rhenium-186(Sn)HEDP for treatment of painful osseous metastases: results of a double-blind crossover comparison with placebo. *Journal of Nuclear Medicine* 1991; **32**:1877–81.

22. Porter AT, McEwan AJ, Powe JE, Reid R, McGowan DG, Lukka H *et al.* Results of a randomized phase-III trial to evaluate the efficacy of strontium-89 adjuvant to local field external beam irradiation in the management of endocrine resistant metastatic prostate cancer. *International Journal of Radiation Oncology Biology, Physics* 1993; **25**:805–13.

23. Quilty PM, Kirk D, Bolger JJ, Dearnaley DP, Lewington VJ, Mason MD *et al.* A comparison of the palliative effects of strontium-89 and external beam radiotherapy in metastatic prostate cancer. *Radiotherapy and Oncology* 1994; **31**:33–40.

24. McQuay HJ, Jadad AR. Incident Pain. Hanks GW, ed. *Cancer surveys*, Vol. 21. *Palliative medicine problem areas in pain and symptom management*. New York: Cold Spring Harbor Laboratory Press, 1994:17–24.

25. Barton R, Hoskin PJ, Yarnold JR *et al.* Radiotherapy for bone pain: is a single fraction good enough. *Clinical Oncology* 1994; **6**:354–5.

Transcutaneous electrical nerve stimulation (TENS) in chronic pain

Summary

Transcutaneous electrical nerve stimulation (TENS) was originally developed as a way of controlling pain through the 'gate' theory [1]. According to the theory, selective stimulation of certain nerve fibres could block, or 'close the gate' on signals carrying pain impulses to the brain.

TENS is widely used. A survey of 50 Canadian hospitals with 200 or more beds [2] indicates that there may be more than 450 000 uses of TENS in Canadian hospitals each year, with many more in private clinics. This carries substantial cost implications. The characteristics of TENS use are given in Table 1, showing predominant use in physiotherapy.

We could find no systematic review of its use in chronic pain other than that of Reeve et al. [2]. This review examined the use of TENS in acute, labour, and chronic pain, and concluded that TENS has not undergone sufficiently strict and rigorous clinical evaluation—especially what they call the 'purifying heat' of randomized controlled trials.

Quality of methods used in clinical trials has been shown to be a key determinant of the eventual results. Schulz and colleagues [12] have demonstrated that trials that are not randomized or are inadequately randomized exaggerate the estimate of treatment effect by up to 40%. Studies that are not fully blinded can exaggerate the estimate of treatment

effect by up to 17%. TENS can almost never be properly blinded [13], and bias is likely from this source alone.

For analgesic drugs, evidence of effectiveness is sought first in standardized acute pain settings, and after it is established there use moves from acute to chronic conditions. This may not be appropriate for TENS.

TENS in chronic pain

Reports were sought of randomized controlled trials (RCTs) for TENS. A number of different search strategies were used to identify eligible published reports in both MEDLINE (1966–1996) using Knowledge Finder 3.3, CINAHL (using MacSPIRS 2.3), the Oxford Pain Relief Database (1950–94) [14], and EMBASE 1980–96. The latest indexing date used was May 1996. The words: 'TENS', 'TNS' and 'transcutaneous electrical nerve stimulation' were used in searching, including single words and combinations of these words. Searching was done using both MeSH terms and free text words. Additional reports were identified from the reference lists of retrieved reports, review articles, and textbooks.

Included were full journal publications of randomized controlled trials in which the analgesic effects of TENS was studied in patients with chronic pain. Reports where TENS was used under experimental pain conditions and where no clinical pain outcome measurements were used were excluded.

Each report that could possibly meet the inclusion criteria was read by each author independently and scored for inclusion and quality using the three item scale [15].

Several types of controls were found, comparing TENS with sham TENS (no current, distant control points), active interventions (e.g. oral non-steroidal anti-inflammatory drugs), or various combinations of these, and TENS compared to TENS (high vs. low frequency stimulation). Some studies used blinded observers. Although there was no prior hypothesis before the original reports were read that TENS could not be adequately blinded, it was determined at the consensus meeting that, despite the considerable efforts documented in some reports, adequate blinding was practically impossible. Consequently, no report was given any points for blinding, even if they were described as double-blind or used blinded observers. Thus, an included report could have a maximum score of 3 and a minimum score of 1.

Information about the pain condition, the number of patients, study design, and year of publication was extracted from the reports. Type of TENS equipment, duration of each

Table 1   TENS usage in Canadian hospitals

	No. of hospitals	%
Users		
Physiotherapists	43	98
Nurses	7	16
Physicians	2	5
Others	5	11
Departments		
Physiotherapy	39	89
Rehabilitation medicine	6	14
Pain clinics	2	5
Labour and delivery	3	7
Application		
Chronic pain	42	96
Acute pain	41	93
Labour and delivery	19	43
All three	16	36

treatment period, hours of TENS per week, and number of TENS sessions were recorded. High frequency TENS (>10 Hz), low frequency TENS (<10 Hz), continuous or pulse stimulation, intensity of stimulation above or below the sensory threshold, and sites of electrode were identified. Control group design and the use of TENS in these controls was similarly noted. Pain outcomes, overall findings, and conclusions were noted for each report, together with any adverse effect or drop-out information.

A judgement was then made by the authors as to whether the overall conclusion of the report was positive or negative for the analgesic effectiveness of TENS. *Post-hoc* subgroup analysis in the original reports was not considered in our judgement of overall effectiveness.

TENS in chronic pain: results

Thirty-eight randomized control trials (RCTs) on chronic pain were included [16–24, 25 duplicate publication with 26, 27–52, 53 duplicate publication with 54, 55–57]

TENS exposure in these trials was low: duration of treatment was less than four weeks in 83% of the trials. In 85% of trials stimulation was for less than 10 hours per week and 67% of the patients had less than 10 TENS sessions in their trial (Fig. 1).

Ten out of 24 trials comparing TENS with a control (no current, placebo tablets, or control points) were regarded having a positive outcome.

In 3 out of 15 trials comparing TENS with active treatment a positive outcome was noted.

In 10 reports a comparison between frequency and mode was done. In 4 out of 5 trials conventional high frequency TENS equalled low frequency pulsed TENS.

Comment

Methods used in trials of TENS

Although randomization should exclude selection bias in trials, blinding should exclude observer bias. Inadequacy of

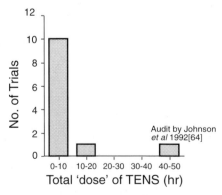

Fig. 1 Number of trials studying different duration (dose) of TENS use.

blinding in clinical trials of analgesic interventions continues to be of concern [61], although this may be less of an issue with pharmacological interventions [62]. Blinding of procedures is much more difficult than blinding of drug studies. Most of the TENS studies did make attempts at blinding, for instance, by removing batteries from the TENS apparatus (sham TENS) or by using staff with no knowledge of the study or allocation to conduct the patient assessments. Lack of blinding has been estimated to exaggerate the estimate of treatment effect of trials by some 17% [12]. Adequate blinding of TENS for both carers and patients is particularly difficult [13].

None of the reports of TENS in chronic pain was judged to have been blinded, and this lowered the quality scores given to the randomized studies. The fact that less than half of the reports showed any positive effect of TENS in acute postoperative pain is all the more striking because of this potential overestimation of treatment effect due to lack of blinding. It is extremely difficult to exclude observer bias in trials of TENS [13], and results must be so judged.

Classic analgesic trial methods study patients given placebo and those given a standard analgesic to establish that the study has sensitivity—that it can actually measure an analgesic response. An analgesic response with a new treatment measured in the same study then has validity. This approach has been found important because group sizes in analgesic trials are usually fewer than 50, so that small differences in the number of responders in placebo or analgesic groups can affect results profoundly. Studies with an A versus B design, as were all those identified with TENS in acute pain and labour, do not have measures of internal sensitivity and this makes the results more difficult to interpret, especially where comparators are not known themselves to be effective (as with comparisons of TENS and sham TENS).

The choice of outcome measure is also an important determinant of how studies are to be judged. TENS is considered to produce pain relief. The most important outcome should therefore be lower pain intensity or greater pain relief. Use of other analgesic interventions is a secondary outcome measure, but one used commonly in these studies. Reduction in analgesic consumption, for example, is an even less direct measure of analgesic effectiveness.

What we are left with, therefore, is the lowest common denominator of information, essentially vote counting rather than a more sophisticated analysis, reflecting the nature of the analgesic scoring methods that predominated in the original reports. Pain scoring using analogue or categorical scales was reported as means (an unreliable statistic [62]), or mean analgesic consumption or time to first analgesic was used. None of these allowed data extraction for further statistical analysis or comparison between reports. While more rigorous pain scoring might have been used, there is no evidence that all of the reports suffered a systematic failure in analgesic measurement.

For TENS in chronic pain, the situation is different. Here we have lack of evidence of effect rather than evidence of lack of effect. The issue is one of dose. Many, perhaps most, chronic pain physicians who use TENS prescribe at least 30 minutes use twice a day for at least a month before any effect may be felt [64]. This pragmatism is supported by the important study of Nash *et al.* [47], who demonstrated a clear improvement in analgesic effects of TENS in a large number of chronic pain patients over a long period of time, and by the audit in Newcastle [64].

None of the randomized trials used doses of TENS which approached this (Fig. 1). Duration of treatment was less than 4 weeks in 83% of the trials and in 85% of the trials stimulation occurred less than 10 hours a week, with 67% of the patients having less than 10 sessions of TENS. Even anecdotal reports of the success of TENS suggest that dose is important; a report in *The Times* by Thomas Stuttaford quoted Grahame Le Saux (then a Blackburn footballer) as using TENS for at least 30 minutes before and after every training session and match to achieve benefit, as well as at other times.

The use of TENS in chronic pain may well be justified, but it cannot be proved. There is a requirement for a randomized trial to address the issue. It will be difficult to design and organize, it will need to be multicentre in the United Kingdom and possibly other European countries, it will require large numbers of patients, and simple outcome measures. Without it a potentially valuable intervention may be under-used, or a useless intervention may continue in use.

Conclusion

TENS may be useful in chronic pain, but there is no useful evidence. A large multicentre randomized trial of TENS with sufficient dose and duration is needed.

References

1. Melzack R, Wall PD. Pain mechanisms: a new theory. *Science* 1965; **150**:971–8.
2. Reeve J, Menon D, Corabian P. Transcutaneous electrical nerve stimulation (TENS): a technology assessment. *International Journal of Technology Assessment in Health Care* 1996; **12**:299–324.
3. Acute Pain Management Guideline Panel. *Acute pain management: operative or medical procedures and trauma.* Clinical Practice Guideline No. 1. Agency for Health Care Policy and Research, U.S. Department of Health and Human Services. *AHCPR* Publication No. 92-0032. Rockville, MD: Public Health Service, 1992:24–5.
4. Royal College of Surgeons of England, the College of Anaesthetists. *Report of the working party on pain after surgery.* London: Royal College of Surgeons, 1990.
5. McCaffery M, Beebe A. *Pain: a clinical manual for nursing practice.* St. Louis, MD: C.V. Mosby 1989.
6. Charman RA. Physiotherapy for the relief of pain. In: Carroll D, Bowsher D, ed. *Pain management and nursing care.* Oxford: Butterworth-Heinemann, 1993:146–65.
7. Chaney ES. The management of postoperative pain. In: Wells P, Frampton V, Bowsher D, ed. *Pain: management and control in physiotherapy.* Oxford: Heinemann, 1988:253–68.
8. Park G, Fulton B. *The management of acute pain.* Oxford University Press, 1991.
9. Woolf CJ, Thomson JW. Stimulation-induced analgesia: transcutaneous electrical nerve stimulation (TENS) and vibration.

In: Wall PD, Melzack R, ed. *Textbook of pain*, (3rd ed). Edinburgh: Churchill Livingstone, 1994:1191–1217. [1671]
10. Justins DM, Richardson PH. Clinical management of acute pain. *British Medical Bulletin* 1991; **47**:561–83.
11. Carroll D, Tramer M, McQuay H, Nye B, Moore A. Transcutaneous electrical nerve stimulation in labour pain: A systematic review. *British Journal of Obstetrics and Gynaecology* 1997; **104**:169–75.
12. Schulz KF, Chalmers I, Hayes RJ, Altman DG. Empirical evidence of bias: dimensions of methodological quality associated with estimates of treatment effects in controlled trials. *Journal of the American Medical Association* 1995; **273**:408–12.
13. Deyo RA, Walsh NE, Schoenfeld LS, Ramamurthy S. Can trials of physical treatments be blinded? The example of transcutaneous electrical nerve stimulation for chronic pain. *American Journal of Physical Medicine and Rehabilitation* 1990; **69**:6–10.
14. Jadad AR, Carroll D, Moore A, McQuay H. Developing a database of published reports of randomised clinical trials in pain research. *Pain* 1996; **66**:239–46.
15. Jadad AR, Moore RA, Carroll D, Jenkinson C, Reynolds DJM, Gavaghan DJ *et al.* Assessing the quality of reports of randomized clinical trials: is blinding necessary? *Controlled Clinical Trials* 1996; **17**:1–12.
16. Abelson K, Langley GB, Sheppeard H, Vlieg M, Wigley RD. Transcutaneous electrical nerve stimulation in rheumatoid arthritis. *New Zealand Medical Journal* 1983; **96**:156–8.
17. Annal N, Soundappan SV, Palaniappan KMC, Chandrasekar S. Introduction of transcutaneous, low-voltage, non-pulsatile direct current (DC) therapy for migraine and chronic headaches. A comparison with transcutaneous electrical nerve stimulation (TENS). *Headache Quarterly* 1992; **3**:434–7.
18. Ballegaard S, Christophersen SJ, Dawids SG, Hesse J, Olsen NV. Acupuncture and transcutaneous electric nerve stimulation in the treatment of pain associated with chronic pancreatitis. A randomized study. *Scandinavian Journal of Gastroenterology* 1985; **20**:1249–54.
19. Cheng RSS, Pomeranz B. Electrotheraphy of chronic musculoskeletal pain: Comparison of electroacupuncture and acupuncture-like transcutaneous electrical nerve stimulation. *Clinical Journal of Pain* 1986; **2**:143–9.
20. Coletta R, Maggiolo F, Di Tizio S. Etofenamate and transcutaneous electrical nerve stimulation treatment of painful spinal syndromes. *International Journal of Clinical and Pharmacology Research* 1988; **8**:295–8.
21. Crockett DJ, Foreman ME, Alden L, Blasberg B. A comparison of treatment modes in the management of myofascial pain dysfunction syndrome. *Biofeedback and Self-Regulation* 1986; **11**:279–91.
22. Dawood MY, Ramos J. Transcutaneous electrical nerve stimulation (TENS) for the treatment of primary dysmenorrhea: a randomized crossover comparison with placebo TENS and ibuprofen. *Obstetrics and Gynecology* 1990; **75**:656–60.
23. Deyo RA, Walsh NE, Martin DC, Schoenfeld LS, Ramamurthy S. A controlled trial of transcutaneous electrical nerve stimulation (TENS) and exercise for chronic low back pain. *New England Journal of Medicine* 1990; **322**:1627–34.
24. Di Benedetto P, Iona LG, Zidarich V. Clinical evaluation of S-adenosyl-l-methionine versus transcutaneous electrical nerve stimulation in primary fibromyalgia. *Current Therapeutic Research: Clinical and Experimental* 1993; **53**:222–9.
25. Fargas-Babjak A, Rooney P, Gerecz E. Randomized trial of codetron for pain control in osteoarthritis of the hip/knee. *Clinical Journal of Pain* 1989; **5**:137–41.
26. Fargas-Babjak AM, Pomeranz B, Rooney PJ. Acupuncture-like stimulation with codetron for rehabilitation of patients with

chronic pain syndrome and osteoarthritis. *Acupuncture and Electrotherapy Research* 1992; 17:95–105.

27. Grimmer K. A controlled double blind study comparing the effects of strong burst mode TENS and High Rate TENS on painful osteoarthritic knees. *Australian Journal of Physiotherapy* 1992; 38:49–56.

28. Herrera-Lasso I, Mobarak L, Fernandez Dominguez L, Cardiel MH, Alarcon Segovia D. Comparative effectiveness of packages of treatment including ultrasound or transcutaneous electrical nerve stimulation in painful shoulder syndrome. *Physiotherapy* 1993; 79:251–3.

29. Heydenreich A, Thiessen M. [Comparison of the effectiveness of drug therapy, invasive and non invasive acupuncture in migraine] Effektivitatsvergleich zwischen medikamentoser Therapie, invasiver und nichtinvasiver Akupunktur bei der Migrane. *Zeitschrift fur Arztliche Fortbildung Jena* 1989; 83:877–9.

30. Heydenreich A. [Single point transcutaneous electric nerve stimulation in a simple placebo comparison in migraine (a prospective randomized study)] Punktformige transkutane elektrische Nervenstimulation (PuTENS) im einfachen Placebovergleich bei der Migrane (Eine prospektive randomisierte Studie). *Zeitschrift fur Arztliche Fortbildung Jena* 1989; 83:881–3.

31. Jensen H, Zesler R, Christensen T. Transcutaneous electrical nerve stimulation (TNS) for painful osteoarthrosis of the knee. *International Journal of Rehabilitation Research* 1991; 14:356–8.

32. Langley GB, Sheppeard H, Johnson M, Wigley RD. The analgesic effects of transcutaneous electrical nerve stimulation and placebo in chronic pain patients. A double blind non crossover comparison. *Rheumatology International* 1984; 4:119–23.

33. Lehmann TR, Russell DW, Spratt KF. The impact of patients with nonorganic physical findings on a controlled trial of transcutaneous electrical nerve stimulation and electroacupuncture. *Spine* 1983; 8:625–34.

34. Leo KC, Dostal WF, Bossen DG, Eldridge VL, Fairchild ML, Evans RE. Effect of transcutaneous electrical nerve stimulation characteristics on clinical pain. *Physical Therapy* 1986; 66:200–5.

35. Lewers D, Clelland JA, Jackson JR, Varner RE, Bergman J. Transcutaneous electrical nerve stimulation in the relief of primary dysmenorrhea. *Physical Therapy* 1989; 69:3V, 19–9V,23.

36. Lewis B, Lewis D, Cumming G. The comparative analgesic efficacy of transcutaneous electrical nerve stimulation and a non-steroidal anti-inflammatory drug for painful osteoarthritis. *British Journal of Rheumatology* 1994; 33:455–60.

37. Lewis D, Lewis B, Sturrock RD. Transcutaneous electrical nerve stimulation in osteoarthrosis: a therapeutic alternative? *Annals of Rheumatic Disease* 1984; 43:47–9.

38. Lundeberg T. A comparative study of the pain alleviating effect of vibratory stimulation, transcutaneous electrical nerve stimulation, electroacupuncture and placebo. *American Journal of Clinical Medicine* 1984; 12:72–9.

39. Lundeberg T, Bondesson L, Lundstrom V. Relief of primary dysmenorrhea by transcutaneous electrical nerve stimulation. *Acta Obstetrics Gynaecologica Scandinavica* 1985; 64:491–7.

40. Mannheimer C, Carlsson C. The analgesic effect of Transcutaneous electrical nerve stimulation (TENS) in patients with rheumatoid arthritis. A comparative study of different pulse patterns. *Pain* 1979; 6:329–34.

41. Mannheimer JS, Whalen EC. The Efficacy of Transcutaneous Electric Nerve Stimulation in Dysmenorrhea. *Clinical Journal of Pain* 1985; 1:75–83.

42. Marchand S, Charest J, Li J, Chenard J, Lavignolle B, Laurencelle L. Is TENS purely a placebo effect? A controlled study on chronic low back pain. *Pain* 1993; 54:99–106.

43. Melzack R, Katz J. Auriculotherapy fails to relieve chronic pain. A controlled crossover study. *Journal of the American Medical Association* 1984; 251:1041–3.

44. Melzack R, Vetere P, Finch L. Transcutaneous electrical nerve stimulation for low back pain. A comparison of TENS and massage for pain and range of motion. *Physical Therapy* 1983; 63:489–93.

45. Milsom I, Hedner N, Mannheimer C. A comparative study of the effect of high-intensity transcutaneous nerve stimulation and oral naproxen on intrauterine pressure and menstrual pain in patients with primary dysmenorrhea. *American Journal of Obstetrics and Gynecology* 1994; 170:123–9.

46. Møystad A, Krogstad BS, Larheim TA. Transcutaneous nerve stimulation in a group of patients with rheumatic disease involving the temporomandibular joint. *Journal of Prosthetic Dentistry* 1990; 64:596–600.

47. Nash TP, Williams JD, Machin D. TENS: Does the Type of Stimulus Really Matter? *Pain Clinic* 1990; 3:161–8.

48. Neighbors LE, Clelland J, Jackson JR, Bergman J, Orr JJ. Transcutaneous electrical nerve stimulation for pain relief in primary dysmenorrhea. *Clinical Journal of Pain* 1987; 3:17–22.

49. Rutgers MJ, Van Romunde LKJ, Osman PO. A small randomized comparative trial of acupuncture versus transcutaneous electrical neurostimulation in postherpetic neuralgia. *Pain Clinic* 1988; 2:87–9.

50. Smith CR, Lewith GT, Machin D. Preliminary study to establish a controlled method of assessing transcutaneous nerve stimulation as treatment for the pain caused by osteo-arthritis of the knee. *Physiotherapy* 1983; 69:266–8.

51. Sunshine W, Field TM, Quintino O, Fierro K, Kuhn C, Burman I et al. Fibromyalgia benefits from massage therapy and transcutaneous electrical stimulation. *Journal of Clinical Rheumatology* 1996; 2:18–22.

52. Taylor P, Hallett M, Flaherty L. Treatment of osteoarthritis of the knee with transcutaneous electrical nerve stimulation. *Pain* 1981; 11:233–40.

53. Thorsteinsson G, Stonnington HH, Stillwell GK, Elveback LR. The placebo effect of transcutaneous electrical stimulation. *Pain* 1978; 5:31–41.

54. Thorsteinsson G, Stonnington HH, Stillwell GK, Elveback LR. Transcutaneous electrical stimulation: a double blind trial of its efficacy for pain. *Archives of Physical Medicine Rehabilitation* 1977; 58:8–13.

55. Tulgar M, McGlone F, Bowsher D, Miles JB. Comparative effectiveness of different stimulation modes in relieving pain. Part I. A pilot study. *Pain* 1991; 47:151–5.

56. Tulgar M, McGlone F, Bowsher D, Miles JB. Comparative effectiveness of different stimulation modes in relieving pain. Part II. A double-blind controlled long-term clinical trial. *Pain* 1991; 47:157–62.

57. Vinterberg H, Donde R, Andersen RB. [Transcutaneous nerve stimulation for relief of pain in patients with rheumatoid arthritis]. *Ugeskrift for Laeger* 1978; 140:1149–50.

58. Chalmers TC, Matta RJ, Smith JJ, Kunzler AM. Evidence favoring the use of anticoagulants in the hospital phase of acute myocardial infarction. *New England Journal of Medicine* 1977; 297:1091–6.

59. Cooperman AM, Hall B, Mikalacki K, Hardy R, Sadar E. Use of transcutaneous electrical stimulation in the control of postoperative pain. *American Journal of Surgery* 1977; 133:185–7.

60. Rooney SM, Jain S, Goldiner PL. Effect of transcutaneous nerve stimulation on postoperative pain after thoracotomy. *Anesthesia and Analgesia* 1983; **62:**1010–12.

61. Wall PD. The placebo effect: an unpopular topic. *Pain* 1992; **51:**1–3.

62. McQuay H, Carroll D, Moore A. Variation in the placebo effect in randomised controlled trials of analgesics: All is as blind as it seems. *Pain* 1996; **64:**331–5.

63. Thomas IL, Tyle V, Webster J, Neilson A. An evaluation of transcutaneous electrical nerve stimulation for pain relief in labour. *Australian and New Zealand Journal of Obstetrics and Gynaecology* 1988; **28:**182–9.

64. Johnson MI, Ashton CH, Thompson JW. Long term use of transcutaneous electrical nerve stimulation at Newcastle Pain Relief Clinic. *Journal of the Royal Society of Medicine* 1992; **85:**267–8.

Intravenous regional sympathetic blockade (IRSB) for reflex sympathetic dystrophy

Summary

This systematic review of intravenous regional sympathetic blocks (IRSBs) in patients with reflex sympathetic dystrophy (RSD) used eight randomized controlled trials (RCTs). Six used guanethidine; none showed significant analgesic effect of IRSBs in relieving pain due to RSD. Two reports, one using ketanserin and one bretylium with 17 patients in total, showed some advantage of IRSBs over control. RCT results were not combined because of the variety of different drugs and outcome measures and because of methodological deficiencies in most of the reports.

Our own trial was stopped prematurely because of the severity of the adverse effects. No significant difference was found between guanethidine and placebo on any of the outcome measures. Patients in all groups reported less than 30% of the maximum possible relief during the first week after the injections and on only two occasions (one saline and one guanethidine low dose) was relief reported for longer than a week. There was no evidence of a dose response for guanethidine.

The use of guanethidine in IRSBs for patients with RSD was not supported by the systematic review.

Introduction

More than 120 years ago Weir Mitchell described a syndrome of persistent burning pain and trophic changes in the limbs of soldiers after gunshot wounds; he called it causalgia. Since then several similar syndromes have been described using different names. The term 'reflex sympathetic dystrophy' (RSD) was first used more than 40 years ago and today it is used to describe the constellation of chronic pain conditions associated with hyperactivity of the sympathetic nervous system [2, 3]. The problem with this definition is the implication that it is a disordered sympathetic nervous system that causes the pain; it may be that the pain causes a disorder of the sympathetic nervous system. The clinical reality is a funny pain in a funny looking limb. The pain is usually constant, severe, and unresponsive to conventional analgesics. It is usually confined to a limb, and the limb may show hyperaesthesia, swelling, changes in skin colour and temperature, changes in sweating, and even bone demineralization [4].

The lack of response of these pains to conventional analgesics led to the development of techniques designed specifically to block the sympathetic nervous system. One of these techniques was described more than 15 years ago [5] and is known as intravenous regional sympathetic block (IRSB). This involves giving a drug known to block the sympathetic nervous system (guanethidine in the original report) in high local concentration in a limb isolated with a tourniquet. Since it was described this method has gained considerable popularity, mainly because of its simplicity and relatively low cost. However, even though IRSB is recommended as the simplest, most effective and safest way to relieve pain associated with sympathetic hyperactivity [6, 7], very few randomized controlled trials have assessed its effectiveness.

We did a systematic review of the literature for IRSBs in patients with RSD, and, because of the paucity of controlled data supporting guanethidine use in IRSBs, did a double-blind cross-over randomized study, designed to assess the effectiveness of IRSBs with guanethidine in patients with RSD who had claimed relief after open blocks and to determine whether the analgesic effects (if any) were dose-dependent.

Systematic review

Methods

A MEDLINE (Silver Platter MEDLINE version 3.0 and 3.1) search was done from 1966 to May 1993. The strategy was designed to identify the maximum number of randomized and/or double-blind reports by using a combination of text words, 'wild cards', and MeSH terms as described previously [8].

Medical journals were hand searched. They were selected from a list of the 50 journals with the highest number of reports in MEDLINE using the optimized strategy, and nine specialist journals which were not included in that list or which were not indexed in MEDLINE. The search process included volumes published between 1950 and 1992 and the order in which journals were searched was determined mainly by local availability.

The eligibility of a study was determined by looking only at the methods section. The following criteria had to be met:

The topic discussed in this chapter is also published in full in Jadad *et al.* [1].

1. Inclusion of patients with chronic pain associated with RSD.
2. Random and/or double-blind allocation of treatments.
3. Administration of an IRSB to at least one of the treatment groups.

A letter was sent to the first author of each eligible study requesting individual data in relation to analgesic measures and adverse effects for all the patients included in the study as well as drop-outs. The authors were asked to describe the randomization method used in the study and to send details of other trials fulfilling our inclusion criteria performed by them or by other research groups.

Results

We found 8 controlled trials assessing the analgesic effects of IRSBs [1, 9–15] in patients with RSD (Table 1). Sample size ranged from 6 to 21 patients.

In most reports guanethidine was the active substance, but reserpine, bretylium, droperidol, and ketanserin were used as alternatives.

Of the eight randomized controlled studies, two (17 patients in total) showed some advantage of IRSBs over control treatments [11, 14]. Neither study used guanethidine. The remaining trials failed to show a significant difference in analgesic response between the IRSBs and the control treatments.

Table 1 Randomized controlled trials of intravenous regional sympathetic blocks in reflex sympathetic dystrophy

Trial	No. of patients	Design	Experimental group (s)	Control group	Treatments per group	Outcomes	Results
[9]	19	P, O	Guanethidine 20 mg + heparin 500 U.	Stellate ganglion block with bupivacaine 75 mg.	4 experimental 8 control	Mean daily pain intensity.	NS. Hyperpathia: 2/7 controls & 4/7 IRSB improved after treatment (no follow-up).
[10]	6	C, DB	Droperidol 2.5 mg + heparin 500–1000 U.	Heparin 500–1000 U in normal saline.	1	Description of current and daily VAS-PI.	NA. On 3 occasions relief with control, on 3 relief with droperidol. Only sustained (2 wks) relief after placebo.
[12]	10	C, DB	Guanethidine 20 mg or reserpine 1.25 mg + lignocaine 250 mg.	Lignocaine 250 mg.	Variable	Mean pain intensity.	NS. Pain relief reported for 2 months or more by 2/12 on reserpine, 1/12 on guanethidine.
[11]	9	C, DB	Ketanserin 10–20 mg.	Normal saline.	2	Mean weekly pain intensity.	S. No individual data.
[13]	21	C, DB	Guanethidine 20–30 mg or reserpine 0.5–1.0 mg.	Normal saline.	1	Reduction in VAS-PI > 50%.	NS. After 4 wks 0/21 had relief with saline, 1/21 with reserpine, 3/21 with guanethidine.
[14]	8	C, DB	Bretylium 1.5 mg/kg + lignocaine 200–300 mg.	Lignocaine 200–300 mg.	2	Duration of VAS relief > 30 mm.	S. No individual data.
[15]	15	C, DB	Guanethidine 15 mg + lignocaine 1% 10 ml.	Lignocaine 1% 10 ml.	1	Somato sensory tests and VAS-PI (provoked and on-going).	NS. No individual data.
[1]	8	C, DB	Guanethidine 10 and 30 mg in saline 25 ml (arm) *or* 20 and 30 mg (leg) in saline 50 ml.	Saline 25 ml (arm) or 50 ml (leg).	1	VAS relief, pain diaries.	NS. Study stopped because of hypotension in 2 patients.

For trial Design: P, parallel; C, cross-over; DB, double-blind; O, open. For Results: S, significant; NS, not significant; NA, not applicable. (Statistical analysis was not possible due to the number of withdrawals.)

Only one [1] of the five guanethidine trials was designed to determine if there was a dose-response for the effects of guanethidine.

The analgesic outcome was measured in such a heterogeneous fashion that it was not possible to combine the results mathematically and most studies had serious methodological deficiencies. The major methodological problems of the studies were poorly defined diagnostic criteria [11, 13, 14], inadequate washout periods [11], incomplete cross-over [12, 13], open administration of treatments [9], no description of the technique [15], and a high proportion of withdrawals with no 'intention to treat' analysis [10, 14].

There was no RCT evidence to support guanethidine use in IRSBs to treat RSD, but some evidence for ketanserin and bretylium. All the studies were small, so that there is substantial risk of false negatives and even false positives.

Comment

Persistent pain due to RSD is usually difficult to control and can be very frustrating for both patients and doctors. Although the most widely used management is IRSB, the results of the few RCTs available are conflicting. Two small studies, neither using guanethidine, did show significant relief [11, 14]. There is thus some limited support for the technique, but none for guanethidine as the active drug in the injection to relieve pain associated with RSD. Only one RCT has ever shown analgesic effects of blocks with guanethidine [16]. It was not included in the systematic review because the study patients had rheumatoid arthritis, not RSD.

Two patients had hypotension in our own study, so that we had to stop the study prematurely [1]. The technique is not innocuous. Prolonged arterial hypotension has been described after multiple IRSBs [17] but our experience shows that it can occur after single injections. Another important lesson is that some patients with RSD do not respond to IRSBs. There are no known predictors of poor response. The argument that these patients who do not respond to a sympathetic block did not have RSD is rather circular, particularly because the effectiveness of IRSBs for pain relief in RSD has not been proven. It remains unclear whether the sympathetic hyperactivity is the cause or a result of the pain, or a confounding factor. The poor analgesic response reported by the patients in these trials makes it difficult to justify the use of this technique with guanethidine for the treatment of patients with RSD. The defence that satisfactory results may follow multiple injections [5, 7] is not supported by double-blind RCTs.

Other drugs given by IRSBs may produce pain relief for RSD. Two RCTs (17 patients in total) of IRSBs using ketanserin and bretylium showed significant relief when compared with control. The technique itself may also produce pain relief, although our results provided little evidence of this. One hypothesis is that pain relief after IRSBs could be due to the ischaemia induced by the tourniquet rather than by the contents of the injection [13, 18]. If that is the case, it would be much simpler and safer to use the tourniquet as the treatment and this could be done by the patient at home. That would fail if pain relief is due to the placebo effect of the procedure (including intravenous injections) performed in the hospital.

References

1. Jadad AR, Carroll D, Glynn CJ, McQuay HJ. Intravenous regional sympathetic blockade for pain relief in reflex sympathetic dystrophy: a systematic review and a randomized, double-blind crossover study. *Journal of Pain and Symptom Management* 1995; **10**:13–20.
2. Schutzer SF, Gossling HR. The treatment of Reflex Sympathetic Dystrophy syndrome. *Journal of Bone and Joint Surgery* 1984; **66A**:625–9.
3. Schwartzman RJ, McLellan TL. Reflex Sympathetic Dystrophy: a review. *Archives Neurology* 1987; **44**:555–61.
4. Procacci P, Maresca M. Reflex sympathetic dystrophies and algodystrophies: historical and pathogenic considerations. *Pain* 1987; **31**:137–46.
5. Hannington-Kiff JG. Intravenous regional sympathetic block with guanethidine. *Lancet* 1974; **1**:1019–20.
6. Loh L, Nathan PW, Schott GD. Painful peripheral states and sympathetic blocks. *Journal of Neurology, Neurosurgery and Psychiatry* 1978; **41**:664–671.
7. Hannington-Kiff J. Pharmacological target blocks in painful dystrophic limbs. In: Wall P, Melzack R, ed *Textbook of pain*, 2nd edn. London: Churchill Livingstone, 1989:754–66.
8. Jadad AR, McQuay HJ. A high-yield strategy to identify randomized controlled trials for systematic reviews. *Online Journal of Current Clinical Trials* [serial online] 1993; Doc No 33:3973 words; 39 paragraphs. 5 tables.
9. Bonelli S, Conoscente F, Movilia PG, Restelli L, Francucci B, Grossi E. Regional intravenous guanethidine vs stellate ganglion block in reflex sympathetic dystrophies: a randomized trial. *Pain* 1983; **16**:297–307.
10. Kettler RE, Abram SE. Intravenous regional droperidol in the management of reflex sympathetic dystrophy: a double-blind placebo-controlled, crossover study. *Anesthesiology* 1988; **69**:933–6.
11. Hanna MH, Peat SJ. Ketanserin in reflex sympathetic dystrophy. A double-blind placebo controlled trial. *Pain* 1989; **38**:145–50.
12. Rocco AG, Kaul AF, Reisman RM, Gallo JP, Lief PA. A comparison of regional intravenous guanethidine and reserpine in reflex sympathetic dystrophy: a controlled, randomized, double-blind crossover study. *Clinical Journal of Pain* 1989; **5**:205–9.
13. Blanchard J, Ramamurthy S, Walsh N, Hoffman J, Schoenfeld L. Intravenous regional sympatholysis: a double-blind comparison of guanethidine, reserpine, and normal saline. *Journal of Pain and Symptom Management* 1990; **5**:357–61.
14. Hord AH, Rooks MD, Stephens BO, Fleming LL. Intravenous regional bretylium for the treatment of reflex sympathetic dystrophy. *Anesthesia and Analgesia* 1992; **74**:818–21.
15. Dhar S, McGlone F, Dean J, Klenerman L. The temporal significance of the placebo response in reflex sympathetic dystrophy. *Proceedings of the British Orthopaedic Research Society Meeting*. London, 1992; **16**:16–17.
16. Levine JD, Fye K, Heller P, Basbaum AI, Whiting-O'Keefe Q. Clinical response to regional intravenous guanethidine in patients with rheumatoid arthritis. *Journal of Rheumatology* 1986; **13**:1040–3.

17. Sharpe E, Milaszkiewicz R, Carli F. A case of prolonged hypotension following intravenous guanethidine block. *Anaesthesia* 1987; **42**:1081–4.

18. Casale R, Glynn C, Buonocore M. The role of ischaemia in the analgesia which follows Bier's block technique. *Pain* 1992; **50**:169–75.

27

Epidural corticosteroids for sciatica

Summary

Two systematic reviews have addressed the effectiveness of epidural steroid injections for sciatica and back pain. Both examined the randomized controlled trials published up to the end of 1994.

The analysis by Koes and colleagues from Amsterdam [1] goes into great depth examining methodological quality of the trials and how this has been scored by the reviewers. This type of review is, frankly, disappointing and does not produce any meta-analytic judgements on which to work, and few enlightening ideas about the future research agenda, other than some anodyne comments about possible trial design.

The best that this review can do is to tell us that, of the four studies with the highest methodological quality assessed by their particular scoring system, two had positive outcomes for epidural steroids (judged by their authors) and two had negative outcomes.

In contrast, a meta-analysis of the same trials by Watts and Silagy [2] is an important step forward in showing that epidural corticosteroids have an analgesic effect on sciatica compared with control. Their analysis, using odds ratios, answered the question 'Do epidural steroids work?'

We wished to address the question 'How well do they work?', to try to assess the extent of the benefit given by the steroids. To do this we re-analysed their data, and adding a new trial (Carette *et al* 1997 [5]) used NNT as the measure of clinical benefit (Table 1), using the outcome of at least 75% pain relief for short-term outcomes (1–60 days) and at least 50% pain relief for long-term outcomes (12 weeks to one year). In circumstances where the numbers of patients entered into individual studies is small, this approach is most likely to produce a reliable indication of the clinically relevant outcomes needed by patients, providers, and purchasers in making decisions about the use of a potentially harmful technique. Evidence from other sources places the risk of neurological sequelae after epidural as 1 in 5000 [3].

Short-term relief

There were 11 trials which gave short-term relief data (more than 75% pain relief), with 319 patients given epidural steroids, and 345 given placebo. Only 3 of these studies were themselves statistically significant [7, 13, 14], but overall there was a statistically significant benefit (1.5 with 95% confidence intervals 1.2–1.9).

The NNT for short-term (1–60 days) greater than 75% pain relief from the 10 trials with short-term outcomes combined, was just under 7.3, with 95% confidence intervals from 4.7 to 16. This means that for 7 patients treated with epidural steroid 1 will obtain more than 75% pain relief short-term who would not have done had they received the control treatment (placebo or local anaesthetic).

Long-term relief

There were six trials which gave long-term relief data with 315 patients given epidural steroids, and 395 given placebo. Only one of these studies was itself statistically significant [9], but overall there was a statistically significant benefit (1.3 with 95% confidence intervals 1.1–1.5).

The NNT for long-term (12 weeks up to one year) improvement from the five trials combined, was about 13 for 50% pain relief, with 95% confidence intervals from 6.6 to 314. This means that for 13 patients treated with epidural steroid one will obtain more pain relief over this longer-term period who would not have done had they received the control treatment (placebo or local anaesthetic).

Comment

These NNT values at first sight appear disappointing. Here is an intervention that shows statistically significant improvement compared with control, and yet the clinical benefit, the NNT for one patient to reach the chosen endpoint, is 7 for short-term benefit and 13 for long-term. The short-term endpoint, however, is quite a high hurdle. Using an easier hurdle of 50% relief rather than 75%, the 'best' NNT achieved by drug treatment of neuropathic pain was just under 3. Patients may choose the epidural if it means they do not have to take medication, particularly if it gives a higher level of relief, even though there is a 1 in 7 chance of this level of response.

The long-term NNT of 13 is perhaps not surprising. Occasional patients in most clinics report a 'cure' as a result of a steroid epidural, but the majority of epidural steroid successes return for repeat epidurals. That one patient has relief lasting between 12 weeks and a year for twelve treated with epidural steroid fits with experience.

The message is that we will have inevitably to expose our practice to the searching type of analysis which Watts and Silagy have used for epidural steroid. This intervention has shown a statistically significant benefit over control. Others will not, and will be discarded. For those interventions that do show statistically significant benefit over control there is then a further stage, which is to define the clinical benefit of

Table 1 Epidural corticosteroids for sciatica

Trial ref.	Improved on epidural steroid	Improved on control	Relative benefit (95% CI)	NNT (95% CI)
Short-term relief (1–60 days)				
[10]	18/24	16/24	1.1 (0.8–1.6)	12 (3–∞)
[11]	9/16	5/19	2.1 (0.9–5.1)	3.3 (1.6–∞)
[4]	8/12	2/11	3.7 (0.98–13.7)	2.1 (1.2–7.5)
[5]	25/76	23/78	1.1 (0.5–2.4)	29 (5.5–∞)
[6]	12/19	8/31	1.1 (0.5–2.4)	33 (4–∞)
[7]	21/35	11/36	2.0 (1.1–3.4)	3.5 (1.9–14)
[12]	15/19	32/44	1.1 (0.8–1.5)	17 (3–∞)
[8]	14/21	18/32	1.2 (0.8–1.8)	10 (3–∞)
[13]	18/28	8/30	2.4 (1.3–4.6)	2.6 (1.6–7.2)
[14]	17/19	3/16	4.8 (1.7–13)	1.4 (1.1–2.1)
[15]	8/27	5/24	1.4 (0.5–3.8)	11 (3–∞)
Combined short-term relief (> 75%)	165/319	131/345	1.5 (1.2–1.9)	7.3 (4.7–16)
Long-term relief (12–52 weeks)				
[4]	10/12	7/11	1.3 (0.8–2.2)	5.0 (1.8–∞)
[5]	41/74	43/77	1.0 (0.7–1.3)	∞
[6]	11/46	4/27	1.6 (0.6–4.6)	10.99 (3.66–∞)
[7]	16/43	8/38	1.8 (0.9–3.7)	6.3 (2.8–∞)
[8]	9/23	14/34	0.95 (0.5–1.8)	∞
[9]	76/117	98/208	1.4 (1.1–1.7)	5.6 (3.5–1.4)
Combined long-term relief	163/315	174/395	1.3 (1.1–1.5)	13 (6.6–314)

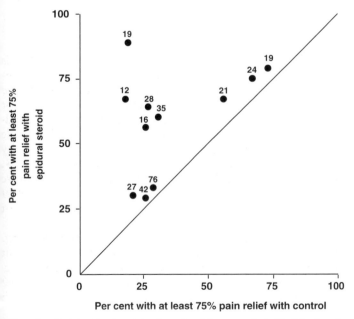

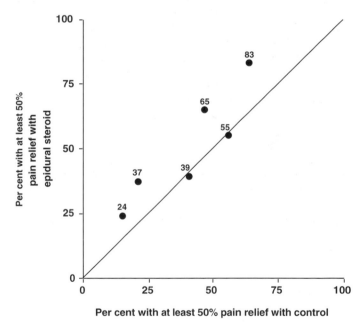

Fig. 1 Epidural steroids for short-term relief (1–60 days). (Numbers next to points indicate number of patients given steroid injections in the trials.)

Fig. 2 Epidural steroids for long-term relief (12–52 weeks). (Numbers next to points indicate number of patients given steroid infections in the trials.)

the intervention. The NNTs for effectiveness are one possible definition, particularly when coupled with NNTs for minor and major harm (NNT of about 40 for dural tap in [2]).

For patients with chronic disease, and in this case chronic painful disease, interventions may be attractive even if their success rate is far lower than would be acceptable in, say, the management of postoperative pain. This means that the interpretation of measures of clinical benefit, such as NNTs, has to be context-dependent. For the moment we need the best possible analysis, as Watts and Silagy have demonstrated, of the data available. If the data is poor then that establishes the clinical research agenda. If the data is reasonable then we can try to define measures of clinical benefit. The art of clinical practice will then come into play, as patient and doctor juggle the risk and benefit of the alternatives, albeit with better data than we have at present.

References

1. Koes BW, Scholten RPM, Mens JMA, Bouter LM. Efficacy of epidural steroid injections for low-back pain and sciatica: a systematic review of randomized clinical trials. *Pain* 1995; **63**:279–88.
2. Watts RW, Silagy CA. A meta-analysis on the efficacy of epidural corticosteroids in the treatment of sciatica. *Anaesthesia and Intensive Care* 1995; **23**:564–9.
3. Kane RE. Neurologic deficits following epidural or spinal anesthesia. *Anesthesia and Analgesia* 1981; **60**:150–61.
4. Bush K, Hillier S. A controlled study of caudal epidural injections of triamcinolone plus procaine for the management of intractable sciatica. *Spine* 1991; **16**:572–5.
5. Carette S, Leclaire R, Marcoux S, Morin F, Blaise GA, St.-Pierre A *et al.* Epidural corticosteroid injections for sciatica due to herniated nucleus pulposus. *New England Journal of Medicine* 1997; **336**:1634–40.
6. Cuckler J, Bernini P, Wiesel S, Booth R, Rothman R, Pickens G. The use of epidural steroids in the treatment of lumbar radicular pain. *Journal of Bone and Joint Surgery* 1985; **67A**:63–66.
7. Dilke T, Burry H, Grahame R. Extradural corticosteroid injection in management of lumbar nerve root compression. *British Medical Journal* 1973; **2**:635–637.
8. Mathews J, Mills S, Jenkins V, Grimes S, Morkel M, Mathews W et al. Back pain and sciatica: controlled trials of manipulation, traction, sclerosant and epidural injections. *British Journal of Rheumatology* 1987; **26**:416–23.
9. Swerdlow M, Sayle-Creer W. A study of extradural medication in the relief of lumbosciatic syndrome. *Anaesthesia* 1969; **23**:341–5.
10. Beliveau P. A comparison between epidural anaesthesia with and without corticosteroid in the treatment of sciatica. *Rheumatology and Physical Medicine* 1971; **11**:40–3.
11. Breivik H, Hesla P, Molnar I, Lind B. Treatment of chronic low back pain and sciatica: comparison of caudal epidural injections of bupivacaine and methyl-prednisolone with bupivacaine followed by saline. In: Bonica JA ed. *Advances in pain research and therapy*, Vol. 1. New York: Raven Press, 1976:927–32.
12. Klenerman L, Greenwood R, Davenport H, White D, Peskett S. Lumbar epidural injections in the treatment of sciatica. *British Journal of Rheumatology* 1984; **23**:35–8.
13. Popiolek A, Domanik A, Mazurkiewicz G. Leczenie sterydowymi ostrzknieciami nadopow owymi chorychz prewlekla rwa kulszowa w przebiegu dyskopatti. *Neurologia i Neurochirurgia Polska* 1991; **25**:640–6.
14. Ridley M, Kingsley G, Gibson T, Grahame R. Outpatient lumbar epidural corticosteroid injection in the management of sciatica. *British Journal of Rheumatology* 1988; **27**:295–9.
15. Snoek W, Weber H, Jorgenson B. Double blind evaluation of extradural methyl prednisolone for herniated lumbar discs. *Acta Orthopaedica Scandinavica* 1977; **48**:635–41.

Spinal cord stimulators for back pain

Summary

Spinal cord stimulation (SCS) for chronic pain, like transcutaneous electrical nerve stimulation (TENS), is based on the 'gate control' theory of pain. Surgically implanted electrodes (usually but not necessarily over the dorsal columns) are stimulated to activate pain inhibitory mechanisms. The number and type of electrodes implanted, and the type of stimulation received, is very variable. Implantation can be at open laminectomy, or may be percutaneous. The neurophysiology is unclear.

Turner et al. [1] have conducted a thorough literature search in an attempt to determine the place of SCS in chronic pain treatment. Their literature search was conducted up to June 1994 and the paper was published in December 1995. They included 39 studies, but none was randomized: all were case series. A majority (82%) did not have planned study protocols. The review does not give the total number of patients treated or reported. Few studies define patient inclusion or exclusion criteria, or give demographic information on patients treated. The source of follow-up data was unclear in most of the studies. Most studies reported on percutaneous electrode implant with single-channel stimulators.

Twenty-nine studies had at least 50% pain relief as an outcome. Across these studies the mean (probably unweighted, but not stated) was 59% of patients achieving this outcome at some follow-up point, with a range of 15% to 100%. Fourteen studies reported one year follow-up with success defined as stimulator in use with at least 50% pain relief. In these, the mean across study success rate was 62%, again with a range of 15% to 100%.

Fewer studies reported success at later follow-up times. At two years five trials reported a mean of 64% success (range 55% to 74%). At five years three studies reported a mean of 53% success (range 50% to 55%). At ten years one study reported 35% success.

Complications were common. In 13 studies there was at least one complication in 42% of patients (range 20%–75%). These were predominantly stimulator or electrode problems (mean 30% and 24% respectively, range 0%–75%). Infection was less common, occurring in 5% of patients in 20 trials that reported it (range 0%–12%). Most complications appeared to be minor.

Turner et al. [1] also report on an ongoing randomized trial, but with limited information and none on pain relief.

It is clear that the evidence on SCS is limited. It is likely to be biased because of lack of randomization and blinding, because it has been conducted by enthusiasts and reporting has been limited. More than half of the studies did not report the number of patients who had been implanted during the study period, for instance.

Turner and colleagues call for a randomized trial or trials with common design, including:

1. Randomization to SCS or control.
2. Follow-up assessment of all patients at uniform times after implantation or entry—six months, and yearly thereafter.
3. Follow-up assessment by independent observer.
4. Description of all relevant clinical and demographic information.
5. Use of common and valid pain and other measures.
6. Assessment of multiple outcomes, including back pain, leg pain, physical functioning, drug use, work status, health care use, and quality of life.

One such trial, of SCS for painful diabetic neuropathy on ten patients who had not responded to conventional treatment, has now been published [2]. The electrode was implanted in the thoracic/lumbar epidural space. Immediate neuropathic pain relief after connecting the electrode was measured using a visual analogue scale (VAS), and exercise tolerance was assessed on a treadmill.

Eight patients had statistically significant pain relief with the electrical stimulator, and the system was made permanent. Seven of these eight had statistically significant relief of pain at 3 months, and this relief was sustained in six till the end of the study at 14 months. These six used the stimulator as the sole treatment for their pain. Exercise tolerance was also improved. One patient died 2 months after the start of the study of unrelated cause while continuing to benefit from treatment and another patient ceased to benefit at 4 months. Baseline pain, checked by turning the system off, was unaltered.

The authors claim that electrical spinal cord stimulation offers a new and effective way of relieving chronic diabetic neuropathic pain, improves exercise tolerance, and should be considered in patients with neuropathic pain who do not respond to conventional treatment.

References

1. Turner JA, Loeser JD, Bell KG. Spinal cord stimulation for chronic low back pain; a systematic literature synthesis. *Neurosurgery* 1995; 37:1088–96.
2. Tesfaye S, Watt J, Benbow SJ, Pang KA, Miles J, MacFarlane IA. Electrical spinal-cord stimulation for painful diabetic peripheral neuropathy. *Lancet* 1996; 348:1698–701.

29
Steroid injections for shoulder disorders

Summary

A systematic review on steroid injections for shoulder disorders [1] indicates that the evidence for the efficacy of these blocks is scarce, and what there is shows poor effect.

The reviewers claim that 10% of the population have one or more episodes of shoulder pain and/or stiffness during their life, and that 5% of all primary care consultations are about shoulder problems. Of new consultations, they estimate that 23% resolve within 1 month, 51% within 6 months, and 59% within one year.

They suggest that (in the Netherlands) 12% of all patient–physician contacts for shoulder disorders involve local steroid injections and that injection therapy is given in 20% of all episodes of shoulder disorders. They also indicate that 40% of the patients still had their shoulder problem after a year which means that a considerable proportion of these (common) shoulder problems are not self-limited. These figures seem high for British practice.

The reviewers found 22 studies that met their inclusion criteria. They put these studies through their rigorous quality scoring system. No study scored more than 60 out of the maximum of 100, with only three scoring more than 50. This is a clear signal that definitive conclusions are unlikely to be possible from the available studies.

A second complexity is that the studies looked at many different treatments, not just at injections. Only three studies compared steroid injection with saline injection, and five compared steroid injection with injection of local anaesthetic. A third difficulty is that the studies used different outcome measures.

Taking the crude criterion of success at four weeks or later after injection, the number-needed-to-treat (NNT) for such success with steroid injection compared with saline injection (three studies) was 17, with a confidence limit which includes no benefit to any patient. For steroid plus local anaesthetic injection versus local anaesthetic alone (five studies), the NNT for success at four weeks or later was 33, again with a confidence limit which includes no benefit to any patient. On this basis one patient in 17 would achieve 'success' with a steroid injection compared with an injection of saline, and one patient in 33 would achieve 'success' with a steroid plus local anaesthetic injection compared with an injection of local anaesthetic alone.

Comment

The evidence that steroid injections for shoulder problems are worthwhile is less than compelling. The onus is on those who wish to continue to offer steroid injections to the shoulder to produce convincing evidence—a starting point would be to use a study design that scored closer to the maximum on the Dutch scale.

Reference

1. van der Heijden CJM, van der Windt DAW, Kleijnen J, Koes BW, Bouter LM. Steroid injections for shoulder disorders: a systematic review of randomized clinical trials. *British Journal of General Practice* 1996; **46**:309–16. [19040]

Summary

This systematic review of the effectiveness and adverse effects of anticonvulsant drugs used randomized controlled trials (RCTs) of anticonvulsants in chronic pain identified by MEDLINE, by manual search, by searching reference lists, and, by contacting investigators. Numbers-needed-to-treat (NNTs) were calculated from dichotomous data for effectiveness, adverse effects and drug-related study withdrawal, for individual studies and for pooled data.

Twenty RCTs of four anticonvulsants were considered eligible. Three placebo controlled studies of carbamazepine in trigeminal neuralgia had a combined NNT for effectiveness of 2.6, for adverse effects 3.4, and for severe effects (withdrawal from study) 24. Three placebo controlled studies of diabetic neuropathy had a combined NNT for effectiveness of 3, for adverse effects 2.5, and for severe effects 20. Three placebo controlled studies of migraine prophylaxis had a combined NNT for effectiveness of 2.4, for adverse effects 2.4, and for severe effects 39.

Phenytoin had no effect in irritable bowel syndrome, and carbamazepine little effect in post-stroke pain. Clonazepam was effective in one study of temporomandibular joint dysfunction.

Although anticonvulsants are used widely in chronic pain surprisingly few RCTs show analgesic effectiveness. No RCT compared different anticonvulsants.

Introduction

Anticonvulsant drugs have been used in pain management since the 1960s, very soon after they were first used in medicine and revolutionized the medical management of epilepsy. The clinical impression is that they are useful for neuropathic pain, especially when the pain is lancinating or burning [2]. Although these disorders are not common (the incidence of trigeminal neuralgia is 4/100 000 per year [3]), they can be very disabling. Carbamazepine is one of few effective interventions for trigeminal neuralgia, for which it is usually the drug of choice [4]. In the United Kingdom, carbamazepine is licensed for paroxysmal pain of trigeminal neuralgia (up to 1600 mg daily); phenytoin is also licensed as second-line to carbamazepine in trigeminal neuralgia if carbamazepine is ineffective or in patients who cannot tolerate effective doses. When anticonvulsants are used as adjuvant drugs in other pain syndromes valproate is often preferred to carbamazepine

because it may be better tolerated [5]. Anticonvulsants are also prescribed in combination with antidepressants, as in the treatment of post-herpetic neuralgia [6]. In the United Kingdom, no anticonvulsant is licensed for a pain indication other than trigeminal neuralgia.

The precise mechanisms of action of anticonvulsant drugs remain uncertain. The two standard explanations are enhanced gamma-aminobutyric acid inhibition (valproate, clonazepam) or a stabilizing effect on neuronal cell membranes. A third possibility is action via N-methyl-D-aspartate (NMDA) receptor sites.

Anticonvulsant drug use is not without risk: serious effects have been reported, including deaths from haematological reactions [7]. The commonest adverse effects are impaired mental and motor function, which may limit clinical use, particularly in the elderly [7–9].

The purpose of this review was to evaluate the analgesic effectiveness of anticonvulsant drugs in order to provide evidence-based recommendations for clinical practice.

Methods

Reports were included in this review if they were randomized controlled trials (RCTs) which investigated the analgesic effects of anticonvulsant drugs in patients, with pain assessment as either the primary or a secondary outcome. Reports excluded were studies which were non-randomized, studies of experimental pain, case reports, clinical observations, or studies of anticonvulsants used to treat pain produced by other drugs.

Reports were identified by several methods. A MEDLINE search (Silver Platter 3.0, 3.1, and 3.11) from 1966 to February 1994 was done using a search strategy designed to identify the maximum number of randomized and/or double-blind reports using a combination of text words, 'wild cards' and MeSH terms [10]. This search strategy was narrowed to include specific anticonvulsant drugs. Forty medical journals were manually searched, chosen from the 50 with the highest number of reports in MEDLINE, and nine specialist journals which were either not on that list or were not indexed [11]. The search process included volumes published between 1950 and 1990. Additional reports were identified from the reference list of the retrieved papers. Eligibility was determined by reading each report identified by the search. A letter was sent to the first author for further information on their published report (method of randomization, double-blinding, outcome measures, and drop-outs) and to ask if

The topic discussed in this chapter is also published in full in McQuay *et al.* [1].

they knew of, any other studies which met our inclusion criteria, either done by them or by other investigators.

Data extraction and analysis

Each report was scored for quality by four of the authors using a three-item scale (maximum 5, minimum 1) [12]; they then met to agree a 'consensus' score for each report. Information about the pain condition and number of patients studied, anticonvulsant drug and dosing regimen, study design (placebo or active control), study duration and follow-up, analgesic outcome measures and results, withdrawals, and adverse effects was taken from each report.

Dichotomous data was used to calculate relative risk (benefit or harm) estimates with 95% confidence intervals using a fixed effects model [13], together with NNT (number-need-to treat [14]). This was done for effectiveness, for adverse effects, and for drug-related study withdrawal. The index of effectiveness varied between reports. In some it was the number of patients improved, in others it was the numbers pain-free at the end of the study. No weighting was used between these different indices. The calculations were done both for the individual reports and by combining single treatment or control arms. For the reports that presented mean data with no significant difference between active and placebo, both treatments were assigned as zero patients improved.

Results

Thirty-seven reports were identified. All were published. Thirty-four were identified by MEDLINE, three from reference lists. Seventeen were excluded (Table 1). One was a duplicate publication [15].

Twenty RCTs were considered eligible. Studies of four anticonvulsant drugs were identified, ten with carbamazepine, five with phenytoin, three with clonazepam, and two with sodium valproate. Seventeen studies were in chronic non-malignant pain, and one each in cancer pain, postoperative pain, and acute herpes zoster. Details of these eligible reports are in Table 2 (placebo controlled) and Table 3 (active controls). The median quality score for the placebo controlled studies was 3 (range 2–5), and for the active controlled studies was 2 (range 1–4). We requested data from 19 authors. Five replied, but only one (Leijon [37]) was able to supply information relevant to this review.

Acute pain

Comparing carbamazepine with prednisolone in the management of acute herpes zoster, the patients treated with prednisolone reported less pain and faster skin healing (3.7 weeks vs. 5.3 weeks) than those treated with 400 mg/day of carbamazepine, and 13/20 carbamazepine patients still had pain at two months compared with 3/20 treated with prednisolone (Table 3) [45].

Table 1 Reports excluded from analysis

Ref.	Anticonvulsant	Condition	Reason for exclusion
[16]	Carbamazepine	Neuralgias	Not RCT
[17]	Carbamazepine	Trigeminal neuralgia	Not RCT
[18]	Carbamazepine	Trigeminal neuralgia	Not RCT
[19]	Carbamazepine	Horton's headache	Not RCT
[20]	Phenytoin	Suxamethonium-induced myalgia	Suxamethonium-induced myalgia
[21]	Flunarizine	NA	Review, not RCT
[22]	Carbamazepine	Drug interaction	Not RCT, drug interaction
[23]	Carbamazepine	Trigeminal neuralgia	Not RCT
[15]	Carbamazepine	Trigeminal neuralgia	Not RCT, dual publication
[24]	Sodium valproate	Chronic headache	Not RCT
[25]	Phenytoin	Rheumatoid arthritis	Not RCT
[26]	Carbamazepine	Facial pain	Not RCT. single-blind
[27]	3,4-hydroxypipridyl 6-(2-chlorophenyl)-pyridazine)	Experimental pain volunteers	Experimental pain
[28]	Carbamazepine	Trigeminal neuralgia	Case report not RCT
[29]	Carbamazepine	Fabry's disease	Case report not RCT
[30]	Carbamazepine	Facial pain	Not RCT
[31]	Clonazepam	Diabetic neuropathy	Not RCT

NA, not applicable.

Chronic pain

Trigeminal neuralgia

Three of the 12 placebo controlled studies in chronic pain were in trigeminal neuralgia, all with carbamazepine [32–34] (Table 2, Fig. 1). Using dose titration to a maximum dose of 1 g/day 19/27 patients had a complete or very good response compared with placebo on five days treatment [33]. Again using dose titration and a cross-over design, but to a maximum dose of 2.4 g/day, 15/20 patients randomized to initial carbamazepine had a good or excellent response compared with placebo on 14 days treatment [33]. The extent to which the pain was relieved may be gauged from the third study [32]. Using doses in the range of 400–800 mg/day for two-week treatment periods, the mean fall in maximum pain intensity was 58% with carbamazepine compared with 26% on placebo. The NNT for effectiveness compared with placebo was 2.6, that for adverse effects 3.4, and that for drug related study withdrawal 24 (Table 4). The relative benefit of two of the three studies, and the overall ratio, showed carbamazepine to be better than placebo.

Table 2 Reports included: trials with placebo control

Ref.	Condition & no. of patients	Design, study duration, & follow-up*	Outcome measures	Dose regimen	Analgesic outcome results	Withdrawals & adverse effects	Quality score
Carbamazepine							
[32]	Trigeminal neuralgia (77)	Multicentre cross-over 8 wks (4 2-wk periods, 2 each on carbamazepine & placebo); no follow-up.	Pain severity, paroxysms, triggers.	100 mg 4 ×/day to 200 mg tds (1 centre) or 200 mg 4×/day (2 centres).	Mean % maximum possible pain intensity fell 58% with carbamazepine, 26% with placebo. Paroxysms & triggers also significantly reduced.	7 withdrawals (1 rash, others logistic). 50% had 1 or more AEs on carbamazepine, 26% on placebo. Giddiness 30%, drowsiness 15%.	5
[33]	Trigeminal neuralgia (30), PHN (6), other chronic neuralgias (6). 36/42 studied double-blind (24/32 TN).	Cross-over 10 days (2 5-day periods); open follow-up, range 2 wks to 36 mths.	Pain relief.	Dose titration 400 mg to 1 g/day.	19/27 TN 'complete or very good' response. Placebo responses 'minimal or absent in all cases'.	3/30 TN withdrawn (rash, leukopenia, abnormal liver function). AE in 23/36 studied double blind; 17 giddiness, 16 drowsiness.	4
[34]	64 facial pain recruited, 54 with trigeminal neuralgia. Results presented on 44 TN only, 'due to insufficient follow-up'.	Partial cross-over (successful first treatment period stayed on that treatment). 20 had carbamazepine only, 7 had placebo only, 17 had placebo then carbamazepine. Follow-up 46 mths.	Global rating (pain intensity & AEs).	Dose titration 100 mg to 2.4 g/day.	15/20 on carbamazepine *ab initio* had good or excellent response. 12/17 switched from placebo to carbamazepine & 6/7 on placebo also had good or excellent response.	2/37 carbamazepine withdrawn, 1 rash, 1 itch. 4/37 on carbamazepine died (of other causes). 10/37 drowsiness, 7/37 staggering gait.	3
[35]	Diabetic neuropathy (30).	Cross-over 6 wks (3 2-wk periods); no follow-up.	Pain intensity.	Dose titration 200 mg– 600 mg/day.	28/30 improved on carbamazepine vs. 19/30 on placebo, 0/30 worse on carbamazepine, 11/30 worse on placebo.	3 withdrawals (2 carbamazepine AEs 1 logistic). 16/30 somnolence, 12/30 dizziness.	4
[36]	Migraine prophylaxis (48).	Cross-over 12 wks (2 6-wk periods); no follow-up.	No. of migraines, global rating.	1 tab 3 × day.	38/45 improved on carbamazepine, 13/48 on placebo. 30 migraines in 45 on carbamazepine, 186 in 48 on placebo.	3 withdrawals, 1 AE on carbamazepine, 2 logistic. 30/45 had AEs with carbamazepine (23 vertigo or dizziness), 11/48 on placebo.	4
[37]	Central post-stroke pain (15).	Cross-over 14 wks (3 4-wk periods with 2 1-wk washouts); no follow-up.	Daily pain intensity, post-treatment, global rating.	Stepped increase to final (day 18) 800 mg daily; amitriptyline 75 mg daily at day 6.	Daily rating: amitriptyline significantly lower pain intensity than placebo on 3/3 wks tested, and carbamazepine on 1/3 wks tested. Global: 10/15 improved on amitriptyline; 5/14 on carbamazepine; 1/15 on placebo.	No withdrawals. 14/15 on amitriptyline and carbamazepine had AEs, 1/15 on placebo. 4 carbamazepine patients had dosage reduction.	4
Phenytoin							
[38]	Irritable bowel (14)	Cross-over 20 wks (4-wk run-in, 6 wks treatment, 4-wk washout, 6 wks treatment); no follow-up.	Bowel movements, pain episodes	Fixed 300 mg/day.	No statistically significant differences between phenytoin & placebo.	2 withdrawals, neither drug-related. No report of AEs.	4

Table 2   *continued*

Ref.	Condition & no. of patients	Design, study duration, & follow-up*	Outcome measures	Dose regimen	Analgesic outcome results	Withdrawals & adverse effects	Quality score
[39]	Diabetic neuropathy (40)	Cross-over 5 wks (2 2-wk periods, 1 wk washout); no follow-up.	Pain intensity & paraesthesiae	Fixed 300 mg/day.	28/38 on phenytoin had at least moderate improvement, 10/38 on placebo.	2 withdrawals 'did not report back'. 4/38 giddiness on phenytoin.	2
[40]	Diabetic poly-neuropathy (12)	Cross-over 46 wks (2 × 23 wks); no follow-up.	Pain intensity	1 capsule 3 ×/day titrated vs. plasma conc.	No statistically significant diff between phenytoin & placebo.	2 drug-related withdrawals on phenytoin, none on placebo. On phenytoin significant increase in plasma glucose and 4 × no. of reports of AEs (16 vs. 4).	2

Sodium valproate

Ref.	Condition & no. of patients	Design, study duration, & follow-up*	Outcome measures	Dose regimen	Analgesic outcome results	Withdrawals & adverse effects	Quality score
[41]	Acute postop (39)	Parallel group (140 min).	Pain intensity	15 mg/kg sodium valproate vs. placebo vs. 2 mg/kg ketoprofen, each IV over 20 min	No significant diff between valproate & placebo. Ketoprofen significant reduction in pain intensity compared with both valproate & placebo	None reported	2
[42]	Migraine prophylaxis (32)	Cross-over 10 wks (2-wk run-in, 2 8-wk periods); no follow-up.	No. of attacks, duration & pain intensity	Fixed 400 mg 2 × day.	Significant reduction in no. of attacks duration and pain intensity on valproate. Valproate effective in 25/29.	3 withdrawals, 1 valproate AEs, 2 placebo. On valproate 2/29 dyspepsia, 2/29 nausea, 2/29 weariness.	3

Clonazepam

Ref.	Condition & no. of patients	Design, study duration, & follow-up*	Outcome measures	Dose regimen	Analgesic outcome results	Withdrawals & adverse effects	Quality score
[43]	Migraine prophylaxis (38)	Cross-over 16 wks (4-wk run-in, 3 4-wk periods; placebo vs. high & low dose clonazepam). Followed up on 2 mg/day for 4 wks.	Headache days	Fixed 1 & 2 mg/day.	Significant reduction in headaches between 2 mg & run-in period, but not between 1 mg & run-in period, or between either 1 or 2 mg & placebo	4 withdrawals, 3 lethargy on 1 mg clonazepam, unclear other. 23/38 drowsy on clonazepam & 10 dizzy.	3
[44]	Tempero-mandibular joint dysfunction (myofascial pain) (20)	Parallel group 60 days; open follow-up.	Pain intensity on palpation & global impression.	Dose titration 0.25–1 mg/day (mean 0.375 mg).	Significantly lower pain intensity and higher global rating at 30 days with clonazepam vs. with placebo.	6/10 clonazepam withdrew; 1 at 1 wk (headache), 5 at 30 days because pain improved. 7/10 placebo withdrew at 30 days because not improved. 3/10 clonazepam drowsy.	3

PHN, post-herpetic neuralgia; TN, trigeminal neuralgia.
*Studies single centre unless otherwise stated.

Three active control studies compared carbamazepine with tizanidine (alpha-2 adrenergic agonist) [46], tocainide (anti-arrhthymic) [47], and pimozide (antipsychotic) [48] (Table 3). Carbamazepine produced better results than tizanidine; there was no significant difference in the tocainide study; pimozide produced better results than carbamazepine.

Diabetic neuropathy

Two placebo controlled studies in diabetic neuropathy (one with carbamazepine [35]. and one with phenytoin [39]), found that with two weeks' treatment between 30% and 50% more patients improved on anticonvulsant than on

Table 3 Reports included: trials with active drug control

Ref.	Condition & no. of patients	Design, study duration, & follow-up[*]	Outcome measures	Dose regimen	Analgesic outcome results	Withdrawals & adverse effects	Quality score
Carbamazepine							
[45]	Acute herpes zoster (40)	Parallel group 4 wks vs. prednisolone; clinic follow-up till no pain (maximum >1 year).	Pain, skin healing, incidence of PHN (> 2 mths)	100 mg 4 ×/day carbamazepine vs. prednisolone 40 mg/day for 10 days then reduced to nought over next 3 wks.	Skin healing significantly faster with prednisolone PHN in 13/20 carbamazepine patients, 3/20 prednisolone.	Not rep.	1
[46]	Trigeminal neuralgia (12)	Parallel group 3 wks vs. tizanidine; no follow-up.	Pain intensity, pain relief, global.	Carbamazepine titrated up to max of 3 × 300 mg/day, tizanidine to 3 × 6 mg/day.	4/6 carbamazepine patients rated treatment as very good, 1/5 tizanidine.	3 withdrawals on tizanidine, 1 not drug-related, 2 because of intolerable pain.	3
[47]	Trigeminal neuralgia (12)	Cross-over 4 wks (2 2-wk periods) vs. tocainide; no follow-up.	Severity, frequency & duration of attacks = TN score.	'Maximum tolerated' dose of carbamazepine vs. tocainide about 20 mg/kg/day' in 3 divided doses.	Tocainide and carbamazepine produced similar improvement compared with placebo: no significant difference between the active treatments.	Tocainide 1/10 nausea, 1/10 paraesthesiae, 1/10 rash (withdrawn).	2
[48]	Trigeminal neuralgia (68)	Multicentre (4) cross-over 24 wks (4-wk placebo run-in then 2 8-wk periods with 4-wk washout) vs. pimozide; open follow-up on pimozide.	Trigeminal neuralgia symptom score.	Step titration carbamazepine 300–1200 mg daily & pimozide 4–12 mg daily in 2 divided doses.	Pimozide lowered symptom score by 78% from baseline compared with 50% on carbamazepine.	68 recruited, 59 randomized, 11 excluded from analysis, 10 protocol deviation, 1 did not returned. 40/48 AEs on pimozide, 21/48 on carbamazepine.	4
Phenytoin							
[49]	Rheumatoid arthritis (60)	Parallel group single-blind 24 wks; no follow-up.	Pain & morning stiffness	Step titration phenytoin 100 mg/day increased by 50 mg/wk to effect or AE. IM gold 10 mg test dose then 50 mg/wk, then, if effective, 50 mg/2 wks.	Mean pain score improvement of 40/100 on gold, 12 on phenytoin.	6 withdrawals phenytoin, 2 no effect, 1 rash, 1 sleep difficulty, 1 lethargy. 1 unrelated death. 6 withdrawals on gold, 2 rash, 1 no effect, 3 proteinuria.	2
[50]	Cancer pain (75)	Parallel group 4 wks vs. buprenorphine & a combination of buprenorphine & phenytoin; no follow-up.	Pain intensity, pain relief.	Phenytoin 2 × 100 mg/day, buprenorphine 2 × 0.2 mg sublingual/day, combin. 0.1 mg sublingual buprenorphine + phenytoin 50 mg 2 ×/day.	Good or moderate relief in 21/25 buprenorphine only, in 18/25 phenytoin only, and in 22/25 combination patients.	13/25 affected in buprenorphine only, 2/25 in phenytoin only, 5/25 in combination.	2

Table 3   *continued*

Ref.	Condition & no. of patients	Design, study duration, & follow-up*	Outcome measures	Dose regimen	Analgesic outcome results	Withdrawals & adverse effects	Quality score
Combinations							
[51]	Post-herpetic neuralgia (29)	parallel group 8 wks carbamazepine + clomipramine (16) vs. TENS (13); no follow-up	Pain intensity, activity, mood.	Carbamazepine 150 mg to 1 g/day, clomipramine 10–75 mg/day; TENS 15 min/wk for 4 wks.	Mean improvement 43/100 mm on drug combination, 0.2 on TENS.	7 withdrawals on drug treatment, 4 (no effect) crossed (successfully) to TENS. 10 withdrawals on TENS (?cause) & 8 crossed to drug treatment 3 successfully.	2

PHN, post-herpetic neuralgia; TN, trigeminal neuralgia; TENS, transcutaneous nerve stimulation.
*Studies single centre unless otherwise stated.

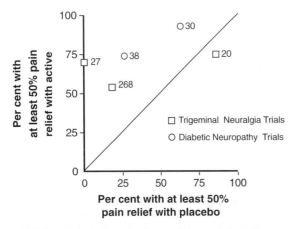

Fig. 1   L'Abbé plot of trigeminal neuralgia and diabetic neuropathy trials with anticonvulsants. (Each point is one trial; numbers are the number of patients treated.)

placebo. A third study using phenytoin for 23 weeks of treatment found no difference in mean pain intensity compared with placebo [40] (Fig. 1). The NNT for effectiveness compared with placebo was 3, for adverse effects 2.5, and for drug-related study withdrawal 20 (Table 4). The combined relative benefit showed a significant effect for anticonvulsant compared with placebo.

There were no eligible active control studies of diabetic neuropathy.

Migraine prophylaxis

Of three placebo controlled studies of migraine prophylaxis, using three different anticonvulsants, two showed greater effect with the anticonvulsant than with placebo (Table 2). Six weeks treatment with carbamazepine 3 tablets per day led to improvement in 38/45 patients compared with 13/48 on placebo [36]. Sodium valproate 800 mg/day for eight weeks produced significant reduction in the number of migraines, in their duration and in pain intensity; valproate was effective in 25/29 patients [42]. The third study used clonazepam at 1 or 2 mg/day for 60 days of treatment, and no significant difference was found between clonazepam and placebo [43]. The NNT for effectiveness compared with placebo was 2.4, for adverse effects 2.4, and for drug-related study withdrawal 39 (Table 4). The combined relative benefit showed a significant effect for anticonvulsant compared with placebo.

There were no eligible active control studies of migraine prophylaxis.

Other pain syndromes

Placebo controlled studies (Table 2). Phenytoin 300 mg/day for six weeks had no effect in the one study of irritable bowel syndrome [38]. In central post-stroke pain four weeks of carbamazepine at a final dose of 800 mg/day was judged to have improved 5/14 patients, compared with 10/15 on 75 mg of amitriptyline and 1/15 on placebo [37]. In a 60-day study of clonazepam (mean daily dose 0.375 mg) in temporomandibular joint dysfunction, analysis at 30 days showed significantly lower pain intensity scores with the anticonvulsant compared with placebo [44].
Active controlled studies (Table 3). In rheumatoid arthritis, a 24-week comparison of phenytoin and intramuscular gold showed significantly better pain relief and morning stiffness on gold at 24 weeks [49]. In cancer pain phenytoin 200 mg/day was compared with buprenorphine alone and a combination of buprenorphine and phenytoin (100 mg/day); all three regimens produced good or moderate relief in more than 60% of patients [50]. A comparison of a combination of carbamazepine and clomipramine with transcutaneous electrical nerve stimulation (TENS) produced improvement for 9/16 on drug treatment and 3/13 on TENS [51].

Adverse effects and drug-related withdrawal

In the placebo controlled studies there were 16 drug-related withdrawals on anticonvulsant treatment compared with 2 on placebo (Table 4C). Where adverse effects were reported the incidence was between 25% and 50% within each study. Drowsiness, dizziness, and gait disturbance were the common problems.

Table 4   Chronic pain reports with placebo control

Ref.	Improved on active drugs	Improved on placebo	Relative benefit (95% CI)	NNT (95% CI)
A. NNT for effectiveness				
Trigeminal neuralgia				
[32]	144/268*	35/190*	2.9 (2.1–4)	2.8 (2.3–3.7)
[33]	19/27	0/27	39 (2.5–614.3)	1.4 (1.14–1.88)
[34]	15/20	6/7	0.9 (0.6–1.3)	–9.3 (4.7–∞)
Combined data	178/315	41/224	3.1 (2.3–4.1)	2.6 (2.2–3.3)
Diabetic neuropathy				
[35]	28/30	19/30	1.5 (1.1–2)	3.3 (2–9.4)
[39]	28/38	10/38	2.8 (1.6–4.9)	2.1 (1.5–3.6)
[40]		(no dichotomous data available)		
Combined data	56/68	29/68	1.9 (1.4–2.7)	2.5 (1.8–4)
Migraine prophylaxis				
[36]	38/45	13/48	3.1 (1.9–5.1)	1.7 (1.4–2.4)
[42]	25/29	4/29	6.3 (2.5–15.7)	1.4 (1.1–1.8)
[43]		(no dichotomous data available)		
Combined data	63/74	17/77	3.7 (2.4–5.9)	1.6 (1.3–2)
Other pain syndromes				
[37]	5/14	1/15	5.4 (0.7–40.4)	3.4 (1.7–105)
[38]		(no dichotomous data available)		
[44]		(no dichotomous data available)		
B. NNT for adverse effects				
Trigeminal neuralgia				
[32]	38/77	20/77	1.9 (1.2–3)	4.3 (2.6–11.7)
[33]	23/36	0/30	39.3 (2.5–620.2)	1.6 (1.3–2.1)
[34]	10/37	0/7	4.2 (0.3–64.2)	3.7 (2.4–7.9)
Combined data	71/150	20/114	2.7 (1.8–4.2)	3.4 (2.5–5.2)
Diabetic neuropath				
[35]	16/30	0/30	33 (2.1–525.8)	1.9 (1.4–2.8)
[39]	4/38	0/38	9 (0.5–161.5)	9.5 (4.9–130)
[40]	10/12	4/12	2.5 (1.1–5.8)	2 (1.2–6.3)
Combined data	30/80	4/80	7.5 (2.8–20.3)	3.1 (2.3–4.8)
Migraine prophylaxis				
[36]	30/45	11/48	2.9 (1.7–5.1)	2.3 (1.6–3.9)
[42]	6/29	2/29	3 (0.7–13.7)	7.3 (3.2–∞)
[43]	23/38	0/38	47 (3–746.6)	1.7 (1.3–2.2)
Combined data	59/112	13/115	4.7 (2.7–8)	2.4 (1.9–3.3)
Other pain syndromes				
[37]	14/15	1/15	14 (2.1–93.5)	1.2 (1–1.5)
[38]	0/12	0/12	NA	NA
[44]	4/10	0/10	9 (0.6–147.1)	2.5 (1.4–10.4)
C. NNT for drug-related withdrawals				
Trigeminal neuralgia				
[32]	1/77	0/77	3 (0.1–72.5)	77 (26.1–∞)
[33]	3/30	0/30	7 (0.4–129.8)	10 (4.8–∞)
[34]	2/37	0/7	1 (0.1–18.8)	18.5 (7.9–∞)
Combined data	6/144	0/114	10.3 (0.6–180.9)	24 (13.5–110.8)

Table 4   *continued*

Ref.	Improved on active drugs	Improved on placebo	Relative benefit (95% CI)	NNT (95% CI)
Diabetic neuropathy				
[35]	2/30	0/30	5 (0.3–99.9)	15 (6.4–∞)
[39]	0/38	0/38	1 (0–49.1)	NA
[40]	2/12	0/12	5 (0.3–94)	6 (2.6–∞)
Combined data	4/80	0/80	9 (0.5–164.5)	20 (10.2–446)
Migraine prophylaxis				
[36]	1/48	0/48	3 (0.1–71.8)	48 (16.3–∞)
[42]	1/32	2/32	0.5 (0.1–5.2)	NA
[43]	3/38	0/38	7 (0.4–131)	12.7 (6.1–∞)
Combined data	5/118	2/118	2.5 (0.5–12.6)	39.3 (14.6–∞)
Other pain syndromes				
[37]	0/15	0/15	1 (0–47.3)	NA
[38]	0/12	0/12	1 (0–46.6)	NA
[44]	1/10	0/10	3 (0.1–65.6)	10 (3.5–∞)

* 77 Patients assessed on multiple cross-over. NA, not applicable or not available.

Discussion

Process

Thirty-seven reports were found: 17 were excluded, 15 because they were not RCTs. Many of the remaining 20 had significant flaws; omission of drug dosage (1), lack of true blinding (1), inappropriate statistical conclusions (1), and omission of statistical testing (7). The quality scores of the placebo controlled studies were higher than those of the active control studies (Tables 2 and 3). Nine of the 20 papers were recent (published in the last decade), but standards of reporting have not improved. The quality of the reporting limited the ability to combine data, because many reports gave insufficient information, used a variety of different outcome measures, and several studies used variable dosing. Although the authors of the original reports were contacted by letter, not all of them replied, and even those who did reply did not have data available.

The numbers-needed-to-treat (NNT) approach was used because the majority of the data was in dichotomous form, which lends itself to this analysis, and because NNTs are more readily clinically interpretable than, for instance, effect sizes. NNTs were calculated for adverse effects, minor and major, as well as for effectiveness, because adverse effects are important for clinical decision making. This approach may be useful in other reviews of long-established interventions. The older the report, the more likely was it to present simple binary data, such as 'improved versus not improved'. More recent reports which restricted data presentation to mean data for treatment and control were not accessible to the NNT method.

Product

Acute pain

Anticonvulsants were ineffective in the one postoperative pain report [41], and similarly in acute herpes zoster [45]. There is no logic in using anticonvulsants to manage acute nociceptive pain when there are other (effective) remedies.

Chronic pain

The overall pattern, of NNT for effectiveness of about 2.5, NNT for adverse effects of about 3, and NNT for drug-related study withdrawal between 20 and 40 was surprisingly similar for the three pain syndromes with more than one RCT (Table 4).

Medical students are often taught that a positive response to carbamazepine is 'diagnostic' for trigeminal neuralgia. If only one patient responds out of two treated this statement needs to be qualified. One caveat is that the study populations may include patients who have had other interventions, such as nerve blocks, and the NNT for effectiveness may be more impressive in trigeminal neuralgia treated with carbamazepine in the initial stages. The statement 'approximately 70% of patients will have significant pain relief' [4] would seem to be about right.

Diabetic neuropathy is perceived as a model for other neuropathic pain syndromes, and results from diabetic neuropathy are often extrapolated to the other syndromes. The results with anticonvulsants reviewed here conflicted, with a negative result in the longest study (46 weeks) balanced by two positive studies. The NNT for effectiveness was the same as the NNT for adverse effects. The usual clinical decision is between antidepressants and anticonvulsants as first-line treatment, and the evidence here does not support the use of anticonvulsants as first-line remedies. Direct evidence comparing antidepressant and anticonvulsant is available from the post-stroke pain study, where the NNT for effectiveness of amitriptyline was 1.7, compared with 3.4 for carbamazepine, with the same NNT for adverse effects and study withdrawal [37].

The three placebo controlled RCTs of anticonvulsants in migraine prophylaxis showed anticonvulsants to be effective. The recent advances in migraine management may reduce the impact of these results.

This review shows that there is a need for high quality studies of the relative effectiveness of different anticonvulsants in chronic pain syndromes, and for comparisons of antidepressants with anticonvulsants. The usefulness of such primary studies would be increased greatly by improvements in the quality of reporting. Investigators presenting data as means for treatment and control should also consider the (simple) presentation of binary data.

References

1. McQuay H, Carroll D, Jadad AR, Wiffen P, Moore A. Anticonvulsant drugs for management of pain: a systematic review. *British Medical Journal* 1995; 311:1047–52.

2. Jacox A, Carr DB, Payne R. *Management of cancer pain.* Clinical Practice Guideline No. 9. Agency for Health Care Policy and Research *AHCPR* Publication No. 94–0592. Rockville, MD: Public Health Service, 1994; 41–74.

3. Rappaport ZH, Devor M. Trigeminal neuralgia: the role of self-sustaining discharge in the trigeminal ganglion. *Pain* 1994; 56:127–138.

4. Loeser JD. Tic douloureux and atypical facial pain. In: Wall P.D., Melzack R, ed *Textbook of pain,* (3rd edn) London: Churchill Livingstone, 1994; 699–710.

5. Twycross R. The management of pain in cancer. In: Nimmo WS, Rowbotham DJ, Smith G, ed. *Anaesthesia* (2nd edn). Oxford: Blackwell Scientific Publications, 1994:1635–51.

6. Monks R. Psychotropic drugs. In: Wall P.D., Melzack R, (ed). *Textbook of pain,* (3rd edn) London: Churchill Livingstone, 1994:963–89.

7. Reynolds JEF. *Martindale: the extra pharmacopoeia,* (30th edn) London: Pharmaceutical Press, 1993:292–314.

8. Grahame-Smith DG, Aronson JK. *Oxford textbook of clinical pharmacology and drug therapy* (2nd edn). Oxford University Press, 1992:433–6; 443–4.

9. Rall TW, Schleifer LS. Drugs effective in the therapy of the epilepsies. In: Goodman Gilman A, Rall TW, Nies AS, Taylor P, ed. *The pharmacological basis of therapeutics* (8th edn). Toronto: McGraw-Hill, 1992:436–62.

10. Jadad AR, McQuay HJ. A high-yield-strategy to identify randomized controlled trials for systematic reviews. *Online Journal of Current Clinical Trials* [serial online] 1993; Doc No 33:3973 words; 39 paragraphs. 5 tables.

11. Jadad AR. Meta-analysis of randomised clinical trials in pain relief. University of Oxford: D. Phil thesis, 1994.

12. Jadad AR, Moore RA, Carroll D, Jenkinson C, Reynolds DJM, Gavaghan DJ *et al.* Assessing the quality of reports of randomized clinical trials: is blinding necessary? *Controlled Clinical Trials* 1996; 17:1–12.

13. Yusuf S, Peto R, Lewis J, Collins R, Sleight P. Betablockade during and after myocardial infarction: an overview of the randomized trials. *Progress in Cardiovascular Disease* 1985; 27:335–71.

14. Cook RJ, Sackett DL. The number needed to treat: a clinically useful measure of treatment effect. *British Medical Journal* 1995; 310:452–4.

15. Kienast HW, Boshes LD. Clinical trials of carbamazepine in suppressing pain. *Proceedings of the Institute of Medicine of Chicago* 1968; 27:50.

16. Arieff A, Wetzel N. Tegretol in the treatment of neuralgias. *Diseases of the Nervous System* 1967; 28:820–3.

17. Farago F. Trigeminal neuralgia: its treatment with two new carbamazepine analogues. *European Neurology* 1987; 26:73–83.

18. Fromm G, Terrence C, Chattha A. Baclofen in the treatment of trigeminal neuralgia: double-blind study and long-term follow-up. *Annals of Neurology* 1984; 15:240–4.

19. Goncikowska M. Treatment of Horton's headache with small doses of pilocarpine and carbamazepine. *Wiadomosci Lekarski* 1984; 37:1093–5.

20. Hatta V, Saxena A, Kaul HL. Phenytoin reduces suxamethonium-induced myalgia. *Anaesthesia* 1992; 47:664–7.

21. Holmes B, Brogden RN, Heel RC, Speight TM, Avery GS. Flunarizine. A review of its pharmacodynamic and pharmacokinetic properties and therapeutic use. *Drugs* 1984; 27:6–44.

22. Hopkins S. Clinical toleration and safety of azithromycin. *American Journal of Medicine* 1991; 91:40S–5.

23. Kienast HW, Boshes LD. Clinical triasl of carbamazepine in suppressing pain. *Headache* 1968; 8:1–5.

24. Mathew NT, Ali S. Valproate in the treatment of persistent chronic daily headache. An open label study. *Headache* 1991; 31:71–4.

25. Naidu MU, Ramesh Kumar T, Anuradha RT, Rao UR. Evaluation of phenytoin in rheumatoid arthritis: an open study. *Drugs Under Experimental Clinical Research* 1991; 17:271–5.

26. Rasmussen P, Riishede J. Facial pain treated with carbamazepin (Tegretol). *Acta Neurologica Scandinavica* 1970; 46:385–408.

27. Schaffler K, Wauschkuhn C, Gierend M. Analgesic potency of a new anticonvulsant drug versus acetylsalicylic acid via laser somatosensory evoked potentials. Randomized placebo controlled double blind (5 way) crossover study. *Arzneimittelforschung* 1991; 41:427–35.

28. Sharav Y, Benoliel R, Schnarch A, Greenberg L. Idiopathic trigeminal pain associated with gustatory stimuli. *Pain* 1991; 44:171–4.

29. Shibasaki H, Tabira T, Inoue N, Goto I, Kuroiwa Y. Carbamazepine for painful crises in Fabry's disease. *Journal of the Neurological Sciences* 1973; 18:47–51.

30. Westerholm N. Treatment of facial pain with G 32 883 (Tegretol Geigy). *Scandinavian Journal of Dental Research* 1970; 78:144–8. 1970; 78:144–8.

31. Young RJ, Clarke BF. Pain relief in diabetic neuropathy: the effectiveness of imipramine and related drugs. *Diabetic Medicine* 1985; 2:363–6.

32. Campbell FG, Graham JG, Zilkha KJ. Clinical trial of carbazepine (Tegretol) in trigeminal neuralgia. *Journal of Neurology, Neurosurgery and Psychiatry* 1966; 29:265–7.

33. Killian JM, Fromm GH. Carbamazepine in the treatment of neuralgia. Use of side effects. *Archives of Neurology* 1968; 19:129–36.

34. Nicol CF. A four year double blind study of tegretol in facial pain. *Headache* 1969; 9:54–7.

35. Rull J, Quibrera R, Gonzalz-Millan H, Lozano CO. Symptomatic treatment of peripheral diabetic neuropathy with

carbamazepine: double-blind crossover study. *Diabetologia* 1969; **5**:215–20.

36. Rompel H, Bauermeister PW. Aetiology of migraine and prevention with carbamazepine (tegretol): results of a double-blind, cross-over study. *South African Medical Journal* 1970; **44**:75–80.

37. Leijon G, Boivie J. Central post-stroke pain—a controlled trial of amitriptyline and carbamazepine. *Pain* 1989; **36**:27–36.

38. Greenbaum DS, Ferguson RK, Kater LA, Kuiper DH, Rosen LW. A controlled therapeutic study of the irritable-bowel syndrome. *New England Journal of Medicine* 1973; **288**:13–16.

39. Chadda V, Mathur M. Double blind study of the effects of diphenylhydantoin sodium on diabetic neuropathy. *Journal of the Association of Physicians of India* 1978; **26**:403–6.

40. Saudek CD, Werns S, Reidenberg MM. Phenytoin in the treatment of diabetic symmetrical polyneuropathy. *Clinical Pharmacology and Therapeutics* 1977; **22**:196–9.

41. Martin C, Martin A, Rud C, Valli M. Comparative study of sodium valproate and ketoprofen in the treatment of postoperative pain. *Annales Françaises d'Anesthesie et de Reanimation* 1988; **7**:387–92.

42. Hering R, Kuritzky A. Sodium valproate in the prophylactic treatment of migraine: a double-blind study versus placebo. *Cephalalgia* 1992; **12**:81–4.

43. Stensrud P, Sjaastad O. Clonazepam (rivotril) in migraine prophylaxis. *Headache* 1979; **19**:333–4.

44. Harkins S, Linford J, Cohen J, Kramer T, Cueva L. Administration of clonazepam in the treatment of TMD and associated myofascial pain: a double-blind pilot study. *Journal of Craniomandibular Disorders* 1991; **5**:179–86.

45. Keczkes K, Basheer AM. Do corticosteroids prevent postherpetic neuralgia? *British Journal of Dermatology* 1980; **102**:551–5.

46. Vilming ST, Lyberg T, Lataste X. Tizanidine in the management of trigeminal neuralgia. *Cephalalgia* 1986; **6**:181–2.

47. Lindström P, Lindblom U. The analgesic effect of tocainide in trigeminal neuralgia. *Pain* 1987; **28**:45–40.

48. Lechin F, van der Dijs B, Lechin ME, Amat J, Lechin AE, Cabrera A *et al*. Pimozide therapy for trigeminal neuralgia. *Archives of Neurology* 1989; **46**:960–63.

49. Richards I, Fraser S, Hunter J, Capell H. Comparison of phenytoin and gold as second line drugs in rheumatoid arthritis. *Annals of Rheumatic Disease* 1987; **46**:667–9.

50. Yajnik S, Singh GP, Singh G, Kumar M. Phenytoin as a coanalgesic in cancer pain. *Journal of Pain and Symptom Management* 1992; **7**:209–13.

51. Gerson GR, Jones RB, Luscombe DK. Studies on the concomitant use of carbamazepine and clomipramine for the relief of post-herpetic neuralgia. *Postgraduate Medical Journal* 1977; **53**:104–9.

31

Antidepressants in neuropathic pain

Summary

This review of the effectiveness and safety of antidepressants in neuropathic pain used randomized controlled trials. The main outcomes were global judgements, pain relief, or fall in pain intensity that approximated to more than 50% pain relief, and information about minor and major adverse effects. Dichotomous data for effectiveness and adverse effects were analysed using relative risk and number-needed-to-treat (NNT) methods.

Twenty-one placebo controlled treatments in 17 RCTs 10 were included, involving 10 antidepressants. In six of thirteen diabetic neuropathy studies the relative risk (benefit) was significant compared with placebo. The combined relative benefit was 1.9 (95% confidence interval 1.6–2.4), with a NNT for benefit of 3 (2.4–4). In two of three post-herpetic neuralgia studies the relative benefit was significant, and the combined relative benefit was 4.8 (2.4–9.4), with a NNT of 2.3 (1.7–3.3). In two atypical facial pain studies the combined relative benefit was 2 (1.5–2.8), with a NNT of 2.8 (2–4.7). Only one of three central pain studies had analysable dichotomous data. The NNT point estimate was 1.7.

Comparisons of tricyclic antidepressants did not show any significant difference between them; they were significantly more effective than benzodiazepines in the three comparisons available. Paroxetine and mianserin were less effective than imipramine.

For 11 of the 21 placebo controlled treatments there was dichotomous information on minor adverse effects; combining across pain syndromes the NNT for minor (noted in published report) adverse effects was 3.7 (2.9–5.2). Information on major (drug-related study withdrawal) adverse effects was available from 19 reports; combining across pain syndromes the NNT for major adverse effects was 22 (13.5–58).

Antidepressants are effective in relieving neuropathic pain. With very similar results for anticonvulsants it is still unclear which drug class should be first choice.

Introduction

Antidepressants have been used for over thirty years to manage neuropathic pain, but in the United Kingdom no antidepressant has a product licence for this indication.

Many of the studies of antidepressants in neuropathic pain are open case reports; interpreting the open studies is difficult because of different drugs and doses used, and because of the simultaneous use of other drugs. The aim of this systematic review was to use the evidence from RCTs of antidepressants in neuropathic pain to address current clinical debates, which include which drug is best, whether selective serotonin re-uptake inhibitors (SSRIs) have any advantage over tricyclic antidepressants, how to manage dose titration, whether benefit is due to analgesic effect rather than mood improvement, and whether the character of the pain is predictive of response, as well as to allow comparison with anticonvulsants—which are the main therapeutic alternative.

In a previous review Onghena and Van Houdenhove looked at placebo controlled studies in chronic non-malignant pain in general, rather than just neuropathic pain, considered papers published up to 1990, and used effect size as the meta-analytic outcome [2]. They concluded that 'the average chronic pain patient who receives an antidepressant treatment is better off than 74% of the chronic pain patients who receive a placebo'. We wished to focus on neuropathic pain, and, by using the number-needed-to-treat (NNT) [3] as the meta-analytic outcome, to produce more precise clinical conclusions, and allow comparison with the effect of anticonvulsants in neuropathic pain [4].

Methods

Reports of randomized controlled trials (RCTs) of antidepressants in chronic pain were sought. From these reports the subset of trials of neuropathic pain (diabetic neuropathy, post-herpetic neuralgia, atypical facial pain and central pain) were selected. Reports were included which were randomized comparisons of antidepressant with placebo, with another antidepressant, or with any other intervention. A number of different search strategies in both MEDLINE (1966–94) and the Oxford Pain Relief Database (1950–92) were used to locate reports, using the individual drug names [5]. Additional reports were identified from the reference lists of retrieved reports and from review articles. Lead authors of identified reports were contacted to provide more details and were asked if they knew of other reports.

Unpublished reports, abstracts and reviews, drugs withdrawn early in development, and studies with fewer than 10 patients per group were excluded. Two of the authors screened all reports to eliminate those that had no pain outcomes, that were definitely not randomized, or were abstracts or reviews.

The topic discussed in this chapter is also published in full in McQuay et al. [1].

Included trials

Each report which could possibly meet the inclusion criteria was read by each author independently and scored for inclusion and quality using a three-item scale [6]. An included report could have a maximum score of 5 and a minimum score of 1. Information about the treatments and controls, type of condition studied, number of patients enrolled and analysed, study design, observation periods, outcome measures used for pain or global evaluation, and their results and minor (noted in published report) and major (drug-related study withdrawal) adverse effects was taken from each report, and agreed by all authors.

Data analysis and extraction

A clinically relevant outcome was defined as a measure equivalent to more than 50% of pain relieved. Dichotomous information was extracted for analysis. The effectiveness measures after the longest duration of treatment were used. A hierarchy of measures was used which approximated in this order:-

1. Patient global judgement (excellent/good).

2. Pain intensity (no pain/slight pain or <50% decrease or from 'neuropathy' scale) or relief (good/excellent).

3. Improved or marked improvement.

Analysis was done separately for placebo and active controlled reports. Relative risk (benefit) estimates, the chance of the intervention being more effective than control, were used to answer the question 'Does this intervention work compared with placebo?', and were calculated for each report, with 95% confidence intervals using a fixed effects model [7]. The NNT, or number-needed-to-harm (NNH), was calculated with its 95% confidence intervals for effectiveness and for minor and major adverse effects, both for the individual reports and by combining the data from the individual reports [3]. A statistically significant improvement over control was assumed when the lower limit of the 95% confidence interval (CI) of the relative risk was <1. In the text NNTs for effectiveness and adverse effects are reported with 95% CI only when the relative risk indicated a statistically significant improvement of the treatment over control. Point estimates of the NNT without 95% CI are reported when the relative risk was not statistically significant. An infinity sign for NNT in the tables indicates a negative or zero value.

Results

The use of the individual drug names (generic and brand) was required for maximum yield from searches of both MEDLINE and the Oxford Pain Relief Database. After excluding a number of reports as obvious reviews, experimental reports in humans or animals, or purely kinetic studies,

another 10 reports were excluded at the final consensus meeting, and the various reasons are given in Table 1. Eighteen reports of antidepressants remained. Several of these reports had multiple treatment arms, so that there were 21 placebo-controlled treatment arms and 11 with active controls. The details of these studies and the quality scores are given in Table 2A (placebo-controlled) and Table 2B (active controlled).

The 21 eligible placebo controlled treatments contained information on over 400 subjects treated with 10 different antidepressants and 373 subjects who received placebo (Table 2). Many of the studies had high scores on the quality scale.

The relative benefit/harm and NNT calculated for each treatment and for treatments combined across pain condition are shown in Table 3. In 6 of 13 reports in diabetic neuropathy there was significant relative benefit compared with placebo. The combined relative benefit for all 13 reports was 1.9 (95% CI 1.6–2.4), with a NNT of 3 (2.4–4). The 13 studies used nine different antidepressants. Some drugs were more effective than others. The NNT for the four imipramine reports combined was 3.7 (2.3–9.5); for the two desipramine reports 3.2 (1.9–9.7), and for eight combined tricyclic reports 3.2 (2.3–4.8). By contrast, the point estimate NNT for paroxetine was 5, for fluoxetine 15.3, and for mianserin there was no difference from placebo. An important feature was the very considerable variation in the improvement seen on placebo (Table 3 and Fig. 1). This variation was from 0% to 75% within the 13 diabetic neuropathy studies.

In two of three studies in post-herpetic neuralgia there was significant relative benefit, and the combined relative benefit was 4.8 (2.4–9.4), with a NNT of 2.3 (1.7–3.3). In both atypical facial pain studies the relative benefit was significant, and the combined relative benefit was 2 (1.5–2.8), with a NNT of 2.8 (2–4.7). Only one of three studies in central pain had analysable dichotomous data. The NNT point estimate for benefit was 1.7 in 15 treated patients. The overall NNT for tricyclic antidepressants, combining the data from 13 reports across pain condition, was 2.9 (2.4–3.7).

Table 1   Trials excluded from analysis

Ref.	Antidepressant	Reason for exclusion
[8]	Trazodone	Inadequate no. of patients (9/group)
[9]	Dothiepin	Dual publication [31]
[10]	Dothiepin	Dual publication [31]
[11]	Imipramine	Dual publication [19]
[12]	Amitriptyline, fluphenazine	Inadequate no. of patients (6)
[13]	Amitriptyline	Mixed musculoskeletal and neurogenic
[14]	Imipramine	Concentration-response study
[15]	Imipramine + paroxetine	No pain outcomes
[16]	L-tryptophan	Inadequate no. of patients (6–8/group)
[17]	Imipramine	Inadequate no. of patients (5)

Table 2 Antidepressant trial details

Ref.	No. of patients	Design, study duration and follow-up	Outcome measures	Dose regimen	Analgesic outcome results	Withdrawals & adverse effects	Quality score & comments
Placebo controlled							
Diabetic neuropathy							
[18]	24	Cross-over, 2 × 30-day periods. Nortriptyline combination with fluphenazine	VAS-PI: decrease in pain as % of initial score.	Wks 1–2: 10 mg nortriptyline + 0.5 mg fluphenazine 3×/day Wks 3–4: 20 mg nortriptyline + 1 mg fluphenazine 3×/day or matching placebo.	≥ 50% decrease in pain at 30 days: 16/18 nortriptyline + fluphenazine, 1/18 placebo (not significant at 15 days).	14/18 had AE on nortriptyline + fluphenazine, 1/18 on placebo. No drug-related withdrawals.	4
[19]	15	Cross-over, 2 × 5-wk periods. Imipramine.	1. 6-item neuropathy scale including pain: 3-point scale. 2. Global rating (patient & investigator).	Wk 1: imipramine 50 mg/day. Wks 2–5: imipramine 100 mg/day.	1. Neuropathy scale: no sig. dif. 2. Patient global rating (improved): 7/12 imipramine, 0/12 placebo.	12/15 had AE on imipramine, 1/15 on placebo. 1/15 drug-related withdrawals on imipramine, 0/15 on placebo.	4
[20]	37	Cross-over, 2 × 6-wk periods. Amitriptyline.	1. Verbal rating scale for pain intensity. 2. Patient global rating: 6-pt scale. 3. Hamilton Depression Scale.	Wks 1–3: dose titration based on AE, dose range: 25–150 mg. placebo. Wks 4–6: maintained on appropriate dose	2. Global rating (complete/virtually complete; a lot of pain relief): 15/29 amitriptyline, 1/29 placebo	28/29 had AE on amitriptyline, 25/29 on placebo. 3/37 drug-related withdrawals on amitriptyline, 3/37 on placebo.	4
[21]	24	Cross-over, 2 × 6-wk periods. Desipramine vs. benztropine placebo.	1. CatPI: 4-pt scale. 2. Patient global rating. 3. Hamilton Depression Scale.	Wks 1–4: desipramine dose titration in 12.5–250 mg/day range, placebo (benztropine) 0.5–1.0 mg/day.	1. CatPI: desipramine sig. better than placebo 2. Global rating (a lot/moderate pain relief): 11/20 desipramine, 2/20 placebo 3. Depression improved on desipramine but not placebo.	18/20 had AE on desipramine, 17/20 on placebo. 2/24 drug-related withdrawals on desipramine, 1/24 on placebo.	4
[22]	46	Cross-over, 2 × 6-wk periods with 2-wk washout fluoxetine vs. benztropine placebo.	1. CatPI: 13-pt scale 2. Patient global rating 3. Hamilton Depression Scale.	Wks 1–4: fluoxetine dose titration in 20–40 mg/day range, placebo (benztropine) 0.125–1.5 mg/day.	1. CatPI: no sig. diff. 2. Global rating (complete/a lot/moderate pain relief): 22/46 fluoxetine, 19/46 placebo 3. Depression improved on fluoxetine but not placebo.	29/46 had AE on fluoxetine, 31/46 on placebo. 3/46 drug-related withdrawals on fluoxetine, 2/46 on placebo.	3
[23]	13	Cross-over, 2 × 3-wk periods. Imipramine.	6-item neuropathy 5-pt scale including pain.	Pre-study dose titration on 50 or 75 mg/day to estimate dose required to achieve target plasma concentration. Final doses ranged from 125 to 200 mg/day given at night.	Imipramine 8/9 scored 6 or less on neuropathy scale, placebo 7/9. 8/9 scores lower on imipramine than on placebo.	AE score sig. higher on imipramine than on placebo. 1/9 drug-related withdrawals on imipramine, 2/9 on placebo, all for dizziness.	4

Table 2 *continued*

Ref.	No. of patients	Design, study duration and follow-up	Outcome measures	Dose regimen	Analgesic outcome results	Withdrawals & adverse effects	Quality score & comments
[24]	26	Cross-over, 3 × 2-wk periods, 1–3 wk washout clomipramine desipramine placebo.	6-item neuropathy 5-pt scale including pain.	Depending on metabolism: clomipramine 50–75 mg/day, desipramine 50–200 mg/day	Clomipramine 14/18 scored 6 or less on neuropathy scale, desipramine 13/18, placebo 10/18.	AE score sig. higher on clomipramine and desipramine than placebo. 3/26 drug related withdrawals on clomipramine, 3/26 on desipramine, 0/26 on placebo.	4
[25]	26	Cross-over, 3 × 2-wk periods, 1–3 wks washout paroxetine imipramine placebo.	1. VAS-PI 2. 6-item neuropathy 5-pt scale including pain. 3. Patient self-rating depression score.	Paroxetine 40 mg/day imipramine adjusted to target plasma concentration (dose 25–350 mg/day).	Paroxetine 18/20 scored 6 or less on neuropathy scale, imipramine 18/19, placebo 14/20 Depression: none of the treatments affected scores.	AE: only dry mouth sig. commoner on imipramine than on paroxetine or placebo. 7/29 drug related withdrawals i mipramine, 0/29 on paroxetine, 0/26 on placebo.	4
[26]	18	Cross-over, 2 × 3-wk periods, at least 1-wk washout citalopram placebo.	6-item neuropathy 5-pt scale including pain.	Citalopram 40 mg/day as a single dose at 8 pm	Citalopram 13/15 scored 6 or less on neuropathy scale, placebo 8/15.	AE scores sig higher on citalopram than placebo, median score 2 on citalopram, 0.04 on placebo. 2/18 drug-related withdrawals on citalopram, 0/18 on placebo.	4
[27]	22	Cross-over, 3 × 2-wk periods, at least 1-wk washout, double dummy mianserin imipramine placebo.	6-item neuropathy 5-pt scale including pain.	Imipramine adjusted to target plasma concentration (dose 25–350 mg/day) mianserin 60 mg/day.	Imipramine 14/18 scored 6 or less on neuropathy scale, mianserin 11/18, placebo 11/18.	AE scores sig higher on mianserin or imipramine than on placebo. 1/22 drug-related withdrawals on imipramine, 0/22 on mianserin, 0/22 on placebo.	4

Post-herpetic neuralgia

Ref.	No. of patients	Design, study duration and follow-up	Outcome measures	Dose regimen	Analgesic outcome results	Withdrawals & adverse effects	Quality score & comments
[28]	26	Cross-over, 2 × 6-wk periods. desipramine placebo (benztropine).	1. CATPI–13-pt scale 2. Global rating: 6-pt scale.	Wks 1–4: dose titration dose range: desipramine 12.5–250 mg/day placebo (benztropine) 0.5–1.0 mg/day.	Desipramine sig better than placebo at wks 3–6 2. Global rating (moderate/a lot/ complete pain relief): 12/19 desipramine, 2/19 placebo; independent of mood.	19/19 AE on desipramine, 15/19 on placebo. 5/26 drug-related withdrawals on desipramine, 3/26 on placebo.	4
[29]	58	Cross-over, 2 × 6-wk periods amitriptyline lorazepam placebo.	1. CATPI–13-pt scale 2. Patient global rating—6-pt scale.	Wks 1–3: amitriptyline dose titration in range 12.5–150 mg/day lorazepam 0.5–6.0 mg/day	1. CATPI: amitriptyline sig better than lorazepam and placebo 2. Global rating (moderate/a lot/ complete pain relief):	30/34 AE on amitriptyline, 18/25 on placebo. 5/34 drug-related withdrawals on amitriptyline, 3/25 on placebo.	3

Table 2 *continued*

Ref.	No. of patients	Design, study duration and follow-up	Outcome measures	Dose regimen	Analgesic outcome results	Withdrawals & adverse effects	Quality score & comments
					15/34 amitriptyline, 7/40 lorazepam, 5/25 placebo.		
[30]	24	Cross-over, 2 × at least 3-wk periods, 1–2-wk washout amitryptyline placebo.	1. VAS-PI 2. Verbal rating of pain intensity 3. VAS depression 4. Beck Depression Inventory.	Amitriptyline dose titration, starting dose 12.5 mg, dose range 25–137.5 mg/day.	1. VAS-PI: amitriptyline sig better than placebo 2. Verbal pain scale (good/excellent): 1 6/24 amitriptyline 1/24 placebo 3. + 4. amitriptyline had no sig effect on depression.	16/24 AE on amitriptyline, 13/24 placebo. 1/24 drug-related withdrawals on amitriptyline, 0/24 placebo	2

Atypical facial pain

Ref.	No. of patients	Design, study duration and follow-up	Outcome measures	Dose regimen	Analgesic outcome results	Withdrawals & adverse effects	Quality score & comments
[31]	95	Parallel group, 3, 6 and 9 wks, follow-up at 12-mths. dothiepin + nocturnal biteguard placebo + nocturnal biteguard dothiepin alone placebo alone.	1. Frequency and severity of pain 2. Reduction in analgesic use 3. Montgomery Asberg Depression Rating scale.	Dothiepin dose titration in range 25–150 mg at night. Mean daily dose 130 mg.	34/48 dothiepin pain free (score 0/1 mild, occasional) at wk 9, 21/45 placebo 2. Reduction in analgesic use: 83% dothiepin 42% placebo 3. No sig dif. in depression rating.	AE and drug-related withdrawals not stated.	4 Extra data available (letter from author).
[32]	40	Cross-over, 2 × 1-mth periods. phenelzine placebo.	1. Degree of pain 2. Hamilton Depression Rating Scale	Phenelzine 3 × 15 mg/day	1. Pain at 1 mth (improvement/marked improvement): 30/40 phenelzine, 9/40 placebo 2. Depression score improved: 6/40 placebo, 12/40 phenelzine. Mood not independent of pain.	AE and withdrawals not stated.	4

Central pain

Ref.	No. of patients	Design, study duration and follow-up	Outcome measures	Dose regimen	Analgesic outcome results	Withdrawals & adverse effects	Quality score & comments
[33]	Post-stroke pain (n. = 15)	Cross-over, 3 × 4-wk periods, 1-wk washout, double dummy amitriptyline carbamazepine placebo	1. CATPI–10-pt scale. 2. Patient global rating: 5-pt scale. 3. Comprehensive Psychopathological Rating Scale.	Amitriptyline day 1: 25 mg day 2–5: 50 mg day 6–28: 75 mg carbamazepine day 1: 200 mg day 2–5: 400 mg day 6–14: 600 mg day 15–17: 700 mg day 18–28: 800 mg.	1. Amitriptyline sig better than placebo at wks 2–4, carbamazepine sig better than placebo at wk 3 only. 2. Global rating 'improved' 10/15 amitriptyline, 5/14 carbamazepine, 1/15 placebo 3. Depression: amitriptyline no sig effect.	14/15 AE on amitriptyline, 13/14 carbamazepine, 7/15 placebo. 0/15 drug-related withdrawals on all treatments.	4
[34]	Central pain. (n = 39)	Cross-over, 3 × 3-wk periods clomipramine nortriptyline placebo	1. VAS-PI 2. investigator global rating—4-pt scale 3. Hamilton Depression Scale	Wk 1: dose titration clomipramine 25–100 mg/day nortriptyline 25–100 mg/day	1. Both sig. better than placebo, clomipramine sig. better than nortriptyline 2. Global rating:	23/24 AE on domipramine, 22/24 nortriptyline, 10/24 placebo. 0/39 drug related	3 extra data available

Table 2 *continued*

Ref.	No. of patients	Design, study duration and follow-up	Outcome measures	Dose regimen	Analgesic outcome results	Withdrawals & adverse effects	Quality score & comments
					clomipramine > nortriptyline > placebo 3. Depression: clomipramine > nortriptyline > placebo	withdrawals on clomipramine, 2/39 nortriptyline, 1/39 placebo	(letter from author).

Active controlled

[35]	Painful mono- and poly neuropathies. (*n* = 48)	Cross-over, 2 × 2-wk periods, 1 wk washout acetylsalicylic acid clomipramine	1. Effect of pain on well being, physical activity, sleep, walking—5-pt scale 2. Global rating (patient & investigator)	Clomipramine day 1: 50 mg/day, day 2: 100 mg/day, day 3–14: 150 mg/day acetylsalicylic acid day 1: 500 mg/day, day 2: 1000 mg/day, day 3–14: 1500 mg/day	doctor global rating 23/40 improved on clomipramine, 6/40 on placebo	37% AE with clomipramine, 17% with aceltylsalicylic acid. Withdrawals not stated	1
[36]	Diabetic neuropathy (*n* = 59)	Parallel group, 3 mths 2 yr open follow-up	1. Painful legs (yes/no) 2. KDS depression scores	Imipramine 100 mg nocte (20) amitriptyline 100 mg nocte (19) diazepam 5 mg tds (20)	1. Complete relief of leg pain in 20/20 on imipramine, 19/19 on amitriptyline and 0/20 on diazepam 2. Mean depression scores reduced significantly by imipramine or amitriptyline not by diazepam	2/20 impotence or frigidity on imipramine, 1/19 diazepam complete cure of all other symptoms by imipramine or amitriptyline, not by diazepam	2
[37]	Post- herpatic neuralgia. (*n* = 35)	Cross-over, 2 × 5-wk periods, 2-wk washout amitriptyline maprotiline	1. VAS-PI 2. CATPI—4-pt scale 3 % pain relief 4. Beck Depression Inventory 5. Clinical effectiveness— 4-pt scale	Wks 1–3: dose titration, starting dose 12.5 mg Wks 4–5: stable dose	1. VAS-PI: amitriptyline sig. better than maprotiline 2. CATPI (mild/no pain): 15/32 amitriptyline 12/32 maprotiline 3. No sig. diff. in % pain relief 4. Depression: no sig. effect of amitriptyline or maprotiline 5. amitriptyline clinically more effective	20/35 AE on amitriptyline, 28/35 maprotiline. 3/35 drug related withdrawals on amitriptyline, 3/35 maprotiline	4

AE, adverse effect; CATPI, categorical paint intensity; VAS-PI, visual analogue scale of pain intensity.

Adverse effects

Dichotomous information on minor adverse effects was available from 11 of the 21 placebo controlled reports (Table 3B). Again there was considerable variation across the placebo treatments, with minor adverse effect incidence varying from 6% to 86%. Combining across pain syndromes (11 reports) the NNT for minor adverse effects was 3.7 (2.9–5.2).

Dichotomous information on major adverse effects was available from 19 of the 21 placebo controlled reports (Table 3C); drug-related withdrawals occurred in 41/498 (8%) of

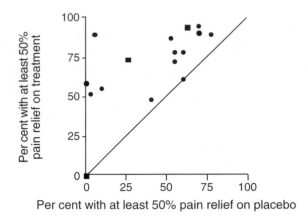

Fig. 1 L'Abbé plot for trials of antidepressants in chronic pain. Relationship between percentage of patients with more than 50% pain relief on placebo (x-axis) and percentage of patients with more than 50% pain relief on active treatment (y-axis). Data points from 13 trials with antidepressants in diabetic neuropathy (circles), and from 3 trials with anticonvulsants (squares), again in diabetic neuropathy [4].

patients treated with active drug compared with 14/303 (5%) of patients treated with placebo. Combining across pain syndromes (19 reports) the NNT for major adverse effects was 22 (13.5–58). This combined figure conceals a lower incidence in the reports for SSRIs (fluoxetine and paroxetine) than with tricyclics.

Active controlled studies

In the three reports that compared tricyclic antidepressants with benzodiazepines, tricyclics were significantly more effective (Table 4). The two reports with dichotomous data on comparisons of different tricyclics did not show any significant difference. The difference between imipramine and paroxetine was not statistically significant and had a NNT point estimate of 21. The comparison between imipramine and mianserin did not show a significant relative risk but had a NNT point estimate of 6. There was no evidence of different minor or major adverse effect incidence for the various drugs.

Table 3A Number-needed-to treat (NNT) for benefit in placebo controlled trials

Trial (ref. no)	Active drug	Improved on active drug	Improved on control	Relative benefit (95% CI)	NNT (95% CI)
Diabetic neuropathy					
[18]	Nortriptyline + fluphenazine	16/18	1/18	16 (2.4–108.2)	1.2 (1–1.5)
[19]	Imipramine	7/12	0/12	15 (0.96–235.4)	1.7 (1.2–3.3)
[20]	Amitriptyline	15/29	1/29	15 (2.1–106.3)	2.1 (1.5–3.5)
[21]	Desipramine	11/20	2/20	5.5 (1.4–21.7)	2.2 (1.4–5.1)
[22]	Fluoxetine	22/46	19/46	1.6 (0.7–1.8)	15.3 (3.7–∞)
[23]	Imipramine	8/9	7/9	1.14 (0.8–1.7)	9 (2.2–∞)
[24]	Clomipramine	14/18	10/18	1.4 (0.9–2.3)	4.5 (1.9–∞)
[24]	Desipramine	13/18	10/18	1.3 (0.8–2.2)	6 (2.1–∞)
[25]	Imipramine	18/19	14/20	1.35 (0.99–1.8)	4 (2.1–43.8)
[25]	Paroxetine	18/20	14/20	1.29 (0.9–1.8)	5 (2.3–∞)
[26]	Citalopram	13/15	8/15	1.63 (0.98–2.7)	3 (1.6–35.9)
[27]	Mianserin	11/18	11/18	1 (0.6–1.7)	∞
[27]	Imipramine	14/18	11/18	1.27 (0.8–2)	6 (2.2–∞)
*Combined data**		180/260	73/205	1.9 (1.6–2.4)	3 (2.4–4)
Post-herpatic neuralgia					
[28]	Desipramine	12/19	2/19	6 (1.56–23.3)	1.9 (1.3–3.7)
[29]	Amitriptyline	15/34	5/25	2.2 (0.9–5.3)	4.1 (2.1–82.1)
[30]	Amitriptyline	16/24	1/24	16 (2.3–111.3)	1.6 (1.2–2.4)
Combined data		43/77	8/68	4.8 (2.4–9.4)	2.3 (1.7–3.3)
Atypical facial pain					
[31]	Dothiepin	34/48	21/45	1.5 (1.1–2.2)	4.1 (2.3–2.1)
[32]	Phenelzine	28/40	9/40	3.1 (1.7–5.7)	2.1 (1.5–3.5)
Combined data		62/88	30/85	2 (1.5–2.8)	2.8 (2–4.7)
Central pain					
[33]	Amitriptyline	10/15	1/15	10 (1.5–68.7)	1.7–(1.1–3)
[34]	Clomipramine		(no dichotomous data available)		
[34]	Nortriptyline		(no dichotomous data available)		

∞, indicates no difference from control.

* Placebo numbers counted once only for [25], [14], [26], and [34]; effectiveness assessed at longest time period recorded.

Table 3B   Number-needed-to-treat (NNT) for minor harm in placebo controlled trials

Trial (ref. no.)	Active drug	Adverse effects on active drug	Adverse effects on control	Relative harm (95% CI)	NNT (95% CI)
Diabetic neuropathy					
[18]	Nortriptyline + fluphenazine	14/18	1/18	14 (2.1–95.6)	1.4 (1.1–2)
[19]	Imipramine	12/15	1/15	12 (1.8–81.1)	1.4 (1–2)
[20]	Amitriptyline	28/29	25/29	1.1 (0.95–1.3)	9.7 (4.1–∞)
[21]	Desipramine	18/20	17/20	1.1 (0.8–1.3)	20 (3.9–∞)
[22]	Fluoxetine	29/46	31/46	0.9 (0.7–1.3)	∞
[23]	Imipramine		(no dichotomous data available)		
[24]	Clomipramine		(no dichotomous data available)		
[24]	Desipramine		(no dichotomous data available)		
[25]	Imipramine		(no dichotomous data available)		
[25]	Paroxetine		(no dichotomous data available)		
[26]	Citalopram		(no dichotomous data available)		
[27]	Mianserin		(no dichotomous data available)		
[27]	Imipramine		(no dichotomous data available)		
*Combined data**		101/128	27/62	1.8 (1.3–2.4)	2.8 (2–4.7)
Post-herpetic neuralgia					
[28]	Desipramine	19/19	15/19	1.3 (1.01–1.6)	4.8 (2.5–36.8)
[29]	Amitriptyline	30/34	18/25	1.2 (0.94–1.6)	6.2 (2.7–∞)
[30]	Amitriptyline	16/24	13/24	1.2 (0.8–2)	8 (2.5–∞)
Combined data		65/77	46/68	1.3 (1.03–1.5)	6 (3.3–33.2)
Atypical facial pain					
[31]	Dothiepin		(no dichotomous data available)		
[32]	Phenelzine		(no dichotomous data available)		
Central pain					
[33]	Amitriptyline	14/15	7/15	2 (1.2–3.5)	2.1 (1.3–5.4)
[34]	Clomipramine	23/24	10/24	2.3 (1.4–3.7)	1.8 (1.3–3)
[34]	Nortriptyline	22/24	10/24	2.2 (1.4–3.6)	2 (1.4–3.7)
Combined data		59/63	17/39	2.2 (1.5–3.1)	2 (1.5–3)

∞, no difference from control

* Placebo numbers counted once only for [25], [14], [26], and [34]; [21–22] omitted from adverse effects (active placebo); harm assessed at longest time period recorded.

Comment

Antidepressants clearly have an analgesic effect when compared with placebo in neuropathic pain. This effect was apparent for several different pain syndromes, and was of a similar magnitude in the different syndromes, despite the presumed differences in the underlying pain mechanisms. Compared with placebo, of a 100 patients with neuropathic pain who are given antidepressants, 30 will obtain more than 50% pain relief, 30 will have minor adverse reactions and 4 will have to stop treatment because of major adverse effects.

Within this overall pattern selective serotonin reuptake inhibitors were less effective in two reports than tricyclic antidepressants (Table 3A). There was insufficient data to say whether SSRIs caused fewer minor adverse effects, but the rate of major adverse reactions was half that seen with the tricyclics (Table 3C).

Antidepressant studies in chronic pain are not easy to do, and one issue is whether to study a fixed dose, avoiding the difficult problem of titrating to an effective dose before embarking on a trial of that effective dose against control, or to do the pre-trial titration. Some reports in this systematic review titrated pre-trial, others used a fixed dose (Table 2). No obvious difference in outcome was apparent for the two approaches. In clinical practice, titration to benefit and minimal adverse effect can be done rapidly with tricyclics, with response evident within five days and perhaps faster [25, 38].

Although controversy has continued as to whether the analgesic effect is separable from effect of the antidepressants on mood, many of these reports showed analgesic benefit without significant change in mood measurements. Another debate, that the character of the pain is predictive of response, may also be resolving. The adage that burning pain should be managed with antidepressant and shooting pain

Table 3C   Number-needed-to-treat (NNT) for major harm in placebo controlled trials

Trial (ref. no.)	Active drug	Withdrawal on active drug	Withdrawal on control	Relative harm (95% CI)	NNT (95% CI)
Diabetic neuropathy					
[18]	Nortriptyline + fluphenazine	0/18	0/18	1 (0.02–47.8)	∞
[19]	Imipramine	1/15	0/15	3 (0.1–68.1)	15 (5.2–∞)
[20]	Amitriptyline	3/37	3/37	1 (0.2–4.6)	∞
[21]	Desipramine	2/24	1/24	2 (0.2–20.6)	24 (5.6–∞)
[22]	Fluoxetine	3/46	2/46	1.5 (0.3–8.6)	46 (8.8–∞)
[23]	Imipramine	1/9	2/9	0.5 (0.05–4.6)	∞
[24]	Clomipramine	3/26	0/26	7 (0.4–129)	8.7 (4.2–∞)
[24]	Desipramine	3/26	0/26	7 (0.4–129)	8.7 (4.2–∞)
[25]	Imipramine	7/29	0/29	885 (477–1642)	4.1 (2.5–11.7)
[25]	Paroxetine	0/29	0/29	1 (0.02–48.8)	∞
[26]	Citalopram	2/18	0/18	5 (0.3–97.2)	9 (3.9–∞)
[27]	Mianserin	0/22	0/22	1 (0.02–48.2)	∞
[27]	Imipramine	1/22	0/22	3 (0.1–69.8)	22 (7.5–∞)
*Combined data**		26/321	5/174	2.3 (1.1–4.9)	19.1 (11–74.4)
Post-herpetic neuralgia					
[28]	Desipramine	5/26	3/26	1.7 (0.4–6.3)	13 (3.7–∞)
[29]	Amitriptyline	5/34	3/25	1.2 (0.3–4.7)	37 (5–∞)
[30]	Amitriptyline	1/24	0/24	3 (0.1–70)	24 (8.2–∞)
Combined data		11/84	6/75	1.6 (0.6–4.2)	19.6 (6.9–∞)
Atypical facial pain					
[31]	Dothiepin	(not stated)			
[32]	Phenelzine	(not stated)			
Central pain					
[33]	Amitriptyline	0/15	0/15	1 (0.02–47.3)	∞
[34]	Clomipramine	0/39	1/39	0.3 (0.01–7.9)	∞
[34]	Nortriptyline	2/39	1/39	2 (0.2–21.2)	39 (9–∞)
Combined data		2/93	1/54	1.2 (0.1–12.5)	334.8 (20.2–∞)

∞ no difference from control
* Placebo numbers counted once only for [25], [14], [26] and [34]; [21–22] omitted from adverse effects (active placebo); harm assessed at longest time period recorded.

with anticonvulsant is not supported. If benefit was found it occurred independent of pain character [22].

The variation in the response to placebo groups in the different trials (Fig. 1) is intriguing. Plotting for each trial the response to treatment (y-axis) against response to placebo (x-axis) shows that a higher proportion of the patients achieved more than 50% relief on active treatment (antidepressant or anticonvulsant [4] than on placebo, so that for most trials the points are plotted in the upper left section of the figure. Both anticonvulsants and antidepressants were effective in diabetic neuropathy, 50% to 85% of patients achieving the hurdle of more than 50% pain relief. The response to placebo, the proportion of patients with more than 50% pain relief, varied from 0% to 75% in trials. Overall, the variation in response to placebo was greater than the response to treatment. We have no simple explanation as to why within this set of trials, on a supposedly homogeneous population of patients, all with diabetic neuropathy, such variation should occur. The Hawthorne effect,

a change in patient behaviour due to participation in a trial [39], may well apply within a particular trial, elevating patient response to placebo because of extra attention, but then there is a variation in the extent of the Hawthorne effect within this set of trials—some had greater response than others.

The aim of systematic reviews should be to guide clinicians to the most effective intervention in a particular condition. In Fig. 1 the points plotted for diabetic neuropathy trials of anticonvulsants [4] and for antidepressants (this review) show similar scatter, suggesting that from the available trials there is no measurable difference in the analgesic benefit of the two drug classes in neuropathic pain. The combined NNT for benefit for antidepressants in diabetic neuropathy was 3 (95% CI 2.4–4), and that for anticonvulsants 2.5 (95% CI 1.8–4). [4] Neither was there substantial difference in the adverse effects, minor or major in the diabetic neuropathy patients. The NNT for minor adverse effects of antidepressants was 2.8 (2–4.7), and that for anticonvulsants 3.1

Table 4 Number-needed-to-treat (NNT) for benefit in active controlled trials

Trial (ref. no.)	Active drug	Improved on active drug	Improved on control	Relative benefit (95% CI)	NNT (95% CI)
Diabetic neuropathy					
[35]	Clomipramine + acetylsalicylic acid	23/40	6/40	3.8 (1.8–8.4)	2.4 (1.6–4.2)
[22]	Amitriptyline + desipramine	28/38	23/38	1.2 (0.9–1.9)	7.6 (2.9–∞)
[24]	Clomipramine + desipramine	14/18	13/18	1.1 (0.7–1.9)	18 (3–∞)
[25]	Imipramine + paroxetine	18/19	18/20	1.1 (0.9–1.3)	21.1 (4.7–∞)
[27]	Imipramine + mianserin	14/18	11/18	1.3 (0.8–2)	6 (2.2–∞)
[36]	Imipramine + diazepam	20/20	0/20	41 (2.7–634)	∞
[36]	Amitriptyline + diazepam	19/19	0/20	41 (2.7–634)	∞
*Combined data**		136/172	71/174	1.9 (1.6–2.3)	2.6 (2.1–3.5)
Post-herpetic neuralgia					
[29]	Amitriptyline + lorazepam	15/34	7/40	2.5 (1.2–5.5)	3.8 (2.1–16.2)
[37]	Amitriptyline + maprotiline	15/32	12/32	1.3 (0.7–2.2)	10.7 (3–∞)
Combined data		30/66	19/72	4.8 (2.4–9.4)	5.3 (2.9–30)
Central pain					
[33]	Amitriptyline + carbamazepine	10/15	5/14	1.9 (0.9–4.1)	3.2 (1.5–∞)
[34]	Clomipramine + nortriptyline	(no dichotomous data available)		NA	NA

∞, no difference from control. Effectiveness assessed at longest time period recorded. NA, not applicable.

(2.3–4.8), and for severe adverse effects with antidepressants 19 (11–74.4), and with anticonvulsants 20 (10–446).

Many clinicians prescribe antidepressants rather than anticonvulsants as first-line in neuropathic pain, either because of perceived greater chance of benefit or lower chance of adverse effects. The only randomized comparison of antidepressant with anticonvulsant showed greater benefit at lower risk with antidepressant [33]. This stratagem is not supported by the systematic reviews, which show little to choose between antidepressant and anticonvulsant. This then is a straightforward research agenda. We need to determine the relative risk and benefit of the best and most appropriate anticonvulsant and the best and most appropriate antidepressant, and then compare them directly in neuropathic pain. A further agenda would be to see if the combination of anticonvulsant and antidepressant performed better than either component alone. Another intriguing enterprise would be to determine which aspects of care increase the proportion of patients taking placebo who achieve more than half relief.

References

1. McQuay HJ, Tramer M, Nye BA, Carroll D, Wiffen PJ, Moore RA. A systematic review of antidepressants in neuropathic pain. *Pain* 1996; **68**:217–27.
2. Onghena P, Van Houdenhove B. Antidepressant-induced analgesia in chronic non-malignant pain: a meta-analysis of 39 placebo-controlled studies. *Pain* 1992; **49**:205–19.
3. Cook RJ, Sackett DL. The number needed to treat: a clinically useful measure of treatment effect. *British Medical Journal* 1995; **310**:452–4.
4. McQuay H, Carroll D, Jadad AR, Wiffen P, Moore A. Anticonvulsant drugs for management of pain: a systematic review. *British Medical Journal* 1995; **311**:1047–52.
5. Jadad AR, McQuay HJ. A high-yield strategy to identify randomized controlled trials for systematic reviews. *Online Journal of Current Clinical Trials* [serial online] 1993; Doc No 33:3973 words; 39 paragraphs. 5 tables.
6. Jadad AR, Moore RA, Carroll D, Jenkinson C, Reynolds DJM, Gavaghan DJ et al. Assessing the quality of reports of randomized clinical trials: is blinding necessary? *Controlled Clinical Trials* 1996; **17**:1–12.
7. Gardner MJ, Altman DG. Statistics with confidence. London: *British Medical Journal* 1989.
8. Davidoff G, Guarracini M, Roth E, Sliwa J, Yarkony G. Trazodone hydrochloride in the treatment of dysesthetic pain in traumatic myelopathy: a randomised, double-blind, placebo-controlled study. *Pain* 1987; **29**:151–61.
9. Feinmann C. Psychogenic facial pain: presentation and treatment. *Journal of Psychosomatic Research* 1983; **27**:403–10.
10. Feinmann C, Harris M, Cawley R. Psychogenic facial pain: presentation and treatment. *British Medical Journal* 1984; **288**:436–8.
11. Kvinesdal B, Molin J, Froland A, Gram LF. Imipramin ved behandling af smerter ved diabetisk ekstremitetsneuropati. *Ugeskrift for Laeger* 1983; **145**:3018–9.
12. Mendel C, Klein R, Chappell D, Dere W, Gertz B, Karam J et al. A trial of amitriptyline and fluphenazine in the treatment of painful diabetic neuropathy. *Journal of the American Medical Association* 1986; **255**:637–9.
13. Sharav Y, Singer E, Schmidt E, Dionne RA, Dubner R. The analgesic effect of amitriptyline on chronic facial pain. *Pain* 1991; **31**:199–209.
14. Sindrup SH, Gram LF, Skjold T, Frøland A, Beck-Nielsen H. Concentration-response relationship in imipramine treatment of diabetic neuropathy symptoms. *Clinical Pharmacology and Therapeutics* 1990; **47**:509–15.

15. Sindrup SH, Bach FW, Gram LF. Plasma beta-endorphin is not affected by treatment with imipramine or paroxetine in patients with diabetic neuropathy symptoms. *Clinical Journal of Pain* 1992; **8**:145–8.

16. Stockstill JW, McCall WDJ, Gross AJ, Piniewski B. The effect of L tryptophan supplementation and dietary instruction on chronic myofascial pain. *Journal of the American Dental Association* 1989; **118**:457–60.

17. Young RJ, Clarke BF. Pain relief in diabetic neuropathy: the effectiveness of imipramine and related drugs. *Diabetic Medicine* 1985; **2**:363–6.

18. Gomez-Perez FJ, Rull JA, Dies H, Rodriquez-Rivera JG, Gonzalez-Barranco J, Lozano-Castañeda O. Nortriptyline and fluphenazine in the symptomatic treatment of diabetic neuropathy. A double blind cross over study. *Pain* 1985; **23**:395–400.

19. Kvinesdal B, Molin D, Froland A, Gram LA. Imipramine therapy of painful diabetic neuropathy. *Journal of the American Medical Association* 1984; **251**:1727–30.

20. Max MB, Culnane M, Schafer SC, Gracely RH, Walther DJ, Smoller B et al. Amitriptyline relieves diabetic neuropathy pain in patients with normal or depressed mood. *Neurology* 1987; **37**:589–96.

21. Max MB, Kishore-Kumar R, Schafer SC, Meister B, Gracely RH, Smoller B et al. Efficacy of desipramine in painful diabetic neuropathy: a placebo-controlled trial. *Pain* 1991; **45**:69.

22. Max MB, Lynch SA, Muir J, Shoaf SF, Smoller B, Dubner R. Effects of desipramine, amitriptyline, and fluoxetine on pain in diabetic neuropathy. *New England Journal of Medicine* 1992; **326**:1250–6.

23. Sindrup SH, Ejlertsen B, Frøland A, Sindrup EH, Brøsen K, Gram LF. Imipramine treatment in diabetic neuropathy: relief of subjective symptoms without changes in peripheral and autonomic nerve function. *European Journal of Clinical Pharmacology* 1989; **37**:151–3.

24. Sindrup SH, Gram LF, Skjold T, Grodum E, Brosen K, Beck-Nielsen H. Clomipramine vs. desipramine vs. placebo in the treatment of diabetic neuropathy symptoms. A double-blind cross-over study. *British Journal of Clinical Pharmacology* 1990; **30**:683–91.

25. Sindrup SH, Gram LF, Brosen K, Eshoj O, Mogensen EF. The selective serotonin reuptake inhibitor paroxetine is effective in the treatment of diabetic neuropathy symptoms. *Pain* 1990; **42**:135–44.

26. Sindrup SH, Bjerre U, Dejgaard A, Brøsen K, Aaes-Jørgensen T, Gram LF. The selective serotonin reuptake inhibitor citalopram relieves the symptoms of diabetic neuropathy. *Clinical Pharmacology and Therapeutics* 1992; **52**:547–52.

27. Sindrup SH, Tuxen C, Gram LF, Grodum E, Skjold T, Brøsen K et al. Lack of effect of mianserin on the symptoms of diabetic neuropathy. *European Journal of Clinical Pharmacology* 1992; **43**:251–5.

28. Kishore-Kumar R, Max MB, Schafer SC, Gaughan AM, Smoller B, Gracely RH et al. Desipramine relieves postherpetic neuralgia. *Clinical Pharmacology and Therapeutics* 1990; **47**:305–12.

29. Max MB, Schafer SC, Culnane M, Smoller B, Dubner R, Gracely RH. Amitriptyline, but not lorazepam, relieves postherpetic neuralgia. *Neurology* 1988; **38**:1427–32.

30. Watson CP, Evans RJ, Reed K, Merskey H, Goldsmith L, Warsh J. Amitriptyline versus placebo in postherpetic neuralgia. *Neurology* 1982; **32**:671–3.

31. Feinmann C, Harris M. Psychogenic facial pain. Part 2: management and prognosis. *British Dental Journal* 1984; **156**:205–8.

32. Lascelles RG. Atypical face pain and depression. *British Journal of Psychiatry* 1966; **112**:651–9.

33. Leijon G, Boivie J. Central post-stroke pain—a controlled trial of amitriptyline and carbamazepine. *Pain* 1989; **36**:27–36.

34. Panerai AE, Monza G, Movilia P, Bianchi M, Francucci BM, Tiengo M. A randomized, within patient, cross over, placebo controlled trial on the efficacy and tolerability of the tricyclic antidepressants chlorimipramine and nortriptyline in central pain. *Acta Neurologica Scandinavica* 1990; **82**:34–8.

35. Langohr HD, Stöhr M, Petruch F. An open and double blind cross over study on the efficacy of clomipramine (Anafranil) in patients with painful mono-and polyneuropathies. *European Neurology* 1982; **21**:309–17.

36. Turkington RW. Depression masquerading as diabetic neuropathy. *Journal of the American Medical Association* 1980; **243**:1147–50.

37. Watson CP, Chipman M, Reed K, Evans RJ, Birkett N. Amitriptyline versus maprotiline in postherpetic neuralgia: a randomized, double-blind, crossover trial. *Pain* 1992; **48**:29–36.

38. McQuay HJ, Carroll D, Glynn CJ. Low dose amitriptyline in the treatment of chronic pain. *Anaesthesia* 1992; **47**:646–52.

39. Spilker B. *Guide to clinical trials*. New York: Raven Press, 1991:699–700.

32

Systemic local anaesthetic-type drugs in chronic pain

Summary

To review the effectiveness of systemically administered local anaesthetic type drugs in chronic pain we sought randomized controlled trials (RCTs) with pain outcomes. Twenty-one RCTs were found in chronic pain. Three duplicate publications were excluded, as was one study where randomization was not stated. Of the remaining 17 studies 10 used intravenous lignocaine, two intranasal lignocaine, four oral mexiletine, and one oral tocainide (450 patients in total).

In pain due to peripheral nerve injury all four studies using intravenous lignocaine were effective, showing either significant pain relief over placebo or a positive dose-response. Oral mexiletine showed efficacy over placebo in all three studies in pain due to peripheral nerve injury, but lacked effect in central pain due to spinal cord injury. Allodynia in pain due to peripheral nerve injury was relieved by intravenous lignocaine as was dysaesthesia due to diabetic neuropathy, in which oral mexiletine also was effective. Intravenous lignocaine showed some efficacy in fibromyalgia but had no effect in all three studies in cancer pain. It was inconsistent in migraine.

The best documented effective dose of intravenous lignocaine was 5 mg/kg, which was well tolerated when infused over 30 minutes. Mexiletine (225–750 mg) caused minor adverse effects that were dose-related. Tocainide should not be used because of toxicity.

Local anaesthetic-type drugs are effective in pain due to peripheral nerve injury but there is little or no evidence to support their use in migraine or cancer-related pain.

Introduction

After peripheral nerve injury neuromas can be formed. Both the neuroma and the dorsal root ganglion display spontaneous activity and increased sensitivity to chemical and mechanical stimuli [2–5]. In experimental models of nerve injury, systemic sodium channel blockers like lignocaine and mexiletine silence spontaneous activity of neuroma and dorsal root ganglion, and reduce their mechanosensitivity at concentrations that do not block nerve conduction [6–8]. Low doses of lignocaine may block glutamate-evoked activity in the dorsal horn of the spinal cord [9].

Lignocaine and related local anaesthetic-type drugs which block sodium channels have therefore been used to relieve clinical pain, as a last resort in cancer-related pain and in other conditions when more traditional treatments failed.

Methods

Randomized control trials (RCTs) of local anaesthetic-type drugs were sought. Reports were included if they were randomized comparisons of local anaesthetic-type drugs with a placebo or/and an active control. A number of different search strategies in EMBASE, MEDLINE Knowledge Server, Silver Platter (1966–1996 September), and the Oxford Pain Relief Database (1950–94) [10] were used without language restriction. Search terms (free text) used included: 'mexiletine', 'mexitil', 'flecainide', 'tambocor', 'lignocaine', 'lidocaine', 'xylocaine', 'xylocard', 'tocainide', 'procainide', 'pronesty', 'encainide', and 'pain', 'painful', 'analgesic', 'analgesia'. Additional reports were identified from the reference lists of retrieved reports and from review articles. Unpublished reports, abstracts, reviews, or reports of experimental pain were not considered. Authors were not contacted.

Included reports and data analysis

Each report was read by each of the authors independently to address methods of randomization and blinding, and description of withdrawals [11]. Authors then met to agree consensus. The minimum quality score of an included RCT was 1, the maximum 5. There was a *pre-hoc* agreement that trials without randomization or with an inadequate randomization method (without concealment of treatment allocation) would be excluded from further analysis.

Information about the treatments and controls, characteristics of the pain condition, number of patients enrolled and analysed, study design, observation periods, outcome measures used for pain intensity, pain relief and consumption of supplementary analgesics, and adverse effects were taken from each report. Quantitative analysis was attempted. Number-needed-to treat (NNT) was calculated [12] when possible and a L'Abbé plot was constructed to analyse the

---

The topic discussed in this is also published in full in Kalso *et al.* [1].

degree of pain relief in different pain conditions [13]. Adverse effects were considered major if they necessitated discontinuation of the treatment or lowering of the dose.

Results

Twenty-one RCTs of systemic local anaesthetic type drugs in pain relief were found. Three reports were published twice, leading to three exclusions [14–16] and one report [17] combined one randomized with one non-randomized study. The remaining 17 reports were in neuropathic pain (9 studies), fibromyalgia (1 study), facial pain (1 study), cancer pain (3 studies), and acute migraine (3 studies) (Table 1).

Four different pain conditions were analysed in 199 patients: peripheral nerve injury, diabetic neuropathy, post-herpetic neuralgia, and trigeminal neuralgia (Table 1). All three reports of peripheral nerve injury showed efficacy for intravenous lignocaine and oral mexiletine over placebo and a dose-response (Fig. 1). One study [19] reported significant reduction of allodynia after intravenous lignocaine.

Both drugs were also effective in diabetic neuropathy but in one study [16] the evidence was weak and confined to certain subgroups (patients who had burning, stabbing, and heat sensations) in a *post-hoc* analysis. Two studies [20, 21] showed a significant relief of dysaesthesia. One study [21] reported a significant effect of lignocaine lasting for eight days.

Lignocaine was also superior to placebo but inferior to morphine in the one study of post-herpetic neuralgia [23].

Mexiletine was without effect compared with placebo in dysaesthetic pain following spinal cord injury. Tocainide was comparable to carbamazepine in trigeminal neuralgia [25].

Two reports [18, 19] studied dose-response and also measured plasma concentrations of lignocaine. The minimum effective lignocaine concentration was 1.5 mg/l and it was achieved with doses of 2–5 mg/kg infused over 30–60 minutes. Dose response was not studied with mexiletine. Dose escalation indicated that 750 mg daily could provide better analgesia [34] but with more adverse effects [16] compared with 450 mg daily.

Fibromyalgia

Eleven women were studied [26]. Pain relief was significant compared with placebo at the end of the infusion and for 15 minutes afterwards. In three of the four responders who had greater than 50% pain relief the effect lasted for 4–7 days. Tender point thresholds were not affected. Effect on sleep was not studied.

Facial pain of mixed origin

In one trial [27] where 28 women with mainly myofascial pain were studied, cocaine 108 mg administered intranasally resulted in significantly better pain relief compared with placebo, whereas lignocaine was without effect as was the higher dose of cocaine (180 mg).

Cancer-related pain

Three studies [28–30] compared intravenous lignocaine 5 mg/kg with saline in cancer-related pain. Most patients (26/30) were on regular analgesics (strong opioids, non-steroidal anti-inflammatory drugs, or both). Each study examined a different pain state: pain due to bony metastases [30], chemotherapy-induced polyneuropathy or radiotherapy-induced plexopathy [29], and tumour invasion of the nerve plexus [28]. Lignocaine had no significant effect.

Migraine

Three reports examined the effect of lignocaine in migraine in 196 patients. Chlorpromazine was significantly better at relieving acute migraine than either intravenous lignocaine (1 mg/kg) or dihydroergotamine [31]. Lignocaine was no better than saline in another study [33]. Intranasal lignocaine (20–80 mg) provided significantly better pain relief than saline [32].

Adverse effects

Electrocardiogram (ECG) was monitored continuously in all but one study [31] during lignocaine infusions. No arrhythmias were noted. A total of 134 lignocaine infusions were given, 21 patients experienced adverse effects which were usually minor (light-headedness, somnolence, nausea, and perioral numbness). The infusion had to be discontinued in five patients and these were considered as major adverse effects. A total of 75 patients received an infusion of 5 mg/kg

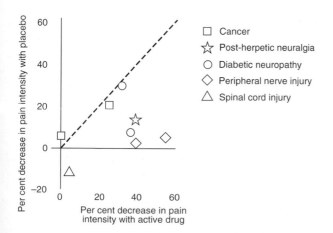

Fig. 1 Analgesic efficacy with active (intravenous lignocaine or oral mexiletine) compared with placebo. Decrease in pain intensity from baseline (before start of treatment) to end of treatment. Each symbol is one trial.

Table 1   Details of randomized controlled trials (RCTs)

Trial (ref. no.)	Condition & no. of patients analysed per group	Design, duration, follow-up	Pain relief	Adverse effects	Quality score
Peripheral nerve injury					
[6]	Peripheral nervous system injury/disease, $n = 11$ (men only) duration of symptoms 1–30 yrs. 5/11 on TCAs 1/11 on NSAID all had failed to receive adequate pain relief after conventional methods.	Cross-over, double-blind, titration to max. tolerable dose, then stable dose for 4 wks oral MEX vs. PL.	MEX 450 mg sig. reduction from baseline, 750 mg sig. diff. from PL, indication of some dose-response.	MEX: 2/11 mild nausea; PL: none rep.	3
[18]	Chronic neuropathic pain, $n = 9$ (allodynia 5/9): polyneuropathy ($n = 6$), local nerve injury ($n = 2$), arachnoiditis ($n = 1$).	Cross-over, double-blind, ≥ 1 wk between treatments L2 mg/kg vs. L5 mg/kg.	VAS-PI: sig. reduction ($P < 0.05$) from baseline with both doses, positive dose-response in VAS-PR but not in VAS-PI.	1/9 withdrew on both doses: heavy feelings & general weakness (conc. 1.1 mg/l), extreme light-headedness & tinnitus (conc. 2.1 mg/l).	4
[19]	Peripheral nerve injury, $n = 11$.	Cross-over, double-blind, 1 wk between treatments LIV vs. NS IV.	Positive concentration dependent reduction in VAS-PI (≥ 1.5 mg/l).	6/11 light-headedness (1.5 ± 0.6 mgl), 1/11 nausea (2.3 mg/l), 2/11 discontinuation of the infusion; PL: 1/11.	2
Diabetic neuropathy					
[20]	Diabetic neuropathy (duration > 6 m), $n = 16$.	Cross-over, double-blind, 4 wks treatment, 1 wk washout po MEX vs. po PL ibuprofen/paracetamol/non-pain med continued, other previous pain med discontinued.	MEX: sig. pain relief, dose response not looked at, no sig. correlation between plasma conc. and clinical effect.	MES: 3/16 mild AE: nausea, hiccup, tremor (1 lowered the dose); PL: none rep.	3
[21]	Diabetic neuropathy, $n = 15$.	Cross-over, double-blind, 2×5 wks, 2-wk washout before study, no other analgesics allowed L IV vs. PL IV.	< 15 mm reduction in VAS-PI: L: 11/15 vs. PL: 4/15	None noted.	2
[22]	Diabetic neuropathy (lasting > 4 mths and < 5 yrs with pain score $\geq 25\%$ on VAS-PI during washout wk) MEX: $n = 47$ PL: $n = 48$.	Parallel group, 1 wk washout, 6 wks treatment, paracetamol allowed po MEX vs. po PL. Multicentre (7 centres).	No overall pain relief but sig. effect in subgroups (burning, stabbing, and heat sensations).	675 mg/day: MEX: 11/47, PL: 6/48 450 mg/day: more AE with PL.	2
Post-herpetic neuralgia					
[23]	Post-herpetic neuralgia (duration > 3 mon), $n = 19$, allodynia: 16/19.	Cross-over, double-blind, 3×3 h, at least 48 h between treatments L IV vs. M IV vs. PL IV.	VAS-PI: L & M sig. better than PL ($P < 0.05$), VAS-PR: M sig. better than PL ($P = 0.01$); L vs. PL ($P = 0.06$).	L:1/19 nausea and light-headedness at 180 mg. conc. 1.33 mg/l; M: 7/19 nausea.	3
Dysaesthetic spinal cord injury					
[24]	Dysaesthetic spinal cord injury, $n = 11$.	Cross-over, double-blind, 4-wk treatment, 1-wk washout oral MEX vs. PL. Ibuprofen/paracetamol/non-pain med continued, other previous pain med discontinued.	No pain relief.	None rep.	3

Table 1 *continued*

Trial (ref. no.)	Condition & no. of patients analysed per group	Design, duration, follow-up	Pain relief	Adverse effects	Quality score
Trigeminal neuralgia					
[25]	Trigeminal neuralgia (several attacks daily, duration of illness 5–19 yrs), n = 12 patients on CARBA before trial, none experienced complete pain relief.	Cross-over, double-blind, 2 × 2 wks– po TOCA vs. po CARBA.	TOCA and CARBA equal,	TOCA: 3/11: pronounced nausea apical paraesthesias, skin rash.	3
Fibromyalgia					
[26]	Fibromyalgia (1990 ACR classification), n = 11 (female).	Cross-over, double-blind, 1 wk between treatments: L IV vs. PL IV follow-up 1 wk 3/11 on paracetamol.	VAS-PI: sig. ($P < 0.05$) better than L vs. PL.	L: 2/11: nausea + perioral numbness, 1/11: drowsiness, dysarthria, tremor; PL: 0/11.	2
Facial pain					
[27]	Facial pain: n = 28 (women) myofascial pain of the face (n = 15) myofascial pain + OA of the TMJ (n = 5) deafferentation neuralgia (n = 4) myofascial pain secondary to deafferentation neuralgia (n = 4) duration of pain 14 mths–18 yrs (mean 4 yrs).	Cross-over, double-blind, 4 × 1 h at least 1 wk between treatments, cotton pledglet L 4% i.n. vs. COCA 15% i.n. vs. COCA 25% i.n. vs. PL i.n.	No sig. effect.	L: insig. decrease in blood pressure, 1/21 nausea.	3
Cancer pain					
[28]	Neuropathic pain in cancer patients (numbness/ allodynia): direct tumour invasion of the nerve plexus. Patients on opioids (mean equivalent daily dose of morphine 231 ± 150 mg) phenytoin, TCAs, corticosteroids already tried n = 10.	Cross-over, double-blind, 2 × 48 h L IV vs. PL IV.	No diff. from baseline, no diff. between L vs. NS.	No sig. AE.	3
[29]	Neuropathic pain with allodynia in cancer patients: n = 10 polyneuropathy (n = 7) plexopathy) (n = 3) co-analgesics: none (n = 4) paracetamol n = (2) NSAID (n = 1) opioid (n = 2) opioid + NSAID (n = 1)	Cross-over, double-blind L IV vs. PL IV 2 × 1 wk at least 1 wk between treatments, follow-up to see how long effect lasted	No diff. between L and NS.	L: 1/10 mild somnolence; PL: none rep.	2
[30]	Painful bone metastases, duration of pain > 3 m n = 10 concomitant analgesics: opioid + peripheral. (n = 8) epidural morphine (n = 1) peripheral (n = 1)	Cross-over, double-blind, 2 × 1 wk L IV vs. NS IV., 1 wk between treatments, if analgesia lasted > 1 wk, 2nd infusion only when pain had returned.	Mean pain relief no diff. from placebo, but > 10 mm relief: L5/10 vs. NS 1/10	L: 4/10: 1. somnolence + nausea, 2 somnolence + circumoral paraesthesias, 3. euphoria, 4. confusion; PL: none rep.	2

Table 1   *continued*

Trial (ref. no.)	Condition & no. of patients analysed per group	Design, duration, follow-up	Pain relief	Adverse effects	Quality score
Migraine					
[31]	Acute migraine (common/classic) L: n = 26 CPZ: n = 24 DHE: n = 26 follow-up: L: n = 17 CPZ: n = 18 DHE: n = 19	Parallel group, single blind (patient), 24 h L IV vs. CPZ IV vs. DHE IV.	Post treatment median score 40 (P < 0.05?), change in severity 50% (P < 0.005?), complete relief 2/26, incomplete relief 15/26, no relief or worse 9/26, additional med 11/26	Non-drug related withdrawals: 19/90; AE: L: minor 5/17 CPZ: minor 4/18 DHE: minor 11/19	2
[32]	Acute migraine with or without aura (IHS), age > 18 yr., pain ≥ moderate L: n = 53 PL: n = 28	Parallel group, double-blind, symptomatic and prophylactic med allowed to continue, follow-up 24 h i.n. vs. PL i.n. multicentre (2 centres)	50% reduction in VAS-PI: L: 26/53 vs. PL: 7/28 Rescue med needed within 4 h: L: 15/53 vs. PL: 20/28 (P < 0.001)	L: minor, local	4
[33]	Acute migraine (headache lasting > 4 h and < 72 h) n = 25L: n = 13 PL: n = 12	Parallel group, double-blind, 2 min infusion, 20 min follow-up, L IV vs. PL IV. paracetamol and/or codeine had been taken before study	reduction in VAS-PI sig. from baseline but not sig. diff. from placebo in 20 min	None	2

AE, adverse effect; CARBA, carbamazepine; CAT, categorical; COCA, cocaine; CPZ, chlorpromazine; DHE, dihydroergotamine; IHS, International Headache; Society; L, lignocaine; M, morphine; MEX, mexiterine; NSAID, non-steroidal anti-inflammatory drug; OA, osteoarthritis; PI, pain intensity; PL, placebo; PR, pain relief; SPID, summed pain intensity difference; TCA, tricyclic antidepressant; TOCA, tocainide; TOTPAR, total pain relief; VAS, visual analogue scale; i.n., intranasal.

over 30–45 minutes. Of these patients 16 had minor and three major adverse effects. In two patients the plasma concentrations were measured at the time of discontinuation. Excessive sedation occurred at 2.42 mg/l and nausea at 2.62 mg/l. One adverse effect was reported during the 100 saline infusions.

Adverse effects were reported in 16 of the 85 patients who were given mexiletine. Adverse effects were dose-related. In three patients they disappeared after the dose was decreased from 10 mg/kg to 8 mg/kg [20] and in another report [22] adverse effects were reported with the low dose (225 mg/day) by 4/47 patients, with the intermediate dose (450 mg/day) by 1/41 patients, and with the high dose (675 mg/day) by 7/21 patients. The adverse effects were considered mild and they did not necessitate withdrawal from the study. Tocainide caused pronounced nausea in 1 patient and apical paraesthesias in another of the 12 patients. A third patient discontinued because of skin rash.

Comment

These results show that sodium channel blockers can reduce pain due to nerve damage. In peripheral nerve injury, diabetic neuropathy, or post-herpetic neuralgia lignocaine was effective at plasma concentrations of 1.5–5 mg/l. The evidence was strongest in pain due to nerve injury where the decrease in pain intensity was 40–60% (Fig. 1). Oral mexiletine 750 mg daily was also effective in these conditions. Allodynia and dysaesthesia were also alleviated. Mexiletine 450 mg had no effect in central pain due to spinal cord injury, perhaps because the effects of these drugs are mainly confined to the peripheral nerves and the dorsal root ganglion. Tocainide has been reported to have caused serious haematological adverse effects including several deaths and should not be used.

Intractable cancer pain is another condition where local anaesthetic-type drugs have been advocated [35]. The result of this review is quite unequivocal. Intravenous lignocaine 5 mg/kg, was without effect. Intravenous lignocaine does not give more relief when combined with high doses of opioids and non-steroidal anti-inflammatory drugs.

Intranasal lignocaine in migraine was significantly more effective than placebo [32]. The NNT for the reduction of pain to mild or none was 3, with intranasal lignocaine compared with placebo. The NNT for the same endpoint with subcutaneous sumatriptan was 2 [36]. Recurrence of headache in 24 hours was 42% after intranasal lignocaine and it varied between 30% and 48% after subcutaneous sumatriptan.

The long-term analgesic effects of intravenous lignocaine were not systematically studied. Only two studies [21, 26] reported that pain relief could last for several days. It is no known if subsequent infusions provide longer relief. Long-term systemic administration of lignocaine is not practical, and no controlled studies have been done on either its efficacy or adverse effects in long-term use.

It is not known if there are patients who benefit from lignocaine who do not benefit from mexiletine. There seems to be little point in using lignocaine infusion to predict response to mexiletine if response could be gauged by taking mexiletine alone.

The encouraging signal from this review is that a difficult subgroup of neuropathic pains can be helped. Delivering and optimizing that benefit will require new approaches. In the meantime the message that all neuropathic pains do not necessarily respond identically is important.

References

1. Kalso E, Tramèr MR, McQuay HJ, Moore RA. Systemic local anaesthetic type drugs in chronic pain: a qualitative systematic review. submitted.

2. Burchiel KJ. Effects of electrical and mechanical stimulation on two foci of spontaneous activity which develop in primary afferent neurons after peripheral axotomy. *Pain* 1984; **18**:249–65.

3. Scadding J. Development of ongoing activity, mechanosensitivity, and adrenaline sensitivity in severed peripheral nerve axons. *Experimental Neurology* 1981; **72**:63–81.

4. Wall PD, Gutnick M. Properties of afferent nerve impulses originating from a neuroma. *Nature* 1974; **248**:740–3.

5. Wall PD, Devor M. Sensory afferent impulses originate from dorsal root ganglia as well as from the periphery in normal and nerve injured rats. *Pain* 1983; **17**:321–39.

6. Chabal C, Russell L, Burchiel K. The effect of intravenous lidocaine, tocainide, and mexiletine on spontaneously active fibers originating in rat sciatic neuromas. *Pain* 1989; **38**:333–58.

7. Devor M, Wall P, Catalan N. Systemic lidocaine silences ectopic neuroma and DRG discharge without blocking nerve conduction. *Pain* 1992; **48**:261–8.

8. Tanelian D, MacIver M. Analgesic concentrations of lidocaine suppress tonic A-delta and C fiber discharges produced by acute injury. *Anesthesiology* 1991; **74**:934–6.

9. Biella G, Sotgui ML. Central effects of systemic lidocaine mediated by glycine spinal receptors: an iontophoretic study in the rat spinal cord. *Brain Research* 1993; **603**:201–6.

10. Jadad AR, Carroll D, Moore A, McQuay H. Developing a database of published reports of randomised clinical trials in pain research. *Pain* 1996; **66**:239–46.

11. Jadad AR, Moore RA, Carroll D, Jenkinson C, Reynolds DJM, Gavaghan DJ *et al.* Assessing the quality of reports of randomized clinical trials: is blinding necessary? *Controlled Clinical Trials* 1996; **17**:1–12.

12. Cook RJ, Sackett DL. The number needed to treat: a clinically useful measure of treatment effect. *British Medical Journal* 1995; **310**:452–4. [11525]

13. L'Abbé KA, Detsky AS, O'Rourke K. Meta-analysis in clinical research. *Annals of Internal Medicine* 1987; **107**:224–33.

14. Kastrup J, Angelo HR, Petersen P, Dejgard A, Hilsted J. Treatment of chronic painful diabetic neuropathy with intravenous lidocaine infusion. *British Medical Journal* 1986; **292**:173.

15. Petersen P, Kastrup J, Zeeberg I. [Intravenous lidocaine in the treatment of chronic pain] Intravenos lidokain i behandling af kroniske smerter. *Ugeskrift for Laeger* 1986; **148**:2158–9.

16. Stracke H, Meyer U, Schumacher H, Armbrecht U, Beroniade S, Buch KD *et al.* [Mexiletine in treatment of painful diabetic neuropathy]. Mexiletin in der Behandlung der schmerzhaften diabetischen Neuropathie. *Medizinische-Klinologie* 1994; **89**:124–31.

17. Petersen P, Kastrup J, Zeeberg I, Boysen G. Chronic pain treatment with intravenous lidocaine. *Neurology Research* 1986; **8**:189–90.

18. Galer B, Harle J, Rowbotham M. Response to intravenous lidocaine infusion predicts subsequent response to oral mexiletine: A prospective study. *Journal of Pain and Symptom Management* 1996; **12**:161–7.

19. Wallace MS, Dyck JB, Rossi SS, Yaksh TL. Computer controlled lidocaine infusion for the evaluation of neuropathic pain after peripheral nerve injury. *Pain* 1996; **66**:69–77.

20. Dejgard A, Petersen P, Kastrup J. Mexiletine for treatment of chronic painful diabetic neuropathy. *Lancet* 1988; **i**:9–11.

21. Kastrup J, Petersen P, Dejgard A, Angelo HR, Hilsted J. Intravenous lidocaine infusion—a new treatment of chronic painful diabetic neuropathy? *Pain* 1987; **28**:69–75.

22. Stracke H, Meyer UE, Schumacher HE, Federlin K. Mexiletine in the treatment of diabetic neuropathy. *Diabetes Care* 1992; **15**:1550–5.

23. Rowbotham MC, Reisner-Keller LA, Fields HL. Both intravenous lidocaine and morphine reduce the pain of postherpetic neuralgia. *Neurology* 1991; **41**:1024–8.

24. ChiouTan F, Tuel S, Johnson J, Priebe M, Hirsh D, Strayer J. Effect of mexiletine on spinal cord injury dysesthetic pain. *American Journal of Physical Medicine and Rehabilitation* 1996; **75**:84–7.

25. Lindström P, Lindblom U. The analgesic effect of tocainide in trigeminal neuralgia. *Pain* 1987; **28**:45–50.

26. Sörensen J, Bengtsson A, Bäckman E, Henriksson KG, Bengtsson M. Pain analysis in patients with fibromyalgia. *Scandinavian Journal of Rheumatology* 1995; **24**:360–5.

27. Marbach JJ, Wallenstein SL. Analgesic, mood, and hemodynamic effects of intranasal cocaine and lidocaine in chronic facial pain of deafferentation and myofascial origin. *Journal of Pain and Symptom Management* 1988; **3**:73–9.

28. Bruera E, Ripamonti C, Brenneis C, Macmillan K, Hanson J. A randomized double-blind crossover trial of intravenous lidocaine in the treatment of neuropathic cancer pain. *Journal of Pain and Symptom Management* 1992; **7**:138–40.

29. Ellemann K, Sjögren P, Banning A-, Jensen TS, Smith T, Geertsen P. Trial of intravenous lidocaine on painful neuropathy in cancer patients. *Clinical Journal of Pain* 1989; **5**:291–4.

30. Sjøgren P, Banning AM, Hebsgaard K, Petersen P, Gefke K. [Intravenous lidocaine in the treatment of chronic pain caused by bone metastases] Intravenos lidokain i behandlingen af kroniske smerter forarsaget af knoglemetastaser. *Ugeskrift for Laeger* 1989; **151**:2144–6.

31. Bell R, Montoya D, Shuaib A, Lee MA. A comparative trial of three agents in the treatment of acute migraine headache. *Annals of Emergency Medicine* 1990; **19**:1079–82.

32. Maizels M, Scott B, Cohen W, Chen W. Intranasal lidocaine for treatment of migraine: a randomized, double-blind, controlled trial. *Journal of the American Medical Association* 1996; **276**:319–21.

33. Reutens DC, Fatovich DM, Stewart Wynne EG, Prentice DA. Is intravenous lidocaine clinically effective in acute migraine? *Cephalalgia* 1991; **11**:245–7.

34. Chabal C, Jacobson L, Mariano A, Chaney E, Britell C. The use of oral mexiletine for the treatment of pain after peripheral nerve injury. *Anesthesiology* 1992; **76:**513–17.

35. Dunlop R, Davies RJ, Hockley J, Turner P. Analgesic effects of oral flecainide. *Lancet* 1988; **1:**420–1.

36. Tfelt-Hansen P. Sumatriptan for the treatment of migraine attacks-a review of controlled clinical studies. *Cephalalgia* 1993; **13:**238–44.

Summary

Capsaicin is an alkaloid derived from chillies and first entered European knowledge after Columbus' second voyage to the New World in 1494. It has been a feature of pharmacopoeias for many years.

Recent interest concerns the use of topical capsaicin as an analgesic for a variety of conditions where pain may not be responsive to classical analgesics. There is evidence that capsaicin can deplete substance P in local nerve sensory terminals. Substance P has been thought to be associated with initiation and transmission of painful stimuli, as well as a number of diseases—arthritis, psoriasis, and inflammatory bowel disease. This has given topical application of capsaicin some degree of logic—remove the neurotransmitter, so remove the pain.

Does capsaicin work?

Zhang and Li Wan Po [1] searched the literature for capsaicin papers using a sensitive strategy. They sought reports of clinical investigations. Only information from randomized, double-blind and placebo controlled studies were used for quantitative analysis by clinical condition.

Results for the 13 trials that fulfilled these criteria and where there were extractable data are shown as a L'Abbé plot (Fig. 1). Each symbol represents the proportion of patients in each trial reaching some clinical endpoint for benefit and the number next to it the number of patients given topical capsaicin. Capsaicin results are plotted against placebo results. Points lying between the line of equality and the capsaicin axis are trials showing benefit. This plot is a simple representation of how similar or dissimilar trial results were found to be.

Diabetic neuropathy

Four trials reported on the use of capsaicin 0.075% cream applied four times daily for 4–8 weeks in diabetic neuropathy in a total of 144 patients treated with capsaicin and 165 with placebo cream. The endpoint was a physician global assessment of pain relief. Clinical improvement was pain completely gone, much better, or better (and not no change, worse, or much worse).

Of the patients 105/144 (73%) responded with capsaicin compared with 81/165 (49%) patients given placebo (Table 1). The relative benefit favouring capsaicin was 1.5 (95% confidence interval 11.2–1.8) and the number-needed-to-treat (NNT) was 4.2 (2.9–7.5).

For every four patients treated with topical capsaicin, one would have had pain of diabetic neuropathy relieved who would not have had they been treated with placebo.

For comparison, oral anticonvulsant therapy for diabetic neuropathy in 66 treated patients in two trials yielded an NNT of 2.5 (1.8–4.0) [2].

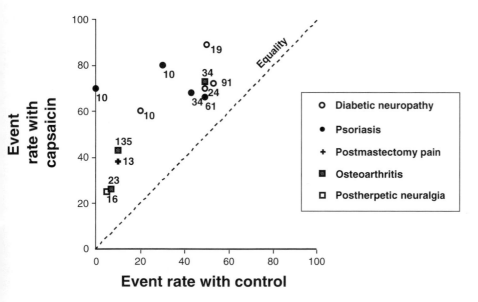

Fig. 1 L'Abbé plot for topical capsaicin in various pain conditions. (Numbers of patients treated are shown by each symbol.)

Table 1   Relative benefit and number-needed-to-treat (NNT) for topical capsaicin in various conditions

No. of trials	No. of patients with > 50% pain relief: capsaicin	No. of patients with > 50% pain relief: placebo	Relative benefit (95% CI)	NNT (95% CI)
Diabetic neuropathy				
4	105/144	81/165	1.5 (1.2–1.8)	4.2 (2.9–7.5)
Osteoarthritis				
3	87/192	30/190	2.9 (2.0–4.1)	3.3 (2.6–4.8)
Post-herpetic neuralgia				
1	4/16	1/16	14 (0.5–32)	NA
Post-mastectomy pain				
1	5/13	1/10	3.9 (0.5–28)	NA
Psoriasis				
4	78/115	55/130	1.6 (1.3–2.0)	3.9 (2.7–7.4)

NA, NNT calculation for efficacy not appropriate (no significant relative benefit).

Osteoarthritis

Three trials reported on the use of capsaicin cream (0.025% in two, and 0.075% in one) four times daily for four weeks in osteoarthritis. The endpoint was articular tenderness or physicians' global assessment of pain relief.

Of the patients 87/192 (45%) responded with capsaicin compared with 30/190 (16%) with placebo (Table 1). The relative benefit favouring capsaicin was 2.9 (2.0–4.1) and NNT was 3.3 (2.6–4.8).

For every three patients treated with topical capsaicin, one would have had pain of osteoarthritis relieved who would not have had they been treated with placebo.

Post-herpetic neuralgia

Only a single trial that fulfilled the inclusion criteria was available. Use of a 0.075% cream three or four times daily for six weeks resulted in pain relief in 4/16 patients with capsaicin compared with 1/16 patients with placebo (Table 1). Relative benefit was 14.0 (0.5–32)—no significant improvement.

Post-mastectomy pain

A single trial of 0.075% cream four times daily for six weeks resulted in pain relief in 5/13 patients with capsaicin compared with 1/10 patients with placebo (Table 1). Relative benefit was 3.9 (0.5–28)—no significant improvement.

Psoriasis

Four trials reported on topical capsaicin 0.025% four times daily for 6–8 weeks in psoriasis. Psoriasis was rated as to the degree of itching, scaling, and erythema. The endpoint was much better or better rating of overall appearance.

Of the patients 78/115 (68%) responded with capsaicin compared with 55/130 (42%) with placebo (Table 1). The relative benefit favouring capsaicin was 1.6 (1.3–2.0) and NNT was 3.9 (2.7–7.4).

For every four patients treated with topical capsaicin, one would have had symptoms of psoriasis relieved who would not have had they been treated with placebo.

Comment

The authors of the review suggested that blinding of trials of capsaicin might be difficult because of its irritant effects when applied to the skin. There may also be suggestions from some of the reports that skin irritation wears off with time, while analgesic effects may improve with time.

How much the placebo effect may influence the results is uncertain. These are difficult clinical conditions, and patients used the creams for up to eight weeks. Variability in the results in placebo groups can be seen from the figure to be from 0% to 50% of patients on placebo getting benefit. All the trials showed benefits over placebo, although not all trials were themselves statistically significant.

The numbers of patients treated in these studies was not great, but that is not unusual in these difficult clinical conditions [2]. The review did not include results of adverse effects, which is a shame, since any treatment choice balances the probability of benefit and the risk of harm.

References

1. Zhang WY, Li Wan Po A. The effectiveness of topically applied capsaicin. A meta-analysis. *European Journal of Clinical Pharmacology* 1994; **46**:517–22.
2. McQuay H, Carroll D, Jadad AR, Wiffen P, Moore A. Anticonvulsant drugs for management of pain: a systematic review. *British Medical Journal* 1995; **311**:1047–52.

Chronic pain: conclusion

Summary

Determining whether a service is worthwhile involves a number of different issues. It involves knowing whether the various components of the service (interventions) are effective, how much they cost, and examining whether their delivery is efficient. The preceding chapters concentrated on trying to determine whether interventions in chronic pain could be shown to be effective through systematic review.

To do this involved developing strategies for finding relevant studies and reviews, and assessing their quality. Over 150 systematic reviews with relevance to chronic pain were found. A system of quality scoring the reviews was applied that shows that high quality reviews are significantly less likely to give a positive result than reviews of lower quality. A simple quality scoring system for randomized trials was devised which has relevance outside pain.

Putting the effectiveness evidence for chronic pain together

Whether we are making decisions for our own patients or for our service or for national or international guidelines, the same principles should apply. The relative efficacy and safety of the possible interventions, and then the cost, have to be the key determinants. The evidence presented here shows that we can, in a simple way, list our effective and ineffective interventions:—

Effective interventions

- Minor analgesics.
- Anticonvulsant drugs.
- Antidepressant drugs.

- Systemic local anaesthetic-type drugs for nerve damage pain.
- Topical non-steroidal anti-inflammatory drugs (NSAIDs) in rheumatological conditions.
- Topical capsaicin in diabetic neuropathy.
- Epidural corticosteroids for back pain and sciatica.

See also McQuay et al. 1997 [1] for evidence of efficacy of psychological interventions.

Interventions where evidence is lacking

- Transcutaneous electrical nerve stimulation (TENS) in chronic pain.
- Relaxation.
- Spinal cord stimulators.

Ineffective interventions

- Intravenous regional sympathetic blockade.
- Injections of corticosteroids in or around shoulder joints for shoulder pain.

We can go further, and try to put some numbers on the levels of efficacy (Table 1).

How well do we do now?

The next step must be to check whether the interventions used in pain clinics reflect these known levels of efficacy. Table 2 shows the attempt the Audit Commission have made to make a matrix of treatment efficacy, determine the percentage of clinics in their sample that offer particular treatments, and to put the percentage offering a particular treatment on the matrix [10].

Table 1 Number-needed-to-treat (NNT) for some analgesic interventions

Condition	Intervention	Outcome	NNT	Ref.	Chapter no.
Postoperative pain	Ibuprofen 400 mg (good)	> 50% pain relief	2.7	[2]	10
	Paracetamol 1 g (good)	> 50% pain relief	4.6	[2]	9
	Codeine 60 mg oral (poor)	> 50% pain relief	> 10	[3]	16
Back pain	Epidural steroid	> 75% relief at 60 days	> 6	[4, 5]	27
Acute sprains, etc.	Topical NSAID (good)	> 50% pain relief	2+	[6]	12
Trigeminal neuralgia	Anticonvulsants	> 50% pain relief	2.5	[7]	30
Diabetic neuropathy	Anticonvulsants	> 50% pain relief	2.5	[7]	30
Diabetic neuropathy	Topical capsaicin	> 50% pain relief	4.2	[8]	33
Neuropathic pain	Antidepressants	> 50% pain relief	2.5	[9]	31

Although all of us may disagree with the particular judgements made about efficacy and safety in Table 2, the approach is the same approach we all use (covertly) in our professional life. What might be perceived as threatening clinical freedom, in that those paying for health care might choose to pay only for treatments in the upper left sections of

Table 2   Chronic pain treatments classified by evidence of effectiveness and risk of side-effects, degree of invasiveness, and cost of the procedure (Audit Commission in [10].)

Clinical risk and/or cost[a]	Evidence of effectiveness					
	Effective[b]		Thought to be effective, but with little formal evidence[c]		Ineffective[d]	
Low	Some minor oral analgesics (e.g. ibuprofen, paracetamol) Topical NSAIDs in rheumatological conditions (e.g single arthritic joint pain) Topical capsaicin in diabetic neuropathy, psoriasis.	90% 95%	TENS provided for use at home. Relaxation therapy.	90%	Some minor oral analgesics (e.g codeine alone)	
Medium	Antidepressant drugs (for, e.g neuropathic pain, post-herpetic neuralgia, diabetic neuropathy). Anticonvulsant drugs (for, e.g trigeminal neuralgia). Systemic local anaesthetic drugs for nerve injury pain.	95% 100% 60%	Outpatient TENS courses. Outpatient psychological intervention programmes. Acupuncture courses by nurse or therapist. Manipulation for back pain. Epidural given once, but abandoned if ineffective. Long-term, low-rate opioids. Surgical intervention for back pain when surgery has not yet been tried (e.g laminectomy for sciatica with positive neurological signs and MRI). Orthopaedic corsets, neck collars used for long periods. Sclerosis injection for low back pain.	60% 70% 50% 50% 21%	Injection of corticosteroids in or around shoulder joints for shoulder pain.	89%
High	Epidural for back pain and sciatica (effects for first 60 days). Inpatient psychological intervention programmes.	25%	Acupuncture courses provided by doctors (higher salary costs). Trigeminal neuralgia treatments using specialized/expensive equipment. (e.g radio frequency block kit). Lignocaine infusion as inpatient. Epidural left *in situ* for several weeks as inpatient. Long-term, high doses of a 'cocktail' of opioids and other drugs. Repeated back pain surgery. Cordotomy. Spinal cord implanted stimulators. Destructive nerve burning, freezing, phenol injections.	65% 30% 45% 84% 11% 25% 95%	Epidural for back pain and sciatica (effects beyond 3 months). IRSB guanethidine.	90%

%, percentage of 20 trusts providing each treatment is listed where known; some treatments may be provided via referral to another clinic.
IRSB, intravenous regional sympathetic blockade; NSAIDs, non-steroidal anti-inflammatory drugs; TENS, transcutaneous electrical nerve stimulation.
[a] Clinical risks could include adverse effects, the degree of invasiveness of the procedure, and whether the effects on the body are reversible. Treatments have been placed into a category according to the professional judgement of consulted practitioners.
[b] Treatments proved to be effective are those with a sufficient number of randomized control trials available to calculate the 'number-needed-to-treat' (NNT), and, in this context, which have values of NNT between 2 and 4.
[c] Many treatments have not been subjected to enough randomized control trials to make a statistical judgement about their effectiveness.
[d] Treatments shown to be without effect in this context are those with NNTs greater than 4.

Table 2, is in reality a matter of judging relative efficacy, safety, and cost.

Primary care prescribing

Another approach is to use the national prescribing data to see to what extent prescribing of oral analgesics in primary care matches the efficacy league table (Chapter 22). We used the Government Statistical Service Prescription cost analysis for England 1996 [11], which provides data on the number of prescriptions for particular categories of drug (Table 3). We then produced a simple scattergram of the number of pre-scriptions for the different drugs against the NNT for single dose analgesia, and the graph is shown in Fig. 1.

Figure 1 shows that prescribing in primary care matches reasonably well to the efficacy of the analgesics. Cost will be a factor, but most analgesics are cheap, so that efficacy should be the primary determinant. Given that there are differences between the single dose efficacy of the different analgesics, safety issues now need to be brought into focus. A problem for us here is that while there may be differences in minor adverse effect incidence on single dosing, with opioids alone or in combination being the worst offenders, the real safety issues are about what happens with multiple or chronic dosing.

For somebody with arthritic pain that requires months or years of taking analgesics, which is the best choice, paraceta-mol or NSAID? At recommended doses paracetamol has minimal safety problems. Using data from four randomized trials, taking NSAIDs for more than two months carries a risk of bleeding or perforating gastroduodenal ulcer of 1 in 228 (150–479), relative risk 2.8 (1.2–6.2), absolute risk 0.69% [12]. We estimate that there is a 1 in 8.3 (12%) risk that these patients with bleed or perforation will die. Using a control event (death) rate of 0.0002% with this experimental death rate of 0.69%/8.3 = 0.083%, we calculate [12] that the average number-needed-to-kill (NNK) for a patient receiving chronic oral NSAIDs for at least two months is 1/(0.083%–0.002%) = 1/0.081% = 1235.

This shows the complexity of what appears at first glance to be a simple choice between NSAID and paracetamol. We conclude that if paracetamol is sufficient to control the pain then the choice should be paracetamol, because of its good long-term safety at recommended doses. Taking NSAIDs for more than two months carries a risk of bleed or perforation, and in turn a risk of death.

A note on acute low back pain

This book has examined the evidence for particular interventions, which are often applicable to a wide variety of pain syndromes. An example of applying evidence to a particular conditions are the Clinical Standards Advisory Group guidelines for the very common problem of acute low back pain. They made firm recommendations for management [13] (Table 4). Prolonged rest is not recommended.

Chronic pain services: evidence on costs

There is little information about the costs and benefits of chronic pain services, and what little there is barely constitutes evidence. Costs may be determined in a bottom-up way—contrasting, for instance, two or more different types of treatment for a condition and working out the costs and benefits for each. This method is precluded by lack of sufficient evidence, for example, the fact that we have no real evidence that TENS works in chronic pain. Evidence of effectiveness must come first. Rational assessment of cost/benefit needs evidence of effectiveness.

The other way is to use a top-down approach, in which the disease burden is examined, changes are estimated, and judgement is made as to whether pain clinics add to costs or reduce them. Here at least there is some evidence, but not very much, and not very recent.

Table 3 UK oral analgesic prescribing and efficacy

Analgesic studied	NNT	Prescriptions (thousands)
Codeine	17.7	657
Dihydrocodeine	9.7	1866
Tramadol	4.7	491
Paracetamol	4.6	6341.4
Dextropropoxyphene HCl 65 mg + paracetamol 650 mg	4.4	10 228.9
Ibuprofen	2.7	5283.4
Diclofenac	2.3	3813.1
Co-codamol (30 mg codeine + 500 mg paracetamol)	1.9	9957.7

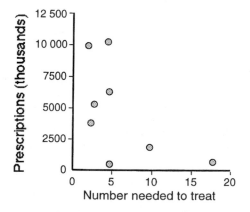

Fig. 1 UK oral analgesic prescribing and efficacy.

Table 4 Management guidelines for acute low back pain. (Clinical Standards Advisory Group 1994 [13].)

Diagnostic triage	
Early management	Simple analgesics
	Physical therapy
	Only 1–3 days' rest
	Encourage early activity
Biopsychosocial assessment at 6 weeks	
Active rehabilitation	

Prevalence

The prevalence of chronic non-malignant pain was estimated for the Oxford Region for the Summer of 1982 [14]. The population served, 2.3 million, had a Regional Pain Relief Unit with 1115 'actively maintained records' of patients with non-malignant pain, records which had not been archived, excluding those who had died or not returned to the unit for 18 months.

This gives an overall prevalence of 485 patients per million population. However, the Unit treated patients from outside the region, and adjusting for that the prevalence would be lower, at 325 patients per million.

Referrals in 1982

Referral patterns for 1982 are shown in Table 5.

Changes since 1982

No documented evidence of change exists. Present patterns of referral and perceived changes include the following:

- Overall workloads have increased since 1982. Medical staffing has increased from one consultant and senior registrar to two consultants, University Reader in Pain Relief (part-time honorary consultant) and senior registrar.
- There are more specialist pain centres in the United Kingdom, and in the former Oxford Region there are consultants (especially anaesthetists) specializing in pain relief.
- More treatment now occurs in primary care, particularly in Oxfordshire. For example, post-herpetic neuralgia will often now be treated by general practitioners with antidepressants.
- Types of patient referred have changed, tending to be more difficult and often with at least some attempt to treat in primary care [15].

Comment

It is likely that the burden of chronic pain as seen at pain clinics has increased substantially in the last decade. Patients are usually in the sixth and seventh decade of life, so demographic imperatives are likely to increase prevalence still further until about 2020.

Cost of chronic pain treatment

A detailed study of the costs incurred by users of specialty pain clinic services [16] has shown that users of the services incur less direct health care expenditure than non users with similar conditions.

Of 626 patients referred to the chronic pain clinic in Hamilton, Ontario, between January 1986 to April 1988, 210 did not attend the clinic (non-attender), 180 had a consultation appointment only (consultation only), 98 had an incomplete treatment programme (incomplete treatment), and 83 had a complete treatment programme (Fig. 2). A sample of 222 of 626 patients was used to compute the use of different types of health services and other costs. This was done by asking patients about their use of five categories of direct health services—primary care, emergency room and specialists, hospital episodes and days, and the use of seven types of other health professionals. Other direct and indirect costs for the patient and associated with their use of health care, were also estimated. Money values in the paper are given in 1991 dollars, but whether these are Canadian or US dollars is unstated.

There was no demographic or condition diagnosed difference between the four groups. The results showed that the direct health care costs were lower for users of chronic pain

Table 5 Referral patterns for the Oxford Regional Pain Relief Unit in 1982

Condition	% of total	Mean age	Mean pain duration
Low back pain	26	52	9
Post-herpetic neuralgia	11	73	3
Post-traumatic neuralgia	9	50	5
Atypical facial neuralgia	6	48	4
Intercostal neuralgia	5	55	4
Trigeminal neuralgia	5	64	9
Perineal neuralgia	4	65	7
Abdominal neuralgia	4	56	6
Stump pain	3	63	13
Osteoarthritic hip	3	74	4
Sympathetic dystrophy	2	59	4
Coccydynia	2	54	6
Cervical spondylosis	2	53	6
Other conditions	19		

Low back pain was the single most prevalent condition treated, although neuralgias together constituted half the total, with 19% of cases of less than 2% of the total individually. Age and pain duration are years.

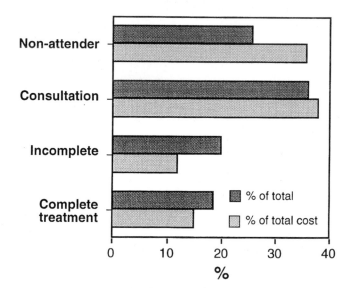

Fig. 2 Total per patient direct health care costs and cost of hospital stay for patients referred to a chronic pain unit using different levels of service (1991 dollars).

services than for non-users. Broken down by type of cost for one year these are shown in Table 6.

The total annual direct health costs were much lower for users of chronic pain services (even if it was only a consultation), and the savings were clearly derived mostly from reduced costs of days spent in hospital (Table 6, Fig. 3).

The 74% of the chronic pain referrals who actually used some chronic pain services used only 64% of the total costs for the referred patients. The 'saving' that came from using chronic pain services derived mainly from the intensive users of the service who had treatments, rather than those who had only a consultation.

Is this true elsewhere? Do chronic pain clinics reduce other NHS expenditure? A case study

From the Canadian study above, it can be argued that attendance at a chronic pain clinic could reduce expenditure elsewhere in the National Health Service NHS so that the cost of the clinics would) more than be covered by savings. To test this idea, the Audit Commission asked a pain clinic to carry out a small study [10]. A randomly selected group of 21

patients who first attended the clinic in October 1996 were asked to take part in a telephone interview. Some of the answers were verified from clinical case notes, but mostly the results relied on the patients' memories. The interviewer (an experienced research nurse) asked the patients about their consultation and treatment histories for the six months before attending the pain clinic, and for the six months since first attending, using a structured questionnaire.

The results (Table 7) suggest that there may be truth in the Canadian study, but to be sure one would need a larger sample of patients, at many more clinics, extending the period before and after the clinics, and preferably tracing patients' records rather than relying on self-report. The implication is that close liaison between the different NHS specialities could reduce excessive referral/treatment and provide a better service for patients.

Comment on costs

These data are the clearest evidence available that chronic pain services not only benefit patients, but are also an efficient way of dealing with chronic pain in the community.

The average direct health care cost of a patient using chronic pain services, even if that was a single consultation, was Can$2947. Referred patients who did not use the service cost more, an average of Can$5181. The difference between these averages was Can$2234.

Using the most conservative estimate—that is no cost inflation since 1991 and assuming that the currency was Canadian dollars with an exchange rate of about Can$2/£— the average difference amounts to a saving in direct health care costs of about £1117 per patient. Using this figure with the 1982 figure of 1115 patients with non-malignant pain on the Oxford Pain Relief Unit books translates to health care savings of £1 250 000.

This compares with the present (1996) running costs (labour, consumables, estates, overheads) of the Pain Relief Unit in Oxford (with a larger workload) of £600 000.

Many, if not most, of the interventions commonly used in chronic pain treatment can be shown to be very effective. Some can be shown not to be effective. Although these findings buttress much of current practice in chronic pain treatment, a common theme is that knowledge remains limited. In particular, information on which to base economic

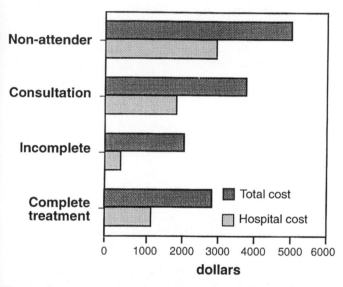

Fig. 3 Percentage of total number and total direct health care costs for patients referred to a chronic pain unit using different levels of service, 1991.

Table 6 Annual per patient direct health care costs for patients referred to a chronic pain unit using different levels of service (1991 dollars)

Service used	Non-attender	Consult only	Incomplete treatment	Complete treatment
Number surveyed	57	80	44	41
Primary care visits	477	422	412	462
Specialists	548	642	862	817
Emergency room	206	439	266	191
Hospital stay	3116	2017	462	1290
Health professional	833	396	226	237
Total	5181	3917	2229	2996

Table 7 Do chronic pain clinics reduced other NHS expenditure? A case study

Average number per patient		In the six months Before After attending the pain clinic		Change
		Before	After	
Outpatient attendances:	NHS pain clinic	0.05	1.6	+97%[b]
	Other NHS medical specialties[c]	2.8	0.9	−222%[b]
	Total	2.8	2.5	−13%
	NHS treatments (e.g. TENS, physiotherapy, surgery)	1.0	0.9	−17%
	Days in hospital	0.2	0.5	+50%
	Accident and emergency attendances	0.1	0.05	−100%
	Different types of drug for pain	2	2.2	11%
	Visits to the GP about pain	5.0	3.0	−64%[b]
	Homes visits by GP	0.1	0.1	−
	Other NHS home visits	0	0	−
	Private treatments	0.4	0.2	−125%[b]
	Patients (%)	Before	After	
Attending outpatient clinics	NHS pain clinic	5%	100%	
	Other NHS medical specialties[c]	81%	38%	
	Either	86%	100%	
Having NHS treatment	Relatively high cost treatments (e.g. surgery)	10%	5%	
	Medium cost (e.g. physiotherapy, nerve block)	62%	43%	
	Low cost (e.g. X-ray)	24%	38%	
	Any treatment	67%	62%	
Hospital inpatient		5%	10%	
Attending accident and emergency		5%	5%	
Taking drugs for pain:	Opioids	14%	16%	
	Antidepressants, tranquillizers, etc.	24%	47%	
	NSAIDS	48%	63%	
	Minor analgesics	71%	74%	
	Any type of drug	90%	90%	
Visiting the GP about pain:	For repeat prescriptions	67%	52%	
	For consultant/advice about pain	62%	24%	
	Any reason to do with pain	86%	71%	
	Having a home visit by GP	5%	5%	
	Other NHS home visits	0	0	
Having private treatment		33%	19%	

[a] +, increase; − reduction
[b] Significant change (paired sample *t*-test, one-tailed, 5% level).
[c] Other NHS specialties include orthopaedics, neurology, vascular surgery, gynaecology, urology, rehabilitation medicine, nephrology.

analysis is missing. However, such information as is available indicates that pain clinics result in direct health care savings of over £1000 per patient per year, and that total savings may be twice the cost of the chronic pain service. Knowing that major demographic changes will affect the NHS over the next several decades, and that aging populations will demand more chronic (and cancer) pain therapy, providing more information on economic as well as humanitarian benefits will be important.

The main conclusion is that recommendations can be made with confidence about the direction of future research in chronic pain, to improve knowledge about the most effective treatments, to determine which patients may benefit best from particular treatments, and to initiate research to determine the most efficient nature and delivery of service.

Conclusion

It is clear that high quality randomized trials are needed in a number of different areas. We simply do not know whether TENS, a widely used intervention in chronic pain (over 500 000 uses each year in Canada [17]), works. Even where there is evidence it is impossible to say, for instance, which is the best antidepressant, or best anticonvulsant, or whether the best antidepressant is better than the best anticonvulsant.

Trials have conventionally used relatively small numbers of patients per group—of the order of 50 or less. These may be enough to demonstrate a statistical difference where effects differ between groups by 30% or more, and are typical of studies carried out with industrial support to establish effectiveness for registration or licensing purposes. Such trials cannot establish the 'true' clinical relevance of an intervention. Work ongoing for a subsequent report shows that for the same difference in effect between groups, a trial to determine the 'true' number-needed-to-treat (plus or minus 0.5 units) would be of the order of 500 patients per group.

These trials would require such large numbers of patients that they would be beyond the capability of any one centre to run. This approach dictates multicentre studies with a common protocol and central randomization, which would need not only to be United Kingdom-wide, but possibly Europe-wide to provide the requisite level of evidence.

References

1. McQuay HJ, Moore RA, Eccleston C, Morley S, de C Williams AC. Systematic review of outpatient services for chronic pain control. *Health Technology Assessment* 1997; **1**(6).
2. Moore A, McQuay H, Gavaghan D. Deriving dichotomous outcome measures from continuous data in randomised controlled trials of analgesics. *Pain* 1996; **66**:229–37.
3. Moore RA, McQuay HJ. Single-patient data meta-analysis of 3453 postoperative patients: Oral tramadol versus placebo, codeine and combination analgesics. *Pain* 1997; **69**:287–94.
4. Watts RW, Silagy CA. A meta-analysis on the efficacy of epidural corticosteroids in the treatment of sciatica. *Anaesthesia and Intensive Care* 1995; **23**:564–9.
5. McQuay H, Moore RA. Epidural steroids (letter). *Anaesthesia and Intensive Care* 1996; **24**:284–6.
6. Moore RA, Nye BA, Carroll D, Wiffen PJ, Tramèr M, McQuay HJ. A systematic review of topically-applied non-steroidal anti-inflammatory drugs. *British Medical Journal*. in press.
7. McQuay H, Carroll D, Jadad AR, Wiffen P, Moore A. Anticonvulsant drugs for management of pain: a systematic review. *British Medical Journal* 1995; **311**:1047–52.
8. Zhang WY, Li Wan Po A. The effectiveness of topically applied capsaicin. A meta-analysis. *European Journal of Clinical Pharmacology* 1994; **46**:517–22.
9. McQuay HJ, Tramer M, Nye BA, Carroll D, Wiffen PJ, Moore RA. A systematic review of antidepressants in neuropathic pain. *Pain* 1996; **68**:217–27.
10. Audit Commission. *No feeling, no pain*. London: Audit Commission, 1997.
11. Government Statistical Service. *Prescription cost analysis for England*, 1996. London: Department of Health, 1997.
12. Tramèr MR, Moore RA, Reynolds DJM, McQuay HJ. Death from gastroduodenal complications due to non-steroidal anti-inflammatory drug use for more than two months—A quantitative systematic review. submitted.
13. Clinical Standards Advisory Group. *Back pain*. London: HMSO, 1994.
14. McQuay HJ, Machin L, Moore RA. Chronic non-malignant pain: a population prevalence study. *Practitioner* 1985; **229**:1109–11.
15. Barsky AJ, Borus JF. Somatization and medicalization in the era of managed care. *Journal of the American Medical Association* 1995; **274**:1931–4.
16. Weir R, Browne GB, Tunks E, Gafni A, Roberts J. A profile of users of speciality pain clinic services: predictors of use and cost estimates. *Journal of Clinical Epidemiology* 1992; **45**:1399–11415.
17. Reeve J, Menon D, Corabian P. Transcutaneous electrical nerve stimulation (TENS): a technology assessment. *International Journal of Technology Assessment in Health Care* 1996; **12**:299–324.

Index

Note: page numbers in *italics* refer to figures and tables